WITHDRAWN

Bisphosphonate *on* Bones

Bisphosphonate
on Bones

Editors:

O.L.M. BIJVOET

Dr. Dirk Bakkerlaan 61
2061 EV Bloemendaal

H.A. FLEISCH

Department of Pathophysiology
University of Bern
Murtenstrasse 35
CH-3010 Bern
Switzerland

R.E. CANFIELD

College of Physians & Surgeons of Columbia University
The Presbyterian Hospital in the City of New York
Irving Center for Clinical Research
New York, NY 10032
USA

R.G.G. RUSSELL

Department of Human Metabolism and Clinical Biochemistry
The University of Sheffield
Medical School
Sheffield S10 2RX, S. Yorkshire
United Kingdom

1995
ELSEVIER
Amsterdam • Lausanne • New York • Oxford • Shannon • Tokyo

ELSEVIER SCIENCE B.V.
Sara Burgerhartstraat 25
P.O. Box 211, 1000 AE Amsterdam, The Netherlands

ISBN: 0 444 89132 3

Preface

During the last quarter of a century, bisphosphonates have become a major tool in the management of bone disease, second only to vitamin D. It is amazing how large a variety of bone-related disorders can be treated with this class of drugs and how efficacious the treatment is.

A great deal of research on these agents has been carried out by investigators from a variety of disciplines, but until now the resulting information had not been presented in a systematic fashion, addressing the needs of clinicians, basic researchers, and their colleagues in the pharmaceutical industry.

To enable physicians to profit optimally from the accumulated experience, to guide pharmacists in their teaching, to help pharmacologist in designing new bisphosphonates and to stimulate biologists in better elucidating their still elusive mechanisms of action, is the scope of this book.

It has been written in its entirety by scientists who have been active and reputed in their different areas from the beginning of bisphosphonate research, and who have been invited by a group of editors who themselves were instrumental in giving the field its form. Every section is written by a major specialist, but the organization is tight, ensuring comprehensiveness and consistency of approach. Particular care has been taken to give insight into the variety of experience and the diversity of sometimes conflicting points of view. This gives the book its unique character.

I will now briefly highlight some of the subjects in order to give you a feeling of the why and how of the book and to wet your appetite.

One tends to forget that bisphosphonates defeat dogma. Previous to their application in medicine, they were known as inhibitors of calcification or as poisons of crystallization. They exert this effect when present in only minute quantities. As such, they find manifold applications. The ability of these and similar substances to modify crystal growth led Neuman to think that, perhaps, the natural polyphosphate-like pyrophosphate might have a role in bone metabolism. The enzyme alkaline phosphatase, presumably a pyrophosphatase, would then regulate this. Pyrophosphate could then be considered as a natural analogue of bisphosphonate. Conversely, bisphosphonates were tried in the hope that they might be useful in arresting excessive and pathological formation of bone in osteopetrosis –the opposite of what happened in fact! Experience teaches that they do locate on bone surface, as expected, but that their action is completely unexpected: they inhibit bone *resorption, not formation.* Results on osteopetrosis and other diseases with excessive ossification or calcification appear disappointing or non-existent. Fortunately, the unexpected effect on bone resorption stimulated investigations in

Paget's disease, a bone disease in which a natural resorption-inhibiting hormone, calcitonin, had been observed to deploy some beneficial activity. The rewarding results led to investigations in more and more diseases with pathological bone loss.

Understanding this interaction with bone resorption, and its mechanisms, is essential for the understanding of the ensuing clinical applications. The bisphosphonate moiety of the drug localizes it on the bone surface, in much the same way as bone scanning agents are localized in bone, but the non-bisphosphonate moiety may be the one that is instrumental in its interaction with resorption. While bisphosphonates localize on bone, perhaps because they are pyrophosphate analogues, their action on bone resorption probably depends partially or totally on the non-bisphosphonate moiety, in this respect they act not as pyrophosphate analogues. This may be one reason why different scientists, using different bisphosphonates with different non-bisphosphonate moieties, discover different mechanisms for this action on bone resorption, a fact that is overlooked all too often. Bisphosphonates do not lend easily to generalization!

One particular property of bone as a tissue should be understood before one starts to grasp not only the clinical and biochemical changes subsequent to the administration of the drug, but also those that occur in bone disease as such. In bone, the various cell types, including the bone-forming and the bone-resorbing cells, combine to one single interacting ecosystem. That is why one has to develop a feeling for other phenomena following pharmaceutical inhibition of bone resorption, for their temporal characteristics. Attention is paid on how to observe these and profit from them.

A second factor of utmost importance in understanding the results of pharmacological intervention is the nature of the pathology. Some conditions follow a rather uniform pattern amongst various patients and may only differ as to severity. An example of this is Paget's disease. In this type of disease, the result of treatment may become quite predictable as one accumulates experience, certainly when the mechanisms of the disease are taken into account. That is why the book not only describes various treatment approaches, but also discusses the relevant pathological mechanisms. The situation is completely different with osteoporosis. Osteoporosis is not only promoted by a large variety of causes, its manifestation is also extremely sensitive to the context of the patients, their age, health, sex, nutrition, activity and environment. It is not useful, therefore, to include a discussion of the condition itself, but we will discuss the results of large trials in which one has tried to modify bone mass and influence fracture.

Patients with conditions that are sensitive to bisphosphonates differ as to dose requirement or advisable type of approach. In some, a single intravenous infusion may suffice, while in others, treatment has to be protracted. In one group of patients, dose and duration of treatment are best guided through individual monitoring; in other groups, adherence to uniform treatment protocols is preferable. Again, with increasing experience and better understanding of the interaction of the drugs with bone physiology, the physicians ability to successfully apply a bisphosphonate in a new condition or to enhance its efficacy in a known one, will improve. The book aims to help the reader acquire that experience.

In this way, the book will review the five areas of bone pathology and calcium metabolism relevant to the multiple conditions amenable to treatment with bisphosphonates. The reader is, moreover, kept completely aware of current variations in approach. Thus, in the clinical sections of the book, attention is given to therapeutic approaches other than those based on bisphosphonate treatment.

Meanwhile, new bisphosphonates are being designed. As it happens, not only the potency or possible side effects and the possible modes of administration, but even the mechanisms of action may differ between drugs. With time, a multiplicity of sometimes simple, but sometimes sophisticated tricks were developed to isolate mechanistic pathways and to distinguish possible forms of interaction between bisphosphonates and physiological mechanisms. This was done in isolated cells, in single or combined organ culture systems and in whole animals. The book not only gives an inspiring insight into the various possibilities, but also offers ways to understand the mutual relevance of basic and clinical work.

The text, therefore, recaptures the history of the bisphosphonates from their beginning (when they were developed on the basis of what later appeared to be a misconception, namely, that they were inhibitors of bone deposition rather than of resorption) to the present (when new potential indications that may be unrelated to bone resorption are emerging in the management of rheumatoid arthritis).

The book is, in a word, multidisciplinary, unbiased with respect to unresolved questions and theories, and written in such a fashion as to allow the reader to relive the history of the bisphosphonates, with its dead-ends and surprises.

Bisphosphonate on Bones is intended for clinical practitioners, specialists, pharmacologists and teachers, alike, as well as for preclinical scientists in pertinent areas of cell biology, physiology, pharmacology, and pharmacy, and workers in the pharmaceutical industry.

O. Bijvoet

Contents

PART B. CHEMISTRY AND PHARMACOLOGY OF THE BISPHOSPHONATES

Origin and Physico-Chemistry

Chapter 7
History of the bisphosphonates: Discovery and history of the non-medical uses of bisphosphonates
Leo J.M.J. Blomen

Chapter 8
Bisphosphonate therapy in acute and chronic bone loss: Physical chemical considerations in bisphosphonate-related therapies
Arman Ebrahimpour and Marion D. Francis

Mechanisms of Action

PART C. THE BISPHOSPHONATES IN THE TREATMENT AND PREVENTION OF BONE PATHOLOGY

Paget's Disease

Malignancy Hypercalcaemia

Metastatic Bone Disease

Rheumatoid Arthritis

Ectopic Calcification and Ossification

PART A

THE PHYSIOLOGY OF BONE-RESORPTION

Bisphosphonate on bones
O. Bijvoet, H.A. Fleisch, R.E. Canfield and G. Russell (eds.)
© 1995 Elsevier Science B.V. All rights reserved.

CHAPTER 1

Normal bone and mineral homeostasis

Elizabeth Shane and John P. Bilezikian

Departments of Medicine and Pharmacology, College of Physicians and Surgeons, Columbia University, 630 West 168th Street, New York, NY 10032, USA

I. Introduction

In a book devoted to the bisphosphonates, a class of drugs that acts to inhibit osteoclast function, it is appropriate to consider first the normal physiology of bone and mineral. This chapter presents an introduction to normal calcium and phosphate homeostasis, the hormones responsible for regulating the metabolism and balance of these ions, and a consideration of how regulation is achieved. This description serves as an introduction to the chapters to follow which will deal specifically with the bisphosphonates.

II. Mineral homeostasis

1. Calcium homeostasis [1–3]

Calcium has many physiologic roles in the organism. In bone, calcium is important for the structural integrity of the skeleton and serves as a reservoir of calcium ion for other physiologic functions. In extracellular fluid (ECF), calcium is a critical factor in several life-defining biochemical processes. Calcium is the coupling factor that links excitation and contraction in skeletal and cardiac muscle. It serves as a cofactor in the coagulation cascade for factors VII, IX, X, and thrombin. It contributes stability to plasma membranes by binding to phospholipids in the lipid bilayer. It also regulates the permeability of plasma membranes to sodium ions. A reduction in ionized calcium increases sodium permeability and enhances the excitability of all excitable tissues; an increase in ionized calcium has the opposite effect. Calcium is essential for the release of cellular secretory products. It serves in several second messenger systems, including cAMP and phosphatidylinositol cell signalling systems. Calcium itself can serve as a key intracellular messenger.

Perhaps because it is so important to so many physiologic processes, the concentration of calcium ion in the extracellular fluid is stringently controlled. A normal adult contains approximately 1000 g of calcium, of which approximately 99% resides within the skeleton, and 1% in the ECF. Approximately 1% of skeletal calcium is freely exchangeable with calcium in the ECF. Although this freely exchangeable pool is small when considered as a proportion of the total skeletal calcium content, it is approximately equal to the total amount of calcium outside the skeleton. This exchangeable pool thus serves as an important reservoir.

The total amount of calcium in the intracellular fluid is much smaller (about 40 mg) than that in the extracellular compartment. Intracellular calcium levels are also much lower (approximately 0.1–1.0 mM) than extracellular calcium, approximately 1 mM. This difference in calcium concentration between the ECF and intracellular fluid is maintained by a system of active transport pumps.

The normal concentration of calcium in plasma averages 10 mg/dl (2.5 mmol/l; 5 mEq/l). About 40% is bound to plasma proteins, primarily albumin. An additional 50% or so circulates as ionized calcium, and 5–10% is complexed to anions such as phosphate, sulfate, and citrate. It is the ionized component that is physiologically important and which is controlled within a very narrow, normal range. Despite this, most laboratories routinely measure the total serum calcium which includes protein-bound, ionized, and complexed components. This is because ionized calcium is technically more difficult to measure and because the total calcium accurately reflects the ionized calcium under normal conditions. In certain circumstances, however, this may not be the case. The most common problem is encountered when the serum albumin concentration is altered by disease. Serum albumin may be low in nephrotic syndrome or in severe liver disease; it may be elevated in states of dehydration. In these instances, total serum calcium will be lower (albumin reduced) or higher (dehydration). However, despite the change in the total calcium level, ionized calcium remains normal. Thus, it is essential to know the albumin level when interpreting a total serum calcium measurement. The general rule is to add or subtract 0.8 mg/dl to or from the measured total calcium concentration for each 1 g/dl by which the albumin concentration is below or above the normal mean (4.0 g/dl), respectively. This is referred to as the 'corrected' serum calcium. For example, if the total serum calcium measures 8.0 mg/dl and the concomitant serum albumin level is 2.0 g/dl, the 'corrected' serum calcium is 9.6 mg/dl.

The ionized calcium concentration is also affected by pH. In this case, the measured total serum calcium remains unchanged. Only the partition between bound and free calcium is altered by pH. Binding of calcium to albumin increases in states of alkalosis and decreases in states of acidosis. In these situations, actual measurement of ionized calcium is necessary in order to determine accurately the concentration of the physiologically active ionized calcium.

Intestinal absorption of calcium (and also phosphate) is the only source of these minerals for the body's needs. The quantity of calcium absorbed by the gastrointestinal tract is determined in part by the amount present in the diet and the absorptive capacity of the intestine. In general, intestinal calcium absorption represents the sum of two processes, namely saturable transcellular absorption that

Calcium Balance

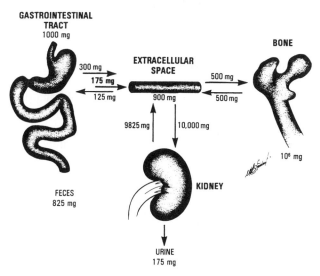

Fig. 1. Overall calcium homeostasis. Three major organs help to regulate calcium homeostasis. Note the dynamic interface between the extracellular space and the gastrointestinal (GI) tract, the kidneys, and the skeleton. (Reproduced with permission from [1].)

is physiologically regulated and nonsaturable paracellular absorption that depends on the concentration gradient between the gut lumen and the blood.

Net intestinal Ca absorption (Fig. 1), which is the difference between dietary calcium intake and fecal calcium excretion, is influenced by the availability of calcium in the diet as well as by a number of other factors, such as the presence of vitamin D and its metabolites. When dietary calcium intake is less than 200 mg/day (5 mmol), the net intestinal calcium absorption is zero. This is because under ordinary circumstances approximately the same amount, 200 mg (5 mmol), of calcium is secreted into the gastrointestinal tract lumen daily. Therefore, under conditions in which the dietary calcium intake is extremely low, even if absorption is 100% efficient, more calcium is excreted than is absorbed. As the dietary calcium intake increases from minimal to higher levels (400–1000 mg/day, 10–25 mmol/day), the net intestinal calcium absorption rises. There is a concomitant decline in absorptive efficiency, such that at calcium intakes above 1000 mg/day, net absorption levels out at approximately 300 mg or 7.5 mmol/day. However, there is a great deal of individual variation in calcium absorption at any level of calcium intake.

Calcium absorption occurs primarily in the duodenum and jejunum [4]. The active metabolite of vitamin D, 1,25-dihydroxyvitamin D [1,25(OH)$_2$D] is the only known hormone that controls calcium absorption. Experimental data in human subjects have shown a direct positive correlation between serum levels of 1,25(OH)$_2$D and absorption of dietary calcium. In the absence of 1,25(OH)$_2$D, only 7% of a normal calcium intake is absorbed. This low percentage reflects the nonhormonally mediated component of calcium absorption. Dietary calcium and $1,25(OH)_2D$ interact in a complex way to determine calcium absorption. Reduced absorption can occur when the dietary calcium intake is low, when $1,25(OH)_2D$ levels are reduced, or when the intestine is unable to respond to $1,25(OH)_2D$. Conversely, increased calcium absorption can occur when the dietary calcium intake is increased or when $1,25(OH)_2D$ levels are increased.

On average, healthy adults require daily calcium intakes well above 400 mg/day to prevent a negative calcium balance. Among healthy adults in steady-state who are eating diets that provide 800 mg (20 mmol) of calcium daily, net intestinal calcium absorption averages about 20–25% of dietary calcium intake or approximately 160–200 mg (4 mmol) daily.

Calcium is continuously gained by and lost from bone in a process called bone remodelling. The major components of this process, bone resorption and bone formation, are tightly coupled both with respect to time and quantity. Thus, bone resorption equals bone formation, and there is no net contribution to the overall calcium balance from the skeleton in adults who are neither gaining nor losing bone. Therefore, in order to sustain a steady-state, in which intake equals output and the net calcium balance is zero, the kidneys will excrete an amount of calcium equal to the net gastrointestinal (GI) tract absorption which is, in this example, 160–200 mg (4–5 mmol) of calcium daily.

The kidneys achieve this goal by reclaiming via tubular reabsorption virtually all the calcium that is filtered through the glomerulus [5, 6]. A normal adult will filter approximately 10,000 mg (250 mmol) of calcium per day. Under normal circumstances, more than 98% of the filtered calcium is reabsorbed by the tubules, and less than 2% is excreted into the urine. This very small percentage of the filtered calcium load is an important element in the regulation of normal calcium homeostasis.

Calcium balance (Fig. 1) is maintained by physiologic alterations in both the amount of calcium absorbed in the small intestine and the amount of calcium expressed by the kidney. However, a minimum intake of calcium in the diet is necessary if these controls are to be effective. Obligate daily losses of calcium occur via the intestine which secretes 200 mg into the gut lumen; via the kidney which is unable to excrete urine that is completely free of calcium; and via the skin through insensible calcium loss. To compensate for these obligate losses of calcium from the body, the daily calcium intake must be greater than 400 mg (10 mmol). However, because of inefficient absorption, a dietary intake of calcium of closer to 800 mg in adult men and premenopausal women is especially necessary in order to maintain calcium balance. Even greater absorptive inefficiencies are believed to be responsible for the higher minimal daily requirement (1500 mg) in postmenopausal women.

The renal handling of calcium is very similar to the renal handling of sodium. For both cations, 65–75% of the filtered load is reabsorbed in the proximal tubule, 20–25% in the loop of Henle, and 5–10% in the distal nephron. There is a good correlation between the fractional excretion of sodium and calcium such that any maneuver which increases sodium excretion (e.g., an increase in dietary sodium intake or an expansion of plasma volume) will also increase calcium excretion. For example, loop diuretics that inhibit sodium reabsorption in the thick ascending limb of the loop of Henle cause calciuresis as well as natriuresis. This relationship is important in the treatment of hypercalcemia with saline and loop diuretics. The prototypical loop diuretic, furosemide, facilitates the saliuresis induced by saline administration. The accompanying increase in urinary calcium excretion will help to lower the serum calcium. There are exceptions to the general rule that urinary sodium and calcium excretion are linked to each other. Thiazide diuretics, for example, increase sodium excretion but decrease calcium excretion. This action of thiazide diuretics is useful in the therapy of hypercalciuric patients who form calcium-containing kidney stones. On the other hand, it makes the thiazide class of diuretics contraindicated in the therapy of hypercalcemic disorders.

2. Phosphate homeostasis

Like calcium, phosphate also has a number of major physiologic roles. In bone, phosphate, along with calcium, is a major component of hydroxyapatite, which is the mineral of the skeleton. Mineralized bone maintains the structural integrity of the skeleton. Phosphate also is an important component of a great number of essential intracellular macromolecules including phospholipids, nucleic acids, phosphoproteins, and glycogen. Phosphorylation of enzymes, receptors, and often key macromolecules is an important regulatory feature of countless intracellular processes. A relatively small amount of inorganic phosphate circulates in plasma. Inorganic phosphate, however, plays a crucial role in normal mineral metabolism, as the major source of phosphate for intracellular processes. It also functions as an important body buffer.

An adult contains approximately 6090 g of phosphorus, of which about 85% is found in bone. The remainder is mostly intracellular, consisting primarily of organic phosphates. A very small amount of phosphate is found in the ECF. Approximately two-thirds of this resides within phospholipids and other plasma proteins. Only the remaining one-third is important in mineral homeostasis. This portion of plasma phosphate is termed 'the acid-soluble phosphate,' or that which remains after plasma is treated with acid to precipitate phospholipids and plasma proteins. It is this acid-soluble phosphate component that is measured by clinical laboratory tests.

Similar to serum calcium, serum phosphate also exists as three fractions. However, the proportional distribution among the three fractions is different: 45% is ionized, 45% is complexed to Na, Ca, and Mg, and 10% is protein-bound. Therefore, in contrast to serum calcium of which only 50% is filterable, approximately 90% of inorganic serum phosphate is filtered at the glomerulus. The major ionic species of phosphate in serum is the divalent anion (HPO_4^{-2}). Also in contrast to serum calcium, the serum phosphate concentration may vary widely (by as much as 30–50%) in the course of a day and is influenced by age, sex, diet, and pH. Normal extracellular phosphate and calcium concentrations are too low for spontaneous precipitation to occur but are high enough to permit deposition of hydroxyapatite $[Ca_{10}(PO_4)_6(OH)_2]$ into the specialized environment of unmineralized bone matrix. An adequate serum phosphate concentration is important to maintain a calcium-phosphate solubility product which is sufficient for normal bone mineralization. Chronic hypophosphatemia may lead to osteomalacia in adults and rickets in children.

The relatively wide daily fluctuations in serum phosphate levels are due primarily to changes in dietary intake. Intestinal phosphate absorption, like calcium absorption, is dependent both on passive phosphate transport related to high intraluminal postprandial phosphate concentrations and on active phosphate transport which occurs in the jejunum and is stimulated by 1,25-dihydroxyvitamin D. Under normal circumstances, phosphate absorption is directly related to intake, averaging about two-thirds of the ingested load. The dietary phosphate intake is 800–900 mg/day in an average diet. Despite the large amounts of phosphate absorbed from the daily diet, under steady-state conditions, intake equals output, and the net phosphate balance is zero. As is the case with calcium, there is no net gain or loss of phosphate from the processes of bone remodelling and intracellular metabolism, under normal circumstances. Therefore, phosphate homeostasis is largely controlled by urinary excretion. An increase in dietary phosphate is associated with the inhibition of renal tubular phosphate reabsorption and vice versa. Phosphate excretion varies directly with phosphate absorption. The control of phosphate excretion is mediated primarily through the actions of parathyroid hormone (see below).

III. The skeleton

The skeleton is a complex organ that is composed mainly of two types of specialized connective tissue, namely, cartilage and bone. The skeleton serves three basic functions — mechanical, protective, and metabolic. It provides support and a site for muscle attachment. It protects the bone marrow and viscera from injury. It is a reservoir of calcium and phosphate ions, which are of critical importance to the many bodily functions outlined in the previous section.

The skeleton is organized into axial and appendicular components [7, 8]. The axial skeleton is comprised mainly of flat bones (skull, scapulae, mandible, pelvis, and vertebrae). The appendicular skeleton includes the long bones such as the femur, tibia, humerus, radius, and ulna. All bones consist of cortical (compact) and cancellous (spongy) components. The exterior part of a bone is composed of a thick dense layer of calcified tissue called the cortex or cortical bone (Fig. 2). The internal space between the cortices is occupied by a network of thin, interconnecting, bony trabeculae or plates that form a honeycomb pattern and is variously termed cancellous, spongy, or trabecular bone. The spaces enclosed by this network of trabeculae are occupied by the bone marrow. While both the axial and the appendicular portions of the skeleton are composed of bone tissue, the relative proportions of cortical and cancellous bone vary. The appendicular skeleton consists largely of cortical bone which fulfils the structural, supportive, and protective roles of the skeleton. The axial skeleton is relatively enriched in cancellous bone, which

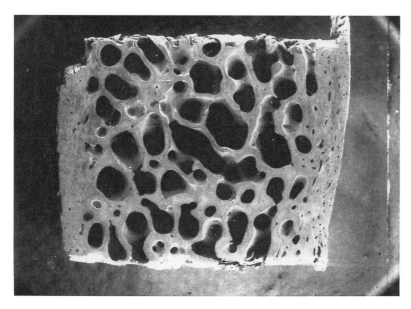

Fig. 2. Scanning electron micrograph of normal bone. The compact bone at the outer margins of the sample are typical of cortical bone. The interlaced honeycombing pattern of trabecular or cancellous bone is seen in the middle. Note the connectivity among the trabecular plates that helps to give cancellous bone its mechanical competence. (Reproduced with permission from Dr. David Dempster.)

is considerably more metabolically active than cortical bone, in part by virtue of its greater surface area. Because of the greater metabolic activity of cancellous bone, it turns over more rapidly (as much as 12% yearly) and thus manifests the effects of certain diseases and therapeutic maneuvers earlier and to a greater extent than cortical bone. For example, cancellous bone is more vulnerable to the effects of both estrogen deficiency and glucocorticoid excess. Bone loss due to these etiologies is detectable at sites predominantly composed of cancellous bone (vertebrae, distal radius) before it appears at primarily cortical sites (proximal radius, femur). In contrast, excessive parathyroid hormone secretion causes cortical bone loss initially, in part because at low doses or when administered intermittently, it is anabolic for cancellous sites.

1. Bone cells and matrix

Existing within and on the surface of the matrix of mineralized and unmineralized bone are three types of bone cells that profoundly influence the development and turnover of the skeleton. These cells (osteoclasts, osteoblasts, and osteocytes) also participate directly in mineral homeostasis.

Osteoclasts are large, multinucleated cells that are responsible for bone resorption. The number of nuclei in the osteoclast may range from 2 to 100, but usually is between 10 and 20. They are formed from bone marrow-derived mononuclear phagocytes which are induced to fuse into osteoclasts by influences that are, at this time, still obscure. Recent observations suggest that protooncogenes such as *c-src* and *c-fos* are essential to normal osteoclast function. Osteoclasts are found in How-ship's lacunae, the depressions in the endosteal surface of mineralized bone that result from their resorptive activity. The membrane at the contact zone between the osteoclast and the bone surface is characterized by the presence of a ruffled border which possesses deep foldings of the plasma membrane in the area facing the bone surface. At this site, the osteoclast creates an acidic microenvironment that is bor-dered by specialized structures in the osteoclast membrane called podosomes that partially seal off the space between the osteoclast membrane and the mineralized bone. Within this space are sequestered a number of enzymes, including carbonic anhydrase, H^+,K^+-ATPases, Na^+–Ca^{2+} exchange systems. The enzyme systems help to solubilize hydroxyapatite crystals, thus releasing calcium and phosphate ions that in turn serve as an available reservoir for maintaining the plasma calcium and phosphate levels. The exposed collagen matrix resulting from osteoclast actions is then subject to degradation by enzymes such as collagenase, lysosomal hydroxylases, and acid phosphatases. Receptors for calcitonin but not for parathyroid hormone or for $1,25(OH)_2D$ are found in osteoclasts.

Osteoclasts are primarily responsible for initiating the process of bone remod-elling (see below) by excavating a unit or packet of bone. They are also critically important in virtually all pathologic states characterized by increased bone resorp-tion such as Paget's disease of bone, hyperparathyroid states, and bone loss related to estrogen deficiency and bony metastases. Because of the underlying premise that many states of accelerated bone resorption are due to excessive osteoclast activity, there has been much interest in developing compounds that specifically impair osteoclast function. The bisphosphonates represent an important class of drugs with this ability.

The cells responsible for bone formation are osteoblasts. Osteoblasts originate from local mesenchymal stem cells. These precursor stem cells can be stimulated to differentiate into mature osteoblasts. Osteoblasts have two functions with respect to bone formation. They synthesize the collagen matrix of new bone, and they also play a pivotal role in the mineralization or calcification of the newly formed matrix. The ultrastructural profile of the osteoblast is typical of a cell involved in protein synthesis and secretion, with an extensive rough endoplasmic reticulum and a well-developed Golgi complex. Osteoblasts are always found as clusters of cuboidal cells lining the endosteal interfaces between bone and marrow space, the site where the majority of bone formation occurs. The plasma membrane of the osteoblast is characteristically rich in alkaline phosphatase, which is a circulating marker of bone formation. Osteoblasts have membrane receptors for parathyroid hormone and cytoplasmic receptors for estrogen. They do not have receptors for calcitonin or $1,25(OH)_2D$. Toward the end of a period of bone formation, an osteoblast will become either a flat lining cell or be incorporated into the bone matrix as an osteocyte.

Osteocytes are the most numerous of the three bone cell types. They are former osteoblasts that have become embedded in the bone matrix that they synthesized.

Osteocytes are completely surrounded by mineralized bone with the exception of a 1–2 μm thick layer of unmineralized matrix that lines the osteocytic lacunae. They maintain contact with each other and with cells lining the bone surface by means of long slender processes that extend through tiny channels in the mineralized matrix called canaliculi. It used to be thought that osteocytes were inactive, end-stage cells. However, it now seems likely that these cells, through their extensive interconnections, are important in maintaining bone integrity. They may additionally play a role in the process of bone remodelling.

Bone matrix (also known as osteoid) consists of collagen fibers and ground substance. Approximately 90% of the noncellular organic matrix is made up of bundles of type I collagen fibers. Type I collagen is distinctive for bone. The individual fibers within a collagen bundle are oriented in an unidirectional manner that alternates from layer to layer. Under normal conditions, this results in the typical pattern of parallel lamellae visualized best by polarized light or electron microscopy. In states characterized by increased bone turnover, when bone is being formed rapidly (for example, Paget's disease, hyperparathyroidism, fracture healing), the collagen bundles are laid down more rapidly and in a less well-organized pattern, resulting in a type called woven bone. The ground substance consists primarily of numerous noncollagenous proteins and highly anionic glycosaminoglycans that are thought to play an important role in the calcification process. The mineral phase of bone is composed of crystals of hydroxyapatite that are generally bound to the collagen fibers and distributed throughout the ground substance. The precise process by which bone matrix is mineralized is not well understood.

2. Bone remodelling

Bone is a very active tissue. In the developing skeleton, these activities are primarily concerned with bone growth and bone modelling — the process by which a bone achieves its characteristic size and shape. In the adult skeleton, the processes of growth and modelling are reserved for repair of gross fractures and microfractures. Normal metabolic activities of the adult skeleton involve predominantly remodelling. Bone remodelling is a life-long and continuous process of destruction and renewal that is intimately related to calcium and phosphate homeostasis [8]. It serves to remove and to replace aged bone with new bone. The process is carried out in individual 'bone remodelling units' as illustrated in Fig. 3 and is characterized by coupling of osteoclast and osteoblast functions with respect to both location and time. The sequence of events within a bone remodelling unit is believed to occur in four distinct phases.

1. *Activation:* During the activation phase of the remodelling cycle, bone marrow precursor cells, responding to as yet unknown hormonal or physical signals, gather on the specific area of bone surface to be resorbed where they fuse to become multinucleated osteoclasts.

2. *Resorption:* The activated osteoclasts excavate a cavity into the bone surface. In cortical bone, the resorption cavity has the appearance of a tunnel within a Haversian canal. In cancellous bone, the cavity is a scalloped pit called a Howship's

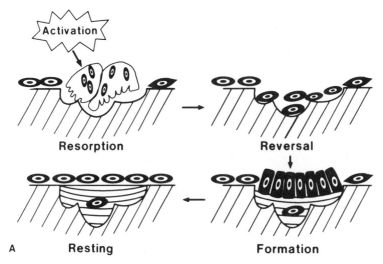

Fig. 3. Bone remodelling. Cellular events associated with bone remodelling are shown. Activation of the osteoclast (upper left hand illustration) is followed by lining of the resorption cavity by mononuclear osteoblast cells. The osteoblast cells then lay down collagen upon which the mineralized surface is formed. Under steady-state conditions, the cavity made by the osteoclast is completely filled by the new bone formed by the osteoblast.

lacuna. From 7 to 15 days is required to excavate a typical resorption pit, which is generally 60 μm deep.

3. *Reversal:* After resorption is completed, the osteoclasts disappear from the resorption pit. During the next 7 to 14 days, a thin cement line is deposited. This consists of a region of randomly organized collagen fibers, in contrast to normal bone in which the deposition of collagen is lamellar. The cement line demarcates the border of the resorption pit and binds newly deposited bone to old bone.

4. *Formation:* Bone formation is intimately coupled to resorption and begins when pre-osteoblasts are attracted to the resorption pit created by the osteoclast. Osteoblasts, which develop from these pre-osteoblasts, then synthesize new collagen and other matrix proteins, filling the resorption cavity with newly formed lamellar osteoid. Mineral deposition then begins at the interface between the newly deposited osteoid and the calcified bone and proceeds toward the bone surface, eventually overtaking matrix deposition and completely calcifying the new packet of bone. The period of time required for the osteoid to mature to the point where it is capable of becoming calcified is called the 'mineralization lag time' and averages 21 days in normal human bone. The complete bone remodelling cycle, from the beginning of bone resorption to mineralization of the newly formed matrix, is generally completed within 8 to 12 weeks.

In young normal individuals, the remodelling cycle is very efficient (Fig. 4). In each bone remodelling unit, the amount of new bone formed is equal to that resorbed. However, with advancing age, osteoblast efficiency declines; the volume of resorbed bone is not completely replaced by an equivalent volume of new bone. Each

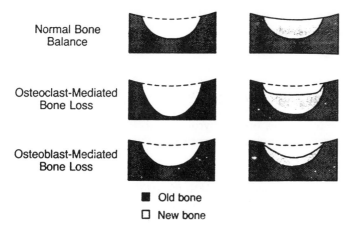

Normal Bone Balance

Osteoclast-Mediated Bone Loss

Osteoblast-Mediated Bone Loss

■ Old bone
□ New bone

Fig. 4. Potential mechanisms of bone loss in osteopenic states. Under normal conditions, the resorption cavity is filled completely by new bone in the shaded area in the top right hand section. In the middle section, the osteoclast has excavated a disproportionately large amount of bone which is not filled by the preprogrammed deposition of new bone by the osteoblast. In the lower section the effect of inadequate osteoblast activity is shown. In this example, the osteoclast has excavated a normal amount of bone but replacement is not complete because of inadequate osteoblast activity. (Reproduced from [15].)

remodelling cycle thus results in a small bone deficit. Age-related bone loss can be regarded as the consequence of the accumulated deficits of many incompletely filled resorption cavities. Any increase in remodelling activity, whether it be due to an increase in the activation rate of new bone remodelling units or an increase in the amount of bone resorbed per unit, will ultimately increase the rate of bone loss.

All physiological, pathophysiologic, or therapeutic processes impact on the skeleton by virtue of their effect upon the remodelling cycle. Since resorption and formation are coupled processes, any hormone or drug that decreases resorption, such as calcitonin, estrogen, or bisphosphonates, will eventually reduce bone formation even though the effects of these agents may not act directly on bone formation. Bone formation, however, may proceed for a time after bone resorption has been inhibited. Since there is a small bone mass deficit (known as the remodelling space) due to the existence of incompletely filled resorption lacunae, initiation of antiresorptive therapy will result in an increase in bone mass as the remodelling space is filled with new bone. With antiresorptive agents, the increase in bone mass will level off as the remodelling space is filled and no more lacunae are formed. An effective agent that leads to increased bone formation, of course, would be associated with more sustained accumulation of bone mass.

IV. Hormonal regulation of mineral metabolism

Parathyroid hormone and $1,25(OH)_2D$ are the two principal regulators of mineral metabolism. These two hormones act in concert to control the concentrations of calcium and phosphorus ions in the blood. They accomplish this primarily by actions in the gastrointestinal tract, skeleton, and kidney.

1. Parathyroid hormone

Parathyroid hormone (PTH) is an 84-amino-acid peptide secreted by the chief cells of the parathyroid glands [9]. The four parathyroid glands, each weighing 25–35 mg, are usually located at the four poles of the thyroid gland. PTH is synthesized as a larger 115-amino-acid precursor molecule (pre-proparathyroid hormone) that is sequentially reduced during intracellular processing. The 84-amino-acid peptide is secreted from storage granules. In general, the amount of stored hormone is quite small, and the secretion rates are closely coupled to the synthetic rates. Intact PTH (1–84) is cleared from the circulation rapidly, with a half-life after secretion on the order of a few minutes. In the liver, a major clearance site, the intact hormone appears to be cleaved within the region of PTH (33–43). Biological activity of PTH can be demonstrated in the amino-terminal (N) 1–34 fragment, whereas the carboxy-terminal (C) fragment is inactive. It is still not clear, however, whether an N-terminal peptide circulates and gains access to target sites. Further, intrahepatic processing may prevent the release of N-terminal peptides into the circulation. It is known, however, that at any given time, intact hormone and inactive C-terminal fragments do circulate. The C-terminal fragments remain in the circulation longer than the intact hormone because the C-terminal fragments are cleared primarily by glomerular filtration. Also, C-terminal fragments are released by the parathyroid cells, which may be a significant source of this fragment. In hypercalcemic states, for example, the ratio of secreted C-terminal fragments to secreted intact hormone rises. In renal insufficiency, C-terminal fragments accumulate because clearance is reduced. The kidney is also responsible for further metabolism of the C-terminal fragments.

A number of assays have been developed to measure PTH in the circulation. Those with the greatest clinical utility measure either intact hormone or the mid-region of the C-terminal fragment. Mid-region assays are less useful when renal function is impaired because these biologically inactive fragments accumulate.

The two principal target organs of PTH are bone and kidney. In both tissues, PTH first binds to specific cell surface receptors, which have been recently characterized and cloned. Binding of PTH to its receptor leads to the formation of 'second messengers' which then mediate the actions of PTH (Fig. 5). Cyclic AMP was the first of these 'second messengers' to be characterized. Cyclic AMP is formed via the activity of adenylyl cyclase, an enzyme that hydrolyzes the substrate Mg-ATP. Adenylyl cyclase activation requires an intact guanine nucleotide transducing protein called Gs. Binding of PTH to its receptor indirectly activates Gs, causing it to interact directly with the catalytic unit of adenylyl cyclase by guanine nucleotide exchange. During this process, the inhibitory nucleotide GDP which is bound to Gs is replaced by the stimulatory nucleotide GTP. The process of GDP–GTP exchange is stimulated when PTH binds to its receptor. GTP-Gs then interacts with adenylyl cyclase, increasing the generation of cyclic AMP. Cyclic AMP binds to the regula-

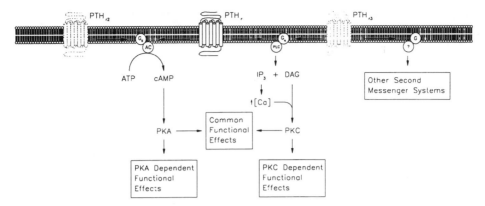

Fig. 5. Model of parathyroid hormone action. The parathyroid hormone receptor interfaces through G-proteins with two transduction systems, adenylate cyclase and phospholipase C leading to the accumulation of cyclic AMP on the one hand and diacylglycerol and inositol triphosphate on the other. These two messenger systems lead to the formation of PKA and PKC, respectively, each of which has its own independent effects as well as ones that are shared. Other messenger systems still to be defined could also be mediated either by the same PTH receptor or PTH receptor subtypes. (Courtesy of Coleman and Bilezikian.)

tory subunit of cyclic-AMP-dependent protein kinase (protein kinase A), causing it to dissociate from the catalytic subunit of protein kinase A. The free catalytic subunit of protein kinase A then phosphorylates specific amino acid residues of certain target proteins. When bone or kidney cells are exposed to PTH, there is a rapid increase in intracellular cyclic AMP levels. In the kidney, this leads to a release of cyclic AMP into the tubular fluid, ultimately to be excreted in the urine. Urinary cyclic AMP can be directly measured and is a well-established marker of PTH bioactivity. In addition to its effect on adenylyl-cyclase-dependent cyclic AMP accumulation, PTH also stimulates the phosphatidylinositol messenger system. This stimulation of phosphatidylinositol turnover in some experimental systems causes rapid increases in inositol phosphate production, cytosolic calcium, and protein kinase C activity. The physiologic significance of this other messenger system as far as PTH action is concerned is unclear.

In bone, PTH increases bone resorption via osteoclast activation. Both the number and the activity of osteoclasts are influenced by PTH. However, the cellular and biochemical mechanisms by which osteoclasts are activated by PTH are not well understood. Osteoclasts do not have PTH receptors, and PTH has no direct effect on isolated mature osteoclasts in vitro. It is believed therefore that PTH leads to osteoclast activation indirectly, by effects on osteoblasts, which do contain PTH receptors. Activated osteoblasts may cause osteoclast activation by generating intercellular signals that 'turn on' the osteoclast. The net effect of these actions of PTH on bone is to cause the release of calcium and phosphate ions, as well as degraded components of collagen, into the ECF. The consequences of sustained hypersecretion of PTH for any reason thus may lead to a decrease in bone mass. These catabolic properties affect cortical bone initially and, over longer periods of time or at higher concentrations, cancellous bone as well. In addition to these catabolic skeletal effects, PTH has been shown to be anabolic for bone under certain circumstances, such as when it is administered intermittently or at low doses. This effect is particularly prominent in cancellous bone. These observations have led to interest in developing ways to use PTH as an agent to increase bone mass in osteoporosis.

In the kidney, PTH exerts three major actions. In the distal tubule, it increases calcium reabsorption against an electrochemical gradient. In the proximal tubule, where phosphate is absorbed along with sodium by an ATP-dependent sodium pump, PTH inhibits phosphate transport, causing phosphaturia. It also stimulates the renal production of $1,25(OH)_2D$ by activating the 1-alpha hydroxylase enzyme located in the mitochondria of the proximal tubule cells.

The ultimate effect of an increase in PTH secretion is to increase the serum calcium level by virtue of an increase in both the release of calcium from bone and the renal tubular reabsorption of calcium. The concomitant increase in $1,25(OH)_2D$ production may contribute to raising the serum calcium level via its effect of increasing calcium absorption from the GI tract. This indirect action of PTH on the GI tract through stimulating $1,25(OH)_2D$ production is not acute and does not contribute to the relatively rapid effects of PTH in raising the serum calcium concentration. Phosphate released into the circulation by PTH-mediated bone resorption is handled by the other effect (causing phosphaturia by decreasing renal phosphate reabsorption). The net effect is a small reduction in the circulating phosphate concentration.

The primary regulator of PTH synthesis and secretion is the concentration of ionized calcium in the serum. When the ionized calcium level falls below its physiological set point (approximately 1.3 mmol), parathyroid cells are stimulated to synthesize and secrete PTH. Conversely, a rise in the ionized calcium level above 1.3 mmol will tend to suppress PTH secretion. These dual actions of calcium on the parathyroid cell help to maintain the serum calcium concentration within narrow normal limits. PTH synthesis is also regulated by $1,25(OH)_2D$. Binding of $1,25(OH)_2D$ to receptors in the parathyroid cell regulates genomic transcription of PTH. The inhibitory actions of $1,25(OH)_2D$ on the parathyroid hormone gene is a feedback mechanism to regulate the influence of PTH on $1,25(OH)_2D$ synthesis.

2. 1,25-Dihydroxyvitamin D

The metabolically active form of vitamin D, 1,25-dihydroxyvitamin D, is derived from two principal sources. Vitamin D_3 or cholecalciferol is formed by the action of ultraviolet light upon its precursor molecule present in skin, 7-dehydrocholesterol. Vitamin D_2 or ergocalciferol is formed by irradiation of its precursor, ergosterol, found primarily in plants. To be available to humans, vitamin D_2 or ergosterol must be ingested in the diet. When there is adequate exposure to ultraviolet light, at the wavelength that can transform 7-dehydrocholesterol, there is no need for dietary supplementation. However, in some situations (northern latitudes, institutionalized individuals), vitamin D stores can be marginal or insufficient. In the USA, milk is routinely fortified with vitamin D to guard against the possibility of vitamin D deficiency, especially in children.

Both vitamin D_2 and vitamin D_3 can be regarded as pro-hormones, in that they require biochemical conversion to become metabolically active [10]. In general, both parent vitamins are processed similarly and can be considered to be biochemically interchangeable. After vitamin D is formed in the skin or absorbed from the GI tract, it is transported to the liver bound to a specific vitamin-D-binding protein that serves as a transport protein for the vitamin D metabolites as well. In the liver, vitamin D is hydroxylated to yield 25-hydroxyvitamin D (25-OHD), the major circulating form. The serum level of 25-OHD is an accurate indicator of body vitamin D stores of this hormone. The average serum concentration is approximately 35 ng/ml, and its half-life is 15 days. The usual range of 25-OHD concentrations is given as 9–52 ng/ml by many laboratories, but values below 15 ng/ml should be considered marginal. Concentrations of 25-OHD tend to show seasonal and geographical variations, tending to be lower in winter months and in northern latitudes.

The final activation of vitamin D occurs in the kidney. A second hydroxylation occurs at this site, producing the active form of the hormone, $1,25(OH)_2D$. The 1-alpha hydroxylase enzyme that catalyzes this conversion constitutes the principal regulatory site of $1,25(OH)_2D$ metabolism. The circulating concentration range of $1,25(OH)_2D$ is approximately 20–50 pg/ml, and its half-life in serum is 15 h. Renal hydroxylation of 25-OHD in the kidney may occur at sites other than position 1 (see below).

Like other steroid hormones, $1,25(OH)_2D$ binds to specific nuclear receptors in classical target tissues, including intestine, bone, and kidney. Receptors have also been identified in many nonclassical tissues such as the immune and hematopoietic systems, pancreas, pituitary, and brain. The effects of $1,25(OH)_2D$ at these sites, not previously thought to be targets for this hormone, are being studied intensively. $1,25(OH)_2D$ alters gene expression in target tissues. More recent evidence has indicated that certain nonclassical actions of $1,25(OH)_2D$ may occur by nongenomic mechanisms: Stimulation of calcium transport soon after cells are exposed to $1,25(OH)_2D$ may represent one of them.

The small intestine is the principal target organ for $1,25(OH)_2D$, where its major effect is to increase absorption of dietary calcium. It does so by increasing the active transport of calcium from the intestinal lumen, across the intestinal epithelial cell, and into the ECF. $1,25(OH)_2D$ mediates this active transport of calcium by stimulating the production of a calcium-binding protein. Although the precise role of this protein has not been completely elucidated, it appears to function in part by sequestering calcium within the intestinal epithelial cell, thus maintaining a low concentration of free ionized intracellular calcium in the cytoplasm. The additional very rapid effect of $1,25(OH)_2D$ to increase calcium transport as noted above may be another important mechanism by which calcium transport is stimulated. Another effect of $1,25(OH)_2D$ on the small intestine is to increase phosphorus absorption, in this case also stimulating active transport of this ion across the intestinal epithelium.

Bone is the second major target organ of 1,25(OH)$_2$D. Despite the absence of 1,25(OH)$_2$D receptors on osteoclasts, 1,25(OH)$_2$D increases mobilization of calcium from bone. It accomplishes this not by interacting directly with individual mature osteoclasts, but rather by promoting osteoclast differentiation from monocytic bone marrow precursors. 1,25(OH)$_2$D also increases osteoblast activity, despite the absence of specific receptors in these cells. It indirectly facilitates bone mineralization via its stimulation of intestinal absorption of calcium and phosphorus, thus providing concentrations of these ions in the ECF that are sufficient to permit mineralization of the osteoid matrix synthesized by osteoblasts.

In the kidney, 1,25(OH)$_2$D does enhance calcium and phosphorus absorption, but these actions do not appear to be of major physiologic importance.

The regulation of vitamin D metabolism occurs primarily at the level of the kidney. Conversion of 25-OHD to either its active metabolite, 1,25(OH)$_2$D, or to its inactive metabolite, 24,25(OH)$_2$D, is regulated by the serum phosphate level and by PTH. Hypophosphatemia directly stimulates 1-alpha hydroxylase activity, which catalyzes the conversion of 25-OHD to 1,25(OH)$_2$D in the kidney and suppresses 24-hydroxylase activity. Conversely, hyperphosphatemia suppresses 1-alpha hydroxylase activity and stimulates 24-hydroxylase activity. Thus, an alteration in the serum phosphate concentration affects intestinal phosphate and calcium absorption indirectly via their influences on the renal production of 1,25(OH)$_2$D. PTH also stimulates 1-alpha hydroxylase activity and increases renal production of 1,25(OH)$_2$D. Conversely, a decline in PTH is associated with a decreased production of 1,25(OH)$_2$D due to lowering of 1-alpha hydroxylase activity. In addition, the level of 1,25(OH)$_2$D itself influences the activity of the 1-hydroxylase enzyme. In the vitamin D replete state, 1-hydroxylase activity is low, and 24-hydroxylase activity is high. This state is regulated further by PTH. When the ionized calcium level is slightly elevated, PTH is suppressed, leading in turn to an inhibition of the 1-alpha hydroxylase activity. The opposite set of effects occurs during the vitamin D deficient state. Ionized calcium levels will tend to fall, and PTH secretion will increase, leading to the generation of active 1,25(OH)$_2$D. Severe hypercalcemia can itself directly suppress renal 1,25(OH)$_2$D production.

3. Calcitonin

A third hormone that may be involved in normal mineral metabolism is calcitonin [11, 12]. This peptide hormone is secreted primarily by parafollicular C-cells of neuroendocrine origin that are located within the thyroid gland. Calcitonin is a single chain, 32-amino-acid peptide with a 1–7 amino terminal disulfide bridge. Tissues other than thyroidal C-cells that produce calcitonin include pituitary cells and the widely distributed neuroendocrine cells.

The major target organs of calcitonin are bone and kidney. Its primary biological effect in bone is to inhibit osteoclast-mediated bone resorption. Within minutes of administration, calcitonin causes the osteoclast to shrink in size and to reduce its bone-resorbing activity. This effect lasts only as long as the osteoclast is exposed to calcitonin; the cell regains its bone-resorbing ability when calcitonin levels decrease. This property has led to the use of calcitonin in the therapy of disorders characterized by increased bone resorption. In the kidney, calcitonin has been reported to increase urinary excretion of calcium and phosphate — albeit at supraphysiologic concentrations. Both these effects are mediated by binding of calcitonin to its receptor in the plasma membrane of the renal target cell. The calcitonin receptor has recently been cloned and shows structural similarities to the PTH/PTHRP and secretin receptors. Calcitonin can stimulate adenylyl cyclase activity and increase intracellular generation of intracellular cyclic AMP. It also can stimulate phosphatidylinositol turnover and increase the intracellular ionized calcium concentration. Other extraskeletal effects have been described — particularly in the pituitary and the central nervous system where it may function as a neurotransmitter. It is these actions that may be responsible for its frequently reported analgesic effect. The central nervous system actions of calcitonin may actually be due to the presence of a closely related peptide, calcitonin gene-related peptide, which is found in great abundance there.

The serum ionized calcium level is the primary regulator of calcitonin secretion. An acute rise in the blood ionized calcium level stimulates calcitonin secretion; conversely, an acute fall in the blood ionized calcium inhibits calcitonin secretion. However, the effects of chronic hypercalcemia and hypocalcemia on calcitonin secretion are not well understood. GI polypeptides such as gastrin and cholecystokinin also stimulate calcitonin secretion when given in pharmacologic doses.

While there are many uncertainties regarding the role of calcitonin in normal mineral and skeletal metabolism in humans, the major action of this hormone (inhibiting osteoclast-mediated bone resorption) has proved useful in the therapy for certain disease states. Calcitonin is used to treat Paget's disease of bone, hypercalcemia of malignancy, and postmenopausal osteoporosis. Like the bisphosphonates, calcitonin is most useful clinically in states characterized by excessive bone resorption via activated osteoclasts.

4. Parathyroid hormone related protein

Parathyroid hormone related protein (PTHRP) was discovered in a search for the secretory product responsible for hypercalcemia in human malignancies [13, 14]. PTHRP has an important but limited primary sequence homology with native PTH. The first 13 amino acids are essentially identical. In part because of this close structural homology in a region of the peptide (1–13) that has full biological activity (1–34), PTHRP can mimic many of the actions of PTH. In many cancers associated with hypercalcemia, especially those characterized by epithelial histology, PTHRP is secreted by the tumor cells and causes osteoclast-mediated bone resorption. In view of the actions of the bisphosphonates in inhibiting osteoclast-mediated bone resorption, they have found a very important clinical application, namely as agents to treat hypercalcemia of malignancy caused by PTHRP.

Although PTHRP was discovered in the abnormal pathophysiological setting of cancer-associated hypercalcemia, efforts to understand its potential as a physiological regulator of calcium metabolism are ongoing. In the adult, there is no evidence at this time to implicate PTHRP in normal calcium homeostasis. Despite the use of sensitive detection methods, PTHRP does not appear to circulate under normal circumstances. However, the presence of large local concentrations of PTHRP in a very wide variety of tissues like keratinocytes, uterine smooth muscle, vascular smooth muscle, placenta, and central nervous system suggest a paracrine or autocrine role for PTHRP in the normal adult. Potential physiologic functions which are currently being investigated may not be limited to calcium metabolism.

In the developing fetus, in contrast to adults, PTHRP may have a very important physiological role. It may actually be the principal circulating calcium-regulating hormone, not relinquishing that role to PTH until after delivery, when PTHRP levels fall and PTH levels rise.

V. Summary

Many hormones, ions, and tissues participate in the complex regulation of mineral homeostasis. The two most important hormones, PTH and $1,25(OH)_2D$, affect the skeleton, kidney, and GI tract to maintain normal concentrations of calcium and phosphate in the blood and ECF. Regulation is achieved by controls at the levels of calcium and phosphate absorption from the diet, reabsorption of these ions from the glomerular filtrate, and regulation of bone turnover. The precise mechanisms by which these hormones affect the handling of calcium depends upon the target organ and the regulatory imperative. The discussion of the bisphosphonates to follow will be more readily understood in the context of this background chapter.

References

1. West, J.B. (Editor), Best and Taylor's physiological basis of medical practice, 12th edn. Hormonal regulation of mineral metabolism, Chapter 56. Williams and Wilkins, Baltimore, 1991.
2. West, J.B. (Editor), Best and Taylor's physiological basis of medical practice, 12th edn. Regulation of calcium, magnesium and phosphate excretion, Chapter 34. Williams and Wilkins, Baltimore, 1991.
3. Stewart, A.F. and Broadus, A.E., Mineral metabolism. In: Felig, P., Baxter, J.D., Broadus, A.E., and Frohman, L.A. (Editors), Endocrinology and Metabo ism, 2nd edn. McGraw-Hill, New York, 1987, pp. 1317–1453.
4. Alpers, D.H., Absorption of vitamins and divalent minerals. In: Sleisenger, M.H. and Fortran, J.S. (Editors), Gastrointestinal disease, 4th edn. W.B. Saunders, Philadelphia, 1989.
5. Suki, W.N. and Rouze, R., Renal transport of calcium, magnesium and phosphorus. In: Brenner, B.M. and Rector, F.C., Jr. (Editors), The kidney, 4th edn. Chapter 10. W.B. Saunders, Philadelphia, 1991.
6. Coe, F.L. and Favus, M.J. (Editors), Disorders of bone and mineral metabolism. Raven, New York, 1992.
7. Parfitt, A.M., Calcium homeostasis. In: Mundy, G.R. and Martins, J.J. (Editors), Physiology and pharmacology of bone. Springer-Verlag, Heidelberg, 1992.
8. Parfitt, A.M., Bone remodelling. In: Riggs, B.L. and Melton, L.J. III (Editors), Osteoporosis. Raven, New York, 1988.
9. Kronenberg, H.M., Parathyroid hormone: Mechanism of action. In: Primer on the metabolic bone diseases and disorders of mineral metabolism, 2nd edn. Raven, New York, 1993.

10. Reichel, H., Koeffler, H.P. and Norman, A.W., The role of the vitamin D endocrine system in health and disease. N. Engl. J. Med. 1989; 320: 980–991.
11. Deftos, L.J., Calcitonin secretion in humans. In: Cooper, C.W. (Editor), Current research on calcium regulating hormones. Univ. of Texas Press, Austin, 1987, pp. 79–100.
12. Deftos, L.J., Calcitonin. In: Primer on the metabolic bone diseases and disorders of mineral metabolism, 2nd edn. Raven, New York, 1993.
13. Halloran, B.P. and Nissenson, R.A. (Editors), Parathyroid hormone-related protein: normal physiology and its role in cancer. CRC Press, Boca Raton, 1992.
14. Orloff, J.J., Wu, T.L. and Stewart, A.F., Parathyroid hormone-like proteins: Biochemical responses and receptor interactions. Endocrinol. Rev. 1989; 10: 476.
15. Riggs, B.L. and Melton, L.J. III, N. Engl. J. Med. 1992; 327: 620–627.

Bisphosphonate on bones
O. Bijvoet, H.A. Fleisch, R.E. Canfield and G. Russell (eds.)
© 1995 Elsevier Science B.V. All rights reserved.

CHAPTER 2

Cell biology of bone: Lineage, cell–cell interactions, cytokines

P.J. Nijweide and R. van 't Hof

Dept. of Cell Biology and Histology, School of Medicine, University of Leiden, Rijnsburgerweg 10,
2333 AA Leiden, The Netherlands

I. Introduction

Bone is a living, continuously self-renewing tissue, perfectly attuned to its many functions. As the most important part of the skeleton, it provides support for the body and sites for muscle attachment. Several vital organs and tissues such as bone marrow are protected by bone. Bone acts as a reservoir for ions such as calcium, phosphate, and magnesium, and helps to regulate the homeostasis of these ions in the blood. It may also act as a sink for circulating or locally produced growth factors and detoxify the body fluids from noxious metal ions. All these functions impose their special requirements on the structure and composition of bone and on the regulation of its metabolism and turnover.

The adaptations of bone tissue to its many functions that change or fluctuate during life are governed and executed by the cells in bone: the osteogenic or bone-forming cells, the osteoclastic or bone-resorbing cells, and a group of cells present in bone but not belonging to either of these proper bone cells. Both groups or families of bone cells consist of the fully differentiated, mature representatives, e.g., osteoblasts and osteoclasts, but also of a cascade of stem, progenitor, and precursor cells. It is not only the activities of the mature forms, but also the generation of these cells by proliferation and differentiation of undifferentiated or less differentiated cells that determine the metabolism and turnover of bone. These stem, progenitor, and precursor cells are not only present in bone but also in bone marrow. Bone and bone marrow are intricately related to each other. The osteoprogenitors on the endosteal surface of long bones form a continuum with the fibrostromal cells of the bone marrow. The stem cell of the osteoclast is none other than the hemopoietic stem cell and is shared with all the different types of circulating blood cells. Regulation of hemopoiesis is therefore also of importance for osteoclastogenesis. Growth factors active in hemopoiesis, the colony-stimulating factors, have been shown to influence the formation of osteoclasts. On the other hand, osteogenic cells are capable of colony-stimulating factor secretion which may regulate hemopoiesis. Several cell types of hemopoietic origin (lymphocytes, macrophages) produce growth factors, especially in pathological situations, which have major effects on bone formation and bone resorption.

The formation and activities of the cells of bone and, in consequence, bone turnover are not constant through life and not of equal rate throughout the skeleton or the individual bones. Bone turnover is highest during the formation and growth of the skeleton and lowest at old age. Within bone, turnover is much higher in the trabecular bone than in cortical bone. The sites at which at any given time bone turnover takes place is probably determined by changes in the local production of a variety of growth factors and cytokines. The production and secretion of these growth factors and cytokines are modulated by humoral factors (hormones), by other local factors, and by environmental factors such as mechanical loading.

The cellular diversity, in cell type and differentiation level, of bone and bone marrow combined with the multitude of humoral, local and environmental factors active in bone creates a complexity of which we learn more each year, but which is still far from being well understood.

II. The cells of bone

Osteoclasts, osteoblasts, and osteocytes, the most prominent, mature differentiation stages of the bone-resorbing and bone-forming cells, are unique to bone. This uniqueness is not so much determined by the cells themselves. Stem or progenitor cells capable of differentiating into osteoclastic or osteoblastic cells are also present elsewhere in the body; osteogenesis may artificially be induced at other sites [1]; osteoclast progenitor cells were shown to circulate in the blood system [2, 3]. Under physiological conditions, however, only bone tissue appears to provide the microenvironment necessary for osteoclastic and osteoblastic differentiation.

1. The osteoclast

Kölliker [4] was the first to observe osteoclasts on bone surfaces and gave them their name. Since that time many investigators have been intrigued by the osteoclast [reviews: 5–9]. Originally, the low frequency of their occurrence hampered the study of their origin, properties and functions. In recent years, the increasing technical possibilities of cell isolation, culture, ion transport measurement, immunocytochemistry, and in situ hybridization have stimulated the pace of information accumulation. Today we are on the verge of the full implementation of molecular biological techniques in osteoclast research [10].

(a) Morphology and markers

The osteoclast is a large multinucleated cell. It is formed by the fusion of mononuclear precursor cells [11–13], may expel old nuclei and refresh its nucleus composition by fusion with other osteoclasts or with additional precursor cells [14, 15]. Ultrastructurally, the osteoclast possesses a number of features which each on its own may not be (completely) osteoclast-specific but which in combination are absolutely determinant. In the cytoplasm lysosomes and mitochondria are abundant. When attached to the bone surface the osteoclast forms a ring structure of strongly attached cell membrane and organelle-free cytoplasm, the clear zone or sealing zone. The part of the cell membrane within this ring, adjacent to the bone surface, shows many foldings or ruffles, the ruffled border [16]. Underneath this area, the bone is demineralized and resorbed.

Cytochemically, the ultrastructural features are expressed as high succinic dehydrogenase (mitochondria) and tartrate-resistant acid phosphatase (lysosomes) activities [17–19]. The demonstration of the first enzyme is nonspecific. The intensity of the reaction in osteoclasts is merely an expression of the high number of mitochondria present. The second enzyme (TRAcP) was at first considered to be osteoclast-specific. However, particularly under in vitro circumstances, TRAcP was recently shown to be induced in other cells, e.g., macrophages [20, 21]. Carbonic anhydrase, a cytosolic enzyme that catalyzes the formation of protons (necessary for osteoclastic bone mineral dissolution) and bicarbonate ions from water and carbon dioxide, is another osteoclast indicator, albeit not an exclusive marker. The enzyme is generally not demonstrated by its cytochemical reaction but immunocytochemically [22].

The lack of an exclusive enzyme marker has led several investigators to raise monoclonal antibodies directed against osteoclasts [23–27; review: 28]. Most of the antigenic determinants concerned are, however, also present in macrophages, especially after cell culture. The most widely applied antibody at this moment is 23C6 [24], elicited by injection of human osteoclasts but cross-reacting with, e.g., rabbit and chick [29]. Antigen 23C6 is also expressed on cultured macrophages [30], but the level of expression is much higher in osteoclasts. Other antibodies used to discriminate especially between osteoclasts and monocytes/macrophages are antibodies that react with the latter cells but not with osteoclasts [28, 31, 32]. In mouse, such an antibody is F4/80 [33]. This marker is often used in combination with TRAcP staining in mouse cell cultures.

Mammalian osteoclasts display a large number of calcitonin receptors [34–36]. In combination with the typical response [37] of osteoclasts to calcitonin (cell movement inhibition, cell contraction), this is considered one of the most specific markers for osteoclasts [38]. However, avian osteoclasts do not express CT receptors [39], and in mammalian species these receptors can be downregulated.

The most convincing marker for osteoclast differentiation remains the ability to resorb bone. Bone resorption can be assessed by various techniques. The formation of resorption pits (Fig. 1) by cells seeded on bone or dentine slices can be studied by light microscopy [40] or electron microscopy [41, 42]. In co-cultures of putative osteoclast precursors and long bones of fetal animals, osteoclastic activity can be visualized either by ^{45}Ca release from prelabeled bones or by light (Fig. 2) or electron microscopy [43, 44].

The need to be able to identify osteoclasts within a multitude of other cell types was especially felt in the search for the ontogeny of the osteoclast and the study

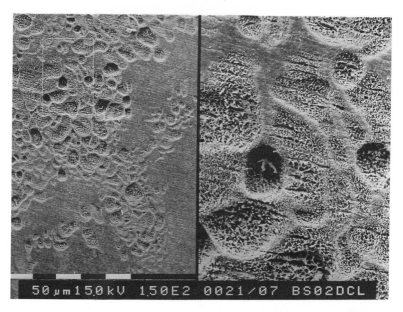

Fig. 1. Isolated chicken osteoclasts were seeded on a thin dentin slice. After two days of culture the cells were removed and the bone slices studied with a scanning electron microscope. The osteoclasts have excavated numerous pits in the surface of the dentin.

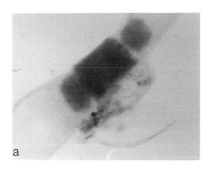
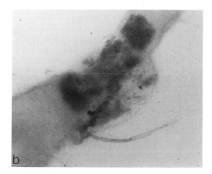

Fig. 2. Bone marrow cells in coculture with a metatarsal bone of a 17-day-old fetal mouse. The bone marrow cells were suspended in a plasma clot which was then placed adjacent to the calcified hypertrophic cartilage area. A: after two days of culture; on both sides of the calcified area calcification has progressed. B: after seven days of culture: the original calcified area is resorbed by osteoclasts induced in the bone marrow cell population.

of the regulation of osteoclast formation. For several decades, investigators have speculated on the possibility of a hemopoietic origin.

(b) Hemopoiesis

In adult mammals, the bone marrow is the main site for hemopoiesis. Bone marrow is a highly vascular connective tissue with a high cell content. It consists

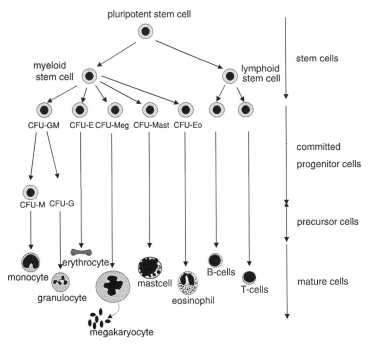

Fig. 3. Hemopoietic differentiation pathways.

of two major cellular components: the hemopoietic cells and the stromal cells. The stromal component contains endothelial cells and reticular (fibrostromal) cells, among others. It provides the microenvironment necessary for hemopoiesis by producing and sequestering growth/differentiation factors and exposing them to hemopoietic cells [45].

All hemopoietic cells are derived from the pluripotent hemopoietic stem cell or PHSC (Fig. 3) [46, 47]. These PHSC have a high capacity of proliferation. Part of the offspring will remain PHSC (self-renewal); the other part may differentiate into many directions: lymphocytes, monocytes, granulocytes, erythrocytes, megakaryocytes, etc. During this process of differentiation from stem cell to mature cell, the progeny of the PHSC gradually loses its capacity to proliferate. Apart from the stem cells and the mature, fully differentiated cells, two other cell compartments are distinguished: the committed progenitor cells, i.e., cells with still high proliferative but not self-renewal capacity, which in contrast to the stem cells are restricted in their differentiation to one or two of the differentiation sublines; and the precursor cells, i.e., cells in a late stage of differentiation which already carry to some extent recognizable morphological and cytochemical features of the nonproliferating end cells. The precursor cells have only limited proliferative capacity [48].

The proliferation and differentiation of hemopoietic stem, progenitor, and precursor cells is regulated by a group of growth factors known as colony-stimulating factors (CSFs) [49]. Some of these factors are more or less specific for one differentiation subline: macrophage CSF (M-CSF), granulocyte CSF (G-CSF), ery-thropoietic (EPO), etc. Others have a more general effect or particularly stimulate stem cell proliferation: GM-CSF, interleukin 3 (IL-3), IL-1, IL-6, etc.

In vitro in bone marrow culture, hemopoiesis will quickly cease unless sufficient stromal cells are present or CSFs are added to the culture medium. The finding that CSFs alone may support hemopoiesis in vitro has led to the development of the colony assay in semisolid media [47]. In this assay, hemopoietic cells are very sparsely seeded in 1% methylcellulose-enforced culture medium. Each proliferative cell (stem or progenitor cell) will give rise to the formation of a colony within the semisolid medium. Analysis of the colonies (mono-, bi-, or multilineage) provides a semiquantitative impression of the number and nature of the stem and progenitor cells present in the original cell suspension. The stem and progenitor cells that give rise to multilineage, monocyte/granulocyte, monocyte, granulocyte, etc. colonies are called, respectively, colony forming unit–stem cell (CFU-S), CFU-GM (the shared committed progenitor of both monocyte and granulocyte sublines), CFU-M, CFU-G, etc.

(c) Hemopoietic origin of the osteoclast

In vivo experiments in the late 1970s provided the first direct evidence for the hemopoietic origin of the osteoclast. Göthlin and Ericsson [50] showed that osteoclast progenitors are present in the blood by parabiotically linking the blood-stream of irradiated rats to that of nonirradiated ^{3}H-thymidine-labeled rats. The left femora of the irradiated rats were fractured. When the animals were killed one to four weeks later, the osteoclasts and macrophages at the fracture site in the irradiated rats were labeled with ^{3}H-thymidine, showing that in the absence of local stem/progenitor cells (by irradiation), the other animal furnished the necessary stem/progenitor cells.

Walker demonstrated that osteopetrosis in osteopetrotic mi/mi mice could be cured by parabiosis with a normal littermate [2] or by transplantation of normal bone marrow or spleen cells [51]. Similar successful transplantation studies have been performed in other species, including man [52].

The final proof for the hemopoietic origin of the osteoclast was delivered by Scheven et al. [53] and Hagenaars et al. [54]. Using the co-culture technique [43], they generated osteoclasts from purified [53] and cloned [54] hemopoietic stem cells. These results were confirmed by experiments of Schneider and Relfson [55] and of Kurihara et al. [56].

(d) The osteoclast lineage

Although it is now well established that the osteoclast stems from the pluripotent hemopoietic stem cell, the lineage along which osteoclast progenitor and precursor cells differentiate towards the mature multinucleated osteoclast has not been satisfactorily elucidated. The direct precursor of the osteoclast (the preOc) is a mononuclear, postmitotic cell which has several osteoclastic characteristics such as TRAcP activity [13, 57] and calcitonin receptors [58]. Generally, there is little dispute that the osteoclast belongs to the myeloid branch of the hemopoietic cell

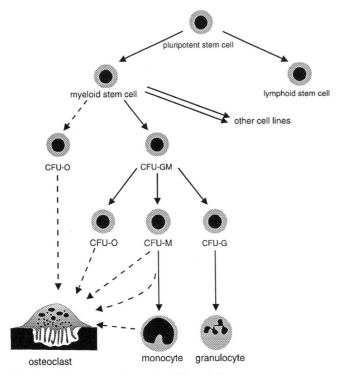

Fig. 4. Possible routes of osteoclast differentiation.

family. Hagenaars et al. [44] showed that the myeloid FDCP-mix cell lines A4 and C2GM [59] are able to differentiate into osteoclasts. Yoneda et al. [60] generated osteoclasts from the promyelocytic cell line HL-60 [61]. There is no unanimity, however, whether the preOc and osteoclast derive from the last stages of the monocyte lineage or whether osteoclast and monocyte differentiation lines bifurcate at a (much) earlier stage (Fig. 4).

Some of the available evidence demonstrates that monocyte precursors, monocytes, and even macrophages are able to differentiate into osteoclasts. Suda and co-workers [62, 63] cultured mouse blood monocytes and alveolar macrophages on a layer of ST2 cells, a bone marrow stroma-derived cell line [64]. In the presence of 1,25-dihydroxy vitamin D_3 [1,25(OH)$_2$D$_3$] and dexamethasone, preOc and osteoclasts were formed. The osteoclast phenotype was determined by staining for TRAcP, binding of calcitonin, and capacity to form pits on dentine slices. These results were confirmed by studies of Alvarez et al. [65] who reported the generation of large numbers of osteoclast-like cells from the monocytic cell fraction in chick bone marrow. More recently, Quin et al. [66] reported that a very large proportion of the strongly adherent fraction of blood monocytes is capable of differentiating into fully functional osteoclasts. Resorption was found on the majority of bone slices when only 200–300 adherent cells/slice were seeded. Indirect support for the monocytic origin of the osteoclast comes from the observations that in fetal organ cultures osteoclast formation is stimulated by M-CSF [67] and that osteopetrosis in the mouse op/op and the rat tl/tl mutants can be cured by administering M-CSF to these animals [68–70]. Takahashi et al. [71] also demonstrated a stimulating activity of M-CSF in the generation of osteoclasts in an in vitro culture system. The stimulating activity of M-CSF was only found on early progenitors, which could subsequently be induced to form osteoclasts on a layer of primary osteoblasts in the presence of $1,25(OH)_2D_3$.

In contrast to these studies, other investigators have supplied evidence for an osteoclast differentiation line much further separated from the monocyte lineage than suggested by the above-mentioned reports. Schneider and Relfson showed that in contrast to CFU-S, CFU-M when transplanted into osteopetrotic rats [72] as well as when co-cultured with fetal rat long bones [73] could not give rise to osteo-clast formation. Similar negative results on osteoclast formation by CFU-M were obtained by Hattersley et al. [74] and Kurihara et al. [75]. These investigators ob-served that monocyte colonies in methylcellulose cultures of hemopoietic cells did not form osteoclasts. Hattersley et al. [74] and Kerby et al. [76] even suggest that the pathways of osteoclasts and monocytes/macrophages bifurcate at a differentiation stage before the CFU-GM. This view is supported by Lee et al. [77], who isolated O-CSF (osteoclast colony-stimulating factor) and studied the progenitor cells stim-ulated by this factor. They concluded that these cells, termed CFU-O, are more immature than CFU-GM. Finally, Kerby et al. [76] cultured alveolar and peritoneal macrophages on ST2 cells but found no evidence for osteoclast differentiation. In sum, the studies mentioned above clearly show that the osteoclast is derived from the hemopoietic stem cell and probably belongs to the myeloid lineage. At present, there is, however, insufficient proof to decide what the relation between the osteo-clast line and monocyte/macrophage line is. Moreover, one should realize that most of the lineage studies are performed in vitro under circumstances different from the in vivo situation (e.g., the high $1,25(OH)_2D_3$ concentration generally used in vitro). The evidence available suggests that osteoclasts may be formed in vitro along different pathways. Which of these pathways represents the lineage along which the osteoclast is formed in vivo awaits further experimentation.

2. The osteogenic cells

The antipodes of the bone-resorbing cells are the osteogenic or bone-forming cells. In contrast to the resorbing cell family in which the mature fully differentiated end cell, the multinucleated osteoclast, is the main executor of the resorption function, the osteogenic cell family contains several highly differentiated forms. Each of these, osteoblast, osteocyte, and lining cell, has its own function in the metabolism of bone tissue. The function of the osteogenic cells is therefore not merely the production of bone matrix, they also play a pivotal role in the regulation of bone formation, bone maintenance, and bone resorption.

(a) Ontogeny

The multipotent stem cell of the osteogenic cell line is the mesenchymal or stromal stem cell [78, 79]. In analogy with the terminology used for the hemopoietic cell system, these cells are also called colony forming units–fibroblasts or CFU-f [80]. The existence of these cells was demonstrated by seeding bone marrow in relatively low concentrations in culture flasks [80]. Single cell-derived colonies of fibroblast-like cells were formed. When these colonies were transplanted in diffusion chambers [81], they gave rise to the formation of either a combination of bone, cartilage, and reticular connective tissues, or bone or reticular tissue alone. In other words, the CFU-f are heterogeneous and include at least three different categories of clonogenic stromal cells: the multipotent CFU-b,c,r and the committed progenitor cells CFU-b and CFU-r [80]. Other experiments with bone marrow stromal cell cultures supplied evidence for a common precursor for adipocytic and osteogenic cells [82].

Similar results were obtained by Aubin and co-workers [83, 84]. They cloned a number of cell lines from cell populations isolated from fetal rat calvariae. One of the cell lines they obtained, RCJ3.1, could give rise to four morphologically distinct cell types: muscle cells, adipocytes, chondroblastic and osteoblastic cells. RCJ3.1 represents therefore a multipotent or perhaps even a pluripotent stem cell. By subcloning RCJ3.1, Aubin et al. obtained a number of mono-, bi-, and tripotential subclones, i.e., cell lines with more or less stringent commitment to three, two or one differentiation lines [83, 84].

Because of the lack of morphologically distinct features, the various stem and progenitor stages of the stromal cell line are not demonstrable in bone tissue. It is generally assumed, however, that the multipotent stromal stem cell and the various early progenitor stages of the osteogenic subline are present in periosteum, endosteum, and stromal compartment of bone marrow. The committed progenitor of the osteogenic cell line is called the osteoprogenitor (Fig. 5).

The most immature stage of the osteogenic cell line which is readily recognizable in bone is the preosteoblast, the immediate precursor of the osteoblast. The preosteoblasts are located adjacent to the layer of osteoblasts coating the bone surface. They have already acquired some of the characteristics of the mature osteoblast, such as alkaline phosphatase activity, albeit to a lesser degree. The cells are still capable of proliferation [85]. During the process of bone formation, some of the osteoblasts are incorporated in the bone matrix and gradually differentiate into osteocytes. Osteoblasts may also change into lining cells on bone surfaces where bone formation has ceased.

(b) Osteoblast morphology and functions

The osteoblast is a polarized, cuboidal, mononuclear cell. It has an extensive rough endoplasmic reticulum and a large golgi apparatus, characteristic features for a cell with high protein synthetic and secretory activity [86]. Cytochemically, the cell is easily recognized by its high alkaline phosphatase activity. Apart from its major product, collagen type I, the osteoblast synthesizes a large number of noncollagenous proteins which may have functions in cell chemotaxis, cell

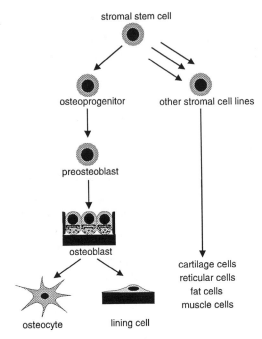

Fig. 5. Osteogenic differentiation.

attachment, and regulation of mineralization [87, 88]. The most osteoblast-specific noncollagenous protein is osteocalcin [89], which appears to be specific to calcified tissues [88–91].

The primary function of the osteoblast is the formation and calcification of bone matrix. A second important function is its apparent pivotal role in the (hormonal) regulation of bone formation and bone resorption. The two major calcium regulating hormones, parathyroid hormone and $1,25(OH)_2D_3$, have their receptors on/in the osteoblasts. Osteoblasts produce a series of local factors which are involved in the local regulation of bone metabolism. Some of these factors are matrix-bound and form an integral part of the bone matrix (e.g., osteopontin and osteocalcin), others are adsorbed to the bone mineral or matrix (bone morphogenic proteins, transforming growth factor ß), while still others are released into the extracellular fluid and remain dissolved (cytokines, prostaglandins).

(c) The lining cell

Relatively little is known about the bone lining cells, although they occupy the major part of the bone surface in the adult. Lining cells are flattened cells containing few organelles [92, 93]. Osteoblasts are thought to change into bone lining cells after bone formation has ceased, and there are some indications that lining cells can be activated to become osteoblasts again [94]. The most important function of the bone lining cell is probably to ensure contact between the cells incorporated in the bone, the osteocytes, and the outside. Secondly, they may serve as nutritional support cells for the osteocytes [92, 93]. The lining cells are coupled to the osteocytes by means of gap junctions between the cell processes of lining cells and connected osteocytes. A third possible important function is the regulation of osteoclastic bone resorption.

(d) The osteocyte

The mature osteocyte is a stellate-shaped cell enclosed within the lacunar-canalicular network of bone. The lacuna contains the cell body, the canaliculi the cytoplasmic processes. Ultrastructurally, recently embedded osteocytes are very similar to osteoblasts [95]. During maturation to mature osteocytes, the cells lose a large part of their cytoplasmic organelles and considerably diminish in size. The localization of the osteocytes within the heavily calcified bone matrix has given rise to many speculations about their function but on the other hand has hampered the study into the role of the osteocyte in bone metabolism. The enormous cell surface which the osteocytes and their cytoplasmic processes represent suggests a role in blood calcium homeostasis. Little evidence has been found, however [96, 97], for the process of osteocytic osteolysis originally proposed by Belanger [98]. An osteocyte-regulated release of mineral without accompanying matrix resorption is perhaps more probable [95]. The fact that within an osteon all osteocytes are connected with each other and with the osteoblasts or bone lining cells on the bone surface suggests that bone possesses an elaborate communication network, or rather two networks: one intracellular from cell to cell, one extracellular from lacuna to lacuna. It is tempting to think that these networks are used to confer messages about the status of the bone inside the osteon to the outside.

III. Regulation of bone turnover

The formation from progenitor/precursor cells and the metabolic activity of the various mature cells of bone are not independent processes within each differentiation line and between cells of different differentiation lines. Bone formation and bone resorption are attuned to each other, leading to the formation and modeling of the skeleton in accordance with the growth of the individual during the growing phase, and to the maintenance and remodeling of the skeleton during the adult phase. A large number of systemic and locally produced factors regulate these processes. Many of these factors appear to have pleiotropic and sometimes even conflicting activities. The apparent inconsistency of some of the actions of factors active in bone is probably the result of artefactual model systems in which the actions of these factors are studied. Systemic hormones, growth factors, cytokines, and cell–cell contact interactions form the orchestra which plays the melody of bone. Listening to only one or a few individual instruments of this orchestra may give a distorted idea of the melody. However, listening to the complete orchestra makes the analysis of the contribution of each individual instrument impossible.

In view of the complexity of the regulatory mechanisms in bone metabolism, we will limit ourselves to what is known about the interactions of the two major cell types of bone, the osteogenic and the osteoclastic cells, and about the production and activities of a number of local factors that are important in these interactions.

1. Osteoblastic regulation of osteoclastic bone resorption

Many of the bone resorption-stimulating agents either exert their activity via the osteoblast or are produced by it. Relatively few agents are known to act directly on the osteoclast itself. Stimulation of resorption may be brought about on three levels: 1. stimulation of proliferation and differentiation of osteoclast progenitor cells; 2. stimulation of differentiation and fusion of postmitotic osteoclast precursor cells; and 3. stimulation of the resorptive activity of existing osteoclasts.

(a) Parathyroid hormone

Parathyroid hormone (PTH) is a potent stimulator of osteoclastic bone resorption. This was first shown by the classic experiments of Gaillard [99] in co-cultures of bone and parathyroid gland. Later experiments have shown that the administration of PTH results in an increased activation of existing osteoclasts as well as a stimulated formation of new osteoclasts, both in vivo and in vitro (review: [8]). The stimulation of new osteoclast formation is primarily caused by a stimulation of precursor differentiation and fusion, not of progenitor proliferation [8].

According to most investigators, the stimulatory effect of PTH must be mediated by osteogenic cells (osteoblasts, lining cells, stromal cells). In contrast to osteogenic cells, osteoclasts were found not to express PTH receptors [100, 101], nor do isolated osteoclasts respond to PTH unless osteogenic cells are also present [102]. Recently, Teti et al. [103] and also Agarwala and Gay [104] reported, however, the presence of PTH receptors on chicken osteoclasts. They showed specific binding of biotinylated PTH, visualized by fluorography, and subsequent rapid internalization of the bound PTH by endocytosis. If this finding is also valid for mammalian osteoclasts, osteoclastic bone resorption may be under dual control.

The mechanism by which the PTH signal is transduced from osteoblast to osteoclast or osteoclast precursor cell is at present not satisfactorily elucidated. Some of the available evidence argues for a cell–cell contact mechanism. Osteoblasts were found to activate osteoclasts in vitro only when they were in close contact with each other [105]. Suda et al. [9] showed that intimate contact between spleen cells and stromal cells was required for the formation of osteoclasts in mixed cell cultures. Another possibility is that the signal from osteoblast to osteoclast is mediated by soluble local factor(s) produced by the osteoblast [104]. A number of recent studies [107–110] have reported the presence of osteoclast-activating activity other than prostaglandins in the supernatant of osteoblast-like cell cultures. Although it has been shown that PTH stimulates prostaglandin production by osteoblasts [111], it is probably not the factor which relates the PTH signal to osteoclasts [112]. The nature of the observed activities is still unclear. As they appear to represent very labile compounds [109, 110], the apparent cell–cell contact-mediated signal transduction pathway mentioned above may in reality be a secreted (very labile) compound-mediated signal transduction.

The bone surface may also play an important role in the interaction between osteoblasts and osteoclasts. PTH causes osteoblasts to retract, thereby exposing bone surface to osteoclasts [113]. Furthermore, PTH stimulates collagenase production and activation by osteoblasts [114–117]. The osteoblasts secrete neutral collagenase in an inactive form and plasminogen activator. Subsequently, plasminogen activator [117] helps, via the activation of plasmin, to convert the inactive collagenase, recently secreted or already present in the bone matrix, into active collagenase. This collagenase may then hydrolyze the collagen present in the thin layer of osteoid that covers the calcified matrix, thereby rendering the calcified matrix surface resorbable for osteoclasts [118–121]. Collagen fragments or compounds adsorbed to the collagen matrix are released by the matrix breakdown and may serve as chemoattractants for osteoclasts [122–124].

(b) 1,25-Dihydroxy vitamin D_3

The active form of vitamin D_3, 1,25-dihydroxy vitamin D_3 ($1,25(OH)_2D_3$) is, like PTH, a potent stimulator of osteoclastic bone resorption [125, 126]. As with stimulation by PTH, stimulation of osteoclast formation and activity by $1,25(OH)_2D_3$ is probably mediated by osteoblasts, since these cells express $1,25(OH)_2D_3$ receptors while osteoclasts do not [127, 128]. Isolated osteoclasts do not respond to $1,25(OH)_2D_3$ [100], but osteoblasts may be activated to produce an osteoclast-activating factor [129].

Although the pattern of resorption-stimulating activities of $1,25(OH)_2D_3$ is in many ways similar to that of PTH, both in vivo and in vitro, the evidence for a role of $1,25(OH)_2D_3$ in the early stages of osteoclast progenitor proliferation and differentiation is much stronger. In bone marrow cultures or in co-cultures of early hemopoietic cells with osteogenic cells (osteoblasts, stromal cells), the addition of $1,25(OH)_2D_3$ to the culture medium is almost obligatory to obtain osteoclast-like cell formation [reviews: 9, 121, 128, 130]. The action of $1,25(OH)_2D_3$ is in part indirect, via the osteogenic cells, but $1,25(OH)_2D_3$ is also known to be able to influence directly differentiation in the myeloid cell lineage [128]. It is also possible that other cells such as monocytes play the role of intermediate cell. Monocytes constitutively express $1,25(OH)_2D_3$ receptors [127]. The production of several cytokines by monocytes is modulated by $1,25(OH)_2D_3$ [130].

(c) Prostaglandins

The prostaglandins are probably the first mentioned candidates for the interaction between osteoblasts and osteoclasts. Virtually all cells, including osteoblasts and osteoclasts have receptors for prostaglandins. Prostaglandins, particularly of the E series, were shown to stimulate bone resorption in bone organ cultures [132]. Prostaglandins are produced by cultured bone [132] and appear to be responsible for the basal rate of resorption in mouse calvariae since addition of indomethacin, an inhibitor of prostaglandin synthesis, blocks basal resorption [133].

Several hormones, growth factors, and cytokines stimulate bone resorption in organ cultures via a prostaglandin-dependent pathway, although the degree of prostaglandin involvement differs from factor to factor and from animal species to animal species [134–139]. Osteoblasts or more generally the osteogenic cells are probably the source of endogenous prostaglandin production in bone [107, 138]. The two classical bone resorption stimulating hormones, PTH and $1,25(OH)_2D_3$, act mainly via a prostaglandin-independent pathway, although both hormones have been shown to stimulate prostaglandin synthesis to a small extent [111, 141].

Prostaglandins stimulate bone resorption by stimulating osteoclast formation from hemopoietic progenitor cells [142]. The resorbing activity of existing osteoclasts, in the absence of osteogenic cells, is inhibited by prostaglandins [143].

(d) Colony-stimulating factors

Colony-stimulating factors (CSFs) play an important role in hemopoiesis. As the osteoclast is derived from the hemopoietic stem cell, these factors may affect the generation of osteoclasts. Effects of several of the CSFs have indeed been found in various in vitro systems, although the reports are sometimes contradictory [review: 130].

Several CSFs (M-CSF, GM-CSF, G-CSF) are secreted by stromal cells [45]. As the amounts of secreted CSFs are quite low and hemopoiesis requires an intimate cell–cell contact between stromal cells and hemopoietic progenitors, it is thought that the CSFs are sequestered by membrane-associated matrix components on the stromal cells and presented in this way to hemopoietic stem and progenitor cells [45].

Osteoclast formation also requires the immediate presence of stromal or osteogenic cells [9]. Calvariae and isolated calvarial cells were shown to produce several CSFs [144]. The M-CSF receptor, a tyrosine kinase encoded by the c-*fms* gene, has been detected on mouse osteoclast-like cells in vitro [145]. It is therefore very likely that at least one of the pathways by which osteogenic cells regulate osteoclast formation and activity is by presenting CSFs on their surfaces. Whether the well-known CSFs are competent to support the complete differentiation pathway of the osteoclast is, however, doubtful. In analogy with the other hemopoietic differentiation lines, one would expect the requirement for a more or less specific osteoclast CSF. The experiments of Lee et al. [146] may have furnished proof for the existence of such an O-CSF.

Little is known whether CSFs may act as intermediates between osteogenic cells and (progenitors of) osteoclasts for the transduction of signals resulting from the binding of hormones and factors to osteogenic cells. Increased release of M-CSF by the osteoblastic cell line MC3T3 in response to IL-1, TNFα, TGFβ, and EGF has been described [147].

(e) Interleukins

Interleukins (ILs) were originally identified as factors important for signalling between leucocytes. IL-1 for instance was described as a mononuclear phagocyte-produced factor which stimulated the formation of T-lymphocytes. Later, it was realized that the production and the action of several interleukins was not limited to the immune system. Although currently there is no direct evidence that interleukins are involved in normal bone remodeling [148], it has been shown that several interleukins are secreted by osteogenic cells and influence the resorption activity or the formation of osteoclasts. So, interleukins may very well be involved in the cross-talk between osteogenic cells and osteoclasts.

Interleukin 1 (IL-1) was the first 'immune' cytokine positively identified as a factor that may influence bone turnover [review: 149]. It is produced by many different cells, e.g., macrophages, but probably also by bone cells [150, 151]. IL-1 is a very potent stimulator of bone resorption [138, 149, 152], although its action is not a direct one, but mediated by other cells, presumably osteoblasts [153]. Part of the action of IL-1 is prostaglandin-mediated, but another part is prostaglandin-independent [139]. How IL-1 stimulates osteoclast activity via the osteoblast in a prostaglandin-independent manner [153] is not known.

IL-1 not only stimulates bone resorption via a stimulation of the activity of existing osteoclasts (in an indirect manner) but also acts on the proliferation and differentiation of the various stem, progenitor, and precursor cell stages of the osteoclast differentiation line. IL-1 in conjunction with IL-3 stimulates hemopoietic stem cell proliferation in a direct manner [154]. IL-1 stimulates the production of prostaglandins in osteoblastic cells, compounds which are known to act on hemopoietic progenitor cell proliferation and differentiation (vide supra). One of the local factors that may mediate the effects of IL-1 is IL-6 [155].

IL-1 stimulates the production of IL-6 by osteogenic cells [153], and IL-6 is known to have an additive effect with IL-3 in the stimulation of hemopoietic stem and progenitor cell proliferation [156]. Furthermore, the effects of IL-1 on bone resorption in organ culture systems are partially impaired by neutralizing antibodies to IL-6 [157]. PTH also stimulates IL-6 production by osteogenic cells [158, 159]. This increased IL-6 production may be responsible for some of the actions of PTH on bone resorption, as is the case in the IL-1-stimulated bone resorption. IL-6 has no effect on existing, mature osteoclasts, either directly or indirectly, but on the differentiation of osteoclast precursors [159, 160]. A report by Girasole et al. describes an inhibitory effect of estrogen on IL-6 production by bone marrow-derived stromal cells and osteoblasts [161]. These results point to IL-6 as an important local factor implicated in the loss of bone during situations with low estrogen levels, such as in postmenopausal women. This was confirmed by experiments during which the loss of bone in ovariectomized animals could be inhibited by the administration of either estrogen or neutralizing antibodies directed against IL-6 [162]. However, in control animals (displaying normal estrogen levels), they did not find any effects on osteoclast formation by the IL-6-neutralizing antibodies, suggesting that under conditions with normal estrogen levels, IL-6 is not essential for osteoclast formation. Recently, the same authors reported that IL-11 is also capable of stimulating osteoclast formation [163]. IL-6 and IL-11 both bind to a heterodimer receptor, consisting of a factor-specific binding peptide and a common signal transduction peptide (gp130). It was shown that PTH and $1,25(OH)_2D_3$ both stimulated IL-11 production by bone marrow cells. Neutralizing antibodies directed against IL-11 did inhibit PTH and $1,25(OH)_2D_3$-stimulated osteoclast formation in both ovariectomized and control mice, whereas anti-IL-6 only inhibited osteoclast formation in the ovariectomized animals. These results indicate that under normal estrogen levels, IL-11 is the more important regulator of osteoclast formation.

2. Genetic control of bone resorption

Over the last years, the development of new techniques have made it possible to investigate the underlying genetic mechanisms that control bone resorption. The analysis of very small quantities of RNA has been made possible by the development of the polymerase chain reaction assay (PCR), which for instance allows the analysis of gene expression in osteoclasts. The function of genes in the organism can now be studied in transgenic animals which either lack or overexpress certain genes. Recently, Chambers et al. reported the isolation of osteoclast inductive stromal cell lines and osteoclast progenitor cell lines from transgenic mice with an inducible immortalizing gene [164]. These cell lines offer great opportunities in the study of osteoclast ontogeny and osteoblast osteoclast interactions. In this section we will describe some of the recent results of the application of molecular biology techniques on bone cells.

(a) fos

One of the early events taking place in osteoblasts after stimulation with PTH, $1,25(OH)_2D_3$ and PGE2 is an increase in c-*fos* mRNA [165, 166]. The protein encoded by the c-*fos* gene is one of the components of the AP-1 transcription factor complex. The AP-1 complex is a heterodimer of the Fos protein with a protein encoded by a member of the *jun* family of proto-oncogenes (c-*jun*, *junB* and *junD*). The AP-1 complex is able to bind to AP-1 consensus sequences in the regulatory domains of target genes and has been shown to be very important in regulating proliferation and differentiation [167]. Genes active in bone with such an AP-1 consensus sequence are the osteocalcin gene [168] and the osteopontin gene [169].

The *fos* gene was originally detected as the transforming gene present in the osteosarcoma-inducing FBJ and FBR murine sarcoma viruses [170–172]. High levels of c-*fos* have also been found in other osteosarcomas [173, 174], indicating an important function for this gene in the control of osteoblast proliferation. C-*fos* expression in normal bone has been observed during embryogenesis and fracture healing [175–178]. Interestingly, the only tissue affected in transgenic mice either overexpressing or lacking c-*fos* appears to be bone. Mice overexpressing c-*fos* develop osteosarcomas and chondrosarcomas [179], while mice lacking c-*fos* develop osteopetrosis [180, 181]. A striking difference between the *fos*-knockout mice and the *fos*-overexpressing mice is the cell type affected. In the *fos*-overexpressing mice, the target cells for the transformation are the osteogenic cells, whereas in the knockout system osteoclast development is blocked by a defect in its hemopoietic progenitor cells. This indicates that c-*fos* does play an important role in both osteoblasts and osteoclasts. Another observation indicating a role for c-*fos* in osteoclasts is that, several hours after PTH stimulation of osteoblasts, high levels of c-*fos* were detected in osteoclasts [165]. These results suggest that the local factors produced by osteoblasts upon stimulation with PTH stimulate c-*fos* expression in osteoclasts and eventually osteoclast activity.

The observations described above clearly indicate that c-*fos* is an important regulator gene in bone. The analysis of the genes switched on or off by c-*fos* in both osteoblasts and osteoclasts may further our understanding of the control of bone turnover.

(b) src

The *src* proto-oncogene was originally identified as the transforming gene in the Rous sarcoma virus. *src* encodes a plasma membrane-bound tyrosine protein kinase and is expressed, in the mouse, in all cells. The only apparent defect in transgenic mice lacking c-*src* is that they show severe osteopetrosis. The effect is different from the osteopetrosis seen in *fos*-knockout mice, because in *src*-knockout, osteoclasts are clearly present, but inactive [182]. *src* is expressed in both osteoblasts and osteoclasts, but transplantation studies in irradiated mice showed that the defect lies with the osteoclasts and not with the osteoblasts [183]. In scr$^-$ mice, osteoclast numbers appear to be normal and are also increased by stimulation of the animals with PTH and $1,25(OH)_2D_3$. However, they form no ruffled border [184]. These results show that *src* does not act on osteoclast formation, but rather on activation. As *src* is normally associated with the plasma membrane at the site of focal adhesion points and to the cytoskeleton, it has been suggested that the defect is the result from impaired adherence to the bone surface of the *src*$^-$ osteoclasts.

(c) Osteopetrotic mutations

Mutations causing osteopetrosis offer an interesting opportunity for studying the genes which are active during bone resorption. Several osteopetrotic mutations have been described. These mutations can be classified into two groups: 1. mutations affecting the stromal cells (environment), and 2. mutations affecting osteoclasts or osteoclast progenitor cells. Examples of the first group are the *op* mutation in the mouse, the *tl* mutation in the rat, and *os* in the rabbit. In both *op* and *tl*, osteopetrosis was shown to be the result of the inability of the stromal cells to synthesize M-CSF [68–70] necessary for osteoclast formation. The defect in the stromal cells of the *os* rabbit is at present unknown [185].

Examples of the second group are *oc* and *mi* mutations in the mouse [186, 187]. In both cases, osteoclasts do develop, but fail to resorb bone. The product of the locus has not yet been identified. The defects observed in *mi/mi* mice closely resemble those caused by defects of either the SCF receptor (the *W* mutation of c-*kit*) or SCF itself (the *Sl* mutation). All three mutation show decreased numbers of mast cells, melanocytes, and basophils [10]. Demulder et al. [188] have reported the stimulation of osteoclast formation by SCF, and it has been shown that the c-*kit* expression in mast cells is decreased in *mi/mi* mice [189]. The *W* and *Sl* mutations, however, do not lead to osteopetrosis. Recently, it was found that the *mi* gene encodes a transcription factor [190]. Therefore, the *mi* gene is thought to play a role in the signal transduction of the stem cell factor.

3. Osteoclastic regulation of osteoblastic bone formation

There are now many indications that osteogenic cells may regulate the formation and activity of osteoclasts. Most of the hormones, growth factors, and cytokines that interfere with the formation and activity of osteoclasts act via the osteogenic cells. It is true that the nature of the molecules that provide the transduction of message from osteoblast to osteoclast is largely unknown, but the general idea is accepted (vide supra). How about the other way around? If osteoblasts may regulate osteoclasts, one would expect the reverse also to take place in bone homeostasis. The observations of Frost [191] suggest such a homeostatic control. They demonstrate that osteoclastic bone resorption and osteoblastic bone formation are closely associated with each other both in space and time [192]. Baron and co-workers [192, 193] developed an experimental system in which the successive stages of the process of local remodeling could be studied. They divided the remodeling sequence into: an activation phase, in which osteoclasts were formed and activated; a resorption phase; a reversal phase, in which the osteoclast left the bone surface; a formation phase, in which osteoblasts were activated to fill up the resorption cavity; and a resting phase during which the osteoblasts stopped the production of new bone and changed into inactive lining cells [192]. Many studies in vivo and in vitro have validated this model. The following questions arise, however: 1. why does resorption start at a particular place; 2. by which mechanism are osteoclasts activated; 3. by which mechanism are osteoblasts activated?

Question 1 will be discussed in the next paragraph. We think that osteocytes play a pivotal role in the choice of the area in which resorption is going to take place. Question 2 is discussed in the preceding paragraphs. Circulating hormones in conjunction with locally produced growth factors and cytokines stimulate osteogenic cells (osteoblasts or lining cells) at the chosen area to secrete another set of cytokines which stimulate in their turn osteoclast progenitor proliferation, differentiation, and fusion, attract the osteoclasts to the bone surface, and activate them. Little information is available at the moment to answer the third question, the coupling between resorption and formation. One of the major reasons is that the number of osteoclasts in bone is small, so that if osteoclasts produce a specific cytokine, it is impossible to recognize and isolate that cytokine from bone conditioned media. Secondly, because the number of osteoclasts in bone is small and there are no osteoclast cell lines available, it is very difficult to isolate enough osteoclasts to obtain conditioned media from osteoclast cultures. It is, however, also possible that osteoclasts do not produce this kind of cytokine, but that other factors are involved.

One of the possible coupling factors is TGFß, as proposed by Mundy and co-workers [194]. TGFß is abundant in bone. It is produced by osteoblasts but also by, e.g., platelets [194]. The TGFß present in the mineralized matrix may be of osteoblastic or another cellular source. It is generally secreted in an inactive form. Acid or enzymatic hydrolysis is necessary for its activation. Osteoblasts have receptors for TGFß. The effects of TGFß on osteogenic cells are not clearly established. Model systems differing in animal species or composition of the cell population have produced sometimes conflicting evidence [194]. In general, however, TGFß appears to stimulate proliferation and differentiation of immature cells. During osteoclastic bone resorption TGFß is liberated from the resorbed bone matrix and activated by the acid milieu of the resorption cavity. The released active TGFß may then, according to Mundy and co-workers, stimulate osteoprogenitors to proliferate and differentiate into active osteoblasts. The finding that TGFß is also chemotactic for cells with the osteoblast phenotype [195] strengthens the possibility of a role for TGFß in coupling of the resorption phase to the formation phase.

An interesting additional mechanism by which osteogenic precursors may be stimulated to become active osteoblasts exactly at the location of prior resorption is proposed by Puzas and co-workers [196]. They noted, as everybody studying the enzyme does, that osteoclast-derived acid phosphatase is deposited by the cell on the surface of the resorption lacuna. More surprisingly, they found that the enzyme stimulates osteoblastic differentiation and activity [197].

4. The role of the osteocyte in bone turnover

Two of the major functions of the skeleton are weight-bearing and providing sites for muscle attachment. During exercise the skeleton will therefore absorb most of the stress caused by exercise. Stress causes strain (distortion) in the bone matrix, the level of which depends on the level of stress but also on the strength of the bone. In 1892 Wolff [198] formulated his law. According to the translation by Heaney [199] the law says: 'every change in the function of a bone is followed by certain definite changes in internal architecture and external conformation' or 'bone mass and structure are driven by mechanical usage'. In other words, every bone or piece of bone will adapt its bone mass and strength to the optimal level of strain. According to the 'bone mass feed back loop' theory described by Heaney [199], the level of strain will be monitored within the bone and compared to a standard, a set point. If the strain level is too high, the bone will adapt itself by instructing the cells responsible for bone remodeling, the osteoblasts and osteoclasts, to strengthen the bone. If the strain level is too low, the remodeling system will cause bone loss. Evidence for such adaptive processes have been found in vivo as well as in vitro [review: 200].

The most obvious candidate as monitor or recorder of the level of strain is the osteocyte. Osteocytes, embedded as they are in the mineralized matrix, are ideally situated to perceive local effects of stress and have been found to be sensitive to strain [201]. Within an osteon, all osteocytes are coupled to each other and to the lining cells or osteoblasts on the bone surface via cell processes and gap junctions. In other words, two communication systems within the bone are open for the transport of signals generated in the bone: the intracellular route from osteocyte to gap junction-coupled other osteocytes and ultimately to the bone surface cells; and an extracellular route via lacunae and connecting canaliculi to the extraosseous fluid [202].

Strain-related adaptation of the skeleton to changes in stress will usually not

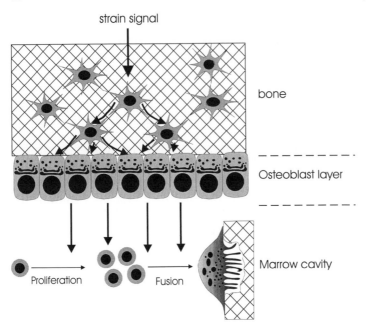

Fig. 6. Hypothetical model of the osteocyte as sensor cell for changes in strain level. Changes in strain level are perceived by the osteocytes and translated into second messengers. These activate osteoblasts or lining cells on the bone surface. Osteoblasts or lining cells may then activate osteoclast formation and activity.

mean a general, overall increase or decrease in bone mass and bone strength but local changes, changes in those locations which will adapt the biomechanical properties of the skeleton optimally with minimal effort. Local defects in the bone, e.g., microfractures, may result in local changes in the strain level at the site of the microfracture. Only the osteocytes in the direct vicinity will sense such a change in the strain level and send out signals to the most nearby cells outside the bone to stimulate a local remodeling process. This will give direction in space and time to the process of remodeling (Fig. 6).

Most of the above is pure conjecture. There is no real solid evidence for a regulatory role of the osteocyte in the processes of adaptation to mechanical loading. The circumstantial evidence available at the moment is, however, convincing enough to stimulate research in this direction [200–206]. Osteocytes were shown to react upon mechanical stimuli [201–203]. Prostaglandin synthesis appears to be involved [207]. Furthermore, osteocytes develop from osteoblasts and may therefore very well have kept intact strain 'receptor' systems and transduction mechanisms that are already present in osteoblasts. A large number of papers describing the effects of mechanical stimuli on osteoblastic cells is available [reviews: 200, 202, 208–210]. Recently, Xia and Ferrier [211] reported on a study in which they showed that mechanical perturbation of one osteoblastic cell may result in a transient increase of intracellular calcium in other osteoblastic cells coupled by cell processes and gap junctions. Finally, a method for the isolation and culture of osteocytes has recently developed in our group [212]. This will enable us to study the role of the osteocyte in bone metabolism, something which hitherto has been very difficult due to the encapsulation of osteocytes in the bone mineral.

References

1. Reddi, A.H., Regulation of bone differentiation by local and systemic factors. In: Peck, W.A. (Editor), Bone and mineral research 3. Elsevier, Amsterdam, 1985, pp. 27–47.
2. Walker, D.G., Osteoporosis cured by temporary parabiosis. Science 1973; 180: 875.
3. Helfrich, M.H., Mieremet, R.H.P., Thesingh, C.W., Osteoclast formation in vitro from progenitor cells present in the adult mouse circulation. J. Bone Miner. Res. 1989; 4: 325–334.
4. Kölliker, A., Die normale Resorption des Knochengewebes und ihre Bedeutung für die Entstehung der typischen Knochen-formen. FCW Vogel, Leipzig, 1873.
5. Hancox, N.M., The osteoclast. Biol. Rev. 1949; 24: 448–469.
6. Hall, B.K., The origin and fate of osteoclasts. Anat. Rec. 1975; 183: 1–12.
7. Marks, S.C., The origin of osteoclasts. J. Pathol. 1983; 12: 226–256.
8. Nijweide, P.J., Burger, E.H., Feyen, J.H.M., Cells of bone: proliferation, differentiation and hormonal regulation. Physiol. Rev. 1986; 66: 855–886.
9. Suda, T., Takahashi, N., Martin, T.J., Modulation of osteoclast differentiation. Endocrine Rev. 1992; 13: 66–80.
10. Noda, M. (Editor), Cellular and molecular biology of bone. Academic Press, San Diego, 1993.
11. Baron, R., Vignery, A., Behaviour of osteoclasts during a rapid change in their number induced by high doses of parathyroid hormone or calcitonin in intact rats. Metab. Bone Dis. Rel. Res. 1981; 2: 339–346.
12. Lorenzo, J.A., Raisz, L.G., Hock, J.M., DNA synthesis is not necessary for osteoclastic responses to parathyroid hormone in cultured fetal rat long bones. J. Clin. Invest. 1983; 72: 1924–1929.
13. Scheven, B.A.A., Wassenaar, A.M., Kawilarang-de Haas, E.W.M., Nijweide, P.J., Differentiation kinetics of osteoclasts in the periosteum of embryonic bones in vivo and in vitro. Anat. Rec. 1986; 214: 418–423.
14. Owen, M., The origin of bone cells. Int. Rev. Cytol. 1970; 28: 213–238.
15. Miller, S.C., Osteoclast cell-surface specializations and nuclear kinetics during egg-laying in Japanese quail. Am. J. Anat. 1981; 162: 35–43.
16. Holtrop, M.E., King, G.I., The ultrastructure of the osteoclast and its functional implications. Clin. Orthop. 1977; 123: 177–195.
17. Hedlund, T., Hulth, A., Johnell, O., Early effects of parathormone and calcitonin on the number of osteoclasts and on serum calcium in rats. Acta Orthop. Scand. 1983; 54: 802–804.
18. Hammarström, L.E., Hanker, J.S., Toverud, S.U., Cellular differences in acid phosphatase isoenzymes in bone and teeth. Clin. Orthop. 1971; 78: 151–167.
19. Minkin, C., Bone acid phosphatase: tartrate-resistant acid phosphatase as a marker of osteoclast function. Calcif. Tissue Int. 1982; 34: 285–290.
20. Hattersley, G., Chambers, T.J., Generation of osteoclastic function in mouse bone marrow cultures: multinuclearity and tartrate-resistant acid phosphatase are unreliable markers for osteoclastic differentiation. Endocrinology 1989; 124: 1689–1696.
21. Modderman, W.E., Tuinenburg-Bol Raap, A.C., Nijweide, P.J., Tartrate-resistant acid phosphatase is not an exclusive marker for mouse osteoclasts in cell culture. Bone 1991; 12: 81–87.
22. Sundquist, K.T., Leppilampi, M., Järvelin, K., Kumpulainen, T., Väänänen, H.K., Carbonic anhydrase isoenzymes in isolated rat peripheral monocytes, tissue macrophages and osteoclasts. Bone 1987; 8: 33–38.
23. Nijweide, P.J., Vrijheid-Lammers, T., Mulder, R.J.P., Blok, J., Cell surface antigens on osteoclasts and related cells in the quail studied with monoclonal antibodies. Histochemistry 1985; 83: 315–324.
24. Horton, M.A., Lewis, D., McNulty, K., Pringle, J.A.S., Chambers, T.J., Monoclonal antibodies to osteoclastomas (giant bone cell tumors): definition of osteoclast specific cellular antigens. Cancer Res. 1985; 45: 5663–5669.

25. Oursler, M.J., Bell, L.V., Clevinger, B., Osdoby, P., Identification of osteoclast specific monoclonal antibodies. J. Cell. Biol. 1985; 100: 1592–1600.

26. Hentunen, T.A., Tuukkanen, J., Väänänen, H.K., Osteoclasts and a small population of peripheral blood cells share common surface antigens. Calcif. Tissue Int. 1990; 47: 8–17.

27. James, I.E., Walsh, S., Dodds, R.A., Gowen, M., Production and characterization of osteoclast-selective monoclonal antibodies that distinguish between multinucleated cells derived from different human tissues. J. Histochem. Cytochem. 1991; 39: 905–914.

28. Horton, M.A., Helfrich, M.H., Antigenic markers of osteoclasts. In: Rifkin, B.R., Gay, C.V., (Editors), Biology and physiology of the osteoclast. CRC Press, Boca Raton, 1992, pp. 33–54.

29. Horton, M.A., Chambers, T.J., Human osteoclast-specific antigens are expressed by osteoclasts in a wide range of non-human species. Br. J. Exp. Pathol. 1986; 67: 95–104.

30. Anthanasou, N.A., Quinn, J., Horton, M.A., McGee, J.O'D., New sites of cellular vitronectin receptor immunoreactivity detected with osteoclast-reacting monoclonal antibodies 13C2 and 23C6. Bone Miner. 1990; 8: 7–22.

31. Horton, M.A., Rimmer, E.F., Moore, A., Chambers, T.J., On the origin of the osteoclast: the cell surface phenotype of rodent osteoclasts. Calcif. Tissue Int. 1985; 37: 46–50.

32. Athanasou, N.A., Heryet, A., Quinn, J., Gatter, K.C., Mason, D.Y., McGee, J.O'D., Osteoclasts contain macrophage and megakaryocyte antigens. J. Pathol. 1986; 150: 239–246.

33. Hume, D.A., Loutit, J.F., Gordon, S., The mononuclear phagocyte system of the mouse defined by immunohistochemical localization of antigen F4/80: macrophages of bone and associated connective tissue. J. Cell. Sci. 1984; 66: 189–194.

34. Rao, L.G., Heersche, J.N.M., Marschuk, L.L., Sturtridge, W., Immunohistochemical demonstration of calcitonin binding to specific cell types in fixed rat bone tissue. Endocrinology 1978; 108: 1972–1978.

35. Warshawsky, H., Goltzman, D., Rouleau, M.F., Bergeron, J.J.M., Direct in vivo demonstration by radio autography of specific binding sites for calcitonin in skeletal and renal tissues of the rat. J. Cell. Biol. 1980; 85: 682–694.

36. Nicholson, G.C., Moseley, J.M., Sexton, P.M., Mendelsohn, F.A.O., Martin, T.J., Abundant calcitonin receptors in isolated rat osteoclasts. J. Clin. Invest. 1986; 78: 355–360.

37. Chambers, T.J., Magnus, C.J., Calcitonin alters behaviour of isolated osteoclasts. J. Pathol. 1982; 136: 27–29.

38. Hattersley, G., Chambers, T.J., Calcitonin receptors as markers for osteoclast differentiation: correlation between generation of bone-resorptive cells that express calcitonin receptors in mouse bone marrow cultures. Endocrinology 1989; 125: 1606–1612.

39. Nicholson, G.C., Moseley, J.M., Sexton, P.M., Martin, T.J., Chick osteoclasts do not express calcitonin receptors. J. Bone Miner. Res. 1987; 2: 53–59.

40. Arnett, T.R., Dempster, D.W., A comparative study of disaggregated chick and rat osteoclasts in vitro: effects of calcitonin and prostaglandins. Endocrinology 1987; 120: 602–608.

41. Chambers, T.J., Revell, P.A., Fuller, K., Athanasou, M.A., Resorption of bone by isolated rabbit osteoclasts. J. Cell. Sci. 1984; 66: 383–399.

42. Boyde, A., Ali, N.N., Jones, S., Resorption of dentine by isolated osteoclasts in vitro. Br. Dent. J. 1984; 156: 216–220.

43. Burger, E.H., van der Meer, J.W.M., Nijweide, P.J., Osteoclast formation from mononuclear phagocytes: role of bone forming cells. J. Cell. Biol. 1984; 99: 1901–1906.

44. Hagenaars, C.E., Kawilarang-de Haas, E.W.M., van der Kraan, A.A.M., Spooncer, E., Dexter, T.M., Nijweide, P.J., Interleukin-3-dependent hematopoietic stem cell lines capable of osteoclast formation in vitro. J. Bone Miner. Res. 1991; 6: 947–954.

45. Allen, T.D., Dexter, T.M., Simmons, P.J., Marrow biology and stem cells. In: Dexter, T.M., Garland, J.M., Testa, N.G. (Editors), Colony stimulating factors. Immunology series, vol. 49. Marcel Dekker, New York, 1990, pp. 1–38.

46. Dexter, T.M., Spooncer, E., Growth and differentiation in the hemopoietic system. Annu. Rev. Cell. Biol. 1987; 3: 423–441.

47. Metcalf, D., The molecular control of cell division, differentiation commitment and maturation in hemopoietic cells. Nature 1989; 339: 27–30.

48. Lajtha, L.G., Haemopoietic stem cells: concepts and definitions. Blood Cells 1979; 5: 447–455.

49. Dexter, T.M., Garland, J.M., Testa, N.G. (Editors), Colony stimulating factors. Immunology series, vol. 49. Marcel Dekker, New York, 1990.

50. Göthlin, G., Ericsson, J.L.E., On the histogenesis of the cells of the fracture callus. Electron microscopic autoradiographic observations in parabiotic rats and studies on labeled monocytes.

Virchows Arch. Abt. B Zellpathol. 1973; 12: 318–329.

51. Walker, D.G., Bone resorption restored in osteopetrotic mice by transplants of normal bone marrow and spleen cells. Science 1975; 190: 784–785.
52. Coccia, P.F., Krivit, W., Cervenka, J. et al., Successful bone marrow transplantation for infantile malignant osteopetrosis. N. Engl. J. Med. 1980; 302: 701–708.
53. Scheven, B.A.A., Visser, J.W.M., Nijweide, P.J., In vitro osteoclast generation from different bone marrow fractions, including a highly enriched haemopoietic stem cell population. Nature 1986; 321: 79–81.
54. Hagenaars, C.E., van der Kraan, A.A.M., Kawilarang-de Haas, E.W.M., Visser, J.W.M., Nijweide, P.J., Osteoclast formation from cloned pluripotent hemopoietic stem cells. Bone Miner. 1989; 6: 179–189.
55. Schneider, G.B., Relfson, M., Pluripotent hemopoietic stem cells give rise to osteoclasts in vitro: effects of rGM-CSF. Bone Miner. 1989; 5: 129–138.
56. Kurihara, N., Suda, T., Miura, Y., Nakauchi, H., Kodama, H., Hiura, K., Hakeda, Y., Kumegawa, M., Generation of osteoclasts from isolated hematopoietic progenitor cells. Blood 1989; 74: 1295–1302.
57. Scheven, B.A.A., Burger, E.H., Kawilarang-de Haas E.W.M., Wassenaar, A.M., Nijweide, P.J., Effects of ionizing irradiation on formation and resorbing activity of osteoclasts in vitro. Lab. Invest. 1985; 53: 72–79.
58. Taylor, L.M., Tertinegg, I., Okuda, A., Heersche, J.N.M., Expression of calcitonin receptors during osteoclast differentiation in mouse metatarsals. J. Bone Miner. 1989; 4: 751–758.
59. Spooncer, E., Heyworth, C.M., Dunn, A., Dexter, T.M., Self-renewal and differentiation of interleukin-3-dependent multi-potent stem cells are modulated by stromal cells and serum factors. Differentiation 1986; 31: 111–118.
60. Yoneda, T., Alsina, M.M., Garcia, J.L., Mundy, G.R., Differentiation of HL-60 cells into cells with the osteoclast phenotype. Endocrinology 1991; 129: 683–689.
61. Collins, S.J., The HL-60 promyelocytic leukemia cell line: proliferation, differentiation, and cellular oncogen expression. Blood 1987; 70: 1233–1244.
62. Udagawa, N., Takahashi, N., Akatsu, T., Tanaka, H., Sasaki, T., Nishihara, T., Koga, T., Martin, T.J., Suda, T., Origin of osteoclasts: mature monocytes and macrophages are capable of differentiating into osteoclasts under a suitable micro-environment prepared by bone marrow-derived stromal cells. Proc. Natl. Acad. Sci. USA 1990; 87: 7260–7264.
63. Suda, T., Takahashi, N., Martin, T.J., Modulation of osteoclast differentiation. Endocrine Rev. 1992; 13: 66–80.
64. Ogawa, M., Nishikawa, S., Ikuta, K. et al., B cell ontogeny in murine embryo studied by a culture system with the monolayer of a stromal cell clone, ST2: B cell progenitor develops first in the embryonal body rather than in the yolk sac. EMBO J. 1988; 7: 1337–1343.
65. Alvarez, J.I., Teitelbaum, S.L., Blair, H.C., Greenfield, E.M., Athanasou, N.A., Ross, F.P., Generation of avian cells resembling osteoclasts from mononuclear phagocytes. Endocrinology 1991; 128: 2324–2335.
66. Quin, J.M.W., McGee, J.O'D., Athanasou, N.A., Cellular and hormonal factors influencing monocyte differentiation to osteoclastic bone-resorbing cells. Endocrinology 1994; 134: 2416–2423.
67. Corboz, V.A., Cecchini, M.G., Felix, R., Fleisch, H., van der Pluijm, G., Löwik, C.W.G.M., Effect of macrophage colony-stimulating factor on in vitro osteoclast generation and bone resorption. Endocrinology 1992; 130: 437–442.
68. Felix, R., Cecchini, M.G., Fleisch, H., Macrophage colony stimulating factor restores in vivo bone resorption in the op/op osteopetrotic mouse. Endocrinology 1990; 127: 2592–2594.
69. Kodama, H., Yamasaki, A., Nose, M., Niida, S., Ohgame, Y., Abe, M., Kumegawa, M., Suda, T., Congenital osteoclast deficiency in osteopetrotic (op/op) mice is cured by injections of macrophage colony stimulating factor. J. Exp. Med. 1991; 173: 269–272.
70. Marks, S.C., Wojtowicz, A., Szperl, M., Urbanowska, E., Mackay, C.A., Wiktor Jedrczak, W., Stanley, E.R., Aukerman, S.L., Administration of colony stimulating factor-1 corrects some macrophage, dental, and skeletal defects in an osteopetrotic mutation (toothless, tl) in the rat. Bone 1992; 13: 89–92.
71. Takahashi, N., Udagawa, N., Akatsu, T., Tanaka, H., Shionome, M., Suda, T., Role of colony-stimulating factors in osteoclast development. J. Bone Miner. Res. 1991; 6: 977–985.
72. Schneider, G.B., Relfson, M., The effects of transplantation of granulocyte-macrophage progenitors on bone resorption in osteopetrotic rats. J. Bone Miner. Res. 1988; 3: 225–232.

73. Schneider, G.B., Relfson, M., A bone marrow fraction enriched for granulocyte-macrophage progenitors gives rise to osteoclasts in vitro. Bone 1988; 9: 303–308.
74. Hattersley, G., Kerby, J.A., Chambers, T.J., Identification of osteoclast precursors in multilineage hemopoietic colonies. Endocrinology 1991; 128: 259–262.
75. Kurihara, N., Chenu, C., Miller, M., Civin, C., Roodman, G.D., Identification of committed mononuclear precursors for osteoclast-like cells formed in long term human marrow cultures. Endocrinology 1990; 126: 2733–2741.
76. Kerby, J.A., Hattersley, G., Collins, D.A., Chambers, T.J., Derivation of osteoclasts from hematopoietic colony-forming cells in culture. J. Bone Miner. Res. 1992; 7: 353–362.
77. Lee, M.Y., Lottsfeld, J.L., Fevold, K.L., Identification and characterization of osteoclast progenitors by clonal analysis of hematopoietic cells. Blood 1992; 80: 1710–1716.
78. Friedenstein, A.J., Precursor cells of mechanocytes. Int. Rev. Cytol. 1976; 47: 327–360.
79. Owen, M., Lineage of osteogenic cells and their relationship to the stromal system. In: Peck, W.A. (Editor), Bone and mineral research 3. Elsevier, Amsterdam, 1985, pp. 1–23.
80. Friedenstein, A.J., Osteogenic stem cells in the bone marrow. In: Heersche, J.N.M., Kanis, J.A. (Editors), Bone and mineral research 7. Elsevier, Amsterdam, 1990, pp. 243–272.
81. Bab, I., Ashton, B., Syftestad, G.T., Owen, M.E., Assessment of an in vivo diffusion chamber method as a quantitative assay for osteogenesis. Calcif. Tissue Int. 1984; 36: 77–82.
82. Beresford, J.N., Bennett, J.H., Devlin, C., Leboy, P.S., Owen, M.E., Evidence for an inverse relationship between the differentiation of adipocytic and osteogenic cells in rat marrow stromal cell cultures. J. Cell. Sci. 1992; 102: 341–351.
83. Grigoriadis, A.E., Heersche, J.N., Aubin, J.E., Differentiation of muscle, fat, cartilage and bone from progenitor cells present in a bone-derived clonal cell population: effect of dexamethasone. J. Cell. Biol. 1988; 106: 2139–2151.
84. Aubin, J.E., Heersche, J.N.M., Bellows, C.G., Grigoriadis, A.E., Evidence for a functional relationship between proliferation and initiation of osteoblast phenotype development. In: Cohn, D.V., Glorieux, F.H., Martin, T.J. (Editors), Calcium regulation and bone metabolism 10. Excerpta Medica, Amsterdam, 1990, pp. 362–370.
85. Scott, B.L., Thymidine-^{3}H electron microscope radio autography of osteogenic cells in the fetal rat. J. Cell. Biol. 1967; 35: 115–126.
86. Scherft, J.P., Groot, C.G., The electronmicroscopic structure of the osteoblast. In: Bonucci, E., Motta, P.M. (Editors), Ultrastructure of skeletal tissues. Kluwer Academic Publishers, Boston, 1990, pp. 209–222.
87. Heinegärd, D., Jirskog-Hed, B., Oldberg, Æ., Remholt, F.P., Wendel, M., Bone macromolecules. In: Cohn, D.V., Glorieux, F.H., Martin, T.J. (Editors), Calcium regulation and bone metabolism 10. Excerpta Medica, Amsterdam, 1990, pp. 181–187.
88. Bianco, P., Ultrastructural immunohistochemistry of noncollagenous proteins in calcified tissues. In: Bonucci, E., Motta, P.M. (Editors), Ultrastructure of skeletal tissues. Kluwer Academic Publishers, Boston, 1990, pp. 63–79.
89. Price, P.A., Vitamin K-dependent bone proteins. In: Cohn, C.V., Martin, T.J., Meunier, P.J. (Editors), Calcium regulation and bone metabolism 9. Excerpta Medica, Amsterdam, 1987, pp. 419–426.
90. Lian, J., Stewart, C., Puchacz, E., Structure of the rat osteocalcin gene and regulation of vitamin D dependent expression. Proc. Natl. Acad. Sci. USA 1989;86: 1143–1147.
91. Groot, C.G., Danes, J.K., Blok, J., Hoogendijk, A., Haushka, P.V., Light and electron microscopic demonstration of osteocalcin antigenicity in embryonic and adult rat bone. Bone 1986; 7: 379–385.
92. Miller, S.C., Bowman, B.M., Smith, J.M., Webster, S.S., Characterization of endosteal bone-lining cells from fatty marrow bone sites in adult beagles. Anat. Rec. 1980; 198: 163–173.
93. Menton, D.N., Simmons, D.J., Chang, S.L., Orr, B.Y., From bone lining cell to osteocyte-a SEM study. Anat. Rec. 1984; 209: 29–39.
94. Miller, S.C., Bowman, B.M., Medullary bone osteogenesis following estrogen administration to mature male Japanese quail. Dev. Biol. 1981; 87: 52–63.
95. Bonucci, E., The ultrastructure of the osteocyte. In: Bonuci, E., Motta, P.M. (Editors), Ultrastructure of skeletal tissues. Kluwer Academic Publishers, Boston, 1990, pp. 221–237.
96. Boyde, A., Jones, S.J., Ashford, J., Scanning electron microscope observations and the question of possible osteocyte bone mini-(re)-modelling. In: Silberman, M., Slavkin, H.C. (Editors), Current advances in skeletogenesis. Excerpta Medica, Amsterdam, 1982, pp. 305–314.
97. Marotti, G., The original contributions of the scanning electron microscope to the knowledge of bone structure. In: Bonucci, E., Motta, P.M. (Editors), Ultrastructure of skeletal tissues. Kluwer

Academic Publishers, Boston, 1990, pp. 19–39.

98. Belanger, L.F., Osteocyte osteolysis. Calcif. Tissue Res. 1969; 4: 1–12.

99. Gaillard, P.J., Parathyroid gland and bone in vitro. Dev. Biol. 1959; 1: 152–181.

100. Silve, C.H., Hradek, G.T., Jones, A.L., Arnaud, C.D., Parathyroid hormone receptor in intact embryonic chicken bone: characterization and cellular localization. J. Cell. Biol. 1982; 94: 379–386.

101. Rouleau, M.F., Mitchell, J., Goltzman, D., In vivo distribution of parathyroid hormone receptors in bone: evidence that the predominant osseous target cell is not the mature osteoblast. Endocrinology 1988; 123: 187–191.

102. Chambers, T.J., McSheehy, P.M.J., Thomson, B.M., Fuller, K., The effect of calcium-regulating hormones and prostaglandins on bone resorption by osteoclasts disaggregated from neonatal rabbit bones. Endocrinology 1985; 116: 234–239.

103. Teti, A., Rizzoli, R., Zambionin-Zallone, A., Parathyroid hormone binding to cultured avian osteoclasts. Biochem. Biophys. Res. Commun. 1991; 174: 1217–1222.

104. Agarwala, N., Gay, C.V., Specific binding of parathyroid hormone to living osteoclasts. J. Bone Miner. Res. 1992; 7: 531–539.

105. Chambers, T.J., Osteoblasts release osteoclasts from calcitonin induced quiescence. J. Cell. Sci. 1982; 57: 247–260.

106. Rodan, G.A., Martin, T.J., Role of osteoblasts in hormonal control of bone resorption — a hypothesis. Calcif. Tissue Int. 1981; 33: 349–351.

107. McSheehy, P.M.J., Chambers, T.J., Osteoblast-like cells in the presence of parathyroid hormone release soluble factor that stimulates osteoclastic bone resorption. Endocrinology 1986; 119: 1654–1659.

108. Morris, C.A., Mitnick, M.E., Weir, E.C., Horowitz, M., Kreider, B.L., Insogna, K.L., The parathyroid hormone-related protein stimulates human osteoblast-like cells to secrete a 9000 Dalton bone resorbing protein. Endocrinology 1990; 126: 1783–1785.

109. Perry, H.M., Skogen, W., Chappel, J.C., Kahn, A.J., Wilner, G., Teitelbaum, S.L., Partial characterization of a parathyroid hormone-stimulated resorption factor(s) from osteoblast-like cells. Endocrinology 1989; 125: 2075–2082.

110. Perry, H.M., Gurbani, S., Development of monoclonal antibodies to parathyroid hormone-induced resorptive factors from osteoblast-like cells. Calcif. Tissue Int. 1992; 50: 237–244.

111. Feyen, J.H.M., van der Wilt, G., Moonen, P., Di Bon, A., Nijweide, P.J., Stimulation of arachidonic acid metabolism in primary cultures of osteoblast-like cells by hormones and drugs. Prostaglandins 1984; 26: 769–781.

112. Raisz, L.G., Koolemans-Deynen, A.R., Inhibition of bone-collagen synthesis by prostaglandin E2 in organ culture. Prostaglandins 1974; 8: 377–385.

113. Jones, S.J., Boyde, A., Scanning electron microscopy of bone cells in culture. In: Copp, D.H., Talmage, R.V. (Editors), Endocrinology of calcium metabolism. Excerpta Medica, Amsterdam, 1978, pp. 97–104.

114. Delaisze, J.M., Eeckhout, Y., Vaes, G., Bone-resorbing agents effect the production and distribution of procollagenase as well as the activity of collagenase in bone tissue. Endocrinology 1988; 123: 264–276.

115. Heath, J.K., Atkinson, S.J., Meikle, M.C., Reynolds, J.J., Mouse osteoblasts synthesize collagenase in response to bone resorbing agents. Biochem. Biophys. Acta 1984; 802: 151–155.

116. Partridge, N.C., Jeffrey, J.J., Ehrlich, L.S., Teitelbaum, S.L., Fliszar, C., Welgus, H.G., Kahn, A.J., Hormonal regulation of the production of collagenase and a collagenase inhibitor activity by rat osteogenic sarcoma cells. Endocrinology 1987; 120: 1956–1962.

117. Hamilton, J.A., Lingelbach, S.R., Partridge, N.C., Martin, T.J., Stimulation of plasminogen activator in osteoblast-like cells by bone-resorbing hormones. Biochem. Biophys. Res. Commun. 1984; 122: 230–236.

118. Sakamoto, S., Sakamoto, M., Biochemical and immunohistochemical studies on collagenase in resorbing bone in tissue culture: a novel hypothesis for the mechanism of bone resorption. J. Periodont. Res. 1982; 17: 523–526.

119. Chambers, T.J., Fuller, K., Bone cells predispose bone surfaces to resorption by exposure of mineral to osteoclastic contact. J. Cell. Sci. 1985; 76: 155–165.

120. Sakamoto, S., Sakamoto, M., Bone collagenase, osteoblasts and cell-mediated bone resorption. In: Peck, W.A. (Editor), Bone and mineral research 4. Elsevier, Amsterdam, 1986, pp. 49–102.

121. Vaes, G., Cellular biology and biochemical mechanisms of bone resorption. Clin. Orthop. Rel. Res. 1988; 231: 239–271.

122. Mundy, G.R., Varani, J., Orr, W., Gondek, M.D., Ward, P.A., Resorbing bone is chemotactic for monocytes. Nature 1978; 275: 132–135.
123. Malone, J.D., Teitelbaum, S.L., Griffin, G.L., Senior, R.M., Kahn, A.J., Recruitment of osteoclast precursors by purified bone matrix constituents. J. Cell. Biol. 1982; 92: 227–230.
124. Mundy, G.R., Poser, J.W., Chemotactic activity of the γ-carboxyglutamic acid containing protein in bone. Calcif. Tissue Int. 1983; 35: 164–169.
125. Raisz, L.G., Trummel, C.L., Holick, M.F., DeLuca, J.F., 1,25-Dihydroxycholecalciferol: a potent stimulator of bone resorption in tissue culture. Science 1972; 175: 768–769.
126. Reynolds, J.J., Pavlovitch, H., Balsan, S., 1,25-Dihydroxycholecalciferol increases bone resorption in thyroparathyroidectomized mice. Calcif. Tissue Res, 1976; 21: 207–221.
127. Merke, J., Klaus, G., Hugel, U., Waldherr, R., Ritz, E., No 1,25-dihydroxyvitamin D3 receptors on osteoclasts of calcium-deficient chicken despite demonstrable receptors on circulating monocytes. J. Clin. Invest. 1986; 77: 312–314.
128. Suda, T., Takahashi, N., Abe, E., Role of vitamin D in bone resorption. J. Cell. Biol. 1992; 49: 53–58.
129. McSheehy, P.J.M., Chambers, T.J., 1,25-Dihydroxyvitamin D3 stimulates rat osteoblastic cells to release a soluble factor that increases osteoclastic bone resorption. J. Clin. Invest. 1987; 80: 425–429.
130. Nijweide, P.J., de Grooth, R., Ontogeny of the osteoclast. In: Rifkin, B.R., Gay, C.V. (Editors), Biology and physiology of the osteoclast. CRC Press, Boca Raton, 1992, pp. 81–104.
131. Skjφdt, H., Russel, G., Bone cell biology and the regulation of bone turnover. In: Gowen, M. (Editor), Cytokines and bone metabolism. CRC Press, Boca Raton, 1992, pp. 1–70.
132. Raisz, L.G., Martin, T.J., Prostaglandins in bone and mineral metabolism. In: Peck, W.A. (Editor), Bone and mineral research 2. Elsevier, Amsterdam, 1983, pp. 286–310.
133. Lerner, U., Indomethacin inhibits bone resorption and lysosomal enzyme release from bone in organ culture. Scand. J. Rheum. 1980; 9: 149–156.
134. Tashjian, A.H., Levine, L., Epidermal growth factor stimulates prostaglandin production and bone resorption in cultured mouse calvaria. BBRC 1978; 85: 966–975.
135. Tashjian, A.H., Hohmann, E.L., Antoniades, H.N., Levine, L., Platelet-derived growth factor stimulates bone resorption via a prostaglandin mediated mechanism. Endocrinology 1982; 111: 118–124.
136. Tashjian, A.H., Voelkel, E.F., Lazzaro, M., Singer, F.R., Roberts, A.B., Derynck, R., Winkler, M.E., Levine, J., α and ß human transforming growth factors stimulate prostaglandin production and bone resorption in cultured mouse calvaria. Proc. Natl. Acad. Sci. USA 1985; 82: 4535–4538.
137. Tashjian, A.V., Voelkel, E.F., Lazzaro, M., Goad, D., Bosma, T., Levine, L., Tumor necrosis factor-α (cachectin) stimulates bone resorption in mouse calvaria via a prostaglandin mediated mechanism. Endocrinology 1987; 120: 2029–2036.
138. Gowen, M., Wood, D.D., Ihrie, E.J., McGuire, M.K.B., Russel, R.G.G., An interleukin 1 like factor stimulates bone resorption in vitro. Nature 1983; 306: 378–380.
139. Garret, R., Mundy, G.R., Relationship between interleukin-1 and prostaglandins in resorbing neonatal calvaria. J. Bone Miner. Res. 1989; 4: 789–794.
140. Rodan, S.B., Rodan, G.A., Simmons, H.A., Walenga, R.W., Feinstein, M.B., Raisz, L.G., Bone resorptive factor produced by osteosarcoma cells with osteoblastic features is PGE2. BBRC 1981; 102: 1358–1365.
141. Shinar, D.M., Rodan, G.A., Biphasic effects of transforming growth factor-ß on the production of osteoclast-like cells in mouse bone marrow cultures: the role of prostaglandins in the generation of these cells. Endocrinology 1990; 126: 3153–3158.
142. Akatsu, T., Takahashi, N., Debari, K., Morita, I., Murota, S., Nagata, N., Takatani, O., Suda, T., Prostaglandins promote osteoclast like cell formation by a mechanism involving cyclic adenosine 3',5'-monophosphate in mouse bone marrow cell cultures. J. Bone Miner. Res. 1989; 4: 29–35.
143. Fuller, K., Chambers, T.J., Effect of arachidonic acid metabolism on bone resorption by isolated rat osteoclasts. J. Bone Miner. Res. 1989; 4: 209–215.
144. Felix, R., Elford, P.R., Stoerckle, C., Cecchini, M., Wetterwald, A., Trechsel, U., Fleish, H., Stadler, B.M., Production of hemopoietic growth factors by bone tissue and bone cells in culture. J. Bone Miner. Res. 1988; 3: 27–36.
145. Kodama, H., Nose, M., Niida, S., Yamasaki, A., Essential role of macrophage colony-stimulating factor in the osteoclast differentiation supported by stromal cells. J. Exp. Med. 1991; 173: 1291–1294.

146. Lee, M.Y., Eyre, D.R., Osborne, W.R.A., Isolation of a murine osteoclast colony-stimulating factor. Proc. Natl. Acad. Sci. USA 1991; 88: 8500–8504.
147. Felix, R., Fleisch, H., Elford, P.R., Bone-resorbing cytokines enhance release of macrophage colony stimulating activity by osteoblastic cell MC3T3-E1. Calcif. Tissue Int. 1989; 44: 356–360.
148. Mundy, G.R., Local factors regulating osteoclast function. In: Rifkin, B.A., Gay, C.V. (Editors), Biology and physiology of the osteoclast. CRC Press, Boca Raton, 1992, pp. 171–185.
149. Gowen, M., Interleukin 1 and tumor necrosis factor. In: Gowen, M. (Editor), Cytokines and bone metabolism. CRC Press, Boca Raton, 1992, pp. 71–91.
150. Lorenzo, J.A., Sousa, S.L., van den Brink-Webb, S.E., Korn, J.H., Production of both interleukin-1α and ß by newborn mouse calvarial cultures. J. Bone Miner. Res. 1990; 5: 77–83.
151. Pfeilschifter, J., Chenu, C., Bird, A., Mundy, G.R., Roodman, G.D., IL-1 and TNF stimulate the formation of human osteoclast-like cells in vitro. J. Bone Miner. Res. 1989; 4: 113–118.
152. Heath, J.K., Saklatvala, J., Meikle, M.C., Atkinson, S.J., Reynolds, J.J., Pig interleukin-1 (catabolin) is a potent stimulator of bone resorption in vitro. Calcif. Tissue Int. 1985; 37: 95–97.
153. Thomson, M.B., Saklatvala, J., Chambers, T.J., Osteoblasts mediate interleukin-1 stimulation of bone resorption by rat osteoclasts. J. Exp. Med. 1986; 164: 104–112.
154. Hagenaars, C.E., van der Kraan, A.A.M., Kawilarang-de Haas, E.W.M., Visser, J.W.M., Nijweide, P.J., Osteoclast formation from cloned pluripotent hemopoietic stem cells. Bone Miner. 1989; 6: 179–189.
155. Roodman, G.D., Interleukin 6: an osteotropic factor? J. Bone Miner. Res. 1992; 7: 475–478.
156. Ikebuchi, K., Wong, G.G., Clark, S.C., Ihle, J.N., Hirai, Y., Ogawa, M., Interleukin-6 enhancement of interleukin-3 dependent proliferation of multipotential hemopoietic progenitors. Proc. Natl. Acad. Sci. USA 1987; 84: 9035–9039.
157. Garret, I.R., Black, K.S., Mundy, G.R., Interactions between interleukin-6 and interleukin-1 in osteoclastic bone resorption in neonatal mouse calvariae. Calcif. Tissue Int. 1990; 46: A37.
158. Feyen, J.H.M., Elford, P., Di Padova, F.E., Trechsel, U., Interleukin-6 is produced by bone and modulated by parathyroid hormone. J. Bone Miner. Res. 1989; 4: 633–638.
159. Löwik, C.W., van der Pluym, G., Bloys, H., Hoekman, K., Aarden, L.A., Bijvoet, O.L.M., Papapoulos, S.E., Parathyroid hormone (PTH) and PTH-like protein (PLP) stimulate interleukin-6 production by osteogenic cells: a possible role of interleukin-6 in osteoclastogenesis. BBRC 1989; 162: 1546–1552.
160. Löwik, C.W.G.M., Differentiation inducing factors: leukemia inhibitory factor and interleukin-6. In: Gowen, M. (Editor), Cytokines and bone metabolism. CRC Press, Boca Raton, 1992, pp. 299–324.
161. Girasole, G., Jilka, R.L., Passeri, G., Boswell, S., Boder, G., Williams, D.C., Manolagas, S.C., 17ß-Estradiol inhibits interleukin-6 production by bone marrow-derived stromal cells and osteoblasts in vitro: a potential mechanism for the anti-osteoporotic effect of estrogens. J. Clin. Invest. 1992; 89: 883–891.
162. Jilka, R.L., Hangoc, G., Girasole, G., Passeri, G., Williams, D.C., Abrams, J.S., Boyce, B., Broxmeyer, H., Manolagas, S.C., Increased osteoclast development after estrogen loss: mediation by interleukin-6. Science 1992; 257: 88–91.
163. Girasole, G., Passeri, G., Jilka, R.L., Manolagas, S.C., Interleukin-11: a new cytokine critical for osteoclast development. J. Clin. Invest. 1994; 93: 1516–1524.
164. Chambers, T.J., Owens, J.M., Hattersley, G., Jat, P.S., Noble, M.D., Generation of osteoclast-inductive and osteoclastogenic cell lines from the H-2KbtsA58 transgenic mouse. Proc. Natl. Acad. Sci. USA 1993; 90: 5578–5582.
165. Lee, K., Deeds, J.D., Chiba, S., Un-No, M., Bond, A.T., Segre, G.V., Parathyroid hormone induces sequential c-fos expression in bone cells in vivo: In situ localization of its receptor and c-fos messenger ribonucleic acids. Endocrinology 1994; 134: 441–450.
166. Candeliere, G.A., Prud'homme, J., St-Arnaud, R., Differential stimulation of fos and jun family members by calcitriol in osteoblastic cells. Mol. Endocrinol. 1991; 5: 1780–1788.
167. Angel, P., Karin, M., The role of Jun, Fos and the AP-1 complex in cell proliferation and transformation. Biochem. Biophys. Acta 1991; 1072: 129–157.
168. Schüle, R., Umesono, K., Mangelsdorf, D., Bolado, J., Pike, J.W., Evans, R.M., Jun-Fos and receptors for vitamins A and D recognize a common response element in the human osteocalcin gene. Cell 1990; 61: 497–504.
169. Craig, A.M., Denhart, D.T., The murine gene encoding secreted phosphoprotein 1 (osteopontin): Promotor structure, activity, and induction in vivo by estrogen and progesteron. Gene 1991; 100: 163–171.

170. Finkel, J.P., Biskis, B.O., Experimental induction of osteosarcomas. Prog. Exp. Tumor Res. 1968; 10: 72–111.
171. Finkel, J.P., Biskis, B.O., Jinkins, P.B., Virus induction of osteosarcoma in mice. Science 1966; 151: 698–701.
172. Finkel, J.P., Reilly, C.A., Biskis, B.O., Viral etiology of bone cancer. Front Radiat. Ther. Oncol. 1975; 10: 28–39.
173. Schon, A., Michiels, L., Janowski, M., Merregaert, J., Erfle, V., Expression of proto-oncogenes in murine osteosarcomas. Int. J. Cancer 1986; 38: 67–74.
174. Wu, J.X., Carpenter, M., Gresens, C., Keh, R., Niman, H., Morris, J.W.S., Mercola, D., The proto-oncogene c-fos is overexpressed in the majority of human osteosarcomas. Oncogene 1990; 5: 989–1000.
175. Dony, C., Gruss, P., Proto-oncogene c-fos expression in growth regions of fetal bone and mesodermal web tissue. Nature 1987; 328: 711–714.
176. Sandberg, M., Vuorio, T., Hirvonen, H., Alitalo, K., Vuorio, E., Enhanced expression of TGF-ß and c-fos mRNA in the growth plates of developing human long bones. Development 1988; 102: 461–470.
177. De Togni, P., Niman, H., Raymond, V., Sawchenko, P., Verma, I.M., Detection of fos protein during osteogenesis by monoclonal antibodies. Mol. Cell. Biol. 1988; 8: 2251–2256.
178. Ohta, S., Yamamura, T., Lee, K., Okomura, H., Kasai, R., Hiraki, Y., Ikeda, T., Iwasaki, R., Kikuchi, H., Konishi, J., Shigeno, C., Fracture healing induces expression of the proto-oncogene c-fos in vivo. Possible role of the fos protein in osteoblastic differentiation. FEBS Lett 1991; 284: 42–45.
179. Grigoriadis, A.E., Schellander, K., Wang, Z.Q., Wagner, E.F., Osteoblasts are target cells for transformation in c-fos transgenic mice. J. Cell. Biol. 1993; 122: 685–701.
180. Wang, Z.Q., Ovitt, C., Grigoriadis, A.E., Mohle-Steinlein, U., Ruther, U., Wagner, E.F., Bone and haematopoietic defects in mice lacking c-fos. Nature 1992; 360: 741–744.
181. Johnson, R.S., Spiegelman, B.M., Papaioannou, V., Pleiotropic effects of a null mutation in the c-fos proto-oncogene. Cell 1992; 71: 577–586.
182. Soriano, P., Montgomery, C., Geske, R., Bradley, A., Targeted disruption of the c-src proto-oncogene leads to osteopetrosis in mice. Cell 1991; 64: 693–702.
183. Lowe, C., Yoneda, T., Boyce, B.F., Chen, H., Mundy, G.R., Soriano, P., Osteopetrosis in src-deficient mice is due to an autonomous defect of osteoclasts. Proc. Natl. Acad. Sci. USA 1993; 90: 4485–4489.
184. Boyce, B.F., Yoneda, T., Lowe, C., Soriano, P., Mundy, G.R., Requirement of pp60src expression for osteoclasts to form ruffled borders and resorb bone in mice. J. Clin. Invest. 1992; 90: 1622–1627.
185. Lenhard, S., Popoff, S.N., Marks, S.C., Defective osteoclast differentiation and function in the osteopetrotic (os) rabbit. Am J Anat 1990; 188: 138–144.
186. Udagawa, N., Sasaki, T., Akatsu, T., Takahashi, N., Tanaka, S., Tamura, T., Tanaka, H., Suda, T., Lack of bone resorption in osteosclerotic (oc/oc) mice is due to a defect in osteoclast progenitors rather than the local microenvironment provided by osteoblastic cells. Biochem. Biophys. Res. Commun. 1992; 184: 67–72.
187. Marks, S.C., Walker, D.G., Mammalian osteopetrosis — a model for studying cellular and humoral factors in bone resorption. In: Bourne, G.H. (Editor), The biochemistry and physiology of bone. Academic Press, New York, 1976, pp. 227–301.
188. Demulder, A., Suggs, S.V., Zsebo, K.M., Scarcez. T., Roodman, G.D., Effects of Stem Cell Factor on osteoclast-like cell formation in long term human bone marrow cultures. J. Bone Miner. Res. 1992; 11: 1337–1344.
189. Ebu, Y., Kanakura, Y., Jippo-Kanemoto, T., Tsujimura, T., Furitsu, T., Ikeda, H., Adachi, S., Kasugai, T., Nomura, S., Kanayama, Y., Yamatodani, A., Nishikawa, S., Matsuzawa, Y., Kitamura, Y., Low c-kit expression of cultured mast cells of mi/mi genotype may be involved in their defective response to fibroblasts that express the ligand for c-kit. Blood 1992; 80: 1454–1462.
190. Hodgkinson, C.A., Moore, K.J., Nakayama, A., Steingrimson, E., Copeland, N.G., Jenkins, N.A., Arnheiter, H., Mutations at the mouse microphthalmia locus are associated with defects in a gene encoding a novel basic-helix-loop helix-zipper protein. Cell 1993; 74: 395–404.
191. Frost, H.M., Mathematical elements of bone remodeling. Charles C. Thomas, Springfield, 1964.
192. Baron, R., Vignery, A., Horowitz, M., Lymphocytes, macrophages and the regulation of bone remodeling. In: Peck, W.A. (Editor), Bone and mineral research 2. Elsevier, Amsterdam, 1984, 175–243.

193. Tran Van, P., Vignery, A., Baron, R., Cellular kinetics of the bone remodeling sequence in the rat. Anat. Rec. 1982; 202: 445–451.
194. Mundy, G.R., Bonewald, L.F., Transforming growth factor beta. In: Gowen, M. (Editor), Cytokines and bone metabolism. CRC Press, Boca Raton, 1992, pp. 93–107.
195. Pfeilschifter, J., Wolf, O., Nauman, A., Minne, H.W., Mundy, G.R., Ziegler, R., Chemotactic response of osteoblast-like cells to transforming growth factor ß. J. Bone Miner. Res. 1990; 5: 825–830.
196. Puzas, J.E., Ishibe, M., Osteoblast/osteoclast coupling. In: Rifkin, B.R., Gay, C.V. (Editors), Biology and physiology of the osteoclast. CRC Press, Boca Raton, 1992, pp. 337–356.
197. Ishibe, M., Rosier, R.N., Puzas, J.E., Human prostatic acid phosphatase stimulates collagen synthesis and alkaline phosphatase content of isolated bone cells. J. Clin. Endocrinol. Metab. 1991; 73: 785–792.
198. Wolff J. Das Gesetz der Transformation der Knochen. Royal Academy, Berlin, 1892.
199. Heaney, R.P., Reality, myth, and model. In: Christiansen, C., Overgaard, K. (Editors), Osteoporosis 1990. Osteopress ApS, Kopenhagen, 1990, pp. 23–29.
200. Burger, E.H., Mechanical effects on osteoclast function. In: Rifkin, B.R., Gay, C.V. (editors), Biology and physiology of the osteoclast. CRC Press, Boca Raton, 1992, pp. 419–432.
201. Skerry, T.M., Bitensky, L., Chayen, J., Lanyon, L.E., Early strain related changes in enzyme activity in osteocytes following bone loading in vivo. J. Bone Miner. Res. 1989; 4: 783–789.
202. Aarden, E.M., Burger, E.H., Nijweide, P.J., Function of osteocytes in bone. J. Cell. Biochem. 1994; 55: 287–299.
203. Rubin, C., Lanyon, L.E., Regulation of bone mass by mechanical strain magnitude. Calcif. Tissue Int, 1985; 37: 411–417.
204. Kufahl, R.H., Saha, S., A theoretical model for stress-generated fluid flow in the canaliculi-lacunae network in bone tissue. J. Biomech. 1990; 23: 171–180.
205. Cowin, S.C., Moss-Salentijn, L., Moss, M.L., Candidates for the mechanosensory system in bone. BED-ASME 1991; 20: 313–316.
206. Weinbaum, S., Cowin, S.C., Zeng, Y., A model for the fluid shear stress excitation of membrane ion channels in osteocytic processes due to bone strain. BED-ASME, 1991; 20: 317–320.
207. Pead, M.J., Suswillo, R., Skerry, T.M., Vedi, S., Lanyon, L.E., Increased ^{3}H-uridine levels on osteocytes following a single short period of dynamic loading in vivo. Calcif. Tissue Int. 1988; 43: 92–96.
208. El Haj, A.J., Minter, S.L., Rawlinson, S.C.F., Suswillo, R., Lanyon, L.E., Cellular responses to mechanical loading in vitro. J. Bone Miner. Res. 1990; 5: 923–932.
209. Burger, E.H., Veldhuyzen, J.P., Influence of mechanical factors on bone formation, resorption and growth in vitro. In: Hall, B.K. (Editor), Bone, vol 7. CRC Press, Boca Raton, 1992, pp. 37–56.
210. Ypey, D.L., Weidema, A.F., Höld, K.M. et al., Voltage, calcium, and stretch activated ionic channels and intracellular calcium in bone cells. J. Bone Miner. Res. 1992; 7 (suppl.2): S367–377.
211. Xia, S.-L., Ferrier, J., Propagation of a calcium pulse between osteoblastic cells. BBRC 1992; 186: 1212–1219.
212. van der Plas, A., Nijweide, P.J., Isolation and purification of osteocytes. J. Bone Miner. Res. 1992; 7: 389–396.

Bisphosphonate on bones
O. Bijvoet, H.A. Fleisch, R.E. Canfield and G. Russell (eds.)
© 1995 Elsevier Science B.V. All rights reserved.

CHAPTER 3

The osteoclast bone interface and bone resorption

Gideon A. Rodan

*Department of Bone Biology and Osteoporosis Research, Merck Research Laboratories, West Point,
PA 19486, USA*

I. Introduction

The previous chapter has described in some detail the origin and differentiation of osteoclasts, the bone-resorbing cells. This chapter will deal with the physiology and biochemistry of the resorptive process in the context of bisphosphonate action. Our knowledge of this subject is still fragmentary, but significant progress has been made over the last few years, and a consensus has developed regarding osteoclastic resorption, albeit many of the specifics still require validation. I shall review the different steps in the process and try to separate between well-established facts and hypotheses, which require further study.

II. How is the bone surface targeted for resorption?

All resorption occurs on bone surfaces, which face either the bone marrow in cancellous and endocortical bone or the Haversian canal in cortical bone. The surfaces are normally covered by lining cells, most likely derived from the osteoblastic lineage. Based on histological evidence, these cells are believed to represent the last stage in osteoblastic differentiation, following the matrix-producing stage. The properties and functions of the lining cells have not been well characterized. Based on their position, they are likely to perceive changes in the strain produced in the matrix by mechanical loads and possibly mediate signals for bone remodeling, which occurs on the bone surface. A change in mechanical load is one of the well-recognized stimuli for bone remodeling [1–3]. It has been shown, for example, that 'osteoblastic' cells, exposed to mechanical stimuli, increase the production of prostaglandin E_2 (PGE_2) [4, 5], which in many studies stimulates both bone resorption and bone formation, thus acting as a potential mediator for the mechanically induced increase in bone turnover.

It is well documented that resorption is increased during estrogen and probably androgen deficiency in women and men, respectively. This is at least in part a result of a larger number of resorption sites. Frost proposed that this is due to a resetting of the 'mechanostat' [6], which anatomically should be located in lining cells and osteocytes. It is not known if these cells have receptors for estrogen or how estrogen may modulate their activity at the biochemical level. Estrogen was shown to downregulate the production of interleukin (IL)-6 in bone-derived and other cells [7] and of IL-1 and tumor necrosis factor (TNFα) in macrophages [8]. IL-6 seems to be necessary for bone loss caused by estrogen deficiency [9, 10]. IL-1 and IL-6 can stimulate osteoclast formation and/or activity, but it is not known if these cytokines are produced by lining cells.

Under normal circumstances, the lining cells may protect the bone surface from osteoclastic resorption, the way endothelial cells protect the blood vessel surface, making the lining cells the likely first target for stimuli which activate bone remodeling. This role for osteoblast-derived cells was proposed in 1981 by Rodan and Martin [11] on the basis of the presence of receptors for resorption stimuli in these cells, such as parathyroid hormone and prostaglandins, and by Chambers, who provided extensive evidence in vitro for the accessory role of osteoblastic cells in bone resorption [12]. The precise factors, which mediate between the lining cells and the osteoclasts, have not been isolated. There are studies which suggest that cell contact is required for osteoclast generation in vitro [13], but resorption activity was also reported to be stimulated by osteoblast conditioned media [14]. Parathyroid hormone, the powerful stimulator of bone resorption, was shown to change the shape of osteoblastic cells [15], probably via cyclic AMP-mediated actin filament depolymerization [16]. This may render the bone surface accessible to osteoclastic action. However, other conditions may have to be fulfilled for activating the resorption surface and lining cells may play a role there, too. It has been observed that at the completion of mineralization, a thin layer of unmineralized matrix remains under the lining cells. It was suggested that this matrix would have to be removed for initiation of osteoclastic resorption and that collagenase, released by the lining cells, would play a role in this process [17]. So far the evidence is indirect, but parathyroid hormone was shown to stimulate collagenase production and secretion in osteoblastic cells [18]. Parathyroid hormone can also promote acid production and secretion in osteoblastic cells [19], which could participate in the preparation of the bone surface for resorption. Another contribution could be made by the noncollagenous proteins, which are incorporated in the matrix and are thus synthesized and secreted along with collagen by the cuboidal osteoblasts. Some of the noncollagenous protein could be released by the lining cells and participate in the attraction or activation of the osteoclasts [20]. These are all important areas of investigation, where further information could enhance understanding at the molecular basis of the resorption activation process and help develop therapy for bone loss.

III. Osteoclast attachment to the bone surface

As described in the previous chapter, the multinucleated osteoclasts are formed by fusion of mononuclear cells, which already possess most of the osteoclast properties, such as calcitonin receptors and tartrate-resistant acid phosphatase, and may be capable of bone resorption themselves [13, 21]. In vitro, this process requires osteoblasts or other inducing cells and is blocked by snake venoms, echistatin and kistrin, which interfere with the binding of arginine-glycine-aspartic acid (RGD)-containing extracellular matrix proteins, such as osteopontin, with integral membrane receptors called integrins. This raises the possibility that the final step of multinucleation and osteoclast differentiation may occur on the bone surface under the influence of local cells and matrix proteins. In vitro studies suggest that osteoblast contact is required for this process, and some of the molecule(s) involved have been identified [13].

Integrins are a large family of heterodimeric receptors, which span the cell membrane, have a large extracellular domain involved in ligand (matrix) binding and an intracellular domain, which is involved in signal transduction [22]. There are many members of both the α and β chains, which can associate with each other in different combinations. The molecular weight of the α chain is about 130 kDa and of β, about 100 kDa. In the mammalian osteoclast, the major integrin is $\alpha_v\beta_3$, known as the vitronectin receptor based on its preferential attachment to that protein. $\alpha_v\beta_3$ was shown to be the antigen of the 'osteoclast-specific' monoclonal antibody, developed by Horton et al. against osteoclastoma [23]. This antibody (23C6) inhibited osteoclast resorption in vitro. Moreover, the snake poison echistatin mentioned above, which inhibits resorption both in vitro and in vivo, was shown to co-localize with $\alpha_v\beta_3$ receptors in rat osteoclasts [24]. It was proposed that the $\alpha_v\beta_3$ integrin is involved in initiating the attachment of the osteoclast to the bone surface. At the site of resorption, this attachment forms a tight seal, histologically identified as the 'clear zone'. Osteopontin, which in vitro mediates the attachment of various cell types [25], was shown to be present at the clear zone [26]. β_3 integrins have also been implicated in osteoclast attachment by the studies of Zambonin-Zallone and Teti [27], and echistatin, the $\alpha_v\beta_3$ ligand, reduced osteoclast attachment in vitro [24]. On the other hand, Lakkakorpi et al. found $\alpha_v\beta_3$ localization in osteoclasts on the basolateral aspects of the membrane and not in the clear zone [28]. There is therefore some conflicting information on the subject, which has to be resolved. It is of interest that osteoclasts themselves can express and synthesize osteopontin, which they may lay down prior to attaching to it [29].

Integrins may have an additional role in osteoclast function by acting as signal transducing receptors. Osteoclast exposure to $\alpha_v\beta_3$ ligands produces a surge in intracellular calcium [30–32]. Further studies will show if this signal transducing ability of the osteoclast integrin plays a role in osteoclast differentiation and multinucleation, in the cessation of function, or in both, and which ligands are involved. This is also an area of very active current investigation.

IV. Acidification of the resorption space

The resorption space defined by the clear zone has a surface of 500–1000 μm^2, thus representing only a small fraction of the osteoclast surface. This localized area of the plasma membrane undergoes substantial changes in order to carry out its resorptive function. The membrane becomes highly convoluted (brush border), increasing its surface area several fold. It has been suggested that the constituents of this part of the membrane differ from the rest of the membrane, as in other polarized cells such as the kidney cells. This small specialized part of the membrane has a functional resemblance to a lysosome [33] and may be produced by the fusion of lysosome-like vesicles with the plasma membrane. Two processes occur in the closed space under the convoluted membrane, sealed by the clear zone: solubilization of the bone mineral hydroxyapatite and digestion of the bone matrix, which is 90% collagen. Mineral dissolution is carried out by acidification of this space. Studies with the pH-sensitive dye acridine orange suggest that the pH in that space can reach 3.5–4 [34, 35]. The tight seal of the clear zone would thus have to maintain a 1000-fold concentration gradient between the resorption space and the extracellular fluid. The osteoclast is endowed with multiple features, which make acidification possible. In the membrane, there is a H^+/ATPase of the vacuolar type [36, 37]. This is an evolutionary conserved enzyme complex, which contains multimers of 5 subunits, ranging in molecular weight between 16 kDa and 100 kDa. Vacuolar ATPases are found in all cells and intracellular vacuoles and lysosomes, but a recent study suggests that the osteoclast H^+/ATPase has some unique features, including vanadate sensitivity and different M_r of some of its subunits [38]. These ATPases are sensitive to an inhibitor called bafilomycin, which was shown to inhibit bone resorption [39]. This powerful acidification requires energy, which should be provided in the form of ATP by the mitochondria, highly abundant in osteoclasts. It also requires compensatory ion fluxes for maintenance of ionic balance in the cell and mechanisms for correcting the alkalinization resulting from the efflux of H^+. The counter-ion of vacuolar ATPases is usually chloride, which is also the case in avian osteoclasts [40]. To handle the alkalinization, the osteoclast has very high levels of carbonic anhydrase type II [41, 42]. This enzyme catalyzes the breakdown of bicarbonate into H^+ and CO_2, which can help generate the protons for restoring the pH and for further proton pumping into the resorption space. Inhibitors of carbonic anhydrase, derivatives of sulfonamides such as acetazolamide and analogues, were shown to inhibit bone resorption, both in vitro and in vivo [43, 44]. The cells are also endowed on the basolateral surface with a chloride bicarbonate exchanger [45], which can further help adjust the concentration of these ions in the osteoclast. Its inhibition also reduced resorption [46, 47]. The cells also have an unusually high level of Na^+/K^+-ATPase in the basolateral membrane, which may be involved in volume regulation and compensate for changes produced in the concentration of these ions, related to membrane potential [48]. These are only a few of a large number of membrane ion channels present in the osteoclast, such as inward rectifying K^+ channels [49, 50], various calcium channels [51, 52], etc., all of which interact in a complex and coordinated fashion to permit its highly specialized function. Most of the details are not yet known, but it is likely that the H^+/ATPase at the brush border plays an important role in the acidification of the resorption space. The regulation of its localization and function remain to be elucidated.

The acid environment is important for the activity of lysosomal enzymes, such as cathepsin L and D, which have been implicated in collagen breakdown and matrix digestion [53–56].

V. Osteoclast activity termination signal

The resorption of a specific lacuna lasts in vitro only several hours. The osteoclast then moves away and resorbs another cavity [57]. The physiological signal, which stops osteoclast resorption in vivo during bone remodeling, is not known, but several agents can inhibit osteoclast activity, and there is some understanding of their mode of action.

A potent physiological inhibitor of osteoclast resorption is the peptide hormone calcitonin. Calcitonin, a 32-amino acid peptide, inhibits bone resorption both in vivo and in vitro, where it acts at subnanomolar concentrations [58]. Calcitonin stimulates cyclic AMP accumulation in osteoclasts. Cyclic AMP analogues and agents which increase cyclic AMP in osteoclasts have similar effects to those of calcitonin on osteoclast shape and activity, but may not mediate all the effects of this hormone [59]. It is not known how cyclic AMP produces osteoclast contraction but, by analogy to smooth muscle, platelets, and other cells, cyclic AMP-dependent phosphorylation of myosin light chain kinase can reduce the activity of this enzyme, and this can lead to the depolymerization of actin filaments [16].

An increase in intracellular calcium produced by calcitonin [60] or by exposing the cells to a high extracellular calcium concentration was also reported to inhibit osteoclastic activity [52, 61]. Extracellular calcium is presumably acting on a calcium sensor, which can mediate the mobilization of calcium from intracellular stores [52, 62]. How calcium may inactivate the cells is not known. As mentioned above, our knowledge of the processes involved in osteoclast inactivation is still limited.

Following cessation of resorption, the osteoclast moves to another site, the resorption surface is populated by cells of the osteoblastic lineage, and bone formation covers that site. It is possible that molecules synthesized by osteoclasts, for example osteopontin, are deposited on the resorbed surface and participate in signalling the reversal phase.

VI. Summary

The bone surface, where resorption takes place, is covered by a layer of lining cells derived from osteoblasts. These cells are separated from the mineralized matrix by a thin layer of nonmineralized material which is removed prior to resorption, probably by collagenase digestion. The lining cells move away, and the mineralized surface is now exposed. Osteoclasts attach to this mineralized surface through a specialized circular area of the membrane called the sealing zone. Resorption occurs in this sealed space of about 1000 μm^3 between the bone surface and the osteoclast membrane. Integrins, specifically $\alpha_v\beta_3$ and their ligands in the bone matrix, particularly osteopontin, have been implicated in osteoclast attachment to bone. Integrins may also be involved in osteoclast activation. Upon attachment to bone, there is an extensive ruffling of the membrane which faces the bone, acidification of the osteoclast bone interface to pH of 3.5 to 4.0, and secretion of lysosomal enzymes and possibly collagenase which digest the matrix. In response to signals which remain to be identified, resorption stops, osteoclasts move away, and the surface will be covered by bone formation.

References

1. Thompson, D.D., Rodan, G.A., Indomethacin inhibition of tenotomy-induced bone resorption in rats. J. Bone Miner. Res. 1988; 3(4): 409–414.
2. Lanyon, L., Functional strain as a determinant for bone remodeling. Calcif. Tissue Int. Suppl. 1984; 36: 56–61.
3. Mori, S., Burr, D.B., Increased intracortical remodeling following fatigue damage. Bone 1993; 14: 103–109.
4. Somjen, D., Binderman, I., Bergen, E., Harell, A., Bone modeling induced by physical stress is prostaglandin mediated. Biochim, Biophys. Acta 1980; 627: 91–100.
5. Yeh, C.K., Rodan, G.A., Tensile forces enhance prostaglandin E synthesis in osteoblastic cells grown on collagen ribbons. Calcif. Tissue Int. 1984; 36: 567–571.
6. Frost, H.M., Perspectives: The role of changes in mechanical usage set points in the pathogenesis of osteoporosis. J. Bone Miner. Res. 1992; 7(3): 253–261.
7. Girasole, G., Jilka, R.L., Passeri, G., Boswell, S., Boder, G., Williams, D.C., Manolagas, S.C., 17-Estradiol inhibits interleukin-6 production by bone marrow-derived stromal cells and osteoblasts in vitro: A potential mechanism for the antiosteoporotic effect of estrogens. J. Clin. Invest. 1992; 89: 883–891.
8. Pacifici, R., Brown, C., Puscheck, E., Friedrich, E., Slatopolsky, E., Maggio, D., McCracken, R., Avioli, L.V., Effect of surgical menopause and estrogen replacement on cytokine release from human blood mononuclear cells. Proc. Natl. Acad. Sci. USA 1991; 88: 5134–5138.
9. Jilka, R.L., Hangoc, G., Girasole, G., Passeri, G., Williams, D.C., Abrams, J.S., Boyce, B., Broxmeyer, H., Manalagas, S.C., Increased osteoclast development after estrogen loss: mediation by interleukin-6. Science 1992; 257: 88–91.
10. Poli, V., Balena, R., Fattori, E., Markatos, A., Yamamoto, M., Tanaka, H., Ciliberto, G., Rodan, G.A., Costantini, F., Interleukin-6 deficient mice are protected from bone loss caused by estrogen depletion. EMBO J. 1994; 13(5): 1189–1196.
11. Rodan, G.A., Martin, T.J., Editorial: Role of osteoblasts in hormonal control of bone resorption — a hypothesis. Calcif. Tissue Int. 1981; 33: 349–351.
12. McSheehy, P.M.J., Chambers, T.J., Osteoblastic cells mediate osteoclastic responsiveness to parathyroid hormone. Endocrinology 1986; 118(2): 824–828.
13. Suda, T., Takahashi, N., Martin, T.J., Modulation of osteoclast differentiation. Endocrine Rev. 1992; 13(1): 66–80.
14. Perry, H.M., Skogen, W., Chappel, J., Khan, A.J., Wilner, G., Teitelbaum, S.L., Partial characterization of a parathyroid hormone stimulated resorption factor(s) from osteoblast-like cells. Endocrinology 1989; 125: 2075–2082.
15. Jones, S.J., Boyde, A., Experimental study of changes in osteoblastic shape induced by calcitonin and parathyroid extract in an organ culture system. Cell. Tissue Res. 1976; 169: 449–465.
16. Egan, J.J., Gronowicz, G., Rodan, G.A., Parathyroid hormone promotes the disassembly of cytoskeletal actin and myosin in cultured osteoblastic cells: Mediation by cyclic AMP. J. Cell. Biochem. 1991; 45: 101–111.

17. Chow, J., Chambers, T.J., An assessment of the prevalence of organic material on bone surfaces. Calcif. Tissue Int, 1992; 50: 118–122.
18. Partridge, N.C., Jeffrey, J.J., Ehlich, L.S., Teitelbaum, S.L., Fliszar, C., Welgus, H.G., Kahn, A.J., Hormonal regulation of the production of collagenase and a collagenase inhibitor activity by rat osteogenic sarcoma cells. Endocrinology 187; 120: 1956–1962.
19. Wong, G., Skeletal actions of parathyroid hormone. Min. Electrolyte Metab. 1982; 8: 188–198.
20. Lian, J.B., Tassinari, M., Glowacki, J., Resorption of implanted bone prepared from normal and warfarin-treated rats. J. Clin. Invest. 1984; 73: 1223–1226.
21. Hattersley, G., Chambers, T.J., Calcitonin receptors as markers for osteoclastic differentiation: correlation between generation of bone-resorptive cells and cells that express calcitonin receptors in mouse bone marrow cultures. Endocrinology 1989; 125(3): 1606–1612.
22. Hynes, R.O., Integrins: versatility, modulation, and signaling in cell adhesion. Cell 1992; 69: 11–25.
23. Davies, J., Warwick, J., Totty, N., Philip, R., Helfrich, M., Horton, M., The osteoclast functional antigen implicated in the regulation of bone resorption is biochemically related to the vitronectin receptor. J. Cell. Biol. 1989; 109: 1817–1826.
24. Sato, M., Sardana, M.K., Grasser, W.A., Garsky, V.M., Murray, J.M., Gould, R.J., Echistatin is a potent inhibitor of bone resorption in culture. J. Cell. Biol. 1990; 111: 1713–1723.
25. Somerman, M.J., Prince, C.W., Sauk, J.J., Foster, R.A., Butler, W.T., Mechanism of fibroblast attachment to bone extracellular matrix: role of a 44 kilodalton bone phosphoprotein. J. Bone Miner. Res. 1987; 2(3): 259–265.
26. Flores, M.E., Norgard, M., Heinegard, D., Reinholt, F.P., Andersson, G., RGD-directed attachment of isolated rat osteoclasts to osteopontin, bone sialoprotein, and fibronectin. Exp. Cell. Res. 1992; 201: 526–530.
27. Zambonin-Zallone, A., Teti, A., Grano, M., Rubinacci, A., Abbadini, M., Gaboli, M., Marchisio, P.C., Immunocytochemical distribution of extracellular matrix receptors in human osteoclasts: A $\beta 3$ antigen is colocalized with vinculin and talin in the podosomes of osteoclastoma giant cells. Exp. Cell. Res. 1989; 182: 645–652.
28. Lakkakorpi, P.T., Horton, M.A., Helfrich, M.H., Karhukorpi, E.-K., Vaananen, H.K., Vitronectin receptor has a role in bone resorption but does not mediate tight sealing zone attachment of osteoclasts to the bone surface. J. Cell. Biol. 1991; 115(4): 1179–1186.
29. Ikeda, T., Nomura, S., Yamaguchi, A., Suda, T., Yoshiki, S., In situ hybridization of bone matrix proteins in undecalcified adult rat bone sections. J. Histol. Cytochem. 1992; 40(8): 1079–1088.
30. Zimolo, Z., Wesolowski, G., Tanaka, H., Hyman, J.L., Hoyer, J.R., Rodan, G.A., Soluble $\alpha_v \beta_3$-integrin ligands raise [Ca2+]i in rat osteoclasts and mouse-derived osteoclast-like cells. Am. J. Physiol. 1994; 266: C376–C381.
31. Shankar, G., Davison, I., Helfrich, M.H., Mason, W.T., Horton, M.A., Integrin receptor-mediated mobilisation of intranuclear calcium in rat osteoclasts. J. Cell. Sci. 1993; 105: 61–68.
32. Paniccia, R., Colucci, S., Grano, M., Serra, M., Zambonin-Zallone, A., Teti, A., Immediate cell signal by bone-related peptides in human osteoclast-like cells. Am. J. Physiol. 1993; 265: C1289–C1297.
33. Baron, R., Neff, L., Brown, W., Courtoy, P.J., Louvard, D., Farquhar, M.G., Polarized secretion of lysosomal enzymes: co-distribution of cation-independent mannose-6-phosphate receptors along the osteoclast exocytic pathway. J. Cell. Biol. 1988; 106: 1863–1872.
34. Baron, R., Neff, L., Louvard, D., Courtoy, P.J., Cell-mediated extracellular acidification and bone resorption: evidence for a low pH in resorbing lacunae and localization of a 100-kD lysosomal membrane protein of the osteoclast ruffled border. J. Cell. Biol. 1985; 101: 2210–2222.
35. Silver, I.A., Murrills, R.J., Etherington, D.J., Microelectrode studies on the acid microenvironment beneath adherent macrophages and osteoclasts. Exp. Cell. Res. 1988; 175: 266–276.
36. Blair, H.C., Teitelbaum, S.L., Ghiselli, R., Gluck, S., Osteoclastic bone resorption by a polarized vacuolar proton pump. Science 1989; 245: 855–857.
37. Vaananen, H.K., Karhukorpi, E.K., Sundquist, K., Roininen, I., Hentunen, T., Tuukkanen, J., Lakkakorpi, P., Evidence for the presence of a proton pump of the vacuolar H+ATPase type in the ruffled borders of osteoclasts. J. Cell. Biol. 1990; 111: 1305–1311.
38. Chatterjee, D., Chakraborty, M., Leit, M., Neff, L., Jamsa-Kellokumpu, S., Fuchs, R., Sensitivity to vanadate and isoforms of subunits A and B distinguish the osteoclast proton pump from other vacuolar H+ATPases. Proc. Natl. Acad. Sci. USA 1992; 89: 6257–6261.
39. Sundquist, K., Lakkakorpi, P., Wallmark, B., Vaananen, K., Inhibition of osteoclast proton transport by bafilomycin A1 abolishes bone resorption. Biochem. Biophys. Res. Commun. 1990; 168(1): 309–313.

40. Blair, H.C., Teitelbaum, S.L., Tan, H.-L., Koziol, C.M., Schlesinger, P.H., Passive chloride permeability charge coupled to H^+-ATPase of avian osteoclast ruffled membrane. Am. J. Physiol. 1991; 260: C1315–C1324.
41. Anderson, R.E., Schraer, H., Gay, C.V., Ultrastructural immunocytochemical localization of carbonic anhydrase in normal and calcitonin-treated chick osteoclasts. Anat. Rec. 1982; 204: 9–20.
42. Vaananen, H.K., Immunohistochemical localization of carbonic anhydrase isoenzymes-I and II in human bone, cartilage and giant cell tumor. Histochemistry 1984; 81: 485–487.
43. Hall, G.E., Kenny, A.D., Bone resorption induced by parathyroid hormone and dibutyryl cyclic AMP: role of carbonic anhydrase. J. Pharmacol. Exp. Ther. 1986; 238(3): 778–782.
44. Kenny, A.D., Role of carbonic anhydrase in bone: partial inhibition of disuse atrophy of bone by parenteral acetazolamide. Calcif. Tissue Int. 1985; 37: 126–133.
45. Teti, A., Blair, H.C., Teitelbaum, S.L., Kahn, A.J., Koziol, C., Konsek, J., Zambonin-Zallone, A., Schlesinger, P.H., Cytoplasmic pH regulation and chloride/bicarbonate exchange in avian osteoclasts. J. Clin. Invest. 1989; 83: 227–233.
46. Hall, T.J., Chambers, T.J., Optimal bone resorption by isolated rat osteoclasts requires chloride/bicarbonate exchange. Calcif. Tissue Int. 1989; 45: 378–380.
47. Klein-Nulend, J., Raisz, L.G., Effects of two inhibitors of anion transport on bone resorption in organ culture. Endocrinology 1989; 125(2): 1019–1024.
48. Baron, R., Neff, L., Roy, C., Boisvert, A., Caplan, M., Louvard, D., Courtoy, P., Evidence for a high and specific concentration of (Na^+, K^+) ATPase in the plasma membrane of the osteoclast. Cell 1985; 46: 311–320.
49. Ravesloot, J.H., Ypey, D.L., Vrijheid-Lammers, T., Nijweide, P.J., Voltage-activated K^+ conductances in freshly isolated embryonic chicken osteoclasts. Proc. Natl. Acad. Sci. USA 1989; 86: 6821–6825.
50. Sims, S.M., Dixon, S.J., Inwardly rectifying K^+ current in osteoclasts. Am. J. Physiol. 1989; 256: C1277–C1282.
51. Miyauchi, A., Hruska, K.A., Greenfield, E.M., Duncan, R., Alvarez, J., Barattolo, R., Colucci, S., Zambonin-Zallone, A., Teitelbaum, S.L., Osteoclast cytosolic calcium, regulated by voltage-gated calcium channels and extracellular calcium, controls podosome assembly and bone resorption. J. Cell. Biol. 1990; 111: 2543–2552.
52. Zaidi, M., 'Calcium receptors' on eukaryotic cells with special reference to the osteoclast. Biosci. Rep. 1990; 10(6): 493–507.
53. Delaisse, J.-M., Vaes, G., Mechanism of mineral solubilization and matrix degradation in osteoclastic bone resorption. In: Rifkin, B.R., Gay, C.V. (Editors), Biology and physiology of the osteoclast. CRC Press, Boca Raton, 1992, pp. 289–314.
54. Wucherpfennig, A.L., Li, Y.-P., Stetler-Stevenson, W.G., Rosenberg, A.E., Stashenko, P., J. Bone Miner. Res. 1994; 4: 549–555.
55. Reponen, P., Sahlberg, C., Munaut, C., Thesleff, I., Tryggvason, K., J. Cell. Biol. 1994; 124: 1091–1102.
56. Delaisse, J.M., Eeckhout, Y., Neff, L., Francois-Gillet, C., Henriet, P., Su, Y., Vaes, G., Baron, R., (Pro)collagenase(matrix metalloproteinase-1) is present in rodent osteoclasts and in the underlying bone-resorbing compartment. J. Cell. Sci. 1993; 106: 1071–1092.
57. Kanehisa, J., Heersche, J.N.M., Osteoclastic bone resorption: in vitro analysis of the rate of resorption and migration of individual osteoclasts. Bone 1988; 9: 73–79.
58. Chambers, T.J., McSheehy, P.M.J., Thomson, B.M., Fuller, K., The effect of calcium regulating hormones and prostaglandins on bone resorption by osteoclasts disaggregated from rabbit long bones. Endocrinology 1985; 116: 234–239.
59. Zaidi, M., Datta, H.K., Moonga, B.S., MacIntyre, I., Evidence that the action of calcitonin on rat osteoclasts is mediated by two G proteins acting via separate post-receptor pathways. J. Endocrinol. 1990; 126: 473–481.
60. Zaidi, M., Pazianas, M., Shankar, V.S., Bax, B.E., Bax, C.M.R., Bevis, P.J.R., Stevens, C., Huang, C.L.-H., Blake, D.R., Moonga, B.S., Alam, A.S.M.T., Osteoclast function and its control. Exp. Physiol. 1993; 78: 721–739.
61. Zaidi, M., Datta, H.K., Patchell, A., Moonga, B.S., MacIntyre, I., 'Calcium-activated' intracellular calcium elevation: a novel mechanism of osteoclast regulation. Biochem. Biophys. Res. Commun. 1989; 163: 1461–1465.
62. Datta, H.K., MacIntyre, I., Zaidi, M., Intracellular calcium in the control of osteoclast function. I. Voltage-insensitivity and lack of effects of nifedipine, BAYK8644 and diltiazem. Biochem. Biophys. Res. Commun. 1990; 167: 183–188.

Bisphosphonate on bones
O. Bijvoet, H.A. Fleisch, R.E. Canfield and G. Russell (eds.)
© 1995 Elsevier Science B.V. All rights reserved.

CHAPTER 4

The assessment of bone metabolism in vivo using biochemical approaches

R.G.G. Russell

Department of Human Metabolism and Clinical Biochemistry, University of Sheffield Medical School, Beech Hill Rd., Sheffield S10 2RX, UK

I. Introduction

The monitoring of organ function by the measurement of tissue-specific biochemical products in body fluids is a well established principle in clinical biochemistry. In the case of bone, such measurements have been routinely limited to only a few assays, notably alkaline phosphatase to provide an indirect measure of osteoblast activity. However, many other products derived from the increased metabolism of bone appear in serum or urine where they can be measured as indicators of bone turnover and disease activity.

There have been a number of significant developments in this area in recent years. This is linked to the increasing interest in metabolic bone diseases particularly osteoporosis, in which the use of biochemical assays for the diagnosis and monitoring of treatment are needed. This brief review will provide an outline of the current status and some anticipated developments in this area.

1. Desirable features of a tissue marker

Biochemical markers of bone turnover measured in plasma or urine are proteins or products derived from them. In general, they are either enzymes derived from osteoblasts involved in bone formation, or from osteoclasts involved in bone resorption, or constituents of the bone matrix, which escape into the circulation during the process of bone formation, or which are released as breakdown products during resorption.

In assessing the value of any marker, several points need to be kept in mind (Table 1). Firstly, an ideal marker should be specific to the tissue being monitored. In the case of bone, this applies to osteocalcin, but not, for example, to hydroxyproline or its peptides. An ideal marker should also be easily measurable by specific, sensitive and precise techniques in either serum or urine. Other criteria

Table 1.

Desirable features of biochemical markers of tissue metabolism

---

– Markers should be tissue specific
– Metabolism of markers should be simple and preferably not influenced by the function of other organs
– Factors controlling the synthesis and degradation of the marker should be well defined
– Sensitive, specific and easy assays need to be available

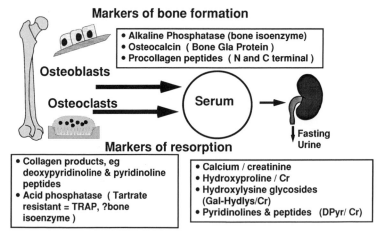

Fig. 1. The major biochemical markers of bone metabolism.

that determine the value of any biochemical marker of tissue metabolism include knowledge of the factors that control its synthesis and metabolism, and its entry into and removal from the circulation. With most markers there is still only limited information available about their metabolism and kinetics, and the factors which influence their production and degradation.

II. Markers of bone formation

The three markers of bone formation in current use are alkaline phosphatase, osteocalcin or bone gla protein, and propeptides derived from type I collagen.

1. Alkaline phosphatase

Alkaline phosphatase in serum has been used for more than 50 years to monitor bone metabolism, and is still the most frequently used marker. It is an ectoenzyme anchored to the cell surfaces of osteoblasts and other cells. The enzyme may be shed initially attached to plasma membrane components. The processes regulating release of the enzyme from cells are poorly understood, but plasma membrane vesicles containing alkaline phosphatase are probably involved in the initiation of mineralisation in skeletal tissues. The clearance from the circulation is relatively slow, with a half-life in the order of 1–3 days for the bone isoenzyme.

Studies of hypophosphatasia, an inherited disease characterised by a deficiency of alkaline phosphatase coupled with defective skeletal mineralisation, gives important clues about its biological function. In this condition the precise genetic defect is most commonly a point mutation that leads to synthesis of a defective enzyme lacking full catalytic activity. There is an accumulation of several phosphorylated metabolites, notably pyridoxal phosphate, phosphoethanolamine and inorganic pyrophosphate, which therefore are probably among the natural substrates for alkaline phosphatase. The accumulation of inorganic pyrophosphate, an inhibitor of crystal growth of hydroxyapatite, may be directly responsible for the defect in skeletal mineralisation.

The values for alkaline phosphatase in plasma and serum are raised in conditions such as Paget's disease, osteomalacia, and after fractures or ectopic bone formation. However, alkaline phosphatase is not specific to bone, and ideally selective measurement of the bone isoenzyme should be used as a marker of bone formation. In clinical practise the major problem for diagnostic purposes is to distinguish between the isoenzymes derived from liver and bone, although the intestinal enzyme may be raised after meals, and the placental isoenzyme during pregnancy.

Only a single gene encodes for the isoenzymes of alkaline phosphatase found in bone, liver and kidney. Fortunately, however, there are different post-translational modifications made to the enzyme from different tissues after synthesis, resulting in glycosylated products. Thus, the bone isoenzyme can be distinguished based on sialic acid residues. The bone isoenzyme can therefore be separated and selectively measured by methods based on differential heat denaturation, electrophoresis, precipitation with wheat germ lectin, and immunoassays with monoclonal or polyclonal antibodies. In this way, specific assays for the bone isoenzyme of alkaline phosphatase are being introduced. Among the best of these are immunoassays, utilising two antibodies, one for capture of the protein and one for its assay. As these specific methods for the bone isoenzyme are becoming more readily available, they are likely to be used more frequently, particularly for distinguishing liver from bone disease, and for population studies or monitoring individuals with bone disease.

In normal individuals about half of the total alkaline phosphatase is derived from bone and the rest from liver. In conditions such as Paget's disease, the changes in alkaline phosphatase are often very substantial, so that the dominant circulating form of the enzyme is from bone, meaning that assays of the total enzyme are often sufficient, and there is no great advantage in using bone-specific assays. The tissue-specific assays come to be much more important in less severely affected patients or in other milder disorders of bone turnover, including osteoporosis, where changes occur predominantly within the normal range.

Values for total alkaline phosphatase show a log-normal distribution. The analytical precision of routine assays for alkaline phosphatase are high, in the order of 1–2%, and the day to day and month to month biological variation is small. Changes

METABOLISM OF OSTEOCALCIN (BONE GLA PROTEIN, BGP)

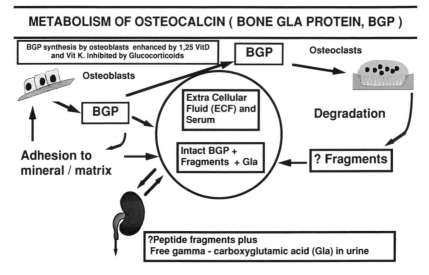

Fig. 2. The synthesis and metabolism of osteocalcin

of 10% or more therefore usually represent significant changes in an individual. However for clinical purposes and in trials of therapies, e.g. in Paget's disease, a fall of 25% or more is usually required to indicate a significant clinical response.

2. Osteocalcin

Osteocalcin, also known as bone Gla protein (BGP), is a bone-specific protein, which has proven to be a sensitive and specific marker of osteoblast activity in a variety of metabolic bone diseases. Factors regulating its production from osteoblasts are known in some detail. Its synthesis is dependent upon the presence of active metabolites of vitamin D, especially 1,25-dihydroxy vitamin D, and it requires vitamin K for the conversion by carboxylation of three glutamate residues to gamma-carboxyglutamate (Gla). These post-translational modifications are similar to those seen in the vitamin K-dependent blood clotting proteins, e.g. prothrombin, and confer calcium-binding properties on osteocalcin. This can be used to differentiate fully carboxylated from partially carboxylated osteocalcin in the circulation, and it has been shown recently that a significant proportion of osteocalcin in osteoporotic elderly patients is incompletely carboxylated. Indeed, the presence of un-decarboxylated osteocalcin is associated with a significantly increased risk of hip fracture in the elderly.

The factors determining the deposition of osteocalcin in the bone matrix and its liberation into the circulation are unclear, and significant metabolism to peptides and even to free Gla occurs. Measurements of the free Gla in plasma and urine have been used in attempts to monitor bone resorption, but appear not to be sufficiently specific or informative.

Measurements of serum osteocalcin by immunoassays show increases in conditions associated with increased bone formation, e.g. hyperparathyroidism, hyperthyroidism, bone metastases. In Paget's disease, however, these increases are less than expected, perhaps reflecting differential incorporation into bone matrix or altered synthesis by osteoblasts. Reduced levels of osteocalcin may reflect lower rates of bone formation, as seen, for example, in myeloma. Osteocalcin values may be substantially reduced during treatment with glucocorticosteroids, although in this case it should be remembered that glucocorticoids specifically suppress osteocalcin synthesis by osteoblasts, while not necessarily similarly depressing collagen synthesis or production of alkaline phosphatase to an equivalent degree.

Serum osteocalcin values can reflect the age-related increase in bone turnover, and the values rise after the menopause and fall after treatment with oestrogens, and also with salmon calcitonin. Such measurements are, therefore, useful in relation to osteoporosis, although many data are based on population studies, rather than changes in individual patients. There are marked differences in the performance of different assays used in different laboratories, some of which are available commercially. New developments include the development of assays utilising antibodies against human rather than bovine osteocalcin, and the use of sandwich assays with two monoclonal antibodies, so that only the intact molecule is measured, rather than fragments. There is also interest in developing non-isotopic methods, and in assays for fragments of osteocalcin that might be released during the resorption of bone matrix.

3. Procollagen peptides

Collagen is the major structural protein of bone and comprises about 90% of the organic material. Collagen clearly contributes to the integrity and strength of bone matrix and defects in its production, e.g. in osteogenesis imperfecta, lead to bone of poor quality, susceptible to fracture. Attempts to measure collagen synthesis represent, therefore, a more logical approach than measuring other less abundant matrix constituents in the assessment of bone formation. During collagen synthesis pro-peptides are released both from the amino-terminal ('N-terminal') and carboxy-terminal ('C-terminal') ends of the procollagen molecule, after the three individual alpha-chains have formed the triple helix, which will become part of the collagen fibril.

Assays for both the N- and C-terminal pro-peptides exist. The C-terminal peptide has the advantage of not being significantly retained in bone, unlike the N-terminal peptide. There is therefore considerable interest in the use of assays for the collagen type I C-terminal peptide (PICP) to monitor collagen synthesis related to bone formation. The values are increased during growth and in situations of increased bone formation, such as occur in Paget's disease, and in response to growth hormone. However, the values vary within a relatively narrow range, and measurements may be of more use in population studies than in monitoring individual patients. Moreover, pro-peptides from type I collagen are also derived from skin and other tissues, so it is desirable to develop bone-specific assays if this is feasible.

III. Measurements of bone resorption

Biochemical markers used to monitor bone resorption include urinary measurements of hydroxyproline-containing peptides, hydroxylysine glycosides and pyridinoline crosslinks, which are all derived from collagen. In some circumstances, fasting urine calcium can give an indirect measure of bone resorption rates and may be useful in Paget's disease and in patients with metastatic bone disease for following responses to treatment. Other measurements include assays of tartrate-resistant acid phosphatase and free Gla (see above).

1. Hydroxyproline

Until a few years ago, the best established and most widely used marker of bone resorption was the measurement of hydroxyproline in urine. Peptides containing hydroxyproline are released into urine from the proteolytic breakdown of collagen in bone and other tissues. Since hydroxyproline is one of the abundant amino acids in collagen, its measurement is logical, but hydroxyproline is also found in other proteins and is not specific for collagen in bone. Furthermore, significant amounts of hydroxyproline can be derived from dietary sources of collagen (gelatin), and there is extensive metabolism within the body. For these reasons it is likely that hydroxyproline assays will be eventually replaced by more specific measurements of bone resorption, notably by the use of pyridinoline crosslinks, which do not suffer from these disadvantages.

Nevertheless, measurements of hydroxyproline, particularly in early morning

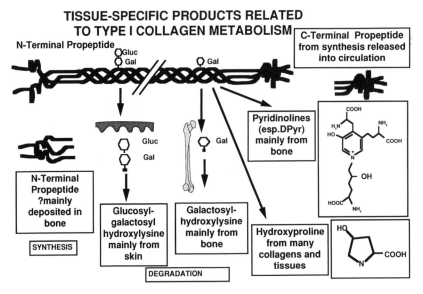

Fig. 3. The major biochemical markers related to the metabolism of type I collagen

fasting urines, have proved to be useful in evaluating responses in trials of new therapies. Their use in individual patients is handicapped by the low precision/ reproducibility of assays, with coefficients of variation (CVs) typically ranging from 10% to 25%. A change of 50% or so may therefore be required in two consecutive measurements before a significant response can be claimed. In Paget's disease the changes that occur are large, and there may be little advantage in using pyridinolines instead of hydroxyproline for practical purposes. Several studies in relation to osteoporosis show that, when measurements are made carefully, urinary hydroxyproline values rise after the menopause and fall again when anti-resorptive drugs such as oestrogens, calcitonins and bisphosphonates are given.

2. Pyridinoline crosslinks

Pyridinoline (Pyr) and deoxypyridinoline (DPyr), also called hydroxylysyl pyridinoline (HL) and lysyl pyridinoline (LP), respectively, are currently receiving considerable attention as the most promising markers of bone resorption. Both are non-reducible crosslinks which stabilise the collagen chains within the extracellular matrix and are formed by the condensation of three lysine and/or hydroxylysine residues in adjacent alpha-chains. Both Pyr and DPyr are present in bone, but DPyr appears to be found in significant quantities only in bone collagen, making it a potentially specific and more robust marker for bone resorption.

About 40% of these crosslinks appear free in urine, and the remainder are in peptide form. The free or total amount after acid hydrolysis is usually measured by reverse-phase HPLC analysis with detection based on the intrinsic fluorescence of these compounds. Although these assays remain the reference methods, they are cumbersome and labour-intensive. Fortunately, there has been recent progress in developing immunoassays against the free amino acids or against peptides containing the crosslinks, and these offer considerable hope for producing more rapid and specific assays. At present, at least three groups of immunoassays have been reported, one for pyridinolines present as free amino acids or in small peptides, another for the crosslinked N-terminal telopeptide in urine, and the third for the C-terminal telopeptide in serum. The CVs for these assays are in the order of 5–15%, and there appears to be significant circadian and other sources of biological variation so that further validation is needed.

The pyridinolines do not appear to be significantly absorbed from the diet. It is thought that they are not metabolised, although this remains to be proven. Excretion in the urine may give a quantitative measure of bone resorption since mature collagen contains about 0.07 mol per mole of collagen. However, more information is needed to determine whether there are differences in pyridinoline crosslink contents of collagen in different parts of the skeleton, since it is clear that there are differences at least between species.

As would be expected from a good marker of bone resorption, the values for pyridinolines in urine are increased in childhood and after menopause. They are also increased in other conditions, e.g. in endocrine (e.g. hyperthyroidism) and neoplastic disorders. There are excellent correlations between excretion of crosslinks

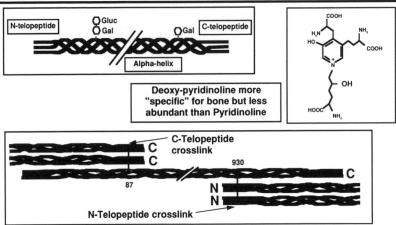

Fig. 4. The position of pyridinoline crosslinks in type I collagen

and bone turnover measured by radioisotope kinetics or bone histomorphometry. There are clear circadian patterns of excretion in these crosslinks with fasting values being of the order of 40% higher than 24-h values, which may reflect increases in bone resorption overnight. These circadian changes are of considerable biological interest but pose problems for choosing appropriate urines for assay. At present, the recommendation should be to use 24-h urines whenever possible, although the use of fasting urine assays (i.e. collections made over defined 2–3 h periods in the morning after the overnight urine is voided) may still be informative if taken under strictly controlled conditions.

In the near future, the current development of fast and reproducible immunoassays, either of free pyridinolines or of degradation peptides containing them, are likely to make measurements of pyridinolines as readily available as alkaline phosphatase. Because of their theoretical advantages, they are therefore likely to become established as the measurements of choice for following changes in bone resorption, particularly when the assays are adapted for use in serum rather than urine.

3. Hydroxylysine glycosides

Hydroxylysine glycosides are also derived from type I collagens. Hydroxylysine, like hydroxyproline derived from proline, is produced by a post-translational hydroxylation. The subsequent glycosylation of hydroxylysine differs in collagens in different tissues. The monoglycosylated galactosyl hydroxylysine is enriched in bone compared with the diglycosylated form, glucosyl galactosyl hydroxylysine, which is the major form in skin.

Assay is by HPLC and is therefore technically demanding and relatively slow.

Reported measurements, however, suggest that this may be a useful marker of bone resorption, for example, in osteoporosis. Some concern exists over whether the glycosylated forms remain intact during passage down the renal tubule. If specific immunoassays could be developed, hydroxylysine glycosides might offer a useful and practical additional measurement of bone resorption.

4. Acid phosphatase

Acid phosphatase is a lysosomal enzyme which exists in several forms in different tissues. The type 5 isoenzyme is the one found in osteoclasts, which appear to be released during bone resorption. Assays of total tartrate-resistant acid phosphatase (TRAP) in the circulation are moderately raised in disorders associated with increased bone resorption, but the assays are difficult to perform because of the instability of the enzyme and the relatively small changes observed in pathological states. The development of immunoassays specific for the type 5 form offer the potential of producing better assays for monitoring bone resorption.

IV. Other assays

A variety of other assays in the past, or of current interest, for measuring bone formation and resorption have been tried.

One interesting observation is that serum proteins such as α_2 HS-glycoprotein, derived from the liver, are deposited in bone, and the values fall when bone formation rates are high. However, although this is of physiological interest, the changes are relatively small, and such measurements do not at present provide a practical method of monitoring bone formation rates in individuals.

As more has become known of specific proteins in bone matrix, other assays have been developed and evaluated, e.g. for osteonectin and osteopontin, and others may be developed in the future, e.g. for other bone sialoproteins and matrix Gla protein. There is also much interest in the measurement of the many cytokines and growth factors now known to influence bone metabolism [e.g. interleukins 1 and 6, tumour necrosis factors (TNFs), insulin-like growth factors I and II and their binding proteins], and in some cases their soluble antagonists (e.g. the IL-1-receptor antagonist) or receptors (e.g. the soluble p55 and p75 TNF receptors).

With regard to the current status of work in this area, there is clearly considerable potential for improving existing assays and developing additional specific assays, but more work is needed.

V. General and specific uses of assays

In the past the major uses for these assays have been to help with the diagnosis and management of patients with florid disorders of bone metabolism, such as Paget's disease or vitamin D-deficient osteomalacia. However, there is a need to use such assays to monitor the more subtle changes that occur in conditions such as osteoporosis, where the changes in an individual may occur within the normal reference range.

1. Paget's disease

Paget's disease is the best example of a disease in which biochemical markers of bone metabolism have been extensively used in clinical practice. There have been three major uses for measurements of bone markers:
1. to assess and to monitor disease activity in individual patients;
2. to evaluate dose–response relationships to existing and new drugs in therapeutic trials;
3. to evaluate the value of novel biochemical markers of bone metabolism, compared with established markers.

The major markers in routine use have been alkaline phosphatase and urinary hydroxyproline. Alkaline phosphatase is of proven value in monitoring disease activity in individuals with Paget's disease and is the standard measurement used in clinical trials and for comparison with new markers.

Many other products of bone have been shown to be raised in serum and/or urine in Paget's disease and to be reduced during treatment. These include products associated with bone formation, e.g. osteocalcin, osteonectin, N- and C-terminal pro-peptides of type I collagen, or with bone resorption, e.g. acid phosphatase, free Gla and hydroxylysine glycosides, especially galactosyl-hydroxylysine that appears to be relatively specific for bone. The measurement of these other products of bone metabolism, e.g. osteocalcin, and other collagen-derived peptides and bone matrix proteins often show unexpected deviations from the predicted increases, compared with alkaline phosphatase and hydroxyproline, which may reflect aberrant production and metabolism of these products in untreated Paget's disease. This is an important reminder that different biochemical markers reflect different biological processes. Serum proteins, e.g. α_2 HS-glycoprotein, that have a high affinity for bone may be reduced in the serum of patients with active Paget's disease.

Studies with biochemical markers in Paget's disease have illustrated another very important principle: it is possible to demonstrate the dissociation between effects of drugs on bone formation and bone resorption. The major drugs used in Paget's disease are the calcitonins and bisphosphonates, which are inhibitors of bone resorption. It is therefore not surprising that the earliest biochemical changes that occur are in the resorption markers, which can show full responses within only a few days of starting treatment with potent bisphosphonates such as pamidronate. It is very important to realise that, in the routine management of patients, alkaline phosphatase measurements change more slowly in response to treatment than do markers of bone resorption, and that the full response may not be seen for several weeks or even months. Since the currently used potent treatments for Paget's disease, especially with the bisphosphonates, can induce complete biochemical remissions, it is important to realise that judging responses on early changes in alkaline phosphatase alone may give a misleading picture of how effective treatment has been. For this reason, it is wise to advocate that measurements of both alkaline phosphatase and of appropriate bone resorption markers should become routine in the therapeutic management of Paget's disease to ensure adequate responses to treatment.

2. Osteoporosis

Perhaps the greatest challenge for the future use of markers is in osteoporosis. There are two major needs:
1. to identify the patients at greatest risk, e.g. those with rapid rates of bone loss compared with bone formation;
2. to monitor the effects of specific treatment (e.g. with oestrogens, calcitonins and bisphosphonates, or with bone-forming agents) in individual patients.

Most data related to age or postmenopausal changes in bone metabolism are based on populations. Important work from Christiansen's group has shown that a combination of biochemical assays, including total alkaline phosphatase and osteocalcin in plasma and hydroxyproline and calcium in fasting urine, have strong predictive power in relation to rates of bone loss subsequently measured by bone densitometry techniques. It is of interest that individual biochemical measurements may each add to the power of this prediction. This reminds us that each marker reflects different biochemical and physiological processes and may not, therefore, always show identical changes. More work is needed from other laboratories to evaluate the value of such measurements in the assessment of individual patients.

The use of bone markers to monitor individual patients requires assays of high precision. In the case of bone-specific alkaline phosphatase, where the precision is of the order of a few percent, this requirement may be easier to meet than with urinary assays for hydroxyproline or pyridinolines, where the coefficient of variation for the assays may be of the order of 15% or so, requiring a treatment-induced change in the region of 30% or more before a true response can be claimed. The increasing interest in the prevention and management of osteoporosis make the need for improved methods for measurement of these markers a high priority.

VI. Prospects for the future

In addition to the development of novel assays of greater specificity and sensitivity, particularly using monoclonal antibodies, there is a need for more rapid assays for practical clinical use. In view of the socioeconomic importance of bone disease, there is likely to be a considerable investment in this area, and the eventual development of fast assays may come.

Although there is a major interest in markers of bone disease, there is also considerable interest in extending these possibilities to other connective tissues, notably cartilage and other joint tissues in relation to destructive arthritis. As with bone, several cartilage-specific components exist (e.g. COMP, cartilage oligomeric protein), and there is a prospect of measuring cartilage-specific crosslinked collagen peptides, e.g. between type IX and type II collagen, which contain pyridinoline crosslinks, to monitor cartilage collagen degradation in articular cartilage. Such assays are in their infancy but offer considerable hope for better diagnosis and evaluation of bone and joint disorders.

VII. Conclusions

The processes of bone formation and resorption can be monitored in vivo by measuring enzymes and other protein products released by osteoblasts and osteoclasts, respectively. The major validated biochemical markers of bone formation currently in use include the bone isoenzyme of alkaline phosphatase, osteocalcin (also known as BGP, bone Gla protein) and pro-peptides derived from the N- or C-terminal ends of the type I procollagen molecule. Markers of bone resorption include TRAP and, in particular, breakdown products of collagen. The longest established of these is the measurement in urine of hydroxyproline in collagen peptides, but the assays are cumbersome. Furthermore, hydroxyproline is not specific to bone collagen and is also derived from the diet. There is much current interest in collagen products that are more specific to bone, including galactosyl hydroxylysine, and the collagen crosslinks, pyridinoline and deoxypyridinoline. The pyridinolines appear to be the most promising markers of resorption and may enable quantitative evaluation of rates of bone resorption in man.

These biochemical methods are of use in the diagnosis and evaluation of bone diseases, in population studies, and for monitoring responses to hormones and drugs. It is important to remember that individual markers reflect different biochemical and physiological processes and may not, therefore, always show identical changes.

There is an increasing amount of work being devoted to the study of bone biomarkers, partly because of the current interest in osteoporosis. There are exciting prospects ahead for improvements in technical methods and for the use of new markers derived from bone cells and bone matrix.

References

1. Azria, M., Russell, R.G.G., Biochemical approaches to the measurement of bone metabolism in vivo. In: Andersen, M. (Editor), Current Opinion in Orthopaedics. Metabolic bone disease. Curr. Sci. 1992; 3 (1): 103–109.
2. Black, D., Marabani, M., Sturrock, R.D., Robins, S.P., Urinary excretion of the hydroxypyridinium crosslinks of collagen in patients with rheumatoid arthritis. Ann. Rheum. Dis. 1989; 48: 641–644.
3. Brixen, K., Nielsen, H.K., Eriksen, E.F., Charles, P., Mosekilde, L., Efficacy of wheat germ lectin-precipitated alkaline phosphatase in serum as an estimator of bone mineralization rate: comparison to serum total alkaline phosphatase in serum bone Gla-protein. Calcif. Tissue Int. 1989; 44: 93–98.
4. Charles, P., Mosekilde, L., Risteli, L., Risteli, J., Eriksen, E.F., Assessment of bone remodeling using biochemical indicators of type I collagen synthesis and degradation: relation to calcium kinetics. Bone Miner. 1994; 24: 81–94.
5. Colwell, A., Russell, R.G.G., Eastell, R., Factors affecting the assay of urinary 3-hydroxy pyridinium crosslinks of collagen as markers of bone resorption. Eur. J. Clin. Invest. 1993; 23: 341–349.
6. Delmas, P.D., Clinical uses of biochemical markers of bone remodeling in osteoporosis. Bone 1992;

13: S17–S21.
7. Delmas, P.D., Christiansen, C., Mann, K.G., Price, P.A., Bone Gla protein (osteocalcin) assay standardisation report. J. Bone Min. Res. 1990; 5: 5–11.
8. Delmas, P.D., Schlemmer, A., Gineyts, E., Riis, B., Christiansen, C., Urinary excretion of pyridinoline crosslinks correlates with bone turnover measured on lilac crest biopsy in patients with vertebral osteoporosis. J. Bone Min. Res. 1991; 6: 639–644.
9. Eastell, R., Hampton, L., Colwell, A., Green, J.R., Assiri, A.M.A., Hesp, R., Russell, R.G.G., Reeve, J., Urinary collagen crosslinks are highly correlated with radioisotopic measurements of bone resorption. In: Christiansen, C., Overgaard, K. (Editors), Osteoporosis 1990. Copenhagen Osteopress, 1990, 469–470.
10. Eastell, R.D., Calvo, M.S., Burrit, M.F., Offord, K.P., Russell, R.G.G., Riggs, B.L., Abnormalities in circadian patterns of bone resorption and renal calcium conservation in type I osteoporosis. J. Clin. Endocrinol. Metab. 1992; 74: 487–494.
11. Eastell, R., Robins, S.P., Colwell, T., Assir, A.M.A., Riggs, B.L., Russell, R.G.G., Evaluation of bone turnover in type I osteporosis using biochemical markers specific for both bone formation and bone resorption. Osteoporosis Int. 1993; 3: 255–260.
12. Editorial, Pyridinium crosslinks as markers of bone resorption. The Lancet 1992; 2: 278–279.
13. Elomaa, I., Virkkunen, P., Risteli, L., Risteli, J., Serum concentration of the cross-linked carboxyterminal telopeptide of type I collagen (ICTP) is a useful prognostic indicator in multiple myeloma. Br. J. Cancer 1992; 66: 337–341.
14. Eyre, D.R., Collagen crosslinking amino-acids. Methods Enzymol. 1987; 144: 115–139.
15. Garnero, P., Delmas, P.D., Assessment of the serum levels of bone alkaline phosphatase with a new immunoradiometric assay in the patients with metabolic bone disease. J. Clin. Endocrinol. Metab. 1993; 77: 1046–1053.
16. Garnero, P., Grimaux, M., Seguin, P., Delmas, P.D., Characterisation of immunoreactive forms of human osteocalcin generated in vivo and in vitro. J. Bone Min. Res. 1994; 9: 255–264.
17. Gertz, B.J., Shao, P., Hanson, D.A., Quan, H., Harris, S.T., Genant, H.K., Chesnut, C.H., Eyre, D.R., Monitoring bone resorption in early postmenopausal women by an immunoassay for cross-linked collagen peptides in urine. J. Bone Min. Res. 1994; 9: 135–142.
18. Hanson, D., Weis, M.E., Bollen, A.-M., Maslan, S.L., Singer, F.R., Eyre, D.R., A specific immunoassay for monitoring human bone resorption: quantitation of type I collagen cross-linked N-telopeptides in urine. J. Bone Min. Res. 1992; 7: 1251–1258.
19. Hill, G.S., Wolfert, R.L., The preparation of monoclonal antibodies which react preferentially with human bone alkaline phosphatase and with lover alkaline phosphatase. Clin. Chem. Acta 1989; 186: 315–320.
20. Kraenzlin, M.E., Lau, K.-H.W., Liang, L., Freeman, T.K., Singer, F.R., Stepan, J., Baylink, D.J., Development of an immunoassay for human serum osteoclastic tartrate-resistant acid phosphatase. J. Clin. Endocrinol. Metab. 1990; 71: 442–451.
21. Krane, S.M., Kantrowitz, F.G., Byrne, M., Pinnell, S.R., Singer, F.R., Urinary excretion of hydroxylysine and its glycosides as an index of collagen degradation. J. Clin. Invest. 1977; 59: 819–827.
22. Masters, P.W., Jones, R.G., Purves, D.A., Cooper, E.H., Cooney. J.M., Commercial assays for serum osetocalcin give clinically discordant results. Clin. Chem. 1994; 40: 358–363.
23. Moro, L., Gazzarrini, C., Modricky, C., Rovis, L., de Bernard, B., Galligioni, E., Crivellari, D., Morassut, S., Monfardini, S., High predictivity of galactosyl-hydroxylysine in urine as an indicator of bone metastases from breast cancer. Clin. Chem. 1990; 36: 772–774.
24. Parfitt, A.M., Simon, L.S., Villanueva, A.R., Krane, S.M., Procollagen type I carboxy-terminal extension peptide in serum as a marker of collagen biosynthesis in bone. Correlation with iliac bone formation rates and comparison with total alkaline phosphatase. J. Bone Min. Res. 1987; 2: 427–436.
25. Pratt, D.A., Daniloff, Y., Duncan, A., Robins, S.P., Automated analysis of the pyridinium crosslinks of collagen in tissue and urine using solid-phase extraction and reversed-phase high performance liquid chromatography. Anal. Biochem. 1992; 207: 168–175.
26. Risteli, J., Elomaa, I., Niemi, S., Novamo, A., Risteli, L., Radioimmunoassay for the pyridinoline cross-linked carboxy-terminal telopetide of type I collagen: a new serum marker of the bone collagen degradation. Clin. Chem. 1993; 39: 635–640.
27. Robins, S.P., Crosslinking of collagen: isolation, structural characterisation and glycosylation of pyridinoline. Biochem. J. 1983; 215: 167–173.
28. Robins, S.P., Black, D., Paterson, C.R., Reid, D.M., Duncan, A., Siebel, M.J., Evaluation of urinary

hydroxypyridinium crosslink measurements as resorption markers in metabolic bone diseases. Eur. J. Clin. Invest. 1991; 21: 310–315.

29. Seibel, M.J., Duncan, A., Robins, S.P., Urinary hydroxy pyridinium crosslinks provide indices of cartilage and bone involvement in arthritic disease. J. Rheum. 1989; 16: 964–970.

30. Szulc, P., Chapuy, M.-C., Meunier, P.J., Delmas, P.D., Serum undercarboxylated osteocalcin is a marker of the risk of hip fracture in elderly women. J. Clin. Invest. 1993; 91: 1769–1774.

31. Uebelhart, D., Gineyts, E., Chapuy, M.-C., Delmas, P.D., Urinary excretion of pyridinium crosslinks: a new marker of bone disease. Bone Min. 1989; 8: 87–96.

32. Uebelhart, D., Gineyts, E., Chapuy, M.-C., Delmas, P.D., Urinary excretion of pyridinium crosslinks: a new marker of bone resorption in metabolic bone disease. Bone Min. 1990; 8: 87–96.

33. Uebelhart, D., Schlemmer, A., Johansen, J.S., Gineyts, E., Christiansen, C., Delmas, P.D., Effect of menopause and hormone replacement therapy on the urinary excretion of pyridinium crosslinks. J. Clin. Endocrinol. Metab. 1991; 72: 367–373.

Bisphosphonate on bones
O. Bijvoet, H.A. Fleisch, R.E. Canfield and G. Russell (eds.)
© 1995 Elsevier Science B.V. All rights reserved.

CHAPTER 5

Assessing the effects of treatment

Cyrus Cooper[1] and L. Joseph Melton, III[2]

[1] *MRC Environmental Epidemiology Unit, Southampton General Hospital, Tremona Road, Southampton SO9 4XY, UK;* [2] *Section of Clinical Epidemiology, Department of Health Sciences Research, Mayo Clinic, 200 First Street Southwest, Rochester, MN 55905, USA*

I. Introduction

Ideas about the utility of a particular treatment arise from virtually any activity within medicine. Some therapeutic hypotheses are suggested by insights into the mechanism of disease at the cellular level. Others emerge through astute clinical observation. Occasionally, the effects of a recently suggested treatment are so dramatic that their value is self-evident without any formal testing. However, the effects of most treatments are considerably less obvious, and a stage is reached in development when ideas about a treatment must be put to a formal test. The clinical trial represents the classical experimental setting within which such evaluations are performed. Following initial studies to assess dose levels and toxicity (phase I) and to elicit evidence of a therapeutic effect (phase II), clinical trials are undertaken to assess the efficacy of the new treatment against some suitable alternative (phase III). These classical experiments are the subject of this chapter, the purpose of which is to highlight some theoretical aspects of controlled clinical trials, to delineate practical difficulties entailed in performing clinical trials, and to illustrate alternative epidemiologic strategies for assessing the effectiveness of treatments. Where necessary, this theoretical framework will be illustrated with examples of intervention studies for osteoporosis, the most commonly encountered metabolic bone disorder in Western populations. The principles outlined, however, are generally applicable to treatment and secondary prevention in a wide range of chronic diseases.

II. Controlled clinical trials

A phase III clinical trial is a prospective study in human subjects comparing the effect and value of an intervention against a control [7]. The simplified structure of a controlled clinical trial is shown in Figure 1. The patients to be studied are selected

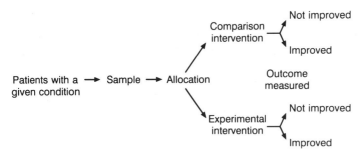

Fig. 1. Structure of a clinical trial. In the classical case, allocation of the intervention is by randomization and comparison is made with a placebo control group.

from a larger group of individuals with the condition of interest. Otherwise identical subjects are then divided into two or more groups with a comparable prognosis: one of the groups is exposed to the intervention, usually by random assignment, while the other (control) group is not exposed but is otherwise treated identically to the intervention group. The subsequent clinical course of both groups is observed, and any differences in outcome are attributed to the intervention.

Clearly, the rigid control of extraneous factors which is possible at the laboratory bench is not achievable in human studies, but the clinical trial provides the closest approximation to this ideal design in human research. Nonetheless, the key stages in this process warrant close attention. These include the selection of study subjects, the choice and allocation of the intervention, the assessment of outcomes, and the analysis and interpretation of results.

1. Subject selection

The patients actually included in a trial determine the extent to which its findings may be generalized to other patients. Generalizability is best assured by selecting the study sample randomly from the general population of appropriate individuals, though this is rarely done. Three important reasons why patients with the condition of interest might not be included in a trial are failure to meet specific entry criteria, refusal to participate, and inability to carry out the intervention.

Inclusion/exclusion criteria for entry into a trial are intended to reduce the heterogeneity of patients in the study, to eliminate subjects whose health is likely to be jeopardized by the treatment, and to improve the chances of patients completing the assigned treatment. As heterogeneity is restricted (for example, by excluding subjects with atypical disease, associated disorders, or an unusually poor prognosis), there is less opportunity for variation in outcome that is unrelated to treatment in the groups being compared. This is especially important in osteoporosis, which is a syndrome involving numerous pathophysiologic mechanisms [18]. However, the results of treatment trials for 'established' disease, in patients who have already experienced an osteoporosis-related fracture, for example, could not be applied to efforts at primary fracture prevention.

A second common reason for lack of inclusion is refusal to participate. Patients who refuse to volunteer may differ systematically from those who agree to enter a trial. Differences may be on the basis of age, gender, and socioeconomic class, the severity of disease, and the prevalence of co-morbid conditions, among others. This potential problem has received little attention, but in one prospective epidemiologic study of bone disease, nonvolunteers were older, more likely to have cardiovascular disease, and less likely to have taken estrogen replacement therapy [9].

Finally, patients who are thought unlikely to comply with the rules of the trial are usually not enrolled. This reduces wasted effort and the analytical problems which occur if patients move in and out of treatment groups or drop out of the trial altogether. However, the results of a trial with such exclusions may seriously overestimate the treatment effectiveness that can be obtained in general medical practice.

For these reasons, the patients who enter clinical trials are usually a highly selected, biased sample of all patients with the condition of interest. This selection process needs to be weighed against the desire to generalize from the results of clinical trials to ordinary practice settings. In many instances, such generalization requires a considerable leap of faith.

A good example of the impact of selection on recruitment is provided by a recently published trial of sodium fluoride for prevention of vertebral fractures among women with established postmenopausal osteoporosis, where only 1 in 6 women initially evaluated ended up fulfilling the entry criteria (Fig. 2). Participants were solicited by a press release, and subsequent enrollment depended upon a screening process by their own physician at which the presence of one or more vertebral fractures was to be verified, and certain exclusion criteria were to be applied [22]. Of 664 women who responded to the press release, only 44% had

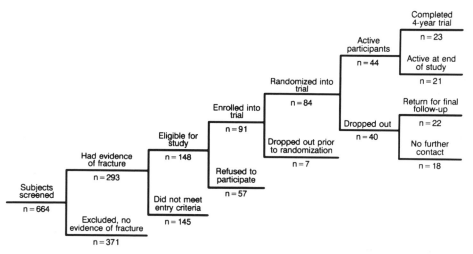

Fig. 2. Recruitment and participation in a clinical trial of sodium fluoride therapy. From [22].

radiographically confirmed vertebral fractures, and half of them had attributes leading to exclusion (most notably the use of widely prescribed drugs such as estrogen and thiazide diuretics). Of the remaining 148 women who were eligible for study, 39% refused to participate, leaving only 91 women (14% overall) to be enrolled. This experience is by no means unique among clinical trials.

2. The intervention and its allocation

Both the type of intervention and the method of its allocation impact upon the design of clinical trials. Most trials have focused on a single, highly specific, pharmacologic intervention which can be described accurately and applied reproducibly. Recent examples in osteoporosis research include trials of bisphosphonate [23], sodium fluoride [19], and calcitonin therapy [17]. Issues like the role of bone density screening and the overall risks and benefits of estrogen replacement therapy are also amenable to investigation within this paradigm [8], although the size of such trials makes them a daunting undertaking. However, the greatest underutilization of controlled trials in osteoporosis research has been in the area of population-based prevention with nonpharmacologic interventions such as dietary change or exercise [21].

Another major issue is the need for a comparison group. While uncontrolled trials may be sufficient for phase I and II studies, several considerations make a comparison group mandatory in assessing the efficacy of therapy in bone disease. First, there is great heterogeneity in bone loss and fracture risk [12], and improvement may result merely from variations in natural history. Figure 3 shows the relation between study duration and apparent fracture rate in the two studies examining the effects of various treatments in osteoporotic fractures. It illustrates that fracture incidence among patients followed for prolonged periods is substantially lower than that in subjects studied for only a short time. This difference is not

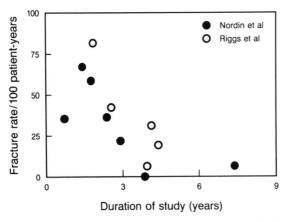

Fig. 3. Relation between apparent fracture rate and duration of study in two studies examining the effects of various treatments in osteoporotic fractures. From [13].

attributable to the interventions used, but results rather from the natural history of vertebral fracture occurrence. Second, apparent improvement can arise through statistical artifact (regression to the mean). For example, women selected for the trial on the basis of particularly low bone density values at baseline are likely to show a rise in bone density upon subsequent measurement, irrespective of any treatment effect. Finally, close attention by the investigators tends to make patients, inadvertently or deliberately, modify their behavior in a beneficial direction upon entering a trial (the Hawthorne effect). There is no way of separating Hawthorne and treatment effects in an uncontrolled trial.

Given the necessity of a comparison group in treatment trials, questions then arise as to the nature of this group. Crossover trials, where each subject is his or her own control, are usually not appropriate in osteoporosis research because treatments may take a long time to work and because the disease process is not stable. Comparisons with patients who are separated in time or place (historical or nonconcurrent controls) are prone to bias in favor of the experimental treatment, and concurrent controls are preferred. They are most often given an intervention that is indistinguishable from the active treatment but has no known mechanism of action (placebo). Ethical concerns arise if novel drug treatments are compared with a completely inactive placebo when treatments of known effectiveness are available, e.g. estrogen replacement therapy in postmenopausal women. A frequent compromise was to use calcium supplementation (a relatively safe measure of uncertain efficacy) as a standard against which newer drugs could be compared. However, evidence of reduced bone loss among controls on calcium led to placebo-controlled trials of calcium supplementation itself [5].

In order to study the unique effects of an intervention, the best way of allocating patients is by means of randomization. The purpose of randomization is to assign patients to experimental treatment or placebo without bias and to justify the use of certain statistical tests. With randomization, relatively large patient groups will, on average, be similar with regard to prognostic factors, including those which are unrecognized. To ensure that the groups are alike with respect to known prognostic factors, stratified (balanced) randomization procedures are often used. Data analysis must be based on this randomized assignment (intention to treat) because the treatment groups so formed are as similar as possible when the decision is made to start therapy. However, the ability to detect real treatment differences may be undermined if subjects subsequently fail to comply with their assigned intervention, especially if compliance is uneven with regard to treatment group.

3. Outcome assessment

Both treatment and control groups in a randomized controlled trial must be monitored to assure compliance with the study protocol and to assess toxicity, as well as to evaluate the outcomes of therapy. The outcome variables must be important (in human terms) and meaningful (in biologic terms). Response to treatment must be defined by the same criteria and sought with equal vigor in both the experimental and control arms of the trial. This is usually insured by

Table 1.

Sample size required to detect a two-fold difference in fracture rate between two populations with different baseline incidence rates for fracture (alpha=0.10; incidence of fracture per 10,000 in two populations). From [14]

Statistical power	1 and 2	10 and 20	100 and 200
0.5	156,000	15,740	1550
0.7	274,000	27,400	2700
0.9	500,000	49,800	4920
0.99	920,000	91,800	9060

'blinding' or masking treatment assignments from the patient and from those who are assessing the outcomes. Great effort is needed to ensure that all subjects remain under study so that the outcomes of interest can be measured, as considerable bias may be introduced with any substantial loss to follow-up [10].

While adverse physiologic effects may occur, bone disease is clinically important mostly because it leads to skeletal fragility and an increased risk of fractures [2]. Thus, an important outcome variable in any trial, especially of osteoporosis therapy, is the incidence of fracture. However, fracture incidence has a number of drawbacks as a primary trial endpoint. Hip fractures have the most devastating economic and morbid consequences, but most hip fractures occur in women over 75 years of age, and incidence rates in middle-aged men and women are low. Because osteoporosis treatments are usually more effective if initiated before extreme bone loss has occurred, i.e. earlier in life, trials using hip fracture incidence as the outcome require large numbers of subjects to be followed for long periods of time. Table 1 shows the change in sample size required to detect a given difference between two populations with various fracture incidence rates. It is clear that the study size needed to achieve a given statistical power (see below) is less when the incidence rates are greater. The incidence of new vertebral fractures in such populations is usually higher than the incidence of hip fractures, but there is considerable controversy regarding the assessment and definition of vertebral fractures [15]. However, recent documentation that most fractures in the elderly are due, at least in part, to low bone mass [20] eases the constraint that hip or vertebral fractures be the only outcomes of interest for therapies aimed at bone.

Sample sizes can be reduced even further by the use of suitable intermediary or surrogate outcomes. For example, if a particular agent slows bone loss, and low bone mass causes fractures, then use of the agent should lead to a reduction in fractures. Unfortunately, as a result of studies showing discordance between drug effects on bone mass and fracture rate [3], this convenient argument is becoming untenable in osteoporosis research. Moreover, increased attention is being paid to the clinical sequelae of fracture as meaningful endpoints. Thus, musculoskeletal pain and functional impairment, particularly as consequences of vertebral or distal forearm fracture, are beginning to be utilized as outcomes in clinical trials. However, the development of valid and reproducible tools for the assessment of these characteristics remains an important issue for future research.

4. Analysis and interpretation

The purpose of any clinical trial is to determine if there is a difference in outcomes between the treatment and placebo groups. In the traditional hypothesis testing approach, tests of statistical significance assess whether observed differences between the groups could conceivably have arisen by chance alone. The P value is a measure of whether the data are consistent with no difference between treatments (the null hypothesis). If P is very small, it is tempting to reject the explanation that the difference arose by chance and to interpret the results as evidence of a real effect. The main objective of a significance test is to quantify and limit the risk of a type I error (α), i.e., of concluding that a difference exists when the null hypothesis is actually true. Using the conventional threshold of $P = 0.05$, there is a 1 in 20 risk of obtaining a false-positive result. Multiple comparisons (for example, comparing treatment groups with respect to several outcome variables) greatly increase the risk of a type I error, but this problem is minimized if the study protocol specifies which comparison is the primary one or if a study design is chosen which provides for repeated testing. Less credibility can be given to tests of post hoc hypotheses which are not specified in advance but derived instead following a review of the data. In osteoporosis research, this often occurs when efficacy is evaluated separately among 'responders' to the treatment.

It is also important to bear in mind that a statistically significant finding is not necessarily biologically significant. Even small differences between groups can attain statistical significance if large numbers are studied. Conversely, a nonsignificant finding is often interpreted as proving the equivalence of two treatments but, in fact, only indicates that the study has failed to establish a difference. This raises the possibility of a type II error, i.e., of concluding that no difference exists when the null hypothesis is actually false. The chance of a type II error (ß) can be judged from the statistical power (1-ß) of the study — the likelihood that a specific difference, if present, will be detected. Statistical power increases with sample size, so that a nonsignificant result from a small trial does not necessarily mean that a treatment is of no benefit. Small trials also do not provide convincing evidence that a treatment is safe since a clinically significant increase in side effects may not prove to be statistically significant. Because the potential for osteoporosis treatments is so widespread [16], even relatively uncommon complications could pose problems in practice. This is one of the concerns of postmarketing surveillance (phase IV studies).

The limitations of significance testing have led to wider use of confidence intervals as a means of presenting results. Instead of testing a specific hypothesis about the magnitude of a treatment effect, confidence intervals give a range which, with a specific probability (say 95%), includes the real treatment difference. Therefore, they provide a range of outcomes with which the observed results are compatible. Regardless of the basic analytic approach chosen, however, numerous (and sometimes arcane) statistical techniques are usually available. Anyone contemplating a clinical trial should insure the availability of an experienced statistical consultant.

III. Alternative strategies for evaluating treatments

While randomized, controlled clinical trials represent the 'gold standard' for assessing treatment efficacy, they may provide misleading information about the likely success of the treatment in actual clinical practice. This relates to nongeneralizability of the trial cohort, to inability to deliver the intervention effectively in the community, and to poor compliance, among others. As a consequence, social costs are often greater than anticipated, as therapeutic indications are expanded, while benefits to society may be much less than expected. Just as with the testing of treatments in individuals, however, clinical trials can be used to assess the effectiveness of preventive strategies within entire populations. This is rarely done because the logistic difficulties in mounting such a trial are often perceived to be insurmountable. Under these circumstances, inferences about the effectiveness of treatments in populations may be made from epidemiologic observations.

1. Analytic epidemiologic studies

Two types of observational designs are used for this purpose: case-control and cohort studies. In a case-control study, patients with the disease in question (e.g., hip fracture) are compared with individuals who do not have the disease (controls). The exposure to a potential protective factor (e.g., previous estrogen replacement therapy) is compared in the two groups, and the risk of disease resulting from the exposure is estimated. In a cohort study, on the other hand, a group of people without the disease is assembled and classified according to exposure status at the outset. After a period of follow-up, disease (hip fracture) incidence is compared among the exposed (estrogen user) and nonexposed (nonuser) groups. A cohort study thus resembles in some ways a clinical trial without the benefit of randomized treatment assignments.

The major deficiency of observational epidemiologic studies, in comparison with randomized controlled trials, is their susceptibility to bias [4]. While randomization serves to balance the arms of a trial with regard to other variables which might influence the outcome, such biases cannot be as effectively controlled within the framework of a case-control or cohort study. For example, in a large cohort study of estrogen replacement therapy, treated women had many fewer fractures than a control cohort [6]. Treatment was not randomized, however, and the beneficial effect may not have been due to estrogen use per se but to some confounding factor which was independently associated with estrogen use. Thus, women who use estrogen replacement tend to be generally healthier than those who do not, to smoke and consume alcohol less, and to engage in more physical activity [1]. Confounding factors may sometimes be adjusted for at the analysis stage, but such studies always leave open the possibility that the findings might be explained by some unmeasured confounder.

Table 2.

Epidemiologic criteria for assessing the possibility that an association is causal. Modified from [11]

Criteria
Strength
Consistency
Specificity
Temporality
Biological gradient
Plausibility
Coherence
Analogy

2. Assessment of causality

Because it is not always possible to obtain unequivocal results from epidemiologic studies, criteria have been established whereby causality may be inferred from an observed association (Table 2). These considerations include the strength of the association between the putative cause and effect, the consistency and specificity of this association from one study to another, the existence of a temporal sequence between cause and effect, a dose-response relationship, the presence of a plausible biological mechanism, and coherence with the generally understood natural history of the disorder; in some instances, it may also be possible to draw analogies with other cause and effect relationships that are more completely understood [11]. When epidemiologic data are used to evaluate the effectiveness of treatments, they are often used in conjunction with other types of evidence, such as small, randomized, controlled trials with intermediary endpoints. The whole body of evidence may then be assessed according to the above criteria. Thus, epidemiologic data suggesting that estrogen replacement therapy reduces the risk of hip fracture are supported by trials demonstrating that estrogens prevent bone loss in the short term, and that they reduce the incidence of age-related fractures at other sites. If used appropriately, the results of such studies may be sufficiently convincing that the widespread use of certain interventions in the general population can be supported.

IV. Conclusions

In the case of osteoporosis treatment, the confusion generated by earlier non-randomized studies of various regimens more than justifies the current emphasis on randomized, controlled clinical trials as the method of choice for evaluating the utility of new interventions. It would be wise to avoid these problems in developing therapies for other bone diseases. However, several facets of the design of clinical trials warrant close attention, particularly the selection of study subjects, the choice of the intervention and the method of its allocation, the assessment of outcomes, and the analysis and interpretation of results. With due care, trials may be designed which effectively answer a wide range of clinical questions. Under some circumstances, however, the size, duration, and cost of a randomized controlled trial become prohibitive, and alternative methods of evaluating treatments are necessary. Epidemiologic studies may provide a less expensive surrogate in such cases, but interpretation of data from case-control or cohort studies must be done with caution.

Acknowledgements The authors would like to thank Mrs. Mary Roberts for assistance in preparing the manuscript.

This work was supported in part by grant AG 04875 from the National Institutes of Health, United States Public Health Service.

References

1. Barrett-Connor, E., Postmenopausal estrogen and prevention bias. Ann. Intern. Med. 1991; 115: 455–456.
2. Cooper, C., Melton, L.J. III, Epidemiology of osteoporosis. Trends Endocrinol. Metab. 1992; 3: 224–229.
3. Cooper, C., Fogelman, I., Melton, L.J. III, Bisphosphonates and vertebral fracture: an epidemiological perspective. Osteoporosis Int. 1991; 2: 1–4.
4. Cummings, S.R., Epidemiologic studies of osteoporotic fractures: methodologic issues. Calcif. Tissue Int. 1991; 49 (Suppl): S15–S20.
5. Dawson-Hughes, B., Dallal, G.E., Krall, E.A., Sadowski, L., Sahyoun, N., Tannenbaum, S., A controlled trial of the effect of calcium supplementation on bone density in postmenopausal women. N. Engl. J. Med. 1990; 323: 878–883.
6. Ettinger, B., Genant, H.K., Cann, C.E., Long-term estrogen replacement therapy prevents bone loss and fractures. Ann. Intern. Med. 1985; 102: 319–324.
7. Friedman, L.M., Furberg, C.D., DeMets, D.L., Fundamentals of clinical trials, 2nd edn. PSG Publishing Company, Littleton, 1985.
8. Goldman, L., Tosteson, A.N.A., Uncertainty about postmenopausal estrogen. Time for action, not debate. N. Engl. J. Med. 1991; 325: 800–802.
9. Heilbrun, L.K., Ross, P.D., Wasnich, R.D., Yano, K., Vogel, J.M., Characteristics of respondents and nonrespondents in a prospective study of osteoporosis. J. Clin. Epidemiol. 1991; 44: 233–239.
10. Heaney, R.P., Perspectives: Lost sampling units and investigational power. J. Bone Miner. Res. 1992; 7: 1119–1121.
11. Hill, A.B., The environment and disease: Association and causation? Proc. R. Soc. Med. 1965; 58: 295–300.
12. Hui, S.L., Slemenda, C.W., Johnston, C.C. Jr., The contribution of bone loss to postmenopausal osteoporosis. Osteoporosis Int. 1990; 1: 30–34.
13. Kanis, J.A., Treatment of osteoporotic fracture. Lancet 1984; 1: 27–33.
14. Kanis, J.A., Caulin, F., Russell, R.G.G., Problems in the design of clinical trials in osteoporosis. In: Dixon, A.St.J. et al. (Editors), Osteoporosis: a multidisciplinary problem. Royal Society of Medicine, London, 1983, pp. 205-221.
15. Kanis, J.A., Geusens, P., Christiansen, C. on behalf of the Working Party of the Foundation, Guidelines for clinical trials in osteoporosis. Osteoporosis Int. 1991; 1: 182–188.
16. Melton, L.J. III, Chrischilles, E.A., Cooper, C., Lane, A.W., Riggs, B.L., How many have osteoporosis? J. Bone Miner. Res. 1992; 7: 1005–1010.
17. Overgaard, K., Hansen, M.A., Jensen, S.B., Christiansen, C., Effect of salcatonin given intranasally on bone mass and fracture rates in established osteoporosis: a dose-response study. BMJ 1992; 305: 556–561.
18. Riggs, B.L., Melton, L.J. III, Involutional osteoporosis. N. Engl. J. Med. 1986; 314: 1676–1686.
19. Riggs, B.L., Hodgson, S.F., O'Fallon, W.M. et al., Effect of fluoride treatment on the fracture rate in postmenopausal women with osteoporosis. N. Engl. J. Med. 1990; 322: 802–809.

20. Seeley, D.G., Browner, W.S., Nevitt, M.C., Genant, H.K., Scott, J.C., Cummings, S.R. for the Study of Osteoporotic Fractures Research Group, Which fractures are associated with low appendicular bone mass in elderly women? Ann. Intern. Med. 1991; 115: 837–842.
21. Smith, E.L., Gilligan, C., Physical activity effects on bone metabolism. Calcif. Tissue Int. 1991; 49 (Suppl): S50–S54.
22. Tilley, B.C., Peterson, E.L., Kleerekoper, M., Phillips, E., Nelson, D.A., Schorck, M.A., Designing clinical trials of treatment for osteoporosis: recruitment and follow-up. Calcif. Tissue Int. 1990; 47: 327–331.
23. Watts, N.B., Harris, S.T., Genant, H.K. et al., Intermittent cyclical etidronate treatment of post-menopausal osteoporosis. N. Engl. J. Med. 1990; 323: 73–79.

Bisphosphonate on bones
O. Bijvoet, H.A. Fleisch, R.E. Canfield and G. Russell (eds.)
© 1995 Elsevier Science B.V. All rights reserved.

CHAPTER 6

The bone scan in diagnosis and treatment

P.J. Ryan and I. Fogelman

Department of Nuclear Medicine, Guy's Hospital, London SE1 9RT, UK

I. Introduction

The radionuclide bone scan is the most widely undertaken procedure in nuclear medicine departments. It is uniquely suited to the investigation of skeletal pathology because of its great sensitivity for lesion detection and its ability to evaluate the whole skeleton rapidly. Moreover, sites which are difficult to assess by routine radiology, such as the ribs, sternum and scapula, are easily seen with scintigraphy. The modern bone scan is almost always performed with technetium-99m-labelled bisphosphonates which have in common a central P-C-P bond and have faster blood clearance and greater bone deposition when compared to other phosphate compounds. The most widely used preparations are ^{99m}Tc methylene bisphosphonate (MDP) and hydroxymethylene bisphosphonate (HMDP).

II. Pathophysiology of bisphosphonate uptake

The bone scan provides a functional measure of metabolic activity and enables study of its relative distribution throughout the skeleton. The mechanism of uptake of bone-seeking radiopharmaceuticals is incompletely understood, but it is thought to occur by chemiadsorption of the phosphonate group onto the calcium of hydroxyapatite in bone [1]. The major factors determining the level of uptake are osteoblastic activity and skeletal vascularity with preferential uptake at sites of active bone formation. The bone scan therefore reflects any metabolic reaction to a disease process, and this ability to detect functional change, which occurs earlier than structural change, is the reason why the bone scan is more sensitive than conventional radiology. For example, for a destructive lesion to be detected in trabecular bone by radiography, it must be greater than 1–1.5 cm in diameter with loss of approximately 50% of the bone mineral content [2]. This greater sensitivity of bone scintigraphy over conventional radiology has led to the replacement of whole-body radiographic skeletal surveys in the assessment of cancer by whole-body bone scanning with spot radiograph views when structural detail is required.

III. Interpretation of the bone scan

Active foci on bone scan are not disease-specific, with nearly all bone pathology producing alterations in osteoblastic activity and flow. Where isolated focal lesions occur, apart from the demonstration of a site of abnormal bone, diagnosis is limited, and correlation with other investigations is required. However, knowledge of the distribution of lesions and pattern of activity associated with disease processes in many cases enables a correct interpretation of the findings, e.g. multiple and randomly distributed areas of increased tracer uptake associated with bone secondaries (Fig. 1), focal rib lesions in a linear pattern seen in rib fractures, and increased tracer uptake throughout an affected bone in Paget's disease. A further advantage of bone scanning is the ability to derive quantitative data most often used in research and in the evaluation of new treatments.

IV. Normal bone scan

Bone scanning is usually performed with a large field-of-view gamma-camera to obtain multiple static views of the skeleton. In some departments a moving gamma-camera is used to produce a single image of the whole skeleton, which is faster to acquire but has lower resolution than the static mode because the camera cannot be kept as close to the body of the patient. Since high resolution is important in most bone imaging studies, static views are generally preferred.

^{99m}Tc-phosphate radiopharmaceuticals are injected intravenously, and most of the skeletal trapping occurs within the first 10 min. The amount remaining in the blood is initially high, so images are delayed until 2–4 h after injection to achieve the best signal-to-noise ratio. In a normal scan the uptake of tracer is both symmetrical and uniform, with the right and left sides of the skeleton being virtual mirror images

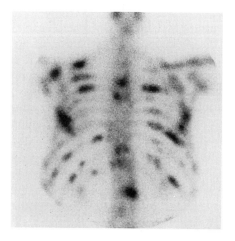

Fig. 1. Multiple bony metastases in carcinoma of the prostate.

of each other. The count rate is higher in the most metabolically active parts of the skeleton, e.g. trabecular bone and epiphyses of growing bones. Excretion of bisphosphonate not taken up by bone is via the kidneys, and in a normal scan both kidneys and bladder are visualised.

In certain conditions it is helpful to obtain information regarding the vascularity of a lesion. An initial dynamic flow study may be performed with rapid sequence images every 2–3 s for 30 s. This can then be followed by a blood pool image at 5 min when much of the radiopharmaceutical is still in the vascular compartment. Blood flow and pool images can help to distinguish soft-tissue disease such as cellulitis (increased vascularity but not bone uptake on later images) from osteomyelitis [3].

1. Normal variants

It is important when interpreting the bone scan to be familiar with the appearances of normal variants and the effects of artifacts. The most common cause of asymmetric activity is malpositioning or rotation of the patient. Physiological curvatures will produce an uneven pattern of uptake, and there may be reduced activity and poor resolution over the anterior ribs due to breast attenuation. Barium from gastrointestinal studies, metallic objects on the patient, prosthetic joints, metallic fixation devices and internal pacemakers will all produce cold areas on the scan. Some increased uptake is commonly seen at the anterior ends and posterior angles of the ribs [4]. Increased uptake is also seen at the sites of epiphyses, which is usually not confusing. However, uptake at the site of the ischiopubic synchondrosis (a fixed joint between the distal end of the inferior pubic ramus and the distal end of the inferior ischial ramus) around the time of fusion (age 4–12 years) is more easily mistaken for an abnormality [5]. There are many 'normal' variants associated with abnormalities in renal position, asymmetry of the bladder and spillages of urine which can cause confusion. Improper preparation of the radiopharmaceutical may lead to free pertechnetate, which will be imaged in the stomach and thyroid, or rarely colloid formation producing activity in the liver, spleen and bone marrow. Bone-scanning agents may also be taken up into diseased soft tissue, and this is thought to relate to the presence of micro-calcification, e.g. areas of acute cerebral infarction, acute myocardial infarction, amyloid deposits, myositis ossificans and a variety of benign and malignant tumours.

2. Drug interactions

Interfering medications are not usually a concern with bone scans. However, there have been recent case reports demonstrating reduced uptake on bone scan following intravenous etidronate [6–8]. False-negative reports have also been demonstrated in patients on long-term oral etidronate for Paget's disease [6]. The probable explanation for this is a direct competition for the skeletal binding sites between the scanning agent and editronate. In practice, the effect of etidronate on the bone scan is seldom of clinical significance, and it must be extremely rare to have any effect from oral therapy. However, nuclear medicine physicians need to be aware of this potential pitfall, particularly when the bone scan is obtained following parenteral bisphosphonate treatment.

V. Single Photon Emission Computed Tomography (SPECT)

SPECT is a valuable addition to bone scintigraphy, offering improved image contrast by reduction in signal-to-noise ratio and improved spatial information. The camera rotates around the body with images generated in multiple planes, and back projection then enables activity from in front and behind the plane of interest to be removed. This technique has led to improved sensitivity for lesion detection, improved localisation and the possibility of display of information in multiple tomographic planes [9]. Various applications have been found for SPECT in bone imaging. Avascular necrosis of the femoral head can be detected with improved sensitivity because the central photon-deficient area can be more clearly identified rather than obscured by surrounding hyperaemia and osteoblastic reaction [10]. Meniscal tears of the knee can be detected with high sensitivity and specificity [11, 12] (Fig. 2), and in the spine separation of activity from the posterior elements and vertebral body has enabled several applications. These include the identification of facetal joint disease [13] (Fig. 3) or spondylolysis as the cause of back pain [14] and the painful pseudoarthrosis [15]. Activity from facetal joints has been shown to occur in about 30% of patients with chronic low-back pain, and it has been suggested that bone SPECT may allow selection of suitable facetal joints for injection with cortisone [16]. Other uses of bone SPECT include the evaluation of malignant otitis externa [17], lesions at the base of the skull [18], temporomandibular joint dysfunction [19] and mandibular condyle disorders [20].

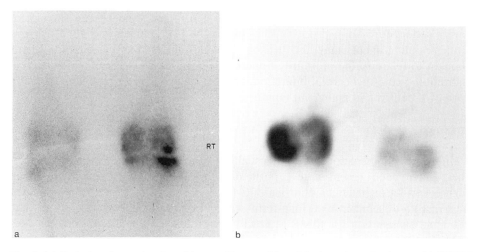

Fig. 2. (a) Posterior planar view in a 24-year-old man with a right lateral meniscal tear. (b) SPECT views of same patient showing a lateral crescent of increased activity on transaxial image.

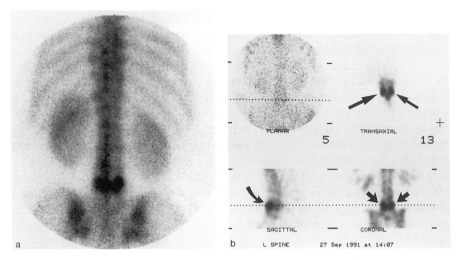

Fig. 3. (a) Posterior planar view in patient with chronic low-back pain showing increased activity at L4/5. (b) SPECT of same patient shows activity localised to the facetal joints.

VI. The bone scan in malignancy

The detection of metastatic disease of the skeleton is the most important indication for performing a bone scan. The most common malignancies metastasising to bone are those of breast and prostate, though bony metastases are also frequently found from tumours of the lung, kidney and thyroid. Metastases are usually seen as multiple, irregularly distributed foci of increased uptake not corresponding to any particular anatomical structure [21]. Generally, they are found in the axial skeleton, but any bone may be affected. The detection of metastases is of importance in the staging of malignancies where the appropriate therapy and prognosis are dependent on this. This particularly applies to tumours of the breast and prostate that have a propensity for early and asymptomatic metastases to bone. In other patients the bone scan can help identify the cause of bone pain or impending fracture sites and may also help in the planning of radiotherapy or identifying suitable sites for bone biopsy. In some cases the presence of a malignancy is only first realised with the detection of a metastasis on bone scan.

1. Bone scan patterns in malignancy

A solitary lesion is a not uncommon scan finding and in general should be further investigated by radiography and on occasion CT scan and bone biopsy. However, sometimes a solitary lesion may remain undiagnosed, and a repeat bone scan 3–6 months later may help clarify the presence or absence of metastases. It should be noted that a solitary rib lesion has only a 10% likelihood of being metastatic [22].

If a metastasis does not produce an osteoblastic response, then the bone scan may be normal. This is uncommon and is best documented in myeloma, although even in this condition the bone scan is usually abnormal (but often less so than with radiographs) [23]. More rarely, a metastasis may be recognised as an area of reduced uptake (cold spot or photopenic lesion). This implies a rapidly growing lytic lesion and occurs most often in myeloma or metastases from a renal carcinoma.

With extensive metastases lesions may coalesce, and diffuse disease can in the extreme case appear normal. The abnormalities on the scan may then be limited to general increased skeletal activity with heightened contrast between bone and soft tissue and with the kidneys often not visualised. This is called a 'superscan' and implies higher than normal extraction of bisphosphonate into bone. This may occur in some benign conditions, e.g. hyperparathyroidism and renal osteodystrophy, but also in malignancy particularly carcinoma of the prostate. If care is not taken, it may be missed, particularly in the early stages. Compared with the 'superscan' of metabolic bone disease, in malignancy the peripheral skeleton is not well seen, and there is often some non-homogeneity of tracer uptake, particularly in the ribs.

On occasion, a characteristic pattern may be seen on the bone scan when diffuse bone marrow involvement by tumour is present. The tracer uptake is increased at the ends of the long bones, often with a typical globular appearance in the humeral and femoral heads and pronounced uptake around the knees.

2. Disease monitoring

The bone scan can be used to monitor the progression of disease and the response to therapy. Radiological changes are slow in response to therapy and may not be detected with sclerotic metastases. Reproducibility of scan technique and in particular image intensity is extremely important. A reduction or increase in the number of lesions indicates successful therapy or worsening disease, respectively. However, interpretation of a change in lesion intensity is more difficult. In general, an increase of activity implies worsening of disease, but healing can also produce an initial increase in activity due to an intense osteoblastic response within the first few months of successful therapy — the flare phenomenon [24]. A decrease in tracer uptake generally implies improvement of disease but can rarely be a feature of a rapidly progressive and aggressive condition [25].

Assessment of the risk of pathological fracture is difficult to obtain from a bone scan, but the presence of long bone involvement, particularly if heavy, should be noted and radiographs obtained. Even if the patient has a poor prognosis, it may still be worthwhile to insert a prophylactic prosthesis to prevent the patient from being confined to bed by a pathological fracture.

3. Breast cancer

Breast cancer is the most frequent cause of bone metastases, and there is extensive literature regarding the use of bone scanning in management. Most recent studies show a low detection rate in clinical stage 1 and 2 disease [26], and the routine use of bone scanning in these stages is not generally appropriate except in research studies. Nevertheless, it is still considered to be useful by some as a baseline, and when positive for metastatic disease will influence management [27, 28]. In larger tumours (greater than 2 cm) and more advanced disease at presentation the pick-up of metastases on bone scan is higher and is more likely to influence management and prognosis [29, 30]. There is little doubt that an abnormal bone scan carries a poor prognosis [31] and the Guy's Hospital experience of a positive bone scan is a median survival of 24 months [32]. The routine value of serial scanning is also controversial but may be useful for the assessment of adjuvant chemotherapy and treatment of early metastatic disease.

4. Prostatic cancer

In prostatic cancer the skeleton is the most common site of metastases. The incidence at presentation is around 30–50% [33–35]. With more advanced clinical staging the frequency of metastases as expected rises [34]. The bone scan is of prognostic value, with an abnormal scan at presentation carrying a 45% mortality at 2 years compared with 20% for a normal scan [35]. Further refinement to prognosis can be made by counting lesions on the initial bone scan [36]. However, it has been observed that the recently identified prostatic-specific antigen (PSA), although not suitable as a screening test for prostatic cancer, is highly predictive for negative bone scans in pre-operative patients if levels are low, and in these patients a staging scan may become unnecessary [37]. The role of serial scans for patient follow-up is less clear, but it has been demonstrated that those with initially negative studies will become positive in 10% at 1 year and 20% at 2 years. Moreover, the scintigraphic changes precede a rise in acid phosphatase in 81% of those in whom the initial bone scan and acid phosphatase value are normal [38]. Other studies have suggested that serial scans have not altered management, and patients mostly presented with bone pain at the time the scan became positive or shortly thereafter [39, 40]. Furthermore, recent studies have shown serial scans provide little extra information over PSA [41].

5. Lung cancer

The skeleton is a common site of metastases in carcinoma of the lung, and at presentation the rate of positive scans is as high as 30–50% [42–44]. Many of these patients have symptoms or evidence of disease at other sites. The incidence of positive scans in asymptomatic patients has been found to be from 8–19% [45, 46]. A bone scan should be obtained in patients with clinical or biochemical evidence of metastases and also in those with potentially resectable tumours because of the poor prognosis associated with surgery once metastases are present. The bone scan can be used to identify the presence of hypertrophic pulmonary osteoarthropathy (HPOA), with the typical appearance being increased activity along the cortical margin of long bones producing a double stripe or tramline appearance [47]. In patients who are symptomatic, imaging of the distal limbs to demonstrate HPOA is useful to confirm the diagnosis, but in asymptomatic patients with lung cancer the low detection rate of HPOA when imaging the distal limbs suggests that it should not be routinely performed.

6. Other cancers

In renal carcinoma, although bone is one of the more common sites of metastases, most studies do not suggest that routine bone scanning is appropriate as the presence of metastases can be suspected clinically or biochemically or from routine radiographs [48]. The bone scan is, however, useful to confirm that metastases are present if suspected and establish their extent. In patients with bladder cancer, there appears to be no role for the bone scan in pre-operative staging, the incidence of metastases at this stage being around 2% [49, 50]. Routine scanning in cervical cancer is probably only required in those with poorly differentiated tumours or locally advanced tumours [51], and in other gynaecological cancers the bone scan should probably be reserved for symptomatic patients. The bone scan is also probably not required for the initial evaluation of testicular cancers but may be of value in stage 4 seminoma and for prognostic information in patients with recurrence after radical treatment for seminoma [52]. Bone scanning is not justified in the management of stage 1 and 2 malignant melanoma but can be useful in more advanced disease. Muss et al. [53] found true-positive results in 14 of 49 patients with advanced melanoma. Thyroid carcinoma may metastasise to bone and if the metastases are functional may be detected by iodine-131 whole body scanning. However, resolution is often poor, and a bone scan is usually required to confirm that metastasis is in bone. In the routine follow-up of asymptomatic patients with treated thyroid cancer, the bone scan is of little value [54], but it is useful in patients complaining of bone pain or who have known metastases elsewhere. In medullary carcinoma of the thyroid, bone scanning may be of value in locating skeletal metastases when there is an elevated serum calcitonin level [55]. In alimentary tumours and those of the head and neck, bone scanning should only be performed when there is clinical evidence of metastases [56, 57].

VII. Primary bone tumours

Bone scanning can be used for both the evaluation of malignant and benign bone tumours. Metastases are rare at presentation in osteogenic sarcoma but more common in Ewing's sarcoma where there is a clear case for bone scanning as part of the initial work-up [58]. Of benign bone lesions, the bone scan is particularly useful in the diagnosis of osteoid osteoma. This tumour accounts for about 10% of benign bone neoplasia and is found generally in adolescents and adults under 30 years of age [59], with the tibia and femur being the most commonly affected sites. The typical bone scan features are of a small intense focus of increased tracer uptake, and a normal scan virtually excludes the diagnosis. Although radiography is usually abnormal with a radiolucent central nidus surrounded by reactive sclerosis, on occasion it may be negative [60]. A variety of benign bone lesions may be active on bone scan including osteoblastomas, chondroblastomas, giant cell tumours and aneurysmal bone cysts. The main indications for scintigraphic imaging of benign bone lesions is to locate an occult cause of pain, to determine the presence of multiple lesions and to evaluate the extent of alteration of skeletal metabolic activity [61]. Other indications can include the pre- and interoperative localisation of certain bone tumours, follow-up for recurrence after treatment, detection of an occult fracture through a benign lesion, locating sites for biopsy and following change in lesion activity.

VIII. Metabolic bone disease

Unlike metastatic bone disease, the bone scan in metabolic bone disease typically involves the whole skeleton. Generalised increased tracer uptake is seen in metabolic disorders where there is high bone turnover and often elevated levels of serum parathyroid hormone. The study will show heightened contrast between the bone and soft tissues, giving an appearance of excellent quality to the extent that it may appear almost too good to be true. The above features are all nevertheless non-specific and, with the exception of absent kidney images, can all be seen in normal subjects, particularly adolescents, in whom the growing skeleton is metabolically active. When mild, diffuse increased tracer uptake may be difficult to detect [62]. However, in more severe cases characteristic patterns of abnormality may be seen [63]. These 'metabolic features' include:
1. increased tracer uptake in the long bones,
2. increased uptake in the axial skeleton,
3. increased uptake in periarticular areas,
4. faint or absent kidney images,
5. prominent calvaria and mandible,
6. 'beading' of the costochondral junctions,
7. 'tie' sternum.
Of various metabolic bone disorders that may cause the above appearances, it is in severe renal osteodystrophy that the most striking bone scan appearances are found. Absence of bladder activity may help to differentiate the bone scan in renal osteodystrophy from other metabolic disorders. The bone scan also provides a sensitive means of detecting sites of ectopic calcification [64]. In addition to renal osteodystrophy the bone scan in renal failure can be used to detect avascular necrosis in patients on steroids and osteomyelitis in the immunosuppressed [65].

1. Primary hyperparathyroidism and osteomalacia

In primary hyperparathyroidism there is a wide range of scan appearances, from normal to those mimicking severe renal osteodystrophy [66]. In mild forms of disease with modest elevation in serum calcium and marginal elevation in serum parathyroid hormone, the bone scan is often normal. The presence of focal abnormalities is unusual in primary hyperparathyroidism, but brown tumours, chondrocalcinosis, vertebral collapse and ectopic calcification may all be detected [67, 68].

Bone scanning in osteomalacia will usually show the classical features of metabolic bone disease, although in the early stages it will be normal [69]. The reason for the increased uptake in osteomalacia, a condition in which there is a mineralisation defect, is uncertain. Suggested explanations are that there may be so much osteoid present that, even though mineralisation is occurring slower than normally at any given site, the total area of mineralisation is increased [70]. Alternatively, there may be increased diffusion of tracer in an extremely large 'osteoid' pool. However, it is most likely to be an effect of secondary hyperparathyroidism as the clinical impression is that the bone scan appearances in osteomalacia reflect the degree of hyperparathyroidism present. Focal abnormalities due to pseudofractures may also be present, and the bone scan provides a sensitive means of their detection, particularly in the ribs where they may be missed on conventional radiology [71]. By contrast, the condition of aluminium-induced osteomalacia produces very poor bone scan images, with high background activity due to failure of tracer uptake by bone [72]. In this condition aluminium is deposited at the calcification front and blocks mineralisation.

2. Paget's disease

Paget's disease is characterised by an initial phase of increased bone resorption followed by an intense osteoblastic response leading to the formation of woven bone [73]. Overall, there is an imbalance in bone remodelling in favour of bone formation, which leads to an increase in the size of bones. Paget's disease is usually polyostotic though 20% of cases are monostotic [74]. The typical appearance is of markedly increased tracer uptake, which is usually distributed evenly throughout the affected bone. An exception to this is osteoporosis circumscripta, where tracer uptake is most intense at the margins of the lesion [75]. The bone scan in Paget's disease shows preservation or even enhancement of the normal anatomical configuration of bone and clear delineation between normal and abnormal bone. In the appendicular skeleton there is generally a progression from the articular end of the bone into the shaft. The distal end of the lesion may have a sharp edge corresponding to the flame-shaped resorption front seen on radiographs. The bone scan is clearly more sensitive for detecting Paget's disease than radiology [76] and enables visualisation of the whole skeleton [77]. There is usually no confusion between metastases and Paget's disease on bone scan, but if the disease is monostotic, the bone scan appearances atypical; or if any doubt about the cause of a bone lesion exists, radiographs of the abnormal areas should be obtained. Single lesions of the spine may sometimes be difficult to diagnose, and a CT scan or bone biopsy is occasionally needed. The bone scan may identify early fracture through pagetic bone when there is focal increased uptake on a background of increased uptake, although identification of a focal increase may not always be possible. Expansion of a lesion on bone scan outside normal anatomical borders or the presence of photopenic areas within a lesion should alert the physician to the presence of sarcomatous change. However, if

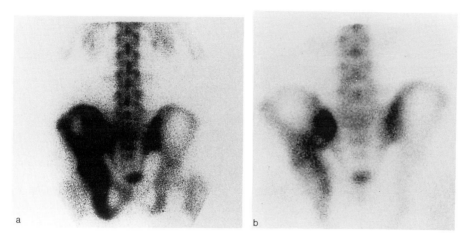

Fig. 4. (a) Posterior pelvis view showing Paget's disease affecting left hemipelvis (before treatment). (b) Same view after Pamidronate therapy.

fracture or sarcomatous change is suspected, radiography and perhaps CT scan with biopsy in the case of sarcoma is necessary.

Scan appearances can improve dramatically after treatment, especially with the newer bisphosphonates [78] (Fig. 4). However, not all lesions respond equally well, and scan appearances may change from generalised uptake to a more focal appearance following therapy. This may be mistaken for metastases if the history of therapy is not known, particularly where there is reactivation of disease. Metabolic activity may persist on bone scan following therapy despite normalisation of the biochemistry values, which implies that the bone scan may be the more sensitive parameter to monitor metabolic activity in lesions. Experience at Guy's Hospital using Pamidronate suggests that the activity on bone scan both before and after therapy can predict the requirement for further therapy [78], though biochemical measures are probably as effective and will be more widely used. The response of biochemical measures to a course of intravenous Pamidronate is difficult to predict from knowledge of pretreatment values [79]. However, recent work has suggested that the bisphosphonate space, a comparison of plasma levels of intravenously injected ^{99m}Tc-HMDP and ^{51}Cr-EDTA (reflecting bisphosphonate uptake into bone) may be a good predictor of the dosage of Pamidronate required to achieve biochemical remission [80].

3. Osteoporosis

The bone scan has little value in the diagnosis of osteoporosis [81]. Scan appearances are often normal, and even when abnormal features are present they are non-specific. These include images of poor quality with a 'washed-out' appearance due to low tracer uptake by the skeleton, loss of spinal height, close proximity of the ribs to each other and of the rib cage to the pelvis [82]. However,

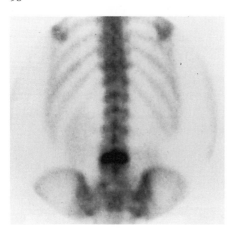

Fig. 5. Linear increased tracer uptake at L4 associated with vertebral collapse.

the bone scan is useful in the patient presenting with back pain who has vertebral collapse on radiographs. The appearance of recent vertebral collapse is intense linear uptake of tracer corresponding to the site or sites of fracture (Fig. 5). This, however, fades over a period of 6 months to 2 years, and therefore the bone scan can help identify whether a vertebral collapse is recent [81]. A normal scan excludes recent fracture, and other causes of back pain should be considered. In osteoporotic patients with multiple collapse on radiographs who subsequently develop further back pain, assessment is difficult without a bone scan. In patients presenting with osteoporosis, one can be concerned about the possibility of co-existent bone disease such as hyperparathyroidism, Paget's disease, metastases or osteomyelitis, and in this context the bone scan is very helpful in evaluating the skeleton. Initial radiographs of fractured bones are sometimes negative, and the bone scan can be used for their detection when radiographs are normal or equivocal. There is much current discussion among researchers into osteoporosis as to what degree of vertebral deformity constitutes a vertebral fracture, and it has been observed that not all new vertebral deformities are accompanied by bone scan changes [83]. This suggests that many deformities seen on radiographs in osteoporotic patients do not arise as a result of fracture. It has been recently proposed that the development of a bone scan abnormality may constitute a better definition of fracture rather than development of vertebral deformity, which may be due to other causes [84]. A clear separation of vertebral fractures and vertebral deformities is important to determine their respective aetiology and significance.

IX. Infection

In osteomyelitis the bone scan has an important role in early diagnosis as it becomes abnormal several days to weeks before conventional radiology shows

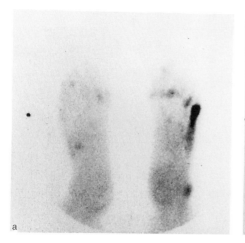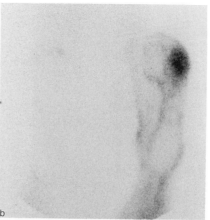

Fig. 6. (a) Increased blood pool in patient with osteomyelitis of head of 5th metatarsal. (b) Increased activity 3 hours after injection of ^{99m}Tc-MDP, at same site in same patient.

changes [85]. The characteristic bone scan pattern is of a focal area of increased uptake in bone. A 3-phase bone scan is now recognised as being superior to static views alone for diagnosis and can also help in distinguishing osteomyelitis from cellulitis. Both will show increased blood flow, but uptake is not present in cellulitis on delayed static imaging [86] (Fig. 6). Sensitivities and specificities for 3-phase bone scanning in acute osteomyelitis range from 83–100% and 73–75%, respectively [87]. A gallium-67 scan or indium-111-labelled white cell scan can be helpful to confirm that the increased activity on bone scan is due to infection. The differentiation from bone infarction is sometimes difficult, especially in sickle cell disease or diabetes mellitus, and negative gallium or white cell scans will exclude infection [88, 89]. The detection of an acute exacerbation of chronic osteomyelitis is less easy with bone scintigraphy, there being a high false-positive rate due to increased bone mass and increased bone turnover from the chronic changes [90]. However, a negative study excludes active infection, and greater activity on gallium scanning than bone scanning yields a high probability of active disease [91].

X. Joint protheses

Patients who undergo arthroplasty are subject to various complications, the most important being infection and loosening. Clinically, these can be difficult to diagnose, though the ESR, radiographic findings and results of joint aspiration can be helpful. However, bone scintigraphy can be of value in both situations, although in the first year after insertion increased uptake of ^{99m}Tc-bisphosphonates may still be seen, and this may persist for up to 2 years in the acetabular component of a total hip replacement [92, 93]. It has been noted that focal increased uptake around the tip

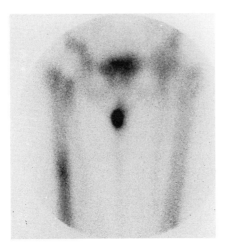

Fig. 7. Focal uptake at tip of right hip prosthesis associated with loosening.

or neck of a femoral prosthesis is more likely to reflect loosening, and diffuse uptake infection [94] (Fig. 7), although not all investigators have been able to separate infection from loosening [95]. However, it has been shown that infected but not loose implants have increased flow on 3-phase imaging [96]. Furthermore, both [67]Ga- and ^{111}In-labelled white cell scans can be used to confirm infection [97, 98].

XI. Arthritis

There is some increase in tracer uptake adjacent to normal joints, which is usually symmetrical. For joints to be recognised as abnormal on bone scan, either increased activity compared with other joints or compared with adjacent non-articular bone is required. Increased joint activity is found in a wide number of arthritic conditions, and the pattern of uptake reflects the typical pattern of joint involvement. Bone scan changes can antedate clinical and radiographic manifestations in inflammatory arthritis [99, 100], and the bone scan can have a role in early diagnosis. Recent work has shown that scintigraphic joint activity in rheumatoid arthritis antedates joint erosions [101]. Furthermore, the level of activity in early disease has predictive value for the development of erosions, with joints inactive on repeated scanning never eroding [102]. Since the development of erosions is an important criterion of progressive arthritis and an indication for second-line anti-rheumatic drugs, the bone scan may assist in planning this form of therapy. However, as a means of monitoring response to therapy in arthritides, the bone scan has not been found to confer advantages over clinical, laboratory and radiological techniques. Studies have also been performed with ^{111}In-labelled white cells, showing it to be a good measure of joint activity in rheumatoid arthritis, though again a role in clinical practice has not been demonstrated [103].

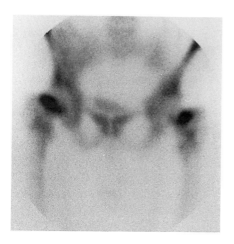

Fig. 8. Bilateral linear increased tracer uptake through the femoral necks of a renal transplant patient due to hip fractures. Patient was thought clinically to have avascular necrosis.

In patients with ankylosing spondylitis, bone scanning can identify radiologically negative sacroiliitis [104]. The sacroiliac joints are more active on bone scan than the pelvis and sacrum in normal subjects, and as sacroiliitis is often bilateral, quantitative techniques have been developed [105]. The sacroiliac joint to sacrum ratio is commonly measured and is high in early disease, falling to normal in more advanced disease. Unfortunately, there are limitations to this test as it may be normal in early disease and elevated in other conditions, e.g. mechanical back pain [106–108]. In the appropriate clinical setting it can nevertheless be an aid to diagnosis, particularly when radiographs are equivocal, and there is strong pretest suspicion [109, 110].

XII. Avascular necrosis

The bone scan is of recognised value in the diagnosis of avascular necrosis and bone infarction. A zone of reduced tracer uptake may be seen in the early stages, followed by increased tracer uptake representing the reaction of the surrounding bone. On occasion, SPECT imaging (see earlier) will reveal a central photon-deficient area in avascular necrosis of the hip even when planar imaging shows diffuse increased uptake [10].

XIII. Trauma

The diagnosis of fracture can usually be made clinically and with radiographs. However, some fractures may not be seen on radiographs for several days following injury, particularly if they are small or incomplete, and the bone scan can be used

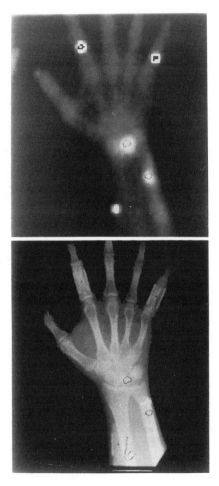

Fig. 9. Wrist registration study in patient with previous fractured ulna and scaphoid. Bone scan shows activity in distal ulna and proximal wrist. Registration enabled activity in proximal wrist to be localised to site of lunate-scaphoid artriculation where osteoarthritic changes were present.

to confirm or exclude significant injury (Fig. 8). It can also be used for locating sites of suspected or unsuspected trauma [111]. In cases of non-accidental injury in childhood, the bone scan can help identify multiple lesions [112]. Fractures of the carpus, navicular and proximal femora may be particularly difficult to see on radiographs, and in these the bone scan is often a valuable tool for diagnosis. In the carpus, digitalisation of the bone scan with the radiograph can be helpful to locate the site of injury precisely by superimposition [113] (Fig. 9). The majority of fractures are detectable by bone scan within hours of injury, with 95% in patients under 65 years old being detectable within 24 h of injury and 95% in those over 65 by 72 h from injury [113]. Various other types of injuries can be usefully investigated by bone scans. These include stress fractures, which may not be detected on radiographs until 1–3 weeks after injury [114], 'shin splints' where typically there is an elongated region of increased tracer uptake on the medial aspect of the posterior portion of the tibia [115], and enthesopathies such as osteitis pubis, plantar fasciitis and Achilles tendonitis, where radionuclide abnormalities may be present without radiological changes [116]. Compartment syndromes can also be usefully imaged, with decreased uptake in the area of increased pressure and increased soft-tissue uptake above and below, and in traumatic rhabdomyolysis there is a large amount of tracer uptake in the damaged muscle within hours of injury [116].

XIV. Quantitative technetium bisphosphonate uptake measurements

Bisphosphonate uptake in the skeleton reflects skeletal metabolic activity, and quantitative techniques can provide a sensitive measure of alteration in skeleton metabolism. The most common, extensively evaluated technique is that of 24-h whole-body retention of technetium-labelled bisphosphonate (WBR) [117]. While 20–40% of the injected bisphosphonate is taken up by the skeleton, the remainder is excreted by the urinary tract, and by 24 h most of the soft-tissue activity has been excreted, with the great majority of bisphosphonate in the body remaining in the skeleton. By using a whole-body counter the activity at injection and at 24 h can then be compared. The technique is only valid if renal function is normal [118]. While WBR has been found to be of clinical value [117, 118] and while an elevated result reflects increased bone turnover, it is not disease-specific and can be found in hyperparathyroidism, osteomalacia and Paget's disease. An indirect measurement of bone uptake can be performed by comparing the clearance of ^{51}Cr-EDTA with ^{99m}Tc-MDP by measuring the ratio of them both in a 4-h sample [119]. Recent work has suggested that a modification of this technique can be useful to predict normalisation of biochemical parameters in Paget's disease following Pamidronate therapy [68].

References

1. Francis, M.D., Fogelman, I., Tc99m diphosphonate uptake mechanism in bone. In: Fogelman, I. (Editor), Bone scanning in clinical practice. Springer-Verlag, Berlin, 1987, pp. 7–17.
2. Edelstyn, G.A., Gillespie, P.J., Grebell, F.S., The radiological demonstration of osseous metastases: experimental observations. Clin. Radiol. 1967; 18: 158–162.
3. Maurer, A.H., Chen, D.C.P., Camargo, E.E., Wong, D.F., Wagner Jr., H.N., Alderson, P.O., Utility of three-phase skeletal scintigraphy in suspected osteomyelitis: concise communication. J. Nucl. Med. 1981; 22: 941–949.
4. Fink-Bennett, D., Johnston, J., Stippled ribs: A potential pitfall in bone scan interpretation. J. Nucl. Med. 1986; 27: 216.
5. Cawley, K.A., Dvorak, A.D., Wilmot, M.D., Normal anatomic variant: Scintigraphy of the ischiopubic synchondrosis. J. Nucl. Med. 1983; 24: 14.
6. Krasnow, A.Z., Collier, B.D., Isitman, A.T., Helman, R.S., Ewey, D., False negative bone imaging due to Etidronate disodium therapy. Clin. Nucl. Med. 1988; 13: 264–267.
7. Chong, W.K., Cunningham, D.A., Case report: Intravenous Etidronate as a cause of poor uptake on bone scanning, with a review of the literature. Clin. Radiol. 1991; 44: 268–270.

8. Hommeyer, S.H., Varney, D.M., Eary, J.F., Skeletal nonvisualization in a bone scan secondary to intravenous etidronate therapy. J. Nucl. Med. 1992; 33: 748–750.

9. Collier, B.D., Hellman, R.S. Jr., Krasnow, A.Z., Bone SPECT. Semin. Nucl. Med. 1987; 17: 247–266.

10. Collier, B.D., Carrera, G.F., Johnson, R.P. et al., Detection of femoral head avascular necrosis in adults by SPECT. J. Nucl. Med. 1985; 26: 979–987.

11. Murray, I.P.C., Dixon, J., Kohan, L., SPECT for acute knee pain. Clin. Nucl. Med. 1990; 15: 828–840.

12. Ryan, P.J., Taylor, M., Allen, P., Clarke, S.E.M., Fogelman, I., SPECT bone imaging of the knees — a comparison with arthroscopic findings. Nucl. Med. Commun. 1992; 13: 224.

13. Ryan, P.J., Evans, P.A., Gibson, T., Fogelman, I., Chronic low back pain: Comparison with radiography and CT. Radiology 1992; 182: 849–854.

14. Collier, B.D., Johnson, R.P., Carrera, G.F. et al., Painful spondylolysis or spondylolisthesis studied by radiography and single-photon emission computed tomography. Radiology 1985; 154: 207–211.

15. Slizofski, W.J., Collier, B.D., Flatley, T.J., Carrera, G.F., Hellman, R.S., Isitman, A.T., Painful pseudoarthroses following lumbar spinal fusion: Detection by combined SPECT and planar bone scintigraphy. Skeletal Radiol. 1987; 16: 136.

16. Ryan, P.J., Gibson, T., Fogelman, I., The identification of spinal pathology in chronic low back pain using bone scintigraphy with SPECT. Nucl. Med. Commun. 1992; 13: 497–502.

17. Strashun, A.M., Nejatheim, M., Goldsmith, S.J., Malignant otitis externa: Early scintigraphic detection. Radiology 1984; 150: 541.

18. Israel, O., Jerushalmi, J., Fremkel, A., Kuten, A., Front, D., Normal and abnormal single photon emission computed tomography of the skull: Comparison with planar scintigraphy. J. Nucl. Med. 1988; 29: 1341.

19. Collier, B.D., Carrera, G.F., Messer, E.J. et al., Internal derangement of the temporomandibular joint: Detection by single photon emission computed tomography. Radiology 1983; 149: 557.

20. Allwright, S.J., Cooper, R.A., Shutter, B., Norman, J., Ede, B., Bone SPECT in hyperplasia of the mandibular condyle. J. Nucl. Med. 1988; 29: 780.

21. Goris, M.L., Bretille, J., Skeletal scintigraphy for the diagnosis of malignant metastatic disease to the bones. Radiother. Oncol. 1985; 3: 319–329.

22. Tumeh, S.S., Beadle, G., Kaplan, W.D., Clinical significance of solitary rib lesions in patients with extraskeletal malignancy. J. Nucl. Med. 1985; 26: 1140.

23. Wahner, H.W., Kyle, R.A., Beabout, J.W., Scintigraphic evaluation of the skeleton in multiple myeloma. Mayo Clin. Proc. 1980; 55: 739–746.

24. Rossleigh, M.A., Lovegrove, F.T.A., Reynolds, P.M. et al., The assessment of response to therapy of bone metastases in breast cancer. Aust. NZ J. Med. 1984; 14: 19–22.

25. Hayward, J.L., Carbone, P.P., Heuson, J.C., Kumoaka, S., Sgaloff, A., Rubens, R.D., Assessment of response to therapy in advanced breast cancer. Eur. J. Cancer 1977; 13: 89–94.

26. Coleman, R.E., Rubens, R.D., Fogelman, I., A reappraisal of the baseline bone scan in breast cancer. J. Nucl. Med. 1988; 29: 1045–1049.

27. McNeil, B.J., Pace, P.D., Gray, E.B., Adelstein, S.J., Wilson, R.E., Preoperative and follow-up bone scans in patients with primary carcinoma of the breast. Surg. Gynaecol. Obstet. 1978; 147: 745–748.

28. Wickerham, L., Fisher, B., Cronon, W., Members of the NSABP Committee for treatment failure. The efficacy of bone scanning in the follow-up of patients with operable breast cancer. Breast Cancer Res. Treat. 1984; 4: 303–307.

29. Lindholm, A., Lundell, L., Martenson, B., Thulin, A., Skeletal scintigraphy in the initial assessment of women with breast cancer. Acta Chir. Scand. 1979; 145: 65–71.

30. Komaki, R., Donegan, W., Manoli, R., Teh, E.L., Prognostic value of pretreatment bone scans in breast carcinoma. AJR 1979; 132: 877–881.

31. McKillop, J.H., Blumgart, L.H., Wood, C.B. et al., The prognostic and therapeutic implications of the positive radionuclide bone scan in clinically early breast cancer. Br. J. Surg. 1978; 65: 649–652.

32. Coleman, R.E., Rubens, R.D., The clinical course of bone metastases from breast cancer. Br. J. Cancer 1987; 55: 61–66.

33. Shafer, R.B., Reinke, D.B., Contribution of the bone scan, serum acid and alkaline phosphatase and radiographic bone survey to the management of newly diagnosed carcinoma of the prostate. Clin. Nucl. Med. 1977; 2: 200–203.

34. O'Donoghue, E.P., Constable, A.R., Sherwood, T. et al., Bone scanning and plasma phosphates in carcinoma of the prostate. Br. J. Urol. 1978; 50: 172–177.

35. Lund, F., Smith, P.H., Suciu, S., Do bone scans predict prognosis in prostatic cancer. Br. J. Urol. 1984; 56: 58–63.
36. Knudson, G., Grinis, G., Lopez-Majeuno, V. et al., Bone scan as a stratification variable in advanced prostate cancer. Cancer 1991; 68: 316–320.
37. Oesterling, J.E., Prostate specific antigen: A critical assessment of the most useful tumour marker for adenocarcinoma of the prostate. J. Urol. 1991; 245: 907–923.
38. Merrick, M.V., Ding, C.L., Chisholm, G.D., Elton, R.D., Prognostic significance of alkaline and acid phosphatase and skeletal scintigraphy in carcinoma of the prostate. Br. J. Urol. 1985; 57: 715–720.
39. Huben, R.P., Schellhammer, P.F., The role of routine follow-up bone scans after definitive therapy of localised prostatic cancer. J. Urol. 1982; 128: 510–512.
40. Corrie, D., Timmons, J.H., Bauman, J.H., Thompson, I.M., Efficacy of follow-up scans in carcinoma of the prostate. Cancer 1988; 61: 195–202.
41. Lighner, D.J., Lange, P.H., Ercole, C.J. et al., Serum prostatic specific antigen (PSA) and the utility of isotopic bone scan (BOS) in the monitoring of patients with carcinoma of prostate (CAD). Proc. Am. Assoc. Clin. Oncol. 1988; 7: 120.
42. Donato, A.T., Ammerman, E.G., Sullesta, O., Bone scanning in the evaluation of the patients with lung cancer. Ann. Thoracic Surg. 1979; 27: 300–304.
43. Kelly, R.J., Cason, R.J., Ferrie, C.B., Efficacy of radionuclide scanning in patients with lung cancer. JAMA 1979; 242: 2855–2857.
44. Merrick, M.V., Merrick, J.M., Bone scintigraphy in lung cancer: a reappraisal. Br. J. Radiol. 1986; 59: 1185–1194.
45. Hooper, R.G., Beechler, C.R., Johnston, M.C., Radioisotope scanning in the initial staging of bronchogenic carcinoma. Am. Rev. Resp. Dis. 1978; 118: 279–286.
46. Kies, M.S., Baker, A.W., Kennedy, P.S., Radionuclude scans in staging of carcinoma of the lung. Surg. Gynaecol. Obstet. 1978; 147: 175–176.
47. Terry, D.W., Isitman, A.I., Holmes, R.A., Radionuclide bone images in hypertrophic pulmonary osteoarthropathy. AJR 1975; 124: 571–576.
48. Blancher, E., Johnston, D.E., Haynie, T.P., Value of routine radionuclide bone scans in renal carcinoma. Urology 1985; 26: 432.
49. Berger, G.L., Sadlowski, R.W., Sharpe, J.R., Finney, R.P., Lack of value of routine preoperative bone and liver scans in cystectomy candidates. J. Urol. 1981; 125: 637–639.
50. Linder, A., Dekernion, J.B., Cost effectiveness of pre cystectomy radiographic scans. J. Urol. 1982; 128: 1181–1182.
51. Basson, J.S., Glasser, M.G., Bony metastases in carcinoma of the uterine cervix. Clin. Radiol. 1982; 33: 623–625.
52. Merrick, M.V., Bone scintigraphy in testicular tumours. Br. J. Urol. 1987; 60: 167–169.
53. Muss, H.B., Richards, F., Barnes, P.L., Willand, V.V., Cowan, R., Radionuclide scanning in patients with advanced malignant melanoma. Clin. Nucl. Med. 1979; 4: 516–518.
54. DeGroot, L.J., Reilly, M., Use of isotope bone scans and skeletal survery x-rays in the follow-up of patients with thyroid carcinoma. J. Endocrinol. Invest. 1984; 7: 175–179.
55. Johnson, D.G., Coleman, R.E., McCook, T.A., Dale, J.K., Wells, S.A., Bone and liver images in medullary carcinoma of the thyroid. J. Nucl. Med. 1984; 25: 419–422.
56. Belson, T.P., Lehman, R.H., Chobanian, D.L., Malin, T.C., Bone and liver scans in patients with head and neck carcinoma. Laryngoscope 1980; 90: 1291–1296.
57. Vider, M., Maruyama, Y., Narvaez, R., Significance of the vertebral venous (Batson's) plexus in metastatic spread in colorectal cancer. Cancer 1977; 40: 67–71.
58. Nair, N., Bone scanning in Ewing's sarcoma. J. Nucl. Med. 1985; 26: 349–352.
59. Lichenstein, L., Bone tumours, 5th edn. Mosby, St Louis, 1977.
60. Swee, R.G., McLeod, R.A., Beabout, J.W., Osteoid osteoma detection, diagnosis and localisation. Radiology 1979; 132: 117–123.
61. Gilday, D.L., Ash, J.M., Benign bone tumours. Semin. Nucl. Med. 1976; 6: 33.
62. Fogelman, I., Citrin, D.L., Bone scanning in metabolic bone disease: a review. Appl. Radiol. 1981; 10: 158–166.
63. Fogelman, I., Citrin, D.L., Turner, J.G., Hay, I.D., Bessant, R.G., Boyle, I.T., Semi-quantitative interpretation of the bone scan in metabolic bone disease. Eur. J. Nucl. Med. 1979; 4: 287–289.
64. DeGraaf, P., Schicht, I.M., Pauwels, E.K., Souverijn, J.H.M., DeGraeff, J., Bone scintigraphy in uraemic pulmonary calcification. J. Nucl. Med. 1979; 20: 201–206.
65. Fogelman, I., Boyle, I.T., Bone scanning in clinical practice. Scott. Med. J. 1980; 25: 45–49.

66. Weigmann, T., Rosenthall, L., Kaye, M., Technetium 99m pyrophosphate bone scans in hyperparathyroidism. J. Nucl. Med. 1977; 18: 213–235.
67. Evens, R.G., Ashburn, W., Bartter, F.C., Strontium-85 scanning of a 'brown tumour' in a patients with parathyroid carcinoma. Br. J. Radiol. 1969; 42: 224–225.
68. Sy, W.M., Mottola, O., Lao, R.S., Smith, A., Freund, H.R., Unusual bone images in hyperparathyroidism. Br. J. Radiol. 1977; 50: 740–744.
69. Fogelman, I., McKillop, J.H., Bessant, R.G., Boyle, I.T., Turner, J.G., Greig, W.R., The role of bone scanning in osteomalacia. J. Nucl. Med. 1978; 19: 245–248.
70. Nordin, B.E.C., Horsman, A., Aaron, J., Diagnostic procedures. In: Nordin, B.E.C. (Editor), Calcium, Phosphate and Magnesium Metabolism. Churchill Livingstone, Edinburgh, 1975, pp. 469–524.
71. Fogelman, I., McKillop, J.H., Greig, W.R., Boyle, I.T., Pseudofracture of the ribs detected by bone scanning. J. Nucl. Med. 1977; 18: 1236–1237.
72. Vanherweghem, J.L., Schoutens, A., Bergmann, P. et al., Usefulness of 99mTc-pyrophosphate bone scintigraphy in aluminium bone disease. Trace Elements Med. 1984; 1: 80–83.
73. Alexandre, C., Meunier, P.J., Edouard, C., Khairi, R.A., Johnston, C.C., Effects of EHDP (5mg/kg/day dose) on quantitative bone histology in Paget's disease of bone. Metab. Bone Dis. Rel. Res. 1981; 23: 309–315.
74. Vellenga, C.J.W.R., Pauwels, E.K.J., Bijvoet, O.L.M., Frilink, W.B., Mulder, J.D., Hermans, J., Untreated Paget's disease of bone studied by scintigraphy. Radiology 1984; 127: 439–443.
75. Rausch, J.M., Resnick, D., Goergen, T.G., Taylor, A., Bone scanning of osteolytic Paget's disease. Case report. J. Nucl. Med. 1977; 18: 699–701.
76. Khairi, M.R.A., Robb, J.A., Wellman, H.N., Johnston, C.C., Radiographs and scans in diagnosing symptomatic lesions of Paget's disease of bone (osteitis deformans). Geriatrics 1974; 29: 49–54.
77. Fogelman, I., Carr, D.L., A comparison of bone scanning and radiology in the assessment of patients with symptomatic Paget's disease. Eur. J. Nucl. Med. 1980; 5: 417–421.
78. Ryan, P.J., Gibson, T., Fogelman, I., Bone scintigraphy following intravenous Pamidronate (APD) for Paget's disease of bone. J. Nucl. Med. 1992; 33: 1589–1593.
79. Ryan, P.J., Sherry, M., Gibson, T., Fogelman, I., Treatment of Paget's disease by weekly infusions of 3 amino-hydroxypropylidene 1-1 bisphosphonate (APD). Br. J. Rheum. 1992; 31: 97–107.
80. Stone, M.D., Marshall, D.H., Hosking, D.J., Perkins, A.C., Evans, A.J., Wastie, M.L., Bisphosphonate space measurement in Paget's disease of bone treated with APD. J. Bone Min. Res. 1992; 7: 295–301.
81. Fogelman, I., Carr, D., A comparison of bone scanning and radiology in the evaluation of patients with metabolic bone disease. Clin. Radiol. 1980; 31: 321–326.
82. Sy, W.M., Osteoporosis. In: Sy, W.M. (Editor), Gamma images in benign and metabolic bone diseases. CRC Press, Boca Raton, 1981, pp. 223–239.
83. Kleerekoper, M., Peterson, E., Nelson, D.A. et al., A randomised trial of sodium flouride as a treatment for postmenopausal osteoporosis. Osteoporosis Int. 1991; 1: 155–161.
84. Kleerekoper, M., Nelson, D.A., Vertebral fracture or vertebral deformity? Calcif. Tissue Int. 1992; 50: 5–6.
85. Handmacher, H., Leonards, R., The bone scan in inflammatory oseous disease. Semin. Nucl. Med. 1976; 6: 95.
86. Mauer, A.H., Chen, D.E.P., Camargo, E.E., Utility of three-phase skeletal scintigraphy in suspected osteomyelitis. Concise communications. J. Nucl. Med. 1981; 22: 941.
87. Alzaraki, N., Dries, D., Datz, F. et al., Value of 24 hour image (four phase bone scan) in assessing osteomyelitis in patients with peripheral vascular disease. J. Nucl. Med. 1985; 26: 711–717.
88. Schauwecker, D.S., Park, H.M., Mock, B.H., Evaluation of complicating osteomyelitis with 99m Tc-MDP, 111In-granulocytes and 67Ga citrate. J. Nucl. Med. 1984; 25: 849.
89. McDougall, I.R., Baumert, J.E., Lantieri, R.L., Evaluation of 111In leukocytes whole body scanning. AJR 1979; 133: 849.
90. Tumeh, S.S., Aliabadi, P., Weissman, B., McNeil, B.J., Radiologic evaluation of chronic osteomyelitis (Abstract). Radiology 1985; 157: 84.
91. Tumeh, S.S., Aliabadi, P., Weissman, B., McNeill, B.J., Chronic osteomyelitis. 99mTc-MDP/67Ga scan patterns associated with active disease. Radiology 1986; 158: 685.
92. Creutzig, H., Bone imaging after total replacement arthroplasty of the hip joint. Eur. J. Nucl. Med. 1976; 1: 177.
93. Browett, J.P., Ostrowski, S., The use of radioscintigraphy in the assessment of the painful total hip replacement. J. Bone Joint Surg. 1980; 62-B: 121.

94. Rushton, N., Wraight, E.P., Tc-99m methylene diphosphonate scanning in Thompson hemiarthroplasties. Br. J. Radiol. 1980; 53: 781.
95. Sauerbaum, B.J.L., Lastra, M.P., Bates, H.R. et al., Bone scanning in prosthetic implants. Proceedings of the 25th annual meeting (Abstract). J. Nucl. Med. 1978; 19: 697.
96. Kroop, S.A., Stone, R.G., Seldin, D.W., Alderson, P.O., Comparison of three-phase bone scintigraphy and Ga-67 imaging in evaluation of painful total hip prostheses (Abstract). J. Nucl. Med. 1983; 24: 84.
97. Rosthenall, L., Lisbona, R., Skeletal imaging. Appleton and Lange, East Norwalk, 1984.
98. Sayle, B.A., Fawcett, H.D., Wilkey, D.J. et al., Indium-111 chloride imaging in the detection of infected prostheses. J. Nucl. Med. 1985; 26: 718.
99. Desaulniers, M., Fuks, A., Hawkins, D., Laciurciere, Y., Rosenthall, L., Radiotechnetium polyphosphate joint imaging. J. Nucl. Med. 1974; 15: 417–423.
100. Rosenthall, L., Lisbona, R., In: Freeman, L.M., Weissman, H.S. (Editors), Nuclear Medicine Annual. Raven Press, New York, 1980.
101. Mottonen, T., Hannonen, P., Rekonen, A., Oka, M., Joint scintigraphy and erosions. Ann. Rheum. Dis. 1986; 45: 966–967.
102. Mottonen, T., Hannonen, P., Toivanen, J., Rekonen, A., Oka, M., Value of joint scintigraphy in the prediction of erosiveness in early rheumatoid arthritis. Ann. Rheum. Dis. 1988; 47: 183–189.
103. Shmerling, R.H., Parker, J.A., Johns, W.D., Trentham, D.E., Measurement of joint inflammation in rheumatoid arthritis with indium-111 chloride. Ann. Rheum. Dis. 1990; 49: 88–92.
104. Lentle, B.C., Russell, A.S., Percy, J.S., Jackman, S.I., The scintigraphic investigation of sacroiliac disease. J. Nucl. Med. 1977; 18: 529–533.
105. Russell, A.S., Lentle, B.C., Percy, J.S., Investigations of sacroiliac disease: comparative evaluation of radiological and radionuclide techniques. J. Rheumatol. 1975; 2: 45–51.
106. Ho, G., Sadownikoff, N., Malhotra, C.M., Claunet, B.C., Quantitative sacroiliac joint scintigraphy. Arthritis Rheum. 1979; 22: 837–844.
107. Lugon, M., Torode, A.S., Travers, R.L., Amaral, A., Lavender, J.P., Hughes, G.R.V., Sacro-iliac joint scanning with technetium-99 diphosphonate. Rheum. Rehab. 1979; 18: 131–136.
108. Chalmers, I.M., Lentle, B.C., Percy, J.S., Russell, A.S., Sacroiliitis detected by bone scintiscanning: a clinical radiological and scintigraphic follow-up study. Ann. Rheum. Dis. 1979; 38: 112–117.
109. Chase, W.F., Houk, R.W., Winn, R.E., Hinzman, G.W., The clinical usefulness of radionuclide scintigraphy in suspected sacro-iliitis; a prospective study. Br. J. Rheum. 1983; 22: 67–72.
110. Diffey, B.L., Pal, B., Gibson, C.J., Clayton, C.B., Griffiths, I.D., Application of Bayes' theorem to the diagnosis of ankylosing spondylitis from radioisotope bone scans. Ann. Rheum. Dis. 1985; 44: 667–670.
111. Matin, P., The appearance of bone scans following fractures, including immediate and long term studies. J. Nucl. Med. 1979; 20: 1227–1231.
112. Haase, G.M., Ovitz, V.N., Sfakianakis, G.N., Morse, T.S., The value of radionuclide bone scanning in the early recognition of deliberate child abuse. J. Trauma 1980; 20: 873–875.
113. Hawkes, D.J., Robinson, L., Crossman, J.E. et al., Registration and display of the combined bone scan and radiograph in the diagnosis and management of wrist injuries. Eur. J. Nucl. Med. 1991; 18: 752–756.
114. Norfray, J.F., Schlachter, L., Kernahan, W.T., Early confirmation of stress fractures in joggers. JAMA 1980; 243: 1647.
115. Brill, D.R., Sports nuclear medicine. Bone imaging of lower extremity pain in athletes. Clin. Nucl. Med. 1983; 8: 101.
116. Matin, P., Basic principles of nuclear medicine techniques for detection and evaluation of trauma and sports medicine injuries. Semin. Nucl. Med. 1988; 18: 90–112.
117. Fogelman, I., Bessent, R.G., Turner, J.G. et al., The use of whole body retention of Tc-99m diphosphonate in the diagnosis of metabolic bone disease. J. Nucl. Med. 1978; 19: 270–275.
118. Fogelman, I., Bessent, R.G., Age related alterations in skeletal metabolism: 24 hour whole body retention of diphosphonate in 250 normal subjects: Concise communication. J. Nucl. Med. 1982; 23: 296–300.
119. Nisbet, A.P., Edwards, S., Lazarus, C.R. et al., Chromium 51 EDTA/technetium 99m plasma ratio to measure total skeletal function. Br. J. Radiol. 1984; 57: 677–680.

PART B

CHEMISTRY AND PHARMACOLOGY OF THE BISPHOSPHONATES

History of the bisphosphonates: Discovery and history of the non-medical uses of bisphosphonates

Leo J.M.J. Blomen

Achtermonde 31, 4156 AD Rumpt, The Netherlands

I. Introduction

Traditionally, bisphosphonates are mainly utilised because of the potential of their molecules and ions to form relatively strong bonds with crystal surfaces, and at the same time their ability to form complexes with positive ions in solutions ('cations') and close to or at a solid-liquid interface. This principal potential is behind most, if not all, of their medical and non-medical applications and actions, both chemical and physical as well as biological in nature.

Although some of them were synthesised long before this principle and any application were known, the major uses only occurred after awareness of the nature of these interactions.

Mirroring this potential, bisphosphonates are most often mentioned in conjunction with crystals, either of calcium carbonates or calcium phosphates of various chemical compositions and mineral forms, or with their (positive) cations in solutions. In organic molecules, the carboxyl group (-COOH) and its derivatives are perhaps the most active biological groups and act similarly to their (in?)organic counterpart, the carbonate ion (CO_3^{2-}). The phosphoric acid and (in?)organic phosphate compounds act as chemically analogous to the carboxyl and carbonate groups, and all of these can provide a strong bond to any cation in/on a crystal surface and/or in a solution. Chemistry mimics nature. All of the interactions in this chapter mimic the basic interaction between Ca^{2+} and CO_3^{2-}, the major substances of biomineralisation, and this, or equivalent, interaction covers all major forms of solid-state formation in living beings, as well as many so-called 'dead' inorganic solidification processes. Similar compounds are involved, and the same reactions. In this way, it is the same slow equilibrium reaction that limits CO_2 removal from the atmosphere to form sea-bottom $CaCO_3$ sediments, and it has the same underlying physico-chemical principles as the bone growth in a human being, or his/her dental stone, kidney stone, or any other solid concretion. One might conclude that the greenhouse effect (carbon dioxide increase in the atmosphere) and extra- or intracellular crystal formation are indeed very fundamentally related, as in a fractal[1] universe, with the globe acting as a microcellular entity. Gaia, mother earth, repeats herself even on the molecular level!

The manifestations of this process are overwhelming in nature and size: the globe contains 5.5 billion people, many millions of fauna species in abundant variety, 40,000 gigatons of C (carbon), a fair percentage of which stored as $CaCO_3$, suspended in the seas and even 50 million gigatons of C stored as $CaCO_3$ in sediments at the bottom of those seas[2] [1]. The biominerals give beauty to coral reefs, shells and pearls, stature to all skeletons and lustre to the teeth. For example, American chickens produce more than 1 million tons of $CaCO_3$ as eggshells for breakfast every year [12]; just think about the huge amounts of limestone these hens eat and dissolve, all deposited long before by geological and biological processes.

This is the background against which bisphosphonates were developed.

II. Inhibition of crystallisation

All crystallisation processes may be influenced by substances present in solution. These processes include:
– nucleation: the origination of new crystals;
– growth: the increase in size and mass of existing crystals;
– agglomeration: the clogging, or lumping together of groups of crystals.
Each of these processes can be promoted (increased) or inhibited (decreased) by those substances, either directly (by adsorption to and blocking active sites on the surface) or indirectly (by modifying the crystal-solution interface). The resulting effect is that the solution 'perceives' a modified crystal surface.

Ever since the turn of the century, the principle of inhibition has been known, although the terminology is of later date. Even in earlier centuries adsorption on porous substances like charcoal was purposely applied for this aim. In 1821 one of the earliest uses of a 'scale inhibitor' was reported by Payen: potato starch reduced deposition in water boilers (reviews in [2]). A citation from A. Payen in 1823:

> Bekanntlich werden die Kessel, in welchen man Brunnen-Wasser längere Zeit über kochen muss, vorzüglich in Dampf-Maschinen, mit einer solchen Kruste überzogen, dass nicht bloss das Wasser nicht mehr gehörig leicht erwärmt werden kann,..., sondern dass die Kessel selbst, deren Metall nicht mehr von Wasser bespült wird, glühend werden, Risse bekommen, und zum grössten Verderben der Gebäude und Menschen springen: das Nachtheiles nicht zu erwähnen, der an

---

[1] Fractals are universal mathematical patterns occurring in nature on different scales, giving nature much of its beauty (e.g. cloud patterns, coastline structures, plant growth forms, snowflake habits, microscopic patterns, but also symmetry patterns such as found in interstellar space, but also in the atomic structure of matter).

[2] Compared to the amounts, the total global fossil fuel reserves, approx. 5000 gigatons of carbon equivalent as coal, oil, gas, etc., form only a small fraction.

den Kesseln durch das Ausschlagen dieser Krusten entsteht. Herr Payen fand auf seiner Reise in England (im Jahr 1821), dass man um allen diesen Nachtheilen vorzubeugen, ungefähr 2/100 des Gewichtes des angewendeten Wassers Erdäpfel daselbst in die Kessel wirft.[3]

The use of adsorption in crystallisation processes in the early years of our century has been reviewed by the famous adsorption scientist Freundlich, among others [4]. As a pioneer in the field the scientist Marc [5] should be considered, who was maybe the first (in 1912) to stress the significance of adsorption for crystallisation and for retardation of kinetics. He developed this idea, by the way, in a suspension experiment, in principle similar to our modern laboratory test systems. It was found that crystallisation rates decreased in the presence of adsorbing dyes, but solution properties remained unchanged. [By the way, Marc was also the first to report a second-order ('parabolic') growth equation such as is common now in most crystallisation experiments, and can thus really be considered a pioneer] [6]. Even complete inhibition was found at a constant supersaturation level. Once again, like in modern crystallisation papers, a simple Langmuir adsorption isotherm [7] was reported in 1918 to describe the measured effects. In the 1920s a general interest arose in the influence of impurities on crystallisation, and the behaviour of inhibitors that had been in common use for a long time was understood (gelatine in ice-cream, arabic gum in confectionery, etc. [8–10]).

The role of phosphate compounds as inhibiting substances was discovered accidentally by Rosenstein: while fertilising orange trees via an irrigation system, he noticed that accidental addition of very little phosphate (1 ppm, or 10^{-6}) was already effective against undesirable crystal formation blocking his irrigation tubes [11]. Due to the diversity of scaling problems in industry, worldwide research efforts followed, and many independent discoveries were made: an explosion in the volume of literature and the number of patents followed [12]. Compounds like metaphosphates and other polyphosphates were developed and applied in practice [13]. The variations in structures became inexhaustible (see e.g. [14]), two of the most important classes being the organic phosphate esters and the phosphonates. The historical path of these developments started in 1938 [15]. Highlights are the development of bisphosphonic acid derivates, as components with the possibility of bi- and tridental binding to crystal surfaces (i.e. two bonds or three, respectively, per molecule). These substances (commonly called di- or bisphosphonates) became widely applied in various fields of technology and medicine. The longest known representative of this group is EHDP [IUPAC name: (1-hydroxyethylidene)-1, 1-bisphosphonic acid, though several names are in common use, such as etidronate, and almost any combination of old and mod-

---

[3] It is of course a well-known fact that boilers in which well water has to be boiled for prolonged periods, in particular in steam engines, become encrusted with scale to such an extent as not only to make it impossible for the water to be heated with the necessary efficiency, ... but also to cause the boiler itself, its metal no longer in contact with the water, to become red hot, develop cracks and bursts to the utmost danger to buildings and persons, not to mention the damage to the boilers from beating out the scale. While visiting England (in the year 1821) Herr Payen found that in order to guard against these ills, it was the custom there to throw potatoes into the boilers, about 2/100 by weight of the water used. [3]

ern nomenclature functional group names; German literature uses HEDP as the abbreviation].[4]

III. The first synthesis of a bisphosphonate

In 1865 N. Menschutkin synthesised a compound closely resembling EHDP as part of a typical synthesis reaction experiment between phosphoric acid and chloroacetyl [16]. Without any particular use or application in mind, he intended to study a reaction and try to understand the products, and it is of particular interest from the point of view of modern 'planned science' to read his observations:

> Man bringt 2 Aeq. phosphorige Säure und 1 Aeq. Chloracetyl in Röhren, welche man vor der Lampe verschliesst und die man während 50 bis 55 Stunden im Oelbad auf 120° erhitzt. Es ist durchaus nothwendig, die Röhren während der Dauer dieses Versuches zwei- oder dreimal zu öffnen. Jedesmal entweichen grosse Mengen Chlorwasserstoffsäure. Nach beendigter Einwirkung ist alles Chloracetyl verschwunden, und man findet in der Röhre eine ganz weisse und krystallinische Masse. Man trocknet diesen Körper bei 100° in einem Kohlen- säurestrom. Die Chlorwasserstoffsäure entweicht vollständig; zugleich destillirt Essigsäure über.
> Die Analysen des auf diese Art erhaltenen Körpers ergaben, dass seine Zusammensetzung bei jeder Darstellung wechselt. Man löst ihn in Wasser und neutralisirt die stark saure Lösung fast vollständig mit Kali. Durch Eindampfen der Flüssigkeit erhält man Krystalle. Eine zweite Krystallisation giebt schöne schief-rhombische Krystalle, welche das Kalisalz einer neuen Säure sind, für die ich die Bezeichnung *acetopyrophosphorige Säure* vorschlage.[5].

It would take quite long before Menschutkin's 'acetopyrophosphoric acid' (C_2P_2 H_6O_6) would be applied in practical situations. In 1897 Von Baeyer and Hofmann described a slightly different reaction procedure at lower temperature and produced acetodiphosphoric acid, with one oxygen atom more per molecule ($C_2P_2H_6O_7$) [17]. In this article, Von Baeyer described his product (the later EHDP) as a very stable compound, hard to decay, and as he described, this stability made him suspect a P-C-P rather than P-O-P or P-O-C bond:

---

[4] The name bisphosphonic acid should be used in order to avoid ambiguity with inorganic diphosphonic acid $H_2P_2H_2O_5$. Information can be found in the IUPAC InformBull 1973; 31: 73–77 (section D-5.5.). The substituted alkyl group is named according to the rules of section A-4.1. of the IUPAC 1957 rules of organic nomenclature (see e.g. R.C. Weast, ed.: *Handbook of Chemistry and Physics*, 57th edn (1976–1977), p. C-7). Even now, in 1992, there is still confusion, although I proposed the consistent use of the bisphosphonate nomenclature in the late 1970s (see e.g. [10]).

[5] Place 2 Eq. phosphoric acid and 1 Eq. chloracetyl into tubes. The latter are to be stoppered below the opening and to be heated for 50 to 55 hours in an oil bath to a temperature of 120°C. It is absolutely essential to open the tubes two or three times in the course of the experiment. Large quantities of hydrochloric acid will escape on each occasion. At the end of the exposure, all the chloracetyl will have disappeared, and the tube will be found to contain a pure white and crystalline mass. The latter is to be dried in a current of carbon dioxide at 100°C. The hydrochloric acid escapes completely; at the same time acetic acid is distilled over.
Analyses of the mass obtained by the above method have shown its composition to be different at every presentation. Dissolve the mass in water and neutralise the strongly acid solution almost completely with potash. By condensing the liquid one obtains crystals. A second crystallisation yields handsome, obliquely rhomboid crystals which represent the potassium salt of a new acid for which I propose the description of *acetopyrophosphoric acid*

Die grosse Beständigkeit unserer Säure zeigt sich auch darin, dass selbst salpetersaure Molybdänlösung beim Erhitzen keine Spur eines Niederschlages giebt, und dass kein Edelmetall reducirt wird. Diese Tathsachen sprechen für die Annahme, dass beide Phosphoratome direct an Kohlenstoff gebunden sind, denn eine P-O-C-Bindung sollte leicht verseifbar sein.[6]

The correct chemical formula was found in that article: $H_3CC(OH)[PO(OH)_2]_2$, and in later years other production routes were devised as well (cited in [5–9] in [18]). Most industrial routes for larger scale production were based on the acetylation of phosphoric acid or phosphorus trichloride [19–22].

The above-mentioned stability of P-C-P over P-O-P and P-O-C bonds is the reason for the greater medical interest in bisphosphonates over the 'more natural' but less stable pyrophosphates.

EHDP has become one of the most applied bisphosphonates in non-medical applications. Most of such applications were described and patented in the 1960s and 1970s. A few were developed in the 1980s, especially in view of the environmental awareness leading to replacement of many phosphorous-containing compounds by alternatives: the stabilities of the compounds were so good that destruction becomes a problem!

With the general formula: $R_1R_2C(PO_3H_2)(PO_3H_2)$ other bisphosphonates were developed. In this formula R1 and R2 were varied in almost any combination of $-H$, $-NH_2$, $-OH$, $-CH_3$ and longer alkyl groups, Cl, $-NR_3R_4$, etc. Together with an analogue series of components, in which one or two of the $-PO_3H_2$ groups were replaced by carboxyl (-COOH) group(s), the two most important classes for non-medical applications have been defined and give rise to a huge number of synthesised components. Even in a 1976 book on organic phosphorus compounds [23], a list of approx. 600 different polyphosphonic acids (most of which are bisphosphonic acids) appear! With each phosphonate group having, moreover, two opportunities to exchange a proton for almost any metal cation, the number of salts one can produce is very large indeed and can be in the hundreds of thousands.[7] Applicability of EHDP, by far, has remained the most significant in non-medical applications.

IV. Main non-medical applications of bisphosphonates

As the last paragraph concluded, the number of bisphosphonate salts is very large indeed. Some of them are in practical use as more or less stable salts or complexes, e.g. the radioactive technetium-tin-EHDP complex used in bone scanning [24]. However, most applications do not require the cations, but the activity is rather due to the (partly deprotonated) acid anions. Because of the fact that bidental

---

[6] The great stability of our acid also shows itself in the fact that even heating of nitric molybdenum solution does not result in any precipitate and that no precious metal is reduced. These facts support the assumption of a direct binding of the two phosphorus atoms to carbon as a P-O-C bond should be easy to saponify.

[7] More recently, other classes of compounds were added to the list, e.g. with $P-(C-P)_2$ or $P-(C-P)_3$ (see p. 578 of [12]), or with branched amino groups attached

Table 1.

Non-medical applications of bisphosphonates

On crystal surfaces
- scale inhibitor in oil, gas, etc.
- inhibitor in boilers, steam systems

On metal surfaces
- corrosion inhibitors for Al, Fe, Cu and alloys, since metal complexes formed with Co, Cr, Pb, Ni, Zn
- pre-treatment of Al surfaces to improve lacquering quality
- favouring electro-deposition by complexing heavy metals

On other surfaces
- glassware cleaning
- coatings

In solutions as complexing agent
- surface active agent
- water softener
- selective rare earth metal complexor
- textile dyeing
- wool softening and stabilising
- synthetic detergents
- soap

Fertilizer industry
- to eliminate undesirable co-precipitation
- fertilizer component

Polymer industry
- stabiliser
- resins
- glues

Household use
- in cosmetics
- in photography
- toothpastes
- tooth powders
- shampoos
- disinfectants
- chelating agent
- dispersing agent

Miscellaneous usage
- insulation materials
- in lubricating oils
- antimicrobiological action
- complexing sorbent constituent
- pasteurisation/sterilisation of food
- anti-decolouriser
- liquefier in cement and ceramic clay
- flame extinguishers
- pesticides

---

bonds are possible with the two phosphonate groups of the bisphosphonate, and even tridental bonds in the presence of other binding sites, e.g. on the $-R_1$ and $-R_2$ groups, the binding of metal ions is possible and strong, both at a surface (interface)

or in solutions (complex formation) [25]. On this basis, most applications can be categorised (see Table 1) into the following classes:
- applications on crystal surfaces and related
- applications on metal surfaces
- applications on other surfaces
- applications in solutions as complexing agent
- applications in the fertilizer industry
- applications in the polymer industry
- applications in household products and
- miscellaneous applications

each of which will be briefly highlighted in the following sections.

1. Applications on crystal surfaces/metal surfaces

The variety of bisphosphonates under study and in use as crystallisation inhibitors is enormous. This has to do with the immense economical interest to prevent undesirable crystallisation ('scale') in the oil industry: concretions in sometimes miles-deep pipelines occur when hot water (often with Ba^{2+} from heavy barium-containing 'kill fluids' to give counterweight pressure in a bore-hole against underground pressure eruptions, and often with Ca^{2+} and sulfates from minerals and sea water) evaporates at high pressure in the hot environment. This sometimes causes calcium and/or barium sulfate deposition (since calcium sulfates and especially barium sulfates have very low solubilities under prevailing conditions), which immediately influences pressure drop in the bore-pipes and which can sometimes block these pipes completely within a few weeks' time, necessitating replacement and long delay.

As for all inhibitors, bisphosphonates act differently on nucleation of crystals (the origination of new crystal phases), on growth of existing crystals, and on agglomeration [10, 26]. The resulting, and desired, action of inhibition is a decrease of the mass accretion of any 'scale' formed.

Mass volume production of bisphosphonates largely accounts for this major area of applications, and a correspondingly large volume of literature on synthesis, test experiments, toxicity, handling and environmental acceptability exists [10, 27–30, 35]. In analogy to the process of medical drugs tests needed before registration and certification, the application areas for inhibitors have developed their own test requirements as well, including studies on bio-accumulation, algae growth, biological and chemical oxygen demands (BOD and COD), acute and long-term fish poisoning tests and adult fish survival curve determinations.

During application as inhibitors in boilers, similar mechanisms are at work (and equally so in kettles, tapwater lines in calcium-rich drinking water regions, etc.). In industrial systems, the problems are aggravated by the extreme conditions: a typical large industrial boiler system can have crystal scale phenomena in conditions varying from ambient temperature to above 700°C at pressures ranging from atmospheric to over 200 bar. Especially under high temperature and pressure conditions, crystallisation occurs at the same sites where corrosion starts: trace amounts [in ppm (10^{-6}) or even ppb (10^{-9}) range in solution] of heavy metals on the surfaces of crystals can start corrosion and crystal formation at the same time. By modifying the crystal habit ('shape' or crystallographic 'form'), the metal traces also influence agglomeration and growth rates, and as such can be responsible for 'life-threatening' actions on the crystal or metal surfaces involved, especially at the liquid/vapour interface of a boiling liquid in metal vessels, containers or pipes.

Even very sophisticated modern energy technologies are influenced by this same effect: as an example in fuel cell systems, a new technology to generate clean electric power by electrochemical reaction of hydrogen with oxygen (or air) to form water, the fuel cells are cooled with tiny stainless steel tubes with boiling water inside, which takes away enough heat generated in the fuel cell as byproduct to keep it at a constant temperature [31–33]. The tiny tubes have a large surface-to-volume ratio, 100–1000 times larger than in large-diameter industrial boilers, and are correspondingly more sensitive to minute traces of heavy metals: so much so that even the most sophisticated methods of producing ultra-low conductivity (ultra-high purity) water are often not sufficient to prevent corrosion. This represents an area for future bisphosphonate application.

The area of corrosion constitutes the second group of applications for bisphosphonates: by binding the traces of heavy metals, the surfaces can be cleansed and corrosion prevented. This principle is being applied in several areas: apart from boilers, it is used to form metal complexes with e.g. Co, Cr, Pb, Zn and Ni to inhibit corrosion of Al, Fe, Cu and their alloys. Bisphosphonates are also used to pretreat Al surfaces in order to have a better attachment and stronger bonding of lacquering layers applied immediately after the process. Similarly, metals are treated with bisphosphonates prior to electro-deposition, e.g. in car and/or bicycle manufacture [34].

The traditional bisphosphonate compound for all these applications is EHDP [35], but many other bisphosphonates and mixtures have been developed for these purposes [36–43].

2. Applications on other surfaces

In the late 1960s, interest arose to find replacement for strong alkaline solutions which were normally applied for washing and rinsing glass articles and objects, but also from metal, rubber, etc, such as in the milk industry and soft drinks bottling factories. The strong alkali was needed to remove grease and fatty substances, but gave rise to undesirable precipitation (stains!) by Fe, Ca and Mg salts from the tapwater. Once again, a perfect application area for EHDP and analogous compounds [43, 44], because of their higher stability over polyphosphates such as pyrophosphates. Similar applications provide better coatings on surfaces of several materials [45].

3. Applications in solutions as complexing agent

The applications referred to in the last section already hint at solution behaviour, at or close to a surface: the metals are 'drawn from the surface' by the bisphosphonate anions and kept in a complex in the solution, or even at the crystal-solution interface. These complexes can be obtained with many metals and with some bisphosphonates can grow to larger sizes and even to relatively high molecular weight 'super complexes', such as the ones commonly referred to as 'polynuclear' complexes [46–48], which in turn have been connected with some biological action hypotheses [10]. Larger complexes close to or at the interface may change the energy, charge distribution and other characteristics of the crystal-solution interface, and thus of the crystal as 'perceived' by the surrounding dissolved species.[8] The one but largest group of bisphosphonate applications is based on complex formation in solution, mostly however, with relatively small 'mononuclear' complexes [49, 50]. Applications range from titrimetric analysis of rare earth metals, scandium, yttrium, bismuth, iron, gallium and indium, etc. [51], to chelating agent forming strong complexes, with applications in e.g. softening tissues of fabrics in which alkaline earth metals have deposited, in softening water directly [15], in detergents and cleaners [in combination with known anionic, cationic or non-ionic (so-called 'amphoteric') wetting agents] and, perhaps more directly but based on the same action again, in textile dyeing, softening and stabilisation of wool, and in soap [18].

As usual in the 1960s, the surprisingly strong ability to form complexes was shown in an experiment by Blaser and Worms, part of the team of the Henkel researchers that produced an immense volume of bisphosphonate patents, both on synthesis and on applications [52], in a surprisingly 'German' experiment: the bisphosphonate complexes were so strong that: 'the blue color characteristic for trivalent iron ions, known as "Berlin blue" or "Prussian blue" does not occur!' Hence the applications in preventing iron hydroxide deposits on textiles and during bottle washing procedures.

Another reason for adding bisphosphonates to products with surface active substances such as soap, body lotions and creams, detergents, etc. is to increase stability, which is not satisfactory for many of those compounds (fats become rancid, stains are formed, colours change, and the odour is influenced). Such processes and therewith the products are being stabilised by the bisphosphonates [41, 42, 53]. In combination with urea and cellulose, EHDP is also used as a strong complexing sorbent [54].

4. Applications in the fertilizer industry

Chemical industry applications range from fine chemicals to base chemicals industry: in fertilizer manufacture bisphosphonates have been applied both as components of fertilizer and as substances to eliminate undesirable coprecipitation in the process of producing the fertilizer: during the manufacture of ammonium phosphate, one of the main components of potassium fertilizers, impurities do precipitate from the phosphoric acid, thus giving rise to co-precipitation and to an

---

[8] In many ways, a crystal with attached 'double layer' of organic complexes is analogous to a cell with surrounding membrane. Further research in this area may give rise to exciting speculations on the analogy between physical and biological actions.

impure crystalline product. The addition of EHDP or any of its water-soluble salts makes it possible to remedy this [18, 65].

5. Applications in the polymer industry

Bisphosphonates are being applied since 1965 as components in polyester-type materials, which are employed as resins, adhesives and glues, coatings and covering layers [55], opening an interesting area of utilisation, including lacquering, which I briefly mentioned before [34]. This section should also mention application as stabiliser [67].

6. Applications in household products

In each household bisphosphonates can be found, in cosmetics, toothpastes, powders and/or mouthwashes, shampoo and disinfectants [56]. Also in photography bisphosphonates are being applied in some film developing processes as a silver-image-nucleus-forming agent [69].

Dental applications have received special interests, even though one could consider them as medical applications rather than household products (but where is the border between those areas, if any?). In dentrifice compositions, such as in toothpastes, powders and mouth water, some compounds age and decompose or solidify over time, making them unsuitable for use, especially in tropical climates. Furthermore, a reaction can occur between acidic components and any carbonate material present in the product to yield carbon dioxide: 'which may generate sufficient pressure within the dentrifice container to cause it to explode...' [57]. Therefore, the calcium phosphates present in those products are stabilised to prevent this decomposition/hydrolysis. Bisphosphonates can be used for this purpose, and at the same time serve to prevent dental stone formation and perhaps act beneficially on caries as well. Calcium salts of bisphosphonates have been developed to serve as the primary polishing agent in dentrifice compositions: a substance hard enough to polish the enamel surface of the tooth, but not too aggressive and too abrasive for the dentin becoming exposed behind receding gums, while also reducing tooth decay [58].

An additional benefit of bisphosphonates is their anti-microbiological effect, one of the earliest patented applications [59], and a 'positive side-effect' of many common applications especially in food, health and cosmetic sectors, or a means of increasing the bacteriostatic effect of other compounds [60]. Excellent microbistatic activity is reported by several bisphosphonates against numerous bacteria [61], and they are active in inhibiting growth of many gram-positive as well as gram-negative bacteria. They can be applied in much lower concentrations than many other microbistatic compositions and are therefore useful to treat hard surfaces to prevent microorganism growth, e.g. for cleaning floors and walls in hospitals, food processing plants, and other private and public buildings [61]. The same effect is beneficial in the dentrifice applications, but also in disinfecting animal skin surfaces, and the reported uses in cosmetic creams, salves, lotions and the like.

7. Miscellaneous usage of bisphosphonates

The list would not be complete without mentioning some other applications of this exciting and versatile class of compounds. Their applicability stretches as far as areas like herbicides, or even as plant growth regulatory substances. As an instance, selective defoliation and leaf growth inhibition while leaving the productive plant parts unaffected can stimulate productivity and at the same time facilitate harvesting, e.g. in flax, cotton, bean crops, etc. [62]. Another application in agriculture is plant regulation by selective retardation of vegetative growth (shorter stems, increased branching), resulting in smaller, bushier plants with increased resistance. This principle is even applied to decrease purposely the frequency of lawn-mowing on golf courses and similar grassy plots. In many plants, such as potatoes, sugar canes, beets, grapes, melons, etc., vegetative growth retardation increases the carbohydrate content at harvest (per weight unit of product). Once again a modern application area for methylammonium salts of (bis)phosphonates.

Finally a few areas should still be referred to, some of which have been briefly looked upon already: the application of bisphosphonates in insulation materials, in lubricating oils, as complexing sorbent constituent [54], in pasteurisation/sterilisation of food, as liquefier in cement and ceramic clays [66], in pesticides [68], flame extinguishers [63], as dispersing agent, for liquefaction of inorganic waste materials [64], as controlled means of supply for trace elements to plants [52], and as an additive to various construction materials.

Epilogue

Imagine the variety described above, which is probably far from complete! It is exciting to see the abundance of applications, affecting everybody's life, even though hardly noticed, if ever. The industrial drive behind the most important applications described here has provided the impetus for industrial support to university clinics and medical institutions to enable these latter groups to add significantly by having imported successfully bisphosphonates into the medical area. Started perhaps as an exciting series of compounds for potential application in medicine, it has developed into a large area of medical research, described in more detail elsewhere in this book, with even more potential for the future. At the base of this success is perhaps the very basic nature of the interactions described at the beginning of this chapter, combined with the added biochemical complexity at cell and cell-organelle level, but being governed by the same principal interaction between divalent cations and the anions of bisphosphonates acting in analogy to the most active organic and inorganic groups available on earth. It is important and surprising to note and understand the similarity with the most significant inorganic equilibrium on earth, that between calcium and carbonate, the solid bone equivalent of the earth shell. On a relative scale thinner than an eggshell, but the basis for an equilibrium, long kept stable, in our biosphere. I will think about that when breaking my eggshell tomorrow morning.

References

1. Blomen, L.J.M.J., Mugerwa, M.N., Introduction. In: Blomen, L.J.M.J., Mugerwa, M.N. (Editors), Fuel Cell Systems. Plenum Publishing, New York, 1992.
2a. Badger, W.L., Critical review of literature on formation and prevention of scale. Res. and Develop. Progr. Rep. Office of Saline Water, U.S. Department of Interior Washington, 1959: 25.
2b. Elliot, J.S., The present state of scale control in sea water evaporators. Desalination 1969; 6: 87–104.
3. Payen, A., Erdäpfel, ein Mittel, die Intkrustierungen in Kesseln zu verhüten. Dingler's Polytech. J. 1823; 10: 254.
4. Freundlich, H., Adsorption and its significance. In: Alexander, J. (Editor), Colloid Chemistry. Chemical Catalog Comp., New York, 1926, Vol. 1: 575–599.
5. Marc, R., Über die Kristallisation aus wässerigen Lösungen. Z. Physik. Chem. VI. Mitteilung 1912; 79: 71–96.
6. Marc, R., Über die Kristallisation aus wässerigen Lösungen. Z. Physik. Chem. II. Mitteilung 1909; 67: 470–500.
7. Langmuir, I., The adsorption of gases on plane surfaces of glass, mica and platinum. J. Am. Chem. Soc. 1918; 40: 1361–1403.
8. Ord, W.M., On the influence of colloids upon crystalline form and cohesion, with observations on the structure and mode of formation of urinary and other calculi. Edward Stanford, London, 1879.
9. Alexander, J., Die Wirkungen von Kolloïden auf die Kristallisation. Koll. Z. 1909; 4: 86–87.
10. Blomen, L.J.M.J., Growth and agglomeration of calcium oxalate monohydrate crystals. Doctoral thesis, University of Leiden, 1982.
11. Rosenstein, L., Process of treating water. U.S. Pat.no. 2038316, 1936; reissue 20360, 1937; 20754, 1938. Shell Development Company, San Francisco.
12. Cowan, C.J., Weintritt, D.J., Water-formed scale deposits. Gulf Publ. Co., Houston, 1976, p. 216.
13. Hall, R.E., Water softening and washing. U.S. Pat.no. 1956515, 1934; reissue 19719, 1935. Hall Labs., Pittsburgh.
14. Van Wazer, J.R., Phosphorus and its compounds. I. Chemistry. Interscience, New York, 1958.
15. Woodstock, W.H., Water-softener. U.S. Pat.no. 2122122, 1938. Victor Chemical Works, Corp. of Illinois.
16. Menschutkin, N., Über die Einwirkung des Chlorazetyls auf phosphorige Säure. Ann. Chem. Pharm. 1865; 133: 317–320.
17. Von Baeyer, H., Hofmann, K.A., Acetodiphosphorige Säure. Ber. Dtsch. Chem. Ges. 1897; 30: 1973–1978.
18. Kabachnik, M.I., Dyatlova, N.M., Medved', T.Ya., Bikhman, B.I., Urinovich, Ye.M., Kolpakova, I.D., Krinitskaya, L.V., Vel'tishchev, Yu.Ye., Yur'eva, E.A., Lastkovskii, R.P., Hydroxyethylidenediphosphonic acid and its applications. Soviet Chem. Ind. 1975; 7: 1034–1038.
19. Worms, K.H., Schmidt-Dunker, M. In: Kosolapoff, G.M., Maier, L. (Editors), Organic phosphorus compounds VII. Wiley and Sons, New York, 1976, Ch.18.
20. Rogovin, L., Brawn, D.P., Nicholas, J., Verfahren zur kontinuierlichen Herstellung von Äthan-1-hydroxy-1,1-diphosphonsäure. GE Pat.no. 1251759, 1967. Proctor and Gamble Co., a corporation of Ohio.
21. Quimby, O.T., Low temperature preparation of ethane-1-hydroxy-1,1-diphosphonic acid. US Pat.No. 3366677, 1968. Proctor and Gamble Co., a corporation of Ohio.
22. Dyer, J.K., Use of amine solvents in the preparation of ethane-1-hydroxy-1,1-diphosphonic acid. US Pat.No. 3366676, 1968. Proctor and Gamble Co., a corporation of Ohio.
23. Kosolapoff, G.M., Maier, L. (Editors), Organic phosphorus compounds VII. Wiley and Sons, New York, 1976.
24. Van den Brand, J.A.G.M., Technetium (TIN) ethane-1-hydroxy-1,1-diphosphonate complexes, preparation, composition and biodistribution. Report no. ECN-98. Netherlands Energy Research Foundation, 1981.
25. Barnett, B.L., Strickland, L.C., Structure of disodium dihydrogen 1-hydroxyethylidenediphosphonate tetrahydrate: a bone growth regulator. Acta Cryst. 1979; B35: 1212–1214.
26. Blomen, L.J.M.J., Bijvoet, O.L.M., Blomen-Kuneken, W., Der Einfluss von HEDP auf Wachstum und Agglomeration von $CaC_2O_4 \cdot H_2O$. Fortschr. Urol. Nephrol. 1983; 20: 416–420.
27. Kabachnik, M.I., USSR Inventor's Certificate 292984. Bynl.izobret, no. 5, 1971.
28. Ralston, P.H., Scale control with aminomethylene-phosphonates. J. Petrol Techn. 1969; 8: 1029–1038.

29. Reddy, M.M., Nancollas, G.H., Calcite crystal growth inhibition by phosphonates. Desalination 1973; 12: 45–61.
30. Huber, L., Studies on the biodegradability and fish toxicity of two organic complexing agents based on phosphonic acid (ATMP and HEDP). Tenside Deterg. 1975; 12: 316–324.
31. Blomen, L.J.M.J., Fuel cells. A review of fuel cell technology and its applications. In: Johansson, T.B., Bodlund, B., Williams, R.H. (Editors), Electricity-efficient end-use and new generation technologies and their planning implications. Lund University Press, Lund, 1990, pp. 627–664.
32. Blomen, L.J.M.J., System development and commercialisation activities by Kinetics Technology International Group (KTI)/Mannesmann. J. Power Sources 1992; 37: 141–154.
33. Fuji Electric Co., Special issue on fuel cells. Fuji Electr. Rev. 1992; 38: 36–72.
34. Haynes, R.T., Irani, R.R., Langguth, R.P., Compositions et procédés pour réactions électrochimiques notamment galvanoplastie ainsi qu'articles conformes àceux obtenus. FR Pat.no. 1458492, 1966. Monsanto Co.
35. Monsanto Industrial Chemicals Co., Dequest^R 2010 phosphonate for scale and corrosion control, chelation, dispersion. Technical Bulletin No. IC/SCS-323.
36. Redmore, D., Paley, W.S., N,N-dimethylene phosphonic acids of alkylene diamines. US Pat.no. 4330487, 1982. Petrolite Corp., St. Louis.
37. Redmore, D., Paley, W.S., N,N-dimethylene phosphonic acids of alkylene diamines. US Pat. no. 4409151, 1983. Petrolite Corp., St. Louis.
38. Cone, C.S., A guide for selection of cooling water corrosion inhibitors. Materials Protection and Performance 1970; 9: 32–34.
39. Hwa, Ch.M., Organic phosphorous acid compound-chromate corrosion protection in aqueous systems. US Pat. no. 3431217, 1969. W.R. Grace and Co., New York.
40. Buckman, J.D., Dialkylamino-N,N bis(phosphonoalkylene)alkylamines and use in aqueous systems as precipitation and corrosion inhibitors. US Pat. no. 4234511, 1980. Buckman Laboratories, Memphis.
41. Redmore, D., Welge, F.T., Hydroxypropylene-amino-phosphonic acids. US Pat.no. 4187245, 1980. Petrolite Corp., St. Louis.
42. Redmore, D., Quaternary aminomethyl phosphonates as scale inhibitors. US Pat.no. 4420399, 1983. Petrolite Corp., St. Louis.
43. Blum, H., Hemmann, S., 4-dimethylamino-1-hydroxybutane-1,1 diphosphonic acid, salts thereof, and processes therefore. US Pat.no. 4624947, 1986. Henkel KG, Düsseldorf.
44. Monsanto Co., Inhibiermittel, Waschzubereitungen, deren Lösungen und Anwendungsverfahren. GE Pat.no. 1937031, 1969, St. Louis.
45. Jacques, J.K., Fabrication de polyuréthanes ignifugés. FR Pat.no. 1455978, 1966. Albright and Wilson Ltd., GB.
46. Wiers, B.W., Polynuclear complex formation in solutions of calcium ion and ethane-1-hydroxy-1,1-diphosphonic acid. II. Light scattering. Sedimentation, mobility and dialysis measurments. J. Phys. Chem. 1971; 75: 682–687.
47. Grabenstetter, E.J., Cilley, W.A., Polynuclear complex formation in solutions of calcium ion and ethane-1-hydroxy-1,1-diphosphonic acid. I. Complexometric and pH titration. J. Phys. Chem. 1971; 75: 676–682.
48. Sillen, L.G., On equilibria in systems with polynuclear complex formation. II. Testing simple mechanisms which give 'core +links' complexes of composition B(AtB)n. Acta Chem. Scand. 1954; 8: 318–335.
49. Irani, R.R., Moedritzer, K., Metal complexing by phosphorus compounds; VI. Acidity constants and calcium and magnesium complexing by mono- and polymethylene diphosphonates. J. Phys. Chem. 192; 66: 1349–1353.
50. Kabachnik, M.I., Lastakovskii, R.P., Medved', T.Ya., Medyntsev, V.V., Kolpakova, I.D., Dyatlova, N.M., The complexing properties of hydroxyethylidenediphosphonic acid in aqueous solutions. Dokl. Akad. Nauk. SSSR 1967; 177: 582–585.
51. Pribil, R., Vesely, V., 1-hydroxy-ethylidene-1,1-diphosphonic acid as a titrimetric agent. Talanta 1967; 14: 591–595.
52. Blaser, B., Worms, K.-H. Process of forming metal ion complexes. US Pat.no. 3214454, 1965. Henkel and Co., Düsseldorf.
53. Blaser, B., Werdelmann, B., Worms, K.-H. Oberflächenaktive Stoffe. GE Pat.no. 1072346, 1959. Henkel and Co., Düsseldorf.
54. Proctor and Gamble Co., Werkwijze voor het bereiden van organo fosforverbindingen. Dutch Pat.no. 6604176, 1966, Cincinnati.

55. Albright and Wilson Ltd., Procédé d'ignifugation de polyesters. FR Pat.no. 1455979, 1966.
57. Smith, R.A., Dixon, J.T., Phosphate compositions. US Pat.no. 1143123, 1967.
58. Irani, R.R., Dentifrice compositions containing insoluble salts of alkylene phosphonic acids. US Pat.no. 3608067, 1969. Monsanto Co., St. Louis.
59. Nösler, H.G., Schnegelberger, H., Bellinger, H. Antimikobielle Mittel. GE Pat.no. 1284041, 1967. Henkel and Co.
60. Irani, R.R., Roberts, H.E. Verwendungen wasserlöslicher Polyphosphonsäureverbindungen als Potenzierungsmittel für Bakterizide. GE Pat.no. 1225818, 1965. Monsanto Co., St. Louis.
61. Blum, H., Hemmann, S., Diphosphonylated oxonitriles, processes and uses thereof, and compositions containing them. US Pat.no. 4719050, 1988. Henkel KG, Düsseldorf.
62. Large, G., Buren, L., Tetra-substituted ammonium salt of N-phosphonomethylglycine and their uses as herbicides and plant growth regulants. PCT/US Pat.no. 83/03608, 1983. Stauffer Chemical Co., Westport.
63. Jacques, J.K., Fabrication de polyuréthanes ignifugés. FR Pat.no. 1455978, 1966. Albright and Wilson Ltd., GB.
64. Blaser, B., Von Freyhold, H., Worms, K.-H., Verfahren zur Verflüssigung von anorganischen Schlämmen. GE Pat.no. 1154028, 1963. Henkel and Co., Düsseldorf.
65. Smith, R.A., Dixon, J.T., Fabrication de phosphate d'ammonium cristallins. FR Pat.no. (addition) 92066, 1968. Albright and Wilson Ltd., UK.
66. Blaser, B., Von Freyhold, H., Worms, K.-H. Verfahren zur Verflüssigung von anorganischen Schlämmen. GE Pat.no. 1154028, 1963. Henkel and Co., Düsseldorf.
67. Dehydag Deutsche Hydrierwerke GmbH, Procédé de préparation de composé's organiques contenant des groupes époxydes. Belgian Pat.no. 635527, 1963.
68. Schmidt, P., Verfahren zur Herstellung von neuen Phosphor enthaltenden organischen Verbindungen. CH Pat.no. 326731, 1956. CIBA, Basel.
69. Bard, C.C., Malloy, R.J., Kuh, A.D., Photographisches Umkehrverfahren. GE Pat.no. 2009693, 1970.

Bisphosphonate on bones
O. Bijvoet, H.A. Fleisch, R.E. Canfield and G. Russell (eds.)
© 1995 Elsevier Science B.V. All rights reserved.

CHAPTER 8

Bisphosphonate therapy in acute and chronic bone loss: Physical chemical considerations in bisphosphonate-related therapies

Arman Ebrahimpour and Marion D. Francis

The Procter and Gamble Company, P.O. Box 538707, Cincinnati, OH 45253, USA

I. Introduction

The bis- or diphosphonates were first recorded in the synthetic literature in Berichte [1]. Sixty-three years were to elapse before the next recorded entry in the literature was made [2]. These authors published in the patent literature the application of 1-hydroxyethylidene bisphosphonate to the soluble complexation of metal ions, primarily calcium and magnesium. Since that time there has been a steady flow of synthetic, chemical, medical, and dental publications on the bisphosphonates. There have also been some interesting structural variants on the bisphosphonates. The general formulas that represent the categories of phosphonic acid compounds are represented in Fig. 1.

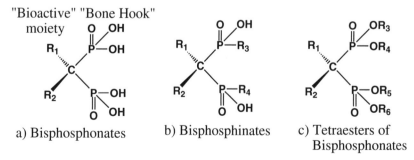

a) Bisphosphonates   b) Bisphosphinates   c) Tetraesters of Bisphosphonates

Fig. 1. Possible structure substitutions (R groups) on the phosphorus (P) atom and geminal carbon (C) atom of the phosphonates which can markedly alter both their physicochemical adsorption to hydroxyapatite (HAP) and their pharmacological action on bone tissue.

The first dental use of a bisphosphonate was for the inhibition or blockage of calculus or tartar deposition. The principle involved was the adsorption of etidronate disodium (1-hydroxyethylidene bisphosphonate disodium salt, EHDP or Didronel) on the tooth surface and to any nuclei of calcium phosphate (calculus) that might form on the tooth surface as a result of diet or the presence of calcifying bacteria [3, 4]. The concentrations of topical solution [5] and dentifrice [6] were such that etidronate saturated the calcium phosphate crystal's growing surfaces, thus inhibiting deposition and accumulation of supragingival calculus. Several bisphosphonates and also pyrophosphate (which has similar crystal-inhibiting properties as the bisphosphonates) are in commercial anticalculus dentifrices today and available to the public in a number of countries. Systemic administration of bisphosphonate was shown to be ineffective in blocking calculus in the oral cavity of rats on a calculus-inducing diet [5].

The first medical use of a bisphosphonate was based on a principle similar to that of calculus inhibition involving the oral dosing of etidronate to a 16-month-old child with ossifying deposition, myositis ossificans progressiva [7]. The principle again was to produce a saturating adsorption of bisphosphonate on the sites of calcium phosphate deposition in the muscle tissues and so block the debilitating effects of the unwanted accretion. In a somewhat similar medical application for heterotopic ossification, etidronate has been used successfully for the inhibition of calcification of soft tissue resulting from hip replacement or spinal chord injury [8]. Again the principle is the same, sites of rapidly forming calcium phosphate (hydroxyapatite or octacalcium phosphate) in muscle tissue can be saturated by oral administration of etidronate and blocked from further deposition which destroys muscle tissue function. Thus, range of motion can be maintained such as in the hip. The application of bisphosphonates that adsorb strongly on hydroxyapatite have the potential to block heterotopic ossification as well as interfere with new bone formation. However, the clinical application of these bisphosphonates for inhibition of heterotopic ossification resides in the ratio of surface capacity of the soft-tissue calcification site relative to the surface capacity of the total calcified bone surface. Bone comprises about 10% of the body weight, and estimates of the differential in the above surface capacity would place it at about 1000 bone to 1 of soft-tissue calcification. Thus, if the bisphosphonate regimen of treatment is followed carefully, minimal bone effects will occur. Subsequently, when the bisphosphonate treatment is terminated, the minor areas of bone involvement will recover [9] as the bisphosphonate desorbs [10] or is buried under the new normal bone formation [11]. Since previously deposited calcified soft tissue is not removed by bisphosphonate therapy, treatment for heterotopic ossification is most effective in patients where no previous heterotopic depositions have occurred. Although bisphosphonate therapy decreases the dissolution rate of previously deposited heterotopic ossification, it also dramatically inhibits the growth rate of such deposition. Thus, bisphosphonate treatment decreases the overall quantity of calcified soft tissue. An example of this was observed in the previously cited myositis ossificans, where calcium phosphate deposits were gradually removed from calcified thigh muscle upon the initiation of etidronate treatment.

The bisphosphonates are best known for their ability to block bone resorption such as in Paget's disease [12, 13] or hypercalcemia of tumor origin [14] or in other bone resorptive processes such as osteoporosis [15, 16]. Several hypotheses have been put forward concerning the mechanism of this antiresorptive effect. These include the inhibited solubility of bisphosphonate adsorbed bone, an antiosteoclastic toxic effect due to phagocytosis of bone particles coated with adsorbed bisphosphonate [17], and possibly site-specific interaction of the bisphosphonates with the cell membrane of the osteoclast producing a functional inactivation [18, 19]. Bisphosphonates may also inactivate osteoclast precursors [20] in addition to influencing mature osteoclasts. To date, the specific mechanism has not been elaborated.

In terms of mechanism, however, one process involved in both the dental and medical activity that has held the test of time is the adsorptive (chemisorptive) activity of all the bisphosphonates for the calcium phosphate phase of both dental enamel and bone. The specific adsorption of ^{3}H-etidronate has been demonstrated on the inorganic components of bone beneath the forming osteoid layer of bare endosteal and periosteal surfaces and in Haversian canals of cortical bone [21]. In addition, if rather than the bisphosphonates (Fig. 1a), bisphosphinates (Fig. 1b) or the tetraesters of bisphosphonates (Fig. 1c) are used, no adsorption of the latter two structures on bone is observed, nor do they have the biological effects of the bisphosphonates. The purpose of this chapter is to discuss the more recent physicochemical data developed for the structural variants of the phosphonates with their hydroxyapatite interactions and the implications for medical application of these changes in physical chemical attributes.

II. Physicochemical processes

Bone modelling and remodelling involves the process of resorption (dissolution/demineralization) of previously mineralized bone and the formation (deposition) of organic matrix and its subsequent mineralization (mineral accretion/growth/formation). Although many calcium phosphate phases such as dicalcium phosphate dihydrate (DCPD) [22] and octacalcium phosphate (OCP) [23, 24] have been suggested as the possible precursors to bone mineral, the mature bone mineral is virtually all in the form of calcium phosphate's most thermodynamically stable phase, hydroxyapatite (HAP). However, stoichiometric HAP [$Ca_{10}(PO_4)_6(OH)_2$] with the Ca/P molar ratio of 1.67 is rarely seen in vivo where calcium-deficient and substituted apatites are often found. Varying amounts of ions such as magnesium, sodium, aluminum, strontium, carbonate, fluoride, and chloride might become substituted in the apatitic crystals depending upon several factors such as the individual's diet and age. Since most of these ions are not often found in large quantities in vivo and in order to avoid possible complications by the above ions, synthetic HAP crystals are widely accepted as the model system in the in vitro investigations of bone mineral growth and dissolution.

Well-characterized physicochemical studies of the calcium phosphates and the bisphosphonates, bisphosphinates, and phosphonoalkylphosphinates are bringing new light into this field. These in vitro kinetic studies of mineralization and re-sorption are especially important since they are conducted under physiologically relevant conditions while the concentration of every involved component is main-tained constant throughout the experiment using the dual constant composition method [25, 26]. Consequently, in these studies the rates of HAP growth and dissolution in the absence (i.e. standard rates) and in the presence of the drugs are measured.

As we have mentioned earlier, the bone affinity or the specific adsorption of bisphosphonates and phosphonoalkylphosphinates on the bone mineral HAP plays a crucial role in the efficacy of these agents on targeting to the mineralizing tissues. Langmuir's derivation of an adsorption isotherm [27] and its related additional refinements [28–30] form a very useful and accurate method for the determination of the affinity of these drugs for the mineralized tissues. Results from adsorption isotherm experiments are given in terms of the equilibrium HAP surface concen-tration of the adsorbed drug as a function of the drug's solution concentration (estimated to represent the drug serum concentration), in units of μmole m^{-2} (Y-axis) and μmole L^{-1} (X-axis), respectively. The subsequent curves in Langmuirian adsorption isotherms reach a plateau at a maximum monolayer surface coverage. In these plots the surface coverage (Y-axis) at the plateau and the slope with which the curve reaches the plateau are indicative of these drugs' affinity for HAP surfaces.

Much of the influence of the phosphonates on the bone mineral HAP is due to their concentration on the mineral surface. Often, small alterations in the drug surface concentration on the HAP surface result in significant changes in the HAP growth and dissolution rates. The combined data from the drug's bone affinity (i.e. adsorption isotherms) and its subsequent influence on the HAP mineralization and resorption rates are needed in order to determine their efficacy in controlling these processes, as shown in Fig. 2.

The mineralization and resorption of bone mineral HAP in vivo are tightly regulated. In young subjects, the overall skeletal mineralization rate exceeds the resorption rate (Fig. 3A i). At peak bone mass in healthy young adults, the rates of these dynamic phenomena are controlled such that growing bones are of good architecture and the net bone accretion and dissolution are balanced (Fig. 3A ii). In adults, there is a small decrease in the skeletal growth and dissolution rates, where the latter might be slightly higher than the former (Fig. 3A iii). However, in the elderly and during the early stages of postmenopause, the rate of skeletal mineralization decreases further while the rate of skeletal resorption remains approximately unchanged, leading to a significant net deficit in the skeletal mineral mass balance (Fig. 3A iv and C). Currently, several bisphosphonate analogues are being investigated in the treatment of skeletal mineral loss and osteoporosis, as illustrated in Fig. 3C. If one chooses an appropriate bisphosphonate analogue at the proper dose regimen for the treatment of osteoporosis, this could lead to the reduction of the deficit in the net skeletal mineral mass balance. In Paget's disease of bone the rates of mineralization and resorption increase drastically (Fig. 3B), and as a result the bone architecture is compromised in a disorganized mosaic of woven and lamellar bone [31]. Paget's disease has been successfully treated [12, 13]

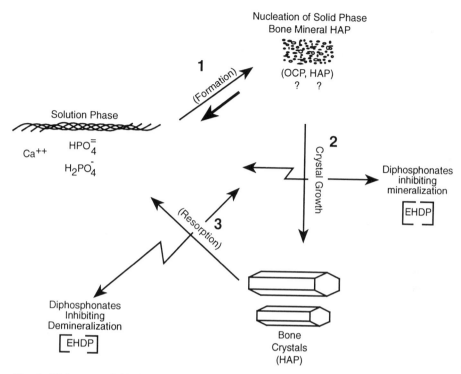

Fig. 2. Dichotomy of bisphosphonate action. A cartoon of the different changes in calcium and orthophosphate of the mammalian system. In step 1, calcium (Ca^{++}) and orthophosphate ($H_2PO_4^-$, HPO_4^{2-}, and PO_4^{3-}) ions in the extracellular fluid form nuclei of dicalcium phosphate dihydrate (DCPD), octacalcium phosphate (OCP) and/or hydroxyapatite (HAP). In step 2, those phases transform into hexagonal crystals of mature HAP unless a significant concentration of metabolite pyrophosphate or geminal bisphosphonate is present to block crystal nucleation and growth. In step 3, mature bone HAP crystals can be dissolved back into its constituent ions (Ca^{++}, $H_2PO_4^-$, HPO_4^{2-}, and PO_4^{3-}) by the action of osteoclastic acid dissolution. The rate of this dissolution can be markedly slowed by the adsorption of metabolite pyrophosphate or bisphosphonates.

with bisphosphonate salts such as etidronate, 3-amino hydroxypropylidene (APD) and dichloromethylene bisphosphonate (Cl_2MDP or clodronate) [32]. Appropriate bisphosphonate therapy can control the rates of bone accretion and dissolution in Paget's disease. Several research groups have focused their attention on different bisphosphonates and the structure-activity relationships among these. In the present discussion we will focus on eight different compounds which we have studied in our physicochemical models.

The structure activity of the bisphosphonate analogues is due to contributions from the two parts of the molecule. Although the so-called 'bioactive moiety' (R_2, Fig. 1) has an important share in the bisphosphonates' bone affinity, the 'bone hook' is the primary contributor to the bone affinity of these molecules. The so-called 'bone hook' itself can be modified by the substitution of different R_1 groups on the geminal carbon. As an example, we may consider the hydroxybisphosphonates

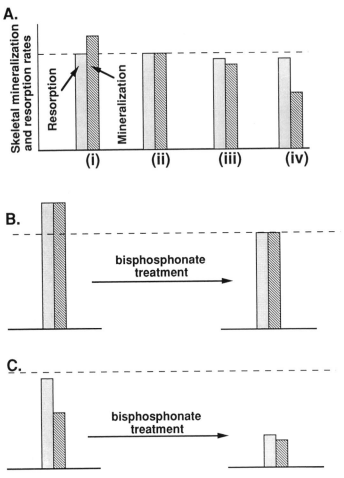

Fig. 3. a. The overall bone information (i) in youth, (ii) at peak bone mass in young adult, (iii) in healthy older adults, (iv) in postmenopausal and elderly adults. b. The overall bone turnover in (i) untreated and (ii) bisphosphonate-treated individuals with Paget's disease. c. The overall bone turnover in (i) untreated and (ii) bisphosphonate-treated osteoporotic individuals.

which are obtained when one substitutes an OH ion for R_1 in Fig. 1. This substitution increases the bone affinity of hydroxybisphosphonates relative to the simple bisphosphonate counterpart. The increased bone affinity is due to the tridentate adsorption of hydroxybisphosphonates (Fig. 4B) on the calcium of the HAP surface compared with the bidentate HAP adsorption (Fig. 4A) of the bisphosphonate molecule.

Alendronate, APD, risedronate, etidronate and clodronate are a few of the compounds that historically demanded much attention. The adsorption isotherms of the last three compounds are compared with each other in Fig. 5a, b and c, respectively. It is interesting to note that the bone affinity of risedronate and

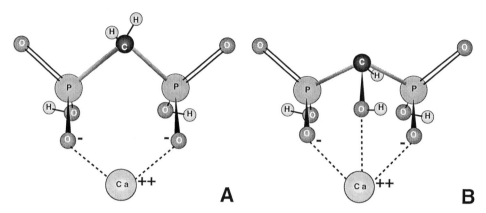

Fig. 4. a. Cartoon of bisphosphonate bidentate binding of calcium (Ca^{++}) in the hydroxyapatite (HAP) surface of bone mineral to the O$^-$ ions on each of the phosphorus (P) atoms of the planar 'W' of the bisphosphonates (O=P-C-P=O).
b. Cartoon of the tridentate binding of Ca^{++} involving in addition to the two O$^-$ groups (a), the hydroxy (OH) group attached to the planar 'W' (O=P-C-P=O) of the hydroxy bisphosphonate. The tridentate binding is stronger than the bidentate binding to the HAP surface.

etidronate is much greater than that of clodronate. This differing affinity can be attributed to the tridentate adsorption of the two hydroxybisphosphonates, risedronate and etidronate, versus the bidentate adsorption of clodronate on the bone mineral HAP surface. Figure 5 a and b also shows the bone affinity of didronel to be significantly greater than that of risedronate, which could be explained by steric factors that are contributed by the size of the 'R$_2$' group (Fig. 1a) on the geminal carbon. Since the 'R$_2$' substituent of risedronate is much bulkier than that of didronel, the adsorption of the former on HAP surfaces would be more sterically hindered than that of the latter. The divergence between the bone affinities of bisphosphonates could also be through contributions from their different calcium salts solubilities. In vitro, much like the in vivo experiments, these drugs encounter calcium ions both in solution and on bone mineral surfaces. It is important to note that adsorption and precipitation are two distinctly different physicochemical events. The calcium salt solubility of various bisphosphonates may be quite different, and the less soluble calcium bisphosphonate salts may actually precipitate in addition to adsorbing on the bone mineral surfaces.

In Fig. 6 the bone affinities of a bisphosphonate (BP) (Fig. 6a), a phosphonoalkylphosphinate (PAP) (Fig. 6b) and a bisphosphinate (BPI) (Fig. 6c) are considered. The 'bioactive moiety' (R$_2$) in these compounds is identical, but the phosphonate groups of the BP are alkyl substituted once (R$_3$=methyl and R$_4$=OH in Fig. 1b) and twice (R$_3$=R$_4$=methyl in Fig. 1b) in the PAP and BPI, respectively. The curves a, b and c in Fig. 6 reach a plateau with decreasing maximums on the Y-axis, respectively, which clearly shows that the substitution of a hydroxyl ion with the alkyl group (R$_3$=CH$_3$) causes a marked reduction in the bone affinity of the PAP compared with that of the BP. Additional alkyl substitution of a second hydroxyl ion in the PAP yields the BPI (R$_3$=R$_4$=CH$_3$) compound where the bone affinity

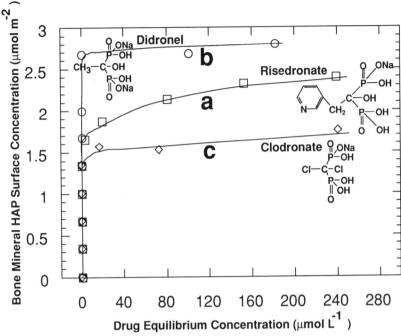

Fig. 5. Risedronate, didronel and clodronate structures and bone mineral hydroxyapatite (HAP) affinities (μmol m^{-2} HAP surface) at physiological concentrations as a function of their equilibrium solution
concentration (μmol L^{-1}).

has all but disappeared. Furthermore, both in vivo and in vitro physicochemical
experiments show the complete inactivity of both the tetraesterified bisphosphonate
(Fig. 1c) and BPI (Fig. 1b) in the treatment of bone loss.

Two BPs with identical 'bone hooks' and different 'bioactive moieties' were also
investigated. The results from their bone mineral adsorption isotherms, shown in
Fig. 7, re-emphasizes the involvement of the entire molecule, including the so-called
'bioactive moiety', in the bone affinity and the efficacy of the molecule. In Fig.
7 the compound with the lower HAP affinity (Fig. 7b) than 2-pyr BP (Fig. 7a)
is conformationally restricted. It is likely that the conformational restriction of
the former compound introduces steric hindrance for the adjacent molecules that
are adsorbed on the bone mineral's surface, resulting in its lower bone affinity.
However, 2-pyr BP molecules can pack more efficiently on the HAP structure, thus
allowing an increased bone affinity.

Using the dual constant composition method [25], the bone mineral growth
and resorption rates and the influence of different HAP surface concentrations of
risedronate on these rates were determined. The results from the bone mineral
HAP growth and resorption are given in Figs. 8 and 9, respectively. The inset
legends in these figures list the surface concentrations in risedronate, in μmol
m^{-2}, on the bone mineral HAP surface. At each risedronate surface concentration,

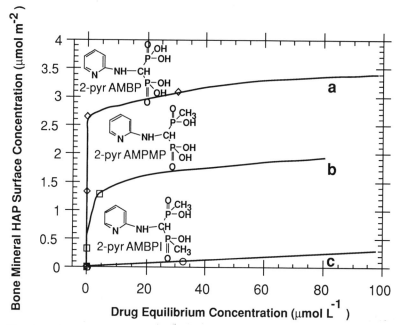

Fig. 6. N-(2-pyridinyl) methylene bisphosphonic acid [2-pyr AMBP], N-(2-pyridinyl) methylene phosphonomethylphosphinic acid [2-pyr AMPMP], and N-(2-pyridinyl) methylene bismethylphosphinic acid [2-pyr AMBP] structures and bone mineral hydroxyapatite (HAP) affinities (μmol m^{-2} HAP surface) at physiological concentrations as a function of their equilibrium solution concentration (μmol L^{-1}).

the mineralization and resorption rates (Figs. 8 and 9, respectively) are obtained from the slope of the corresponding line. Figures 8 and 9 illustrate the remarkable changes in the rate of HAP mineralization and demineralization as a result of changes in the concentration of risedronate on the HAP surface. The mineral growth and dissolution rates are considerably inhibited at risedronate HAP surface concentrations of 1.34 (Fig. 8) and 1.947 (Fig. 9) μmol m^{-2}, respectively. These risedronate HAP surface concentrations (Y-axis in Fig. 5a) are correlated with the risedronate equilibrium concentration (X-axis in Fig. 5a) well below 10 μmol L^{-1}. This suggests that an effective inhibition of the HAP mineral growth rate can be achieved at a risedronate equilibrium concentration of less than 10 μmol L^{-1}.

Although the BP serum concentration is the same as what the osteoblasts are exposed to in vivo, the resorbing osteoclasts may be exposed to a considerably greater BP concentration under their ruffled border. Our calculations, as well as those made by others [33], indicate that surface-adsorbed BP saturation levels on the bone particles result in concentrations as high as 50 μmol L^{-1} or more under the resorbing osteoclastic ruffled border. This differential between the BP serum level (<10 μmol L^{-1}) and the BP concentration in contact with the ruffled border of resorbing osteoclasts (>50 μmol L^{-1}) accounts for the huge differential in vivo between mineralization and resorption of over 1 to 200, respectively.

The results for the bone mineral HAP growth rates at different BP and PAP

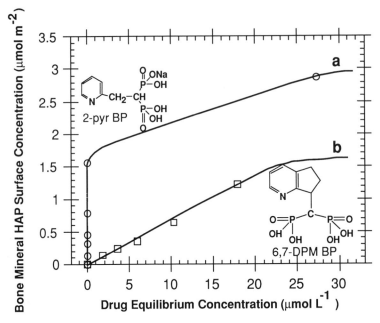

Fig. 7. Monosodium 2-(2-pyridinyl) ethylene bisphosphonate [2-pyr BP] and (6,7-dihydro-5H-1-pyrindine-7-yl) methylene bisphosphonic acid [6,7-DPM BP] structures and bone material HAP affinities (μmol m^{-2} HAP surface) at physiological concentrations as a function of their equilibrium solution concentration (μmol L^{-1}).

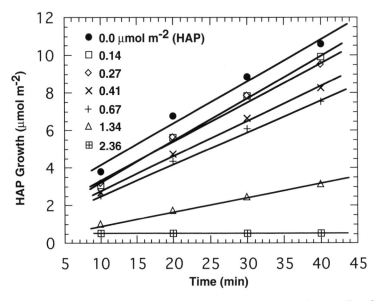

Fig. 8. Bone mineral HAP growth rates at different risedronate [monosodium 2-(3-pyridinyl) hydroxyethylidene bisphosphonate] surface concentrations (μmol m^{-2}) on HAP at physiological conditions.

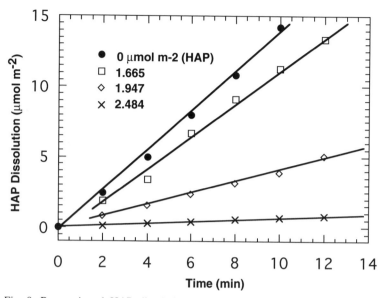

Fig. 9. Bone mineral HAP dissolution rates at different risedronate [monosodium 2-(3-pyridinyl) hydroxyethylidene bisphosphonate] surface concentrations (μmol m^{-2}) on HAP under physiological conditions.

Table 1.

Monosodium 2-(3-pyridinyl) hydroxyethylidene bisphosphonate [risedronate], N-(2-pyridinyl) methylene phosphonomethylphosphinic acid [2-pyr AMPMP], and N-(2-pyridinyl) methylene bismethylphosphinic acid [2-pyr AMBPI] inhibitory influence on the bone mineral HAP mineralization rates at different initial drug concentrations (μmol L^{-1}), and equilibrium in solution (μmol L^{-1}) and on the HAP surfaces (μmol m^{-2}). These in vitro experiments are conducted under physiological conditions.

Compound	Inhibition in HAP mineralization rate (%)	Initial concentration of additive in solution (μmol l^{-1})	Equilibrium conc. additive in solution (μmol l^{-1})	Equilibrium conc. additive HAP (μmol m^{-2})
Risedronate	17.82	60	0	0.41
	68.26	200	0	1.34
2-pyr AMPMP	20.84	60	0	0.40
	76.55	200	9.60	1.25
2-pyr AMBPI	26.15	690	535.04	1.04

concentrations are summarized in Table 1. There the values for the equilibrium concentration of BP, PAP and BPI in the solution are given in the fourth column. It is clearly shown that to obtain a similar HAP surface concentration (Table 1, column 5) of BP, PAP and BPI, the solution concentration of the PAPs and BPI should be significantly greater (many orders of magnitude; Table 1, column 4) than those of the BPs. Moreover, in these physicochemical models, the BPI is virtually inactive at equilibrium serum concentrations greater than 500 μmol L^{-1}.

III. Conclusions

Bisphosphonate and the phosphonoalkylphosphinate interaction with hydroxyapatite, resulting in adsorption on the surface of the inorganic crystals of bone, appears to be the primary mechanism involved in the medicinal and biological action of these compounds. Without significant adsorption of these drugs on the bone mineral, no biological activity is seen either in vivo or in vitro. Once adsorption has been accomplished, variations in the structure of the 'bioactive moiety' (R_2 groups in Fig. 1a) provides the additional changes in the adsorptive and biological activity. Thus, hydroxybisphosphonates such as etidronate and risedronate have an identical 'bone hook' but vary in anti-resorptive activity by about 200- to 1000-fold depending on the assay system. Structure-activity relationship studies are currently being carried out to help further elucidate the stereo-structural and other structural considerations in adsorption, and biological mineralization and resorption activities of bone. It is believed that with careful deliberations regarding the 'bone hook' and the 'bioactive moiety' of the drugs, it would be possible to further improve these classes of compounds in order to obtain even more effective drugs to combat diseases of the bone.

References

1. Von Beyer, H., Hofmann, K.S., Acitodiphosphonige Saure. Berichte, 1897, 30: 1973.
2. Blaser, B., Worms, K.H., Application of organic acylation products of phosphorous acids or their derivatives as complexing agents for metal ions. 1960; May 25, Henkel and Co., 1, 080, 235.
3. Francis, M.D., Briner, W.W., The effect of phosphonate on dental enamel in vitro and calculus formation in vivo. Calcif. Tissue Res. 1973; 11: 1–9.
4. Francis, M.D., Slough, C.L., Briner, W.W., An in vitro and in vivo investigation of melitate and ethane-1-hydroxy-1, 1-diphosphonate in calcium phosphate systems. Calcif. Tissue Res. 1977; 23: 53–60.
5. Briner, W.W., Francis, M.D., In vivo and in vitro calculation of anticalculus agent. Calcif. Tissue Res. 1973; 11: 10–22.
6. Herforth, V.A., Fligge, U., Strassburg, M., Clinical investigation on the reduction of calculus formation by the use of a toothpaste containing 1% EHDP. Dtsch. Zahnaertztl. 1977; 32: 757–759.
7. Bassett, C.A.L., Donath, A., Macagno, F., Preisig, R., Fleisch, H., Francis, M.D., Diphosphonates in the treatment of myositis ossificans. Lancet 1969; 2: 845.
8. Finerman, G.A.M., Stover, M.D., Heterotopic ossification following hip replacement or spinal chord injury. Two clinical studies with EHDP. Metab. Bone Dis. Rel. Res. 1981; 4 and 5: 337–342.
9. King, W.R., Francis, M.D., Michael, W.R., Effect of disodium ethane-1-hydroxy-1, 1-diphosphonate on bone formation. Clin. Orthop. 1971; 78: 251–270.
10. Francis, M.D., Diphosphonates: From old to new-dental calculus through arthritis. In: Russell, R.G.G. (Editor), Bisphosphonates. Current status and future prospects. IBC Technical Services Ltd., London, 1990.
11. Kasting, G.B., Francis, M.D., Retention of etidronate in human, dog, and rat. J. Bone Miner. Res. 1992; 7: 513–522.
12. Altman, R.D., Johnston, C.C., Khairi, M.R.A., Influence of disodium etidronate on clinical and laboratory manifestations of Paget's disease of bone (osteitis deformans). N. Engl. J. Med. 1973; 289: 1379–1384.
13. Smith, R., Russell, R.G.G., Bishop, M., Diphosphonate and Paget's disease of bone. Lancet 1971; 1: 945–947.
14. Ritch, P.S., Hypercalcemia of malignancy. In: Diphosphonates — The first decade. A symposium on diphosphonates in the management of metabolic bone disorders. Virginia Commonwealth

University, 1988, pp. 24–38.

15. Storm, T., Thamsborg, G., Steiniche, T., Genant, H.K., Sorensen, O.H., Effect of intermittent cyclical etidronate therapy on bone mass and fracture rate. N. Engl. J. Med. 1990; 322: 1265–1271.

16. Watts, N.B., Harris, S.T., Genant, H.K., Intermittent cyclical etidronate treatment of postmenopausal osteoporosis. N. Engl. Med. 1990; 323: 73–79.

17. Benedict, J.J., The physical chemistry of the diphosphonates — its relationship to their medical activity. In: Donath, A., Courvoisier, B. (Editors), Symposium CEMO, IV. Diphosphonates and bone. Editions Medicine et Hygiène, Geneva, 1983.

18. Ebetino, F.H., Kass, S.M., Crawford, R.J., Bisphosphonates: Molecular modeling, structure activity relationships and the rational design of new analogs. Phosphorus, Sulfur, Silicon 1993; 76: 151–154.

19. Ebetino, F.H., Dansereau, S.M., Bisphosphonate antiresorptive structure-activity relationships. In: Bijvoet, O.L.M., Russell, R.G.G. (Editors), Bisphosphonate therapy in acute and chronic bone loss. Elsevier Science Publishers, Amsterdam, pp. 1995; 139–153.

20. Boonekamp, P.M., van der Wee-Pals, L.J.A., van Wijk-van Lennep, M.M.L., Thesing, C., Bijvoet, O.L.M., Two modes action of bisphosphonates on osteoclastic resorption of mineralized matrix. Bone Miner. 1986; 1: 27.

21. Francis, M.D., Fogelman, I., ^{99m}Tc Diphosphonate uptake mechanism on bone. In: Fogelman, I. (Editor), Bone scanning in clinical practice. Springer-Verlag, London, 1987, pp. 7–17.

22. Francis, M.D., Webb, N.C., Hydroxyapatite formation from a hydrated calcium monohydrogen phosphate. Calcif. Tissue Res. 1971; 6: 335–342.

23. Christoffersen, J., Christoffersen, M.R., Kibalczyc, W., Andersen, F.A., A contribution to the understanding of the formation of calcium phosphates. J. Crystal Growth 1989; 94: 767.

24. Tomazic, B.B., Tung, T.S., Gregory, T.M., Brown, W.E., Mechanism of hydrolysis of octacalcium phosphate. Scanning Microscopy 1989; 3: 119–127.

25. Ebrahimpour, A., Zhang, J., Nancollas, G.H., Dual constant composition method and its application to studies of phase transformation and crystallization of mixed phases. J. Crystal Growth 1991; 113: 83–91.

26. Zhang, J., Ebrahimpour, A., Nancollas, G.H., Dual constant composition studies of phase transformation of dicalcium phosphate dihydrate into octacalcium phosphate. J. Colloid Interface Sci. 1992; 152: 132–140.

27. Langmuir, I., Evaporation, condensation and reflection of molecules, and the mechanism of adsorption. Phys. Rev. 1916; 8: 149–176.

28. Christoffersen, J., Christoffersen, M.R., Kinetics of dissolution of calcium hydroxyapatite IV. The effect of some biologically important inhibitors. J. Crystal Growth 1981; 53: 42–54.

29. Norde, W., Lyklema, J., Protein adsorption and bacterial adhesion to solid surfaces: a colloid-chemical approach. Colloids and Surfaces 1989; 38: 1–13.

30. Norde, W., Adsorption of proteins from solution and the solid-liquid interface. Adv. Colloid Interface Sci. 1986; 25: 276–340.

31. Siris, E.S., Paget's disease of bone. In: Murray, J.F. (Editor), Primer on the metabolic bone disease and disorder of mineral metabolism. Am. Soc. Bone Miner. Res., Kelseyville, 1990, 253–259.

32. Douglas, D.L., Tuckworth, T.L., Russell, R.G.G., Kanis, J.A., Preston, C.J., Preston, F.E., Preston, M.A., Woodhead, J.S., Effect of dichloromethylene diphosphonate on Paget's disease of bone and hypercalcemia due to primary hyperparathyroidism of malignant disease. Lancet 1980; i: 894–898.

33. Sato, M., Grasser, W., Endo, N., Akins, R., Simmons, H., Thompson, D.D., Golub, E., Rodan, G.A., Bisphosphonate action, alendronate localization in rat bone and effects on osteoclast ultrasctructure. J. Clin. Invest. 1991; 88: 2095–2105.

Bisphosphonate on bones
O. Bijvoet, H.A. Fleisch, R.E. Canfield and G. Russell (eds.)
© 1995 Elsevier Science B.V. All rights reserved.

CHAPTER 9

Bisphosphonate antiresorptive structure-activity relationships

Frank H. Ebetino and Susan M. Dansereau

Procter and Gamble Pharmaceuticals, Miami Valley Laboratories, P.O. Box 538707, Cincinnati, OH 45253, USA

I. Introduction

The elucidation and further development of the structure-activity relationships (SAR) in the bisphosphonate class of compounds has flourished during the past 10 years. The design of this relatively new class of medicinal agents has progressed steadily from alkyl-substituted bisphosphonates to bisphosphonates substituted with a range of heterocyclic and heteroatomic moieties. These new targets have resulted in a wider variety of bone actives, including potent antiresorptive agents. In addition, studies on the effect of variation of the P-C-P backbone of bisphosphonates have led to analogues of varied hydroxyapatite (HAP) affinity, calcium chelation and antimineralization properties.

Although the structure-activity relationships are now clearer, in general, the results of the studies to date have primarily confirmed the overall complexity and potential multiple mechanisms of action by which these interesting agents may be working [1]. This discussion will focus primarily on those key SAR trends which are believed to contribute most significantly to the overall antiresorptive potency of a given bisphosphonate analogue. The emphasis has been placed on those structural features that appear to contribute to the design of antiresorptive agents; however, it is recognized that it would be impossible to completely separate the features of the antiresorptive potency from other activities (such as antimineralization effects) in this series [2].

II. Early generation bisphosphonates

After the initial discoveries that alkyl bisphosphonates such as EHDP (1-hydroxyethylidene bisphosphonic acid) could effect the formation/dissolution of hydroxyapatite crystals in vitro and bone metabolism in vivo [3], the first SAR stud-

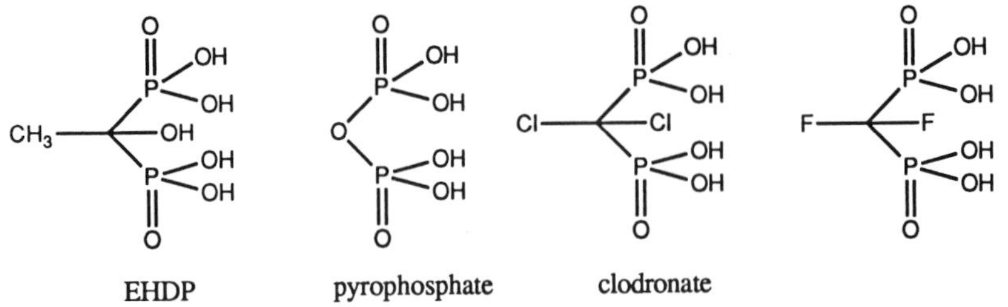

Fig. 1.

ies were undertaken. These studies were aimed primarily at modifying the geminal diphosphonate-substituted carbon by the attachment of a variety of heteroatomic moieties and alkyl chains. These substituents included halogens, amino, hydroxyl, thio and acetyl groups and C1–C20 alkyl chains. Disubstitution was studied in the case of the halogens, and the dichloro and difluoro members of this class received extensive attention (Fig. 1).

Good correlation was generally observed between crystal growth inhibition determined in vitro and inhibition of bone resorption and mineralization determined in vivo [4]. Those analogues that had increased capability for binding to the hydroxyapatite surface were better inhibitors of crystal growth and dissolution. For example, the geminal hydroxyl-substituted bisphosphonates possess high affinity for HAP and are also generally the most potent antiresorptive agents.

The difluoro-substituted methylene bisphosphonates were believed to be more electronically similar to pyrophosphate, and similarly an increased affinity for hydroxyapatite was noted [5,6]. An early discontinuity was the antiresorptive potency observed in vivo with dichloromethane bisphosphonate (clodronate). Although clodronate is a less potent inhibitor of crystal growth than EHDP (etidronate), it is more antiresorptive and is considered the first anomaly in the physicochemical means of predicting antiresorptive activity.

This early work resulted in the clinical application of etidronate disodium and clodronate for the treatment of Paget's disease. Etidronate (Didronel) is an advanced clinical candidate for the treatment of osteoporosis in the USA and is marketed widely for this indication in Europe [7,8]. It is the only member of this first generation of bisphosphonates to find global therapeutic utility [9a]. A number of new bisphosphonates are now under intensive clinical study. These second and third generation bisphosphonates are characterized by nitrogen functionality and increased antiresorptive activity.

III. The design of highly potent antiresorptive bisphosphonates

A discontinuity between crystal growth inhibition and antiresorptive potency became more evident with the discovery of the aminoalkyl-1-hydroxyl-1,1-bisphosphonic acid series. In this series, the compounds are hydroxyl-substituted bisphosphonates,

Table 1.

Compound		Growing Rat Model[a]
		LED[b]
APD pamidronate	NH$_2$ ... P structure	0.03
alendronate	NH$_2$ ... P structure	0.001
Dimethyl APD	(CH$_3$)$_2$N ... P structure	0.01
BM 21.0955	CH$_3$(CH$_2$)$_4$ / CH$_3$ N ... P structure	0.0001

[a] A measure of antiresorptive activity in the growing rat long bone.
[b] Lowest effective dose in mg P/kg

as is EHDP, and possess essentially equivalent affinities for hydroxyapatite. Although these compounds are equipotent inhibitors of crystal growth compared to EHDP, they are one to two orders of magnitude more antiresorptive in acute in vivo rat models [9b]. It should be noted at this point that the scope of this structure-activity discussion is intended to be one of general trends in antiresorptive potencies. It is not intended to be a comprehensive pharmacological review because of the numerous sources of structures and numerous methods of evaluation. However, where a generalization is made between two structures or classes, we have tried to compare data from the same model.

Notable early members of this class include current and past clinical candidates such as APD (pamidronate), alendronate, and dimethyl APD (Table 1). More recently, Boehringer Mannheim has discovered an extremely potent member of this class, N-methyl-N-pentyl APD or BM 21.0955 [10]. Early on, it was thought that the buffering capacity of the basic nitrogen functionality played a key mechanistic role. Research has now expanded to include a wider range of basic nitrogen moieties in search of optimal bisphosphonates for the mediation of bone resorption.

The next wave in SAR studies was approached from essentially two avenues. First, laboratories studying bisphosphonates simultaneously expanded their research to include nitrogen-containing heterocycles. A second approach sought to better

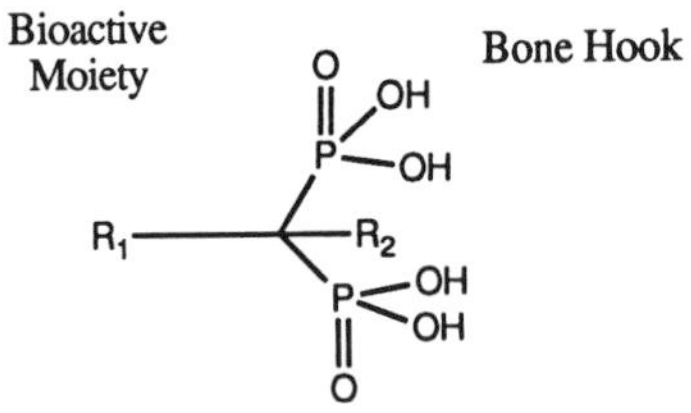

Fig. 2.

understand the biological effect of variation in the P-C-P moiety of the molecule. The primary focus in this regard was to widen the therapeutic index between undesirable antimineralization effects and the desirable antiresorptive potency. One theory that has evolved views the biological activity of bisphosphonates as being comprised of two design components. Molecules are viewed as having a 'bone hook' function (the moiety that is directly responsible for the primary HAP adsorption function) and a 'bioactive moiety' (the appendage that often includes basic nitrogen functionality and imparts varying antiresorptive potency within a given affinity class) (Fig. 2). Within this paradigm one could then attempt to custom design the two functions.

IV. Heterocyclic substituted bisphosphonates

The initial use of a variety of heterocycles included pyridyl substituents such as pyridyl aminoalkane bisphosphonates, pyridyl alkane bisphosphonates, pyridyl thioalkane bisphosphonates and pyridyloxoalkane bisphosphonates. Within the pyridyl-substituted series, crystal growth inhibition decreases in the order hydroxy bisphosphonates, aminomethylene bisphosphonates [$RNHCH(PO_3H_2)_2$], alkylidene bisphosphonates [$RCH(PO_3H_2)_2$], thiomethane bisphosphonates [$RSCH(PO_3H_2)_2$] to oxomethylene bisphosphonates [$ROCH(PO_3H_2)_2$] [11]. Some compounds in this series were found to be three orders of magnitude more potent than EHDP. For example, N-(2-(3-methyl)pyridyl)aminomethane bisphosphonate (NE-97220) was shown to possess a lowest effective dose of 0.001 mg P/kg/day in acute rat models [8]. A more complete list of antiresorptive potencies measured in the thyroparathyroidectomy (TPTX) model [12] and in the growing rat (GR) model are listed in Table 2.

Perhaps the most exciting member of the pyridyl bisphosphonate class was designed by combining the most potent bone affinity hook with this heterocyclic functionality. Thus, NE-58095, or 2-(3-pyridyl)ethane-1-hydroxy-1,1-bisphosphonic acid (risedronate), was found to have an acute potency of 0.0003 mg P/kg (growing rat). This compound has also proven useful for the inhibition of inflammation and bone resorption in the adjuvant arthritic rat at slightly higher dose levels, presumably through antiresorptive mechanisms as well [13]. All members of this series and the other heterocyclic-substituted 1-hydroxy alkane bisphosphonates,

Table 2.

Compound		TPTX[a]	Growing Rat Model[a]
NE-58095		0.001	0.0003
NE-97220		0.01	0.001
diazine AMBP		0.01	0.001
NE-97221		0.01	0.01
pyrAEBP		0.01	-
pyrSMBP		0.1	0.1
pyrOMBP		1.0	0.1

[a] Lowest effective dose in mg P/kg

from a physicochemical point of view, have the same affinity for hydroxyapatite and thus the same theoretical retention on bone and antimineralization capability at common higher doses. The increased antiresorptive potent analogues therefore provide an opportunity to treat patients with low levels of bisphosphonates and avoid the undesired antimineralization effects.

Other researchers have focused on the use of alternative heterocycles and amino-substituted alicyclic bisphosphonates such as compound 1 (Fig. 3) [14]. Heterocyclic substitution has included a variety of imidazoles, pyrazoles, oxazoles, fused bicyclics, pyrindines and quinolines [15, 16]. Interestingly, in the oxazole aminomethylene bisphosphonate series, the most potent analogue, YM-084, was optimized with a

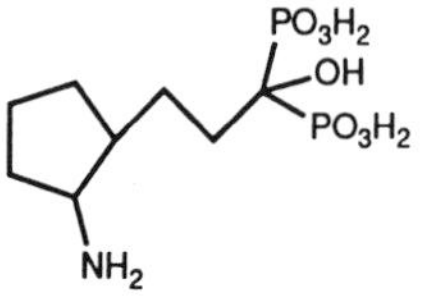

1

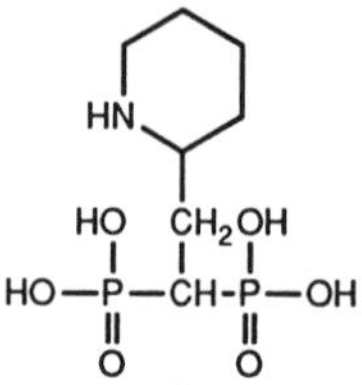

2

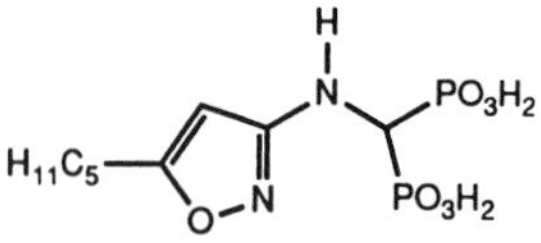

YM-084

Fig. 3.

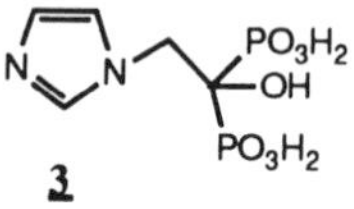

3

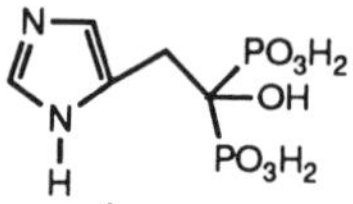

4

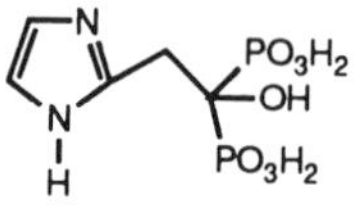

5

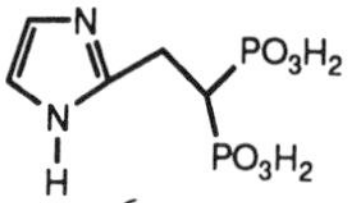

6

	3	4	5	6
TPTX ED$_{50}$ (ug/kg)	0.07	0.5	50	100

Fig. 4.

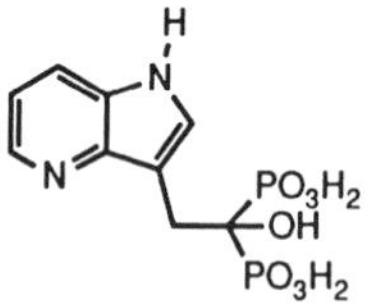

7

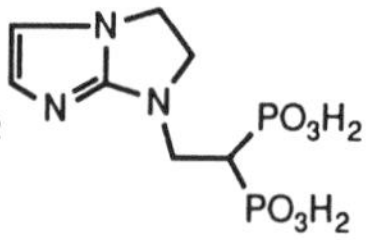

8

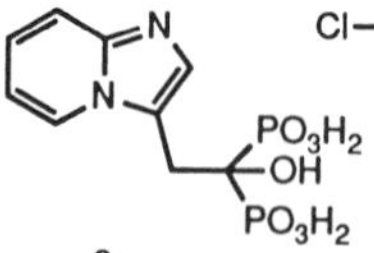

9

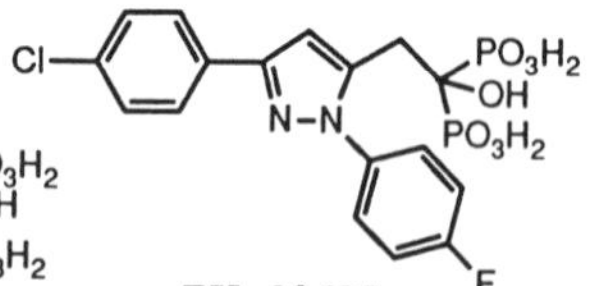

ZK 90695

	7	8	9
LED (TPTX)	0.0001 mgP/kg	0.3 mgP/kg	0.0001 mgP/kg

Fig. 5.

pentyl chain at C5 on the ring [15, 17]. These results suggest a lipophilic requirement for optimal bisphosphonate antiresorptive potency. It has also been demonstrated that the piperidine 2 and other piperidinylidene bisphosphonates are nearly as potent as their corresponding parent pyridine analogues [18].

For many of the new heterocyclic bisphosphonates the data have yet to be published. Preliminary antiresorptive data on the Ciba-Geigy imidazole series [19] has shown that compound 3 is more potent that the structural variants 4, 5 and 6 (Fig. 4).

The Yamanouchi company has recently disclosed a series of fused polyaza unsaturated bicyclic heterocycles 7, 8 and 9 [20]. Several of the compounds in which activity is reported are noted (Fig. 5). It has also been reported that the substituted pyrazole ZK 90695, an analogue of the antiinflammatory agent Pirazolac, demonstrates antiarthritic activity [21].

Non-nitrogen containing heterocyclic substitution generally provides bisphosphonates with less antiresorptive potency (LED > 1.0 mg P/kg) then the correspond-

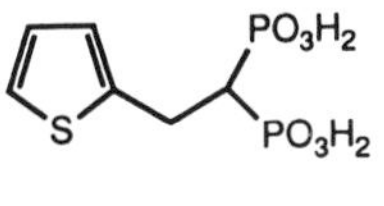

Fig. 6.

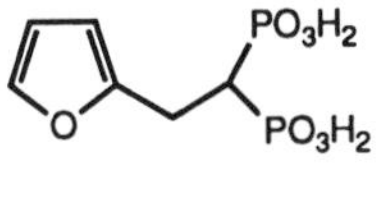

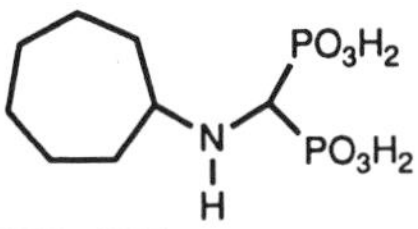

ing nitrogen containing heterocycles. Examples include 2-(2-thiophenyl)ethane-1,1-bisphosphonate 10 and 2-(2-furanyl)ethane-1,1-bisphosphonate 11 (Fig. 6). The most potent alkyl-substituted bisphosphonates discovered to date are the cycloalkane-substituted aminoalkane bisphosphonates. Researchers have found increasingly potent analogues by substitution of lipophilic hydrocarbons onto the aminomethylene bisphosphonate moiety. For example, YM-175 [22], or cycloheptane aminomethane bisphosphonate, demonstrated acute in vivo potencies as low as 0.001 mg P/kg. This series of compounds apparently optimize a lipophilic or hydrophobic interaction or a component of bisphosphonate antiresorptive potency [23].

V. Modifications in the P-C-P physical chemistry

1. Cyclic bisphosphonates

With first generation bisphosphonates, mineralization defects have closely paralleled antiresorptive potencies. Attempts to widen the index between the positive antiresorptive potency and negative mineral defects have followed generally one of two courses. Variations in the side chain, i.e. nitrogen-containing heterocycles (vida supra), have provided more potent antiresorptive analogues without a significant increase in mineralization defects. Another approach has sought to decrease mineralization defects by decreasing the hydroxyapatite affinity.

The first series that demonstrated leads in this regard was the cycloalkyl bisphosphonates. Early members of this series included saturated and unsaturated hydrocarbon ring systems. Representative examples include cyclopentane bisphosphonate, indan bisphosphonate, and hexahydroindan bisphosphonate [24]. Table 3 lists the antiresorptive potencies found in this series. Only the indan analogues reached potencies significantly lower than 1 mg P/kg. All members of this series did, however, demonstrate reduced affinity for bone in preliminary assays [25].

Finally, because a wider disparity between the hydroxyapatite affinity and the antiresorptive potency was desired in this structural class, attempts to find more potent inhibitors of resorption were made incorporating the heterocyclic functionality. With the discovery of high potency in the pyridyl alkane bisphosphonate class, the nitrogen-containing cyclic bisphosphonates were designed. Antiresorptive potency better than other non-nitrogen-containing cyclic bisphosphonates was not observed with these pyrindine analogues, including NE-58086, the quinoxoline bisphosphonate [26], and the azacyclopentane bisphosphonate (Fig. 7) [27].

Table 3.

	TPTX[a]	Growing Rat Model[a]
	NA[b]	NA
	0.50	1.0
	1.0	1.0
	1.0	0.1
	0.1	1.0

[a] Lowest effective dose in mg P/kg
[b] Not active

2. Bisphosphonate esters

Recently, workers at Upjohn published a new class of cyclic bisphosphonates with potential antiarthritic activity [28a]. No antiresorptive data are available yet in the class. This series is characterized by nitrogen functionality beta to the geminal bisphosphonate (Table 4). These bisphosphonates have been administered in preclinical animal models in the tetraester form [28b]. It is known that tetra-alkyl bisphosphonates do not possess affinity for hydroxyapatite. Since HAP binding is most certainly a component of the antiresorptive mechanism of action for bisphosphonic acids, the pyrazolindinones reported by Upjohn are either prodrugs for acids or owe their antiarthritic activity to a HAP-binding-independent mechanism.

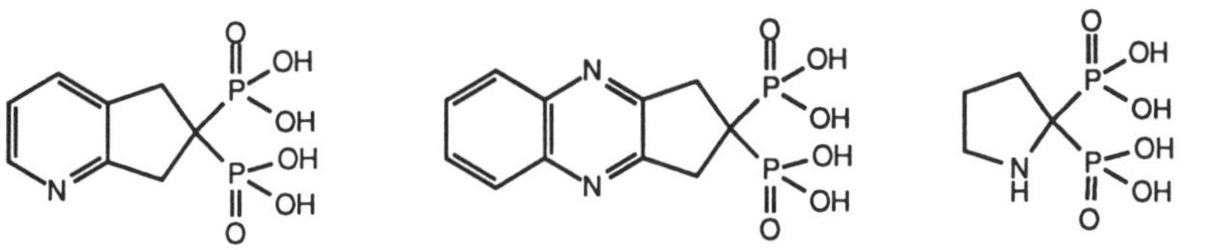

NE-58086 Quinoxoline BP Azacyclopentane BP

Fig. 7.

3. Phosphinic acid variations

Although numerous studies had been conducted on the modification of the P-C-P bond angles through geminal carbon substitution, until our recent work [29] bone metabolic studies had not been reported on analogues in which the phosphorus nucleus had been modified. To most effectively study the scope of variation within the 'bone hook' function of these molecules, we viewed varying the phosphorus nucleus as a necessary step in a rational drug design approach. For example, phosphinic acid substituents had not been screened for bone activity. As we began our study of phosphinic acid analogues, it became apparent that a reduction in bone affinity was likely because there is a reduced potential for tridentate hydroxyapatite binding. We anticipated the discovery of new pharmacology and new safety levels since theoretically a wider index between antiresorptive activity and mineralization defects could be obtained.

Early efforts in this approach led to the synthesis of members of the bisphosphinic acid series in which both phosphonic acid residues were modified as shown in

Table 4.

Effect of pyrazoline diphosphonates on a 28-day model of adjuvant-induced polyarthritis in male wistar rats

Hindpaw arthritis[a,b] compound	Dose (mg/kg)	Inhibition (%)
R = phenyl	15	38
R = cyclohexyl	15	14
R = tert-butyl	15	54
R = 3-fluoro phenyl	15	45

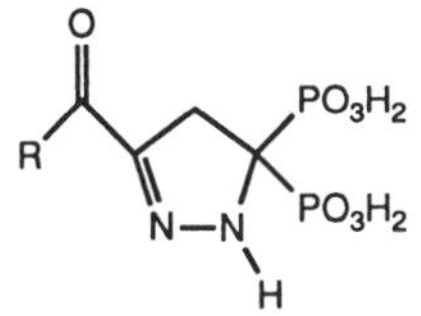

Pyrazoline Diphosphonate

[a] Compounds were administered subcutaneously, once daily for 28 days. The capacity of the test compound to affect hindpaw arthritis was quantitated with mercury displacement plethysmography.
[b] Data are the means of 10 to 20 rats.

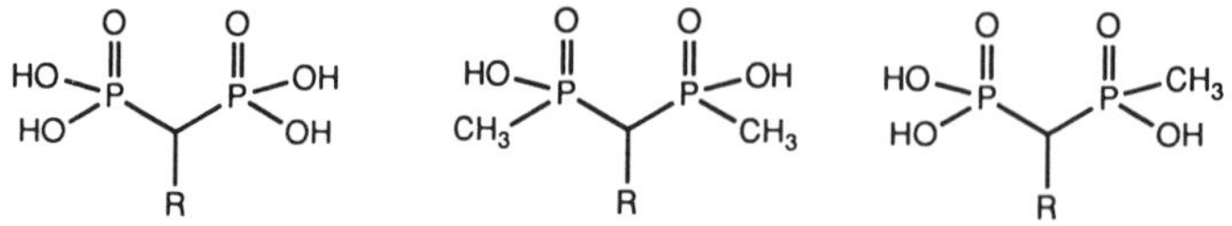

Bisphosphonate   Bisphosphinate   Alkylphosphonomethylphosphinate
                                                          (APMP)
                                              an alkylphosphonoalkylphoshpinate
                                                          (APAP)

Fig. 8.

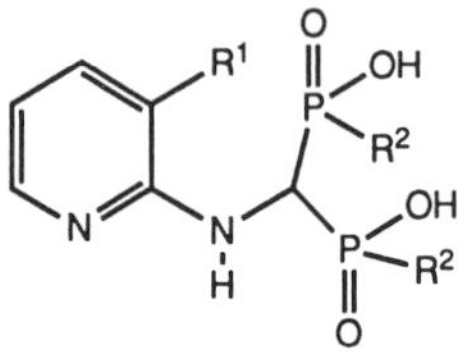

12 $R^1=R^2=CH_3$
13 $R^1=H, R^2=CH_3$
14 $R^1=CH_3, R^2=n$-butyl
15 $R^1=H, R^2=n$-butyl

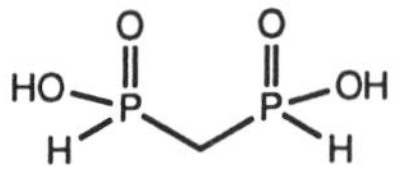

Methylenebisphosphonous acid
16

Fig. 9.

Figure 8. Drawing from one of the most potent antiresorptive bisphosphonate series, pyridyl aminomethane bisphosphinic acids were synthesized and screened. These compounds are characterized by extremely low HAP affinity properties relative to the bisphosphonates [4].

Bisphosphinic acids 12–15 (Fig. 9) were investigated in both the HAP crystal growth and antiresorptive assays. With the HAP-seeded crystal growth model, no inhibition of crystallization was observed with this series even at concentrations 100-fold higher than effective inhibitory doses for the corresponding bisphosphonates. We also studied representatives of this series in vivo and found them to be inactive even at levels of 10 mg P/kg (TPTX and GR models). To better understand the contribution of steric bulk to the inactivity of bisphosphinic acids, methylenebis-phosphonous acid 16, the sterically least demanding member of the class, was prepared. In the crystal growth inhibition model methylenebisphosphonous acid also demonstrated no activity.

Analogues intermediate in bone affinity relative to the bisphosphinates and bisphosphonates were designed [30]. One phosphorus moiety is a phosphinate [-P(O)(OH)(alkyl)], and one is a phosphonate [-P(O)(OH)$_2$] in the phospho-noalkylphosphinate (PAP) class. It was anticipated that analogues within this class would be discovered with high antiresorptive potency and reduced HAP binding. PAPs therefore provided an opportunity to widen the index between antiresorptive potency and antimineralization defects [26].

PAPs screened in vitro generally demonstrated reduced HAP affinity, and some analogues showed reduced antiresorptive activity in in vivo rat models, e.g. analogues 17 and 20 [29]. A tolerance for steric bulk may exist in the phosphinate alkyl substituent since the phosphononbutylphosphinate 19 and the phosphono-hexylphosphinate 21 inhibit crystal formation at comparable concentrations to the

Table 5.

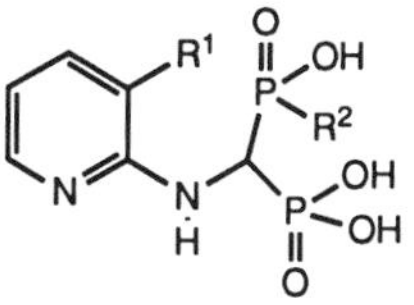

17 R^1=CH_3, R^2=CH_3
18 R^1=H, R^2=CH_3
19 R^1=CH_3, R^2=n-butyl
NE-97220 R^1=CH_3, R^2=OH

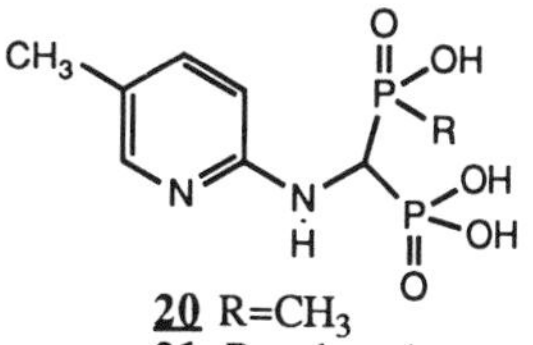

20 R=CH_3
21 R=n-hexyl
22 R=OH

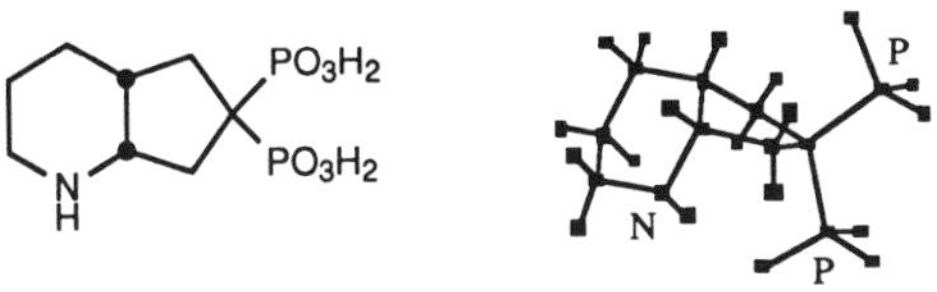

Fig. 10.

corresponding phosphonomethylphosphinates 17 and 20. For comparison, the inhibitory concentrations obtained for the corresponding bisphosphonate 22 and for NE-97220 are shown. Finally, an aminomethane phosphonomethylphosphinate has been tested at 100 mg P/kg in the acute growing rat model, and no antimineralization effects were observed [31], again suggesting that a wider index between antimineralization properties and antiresorptive properties may be available with this new 'bone hook' class. Work is in progress to better define the antiresorptive and P-C-P physicochemical properties of these agents [4].

V. A Receptor mechanism theory

The mechanism of action for the antiresorptive activity achieved with bisphosphonates is still unknown. Possibly a binding site for bisphosphonates (other than HAP) exists and mediates one of the potential mechanisms of antiresorptive potency. From a medicinal chemistry structure-activity point of view, the evidence is growing for this possibility. First, the wide range of potencies that have been obtained within a relatively structurally simple class of compounds is suggestive of such a receptor/binding site mechanism. Secondly, large potency variations observed from relatively minor structural modifications are suggestive of the involvement of a stereospecific recognition step in the mechanism of action. For example, compare the significant potency differences in the pyridylalkyl analogues 29 versus 30 and in the hydroxyl bisphosphonic acids NE-58095 versus NE-58051 (Table 6). Minor changes in chain length can dramatically affect the antiresorptive activity.

The structure-activity relationships of bisphosphonates are being studied using computer-aided molecular design techniques, as has been reported by at least two

Table 6.

Structure	TPTX LED in mg P/kg
29	0.01
30	NA[a] (10)
NE-58095	0.001
NE-58051	1.0

[a] Not active at 10 mg P/kg

laboratories. The recent discovery of the first highly antiresorptive potent cyclic BP, NE-58025, a conformationally restricted active bisphosphonate (LED=0.01 mg P/kg), proved to be an extremely valuable design tool in this regard [32]. Its 3D structure was elucidated by single crystal X-ray crystallography, and its solution conformation was demonstrated by 2D NMR techniques at physiological pH. The good correlation between the solid-state conformation and the solution conformation with this analogue provided a rigid template to design other predicted active and inactive analogues through conformational analysis (Fig. 10) [33].

Researchers at the Yamanouchi company [34] recently published a computational mapping of the geometry of the hydrophobic requirement for improved antiresorptive potencies. Also, they have found a 10-fold difference in potencies for two stereoisomers (Fig. 11).

As this type of work continues to offer rational design possibilities and to further our understanding of the bisphosphonate structure activity, additional evidence for the role of a stereospecific recognition event in the bisphosphonate mechanistic cascade may follow. The structure-activity to date continues to be consistent with

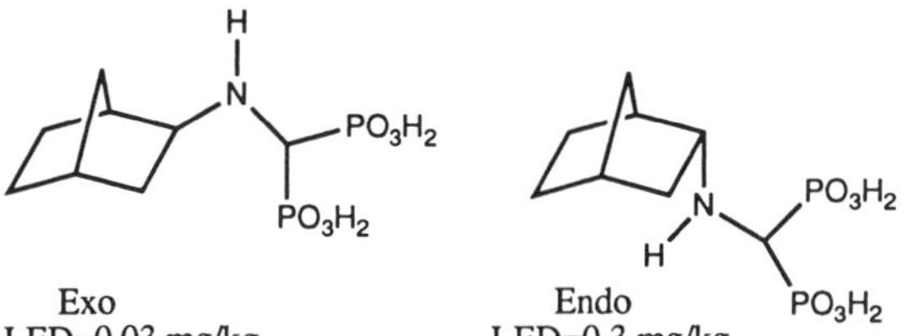

Exo
LED=0.03 mg/kg

Endo
LED=0.3 mg/kg

Fig. 11.

multiple mechanisms of action occurring with the bisphosphonates. Thus, probably no single descriptor exists to precisely predict the overall potency of each drug.

VI. Conclusion

The structure-activity data being published in the field has increased significantly in the last few years. In fact, with the growing evidence for the implication of receptors in the bisphosphonate mechanism of action, we may have only begun to 'scratch the surface' in our understanding of the SAR. For example, reports of some work in the field of peptido-bisphosphonates [35, 36] and other targeting examples have begun to appear in the literature but stretch beyond the scope of this report. Therefore, the design and synthesis of novel bisphosphonates for the treatment of bone resorption and other bone disorders have become a viable field in medicinal chemistry that should see important growth in the future.

References

1. Geddes, A.D., D'Souza, S.M., Ebetino, F.H., Ibbotson, K.J., Bisphosphinates: structure-activity relationships and therapeutic implications. In: Heersche, J.N.M., Kanis, J.A. (Editors), Bone and Mineral Research/8. Elsevier Science Publishers, London, 1994, pp. 265–306.
2a. Fleisch, H., Bisphosphonates: mechanisms of action and clinical use. In: Mundy, G.R., Martin, T.J. (Editors), Physiology and pharmacology of bone. Springer-Verlag, Berlin, 1993, pp. 377–418.
2b. Ebetino, F.H., Russell, R.G.G., Metabolic bone disease; current therapies and future prospect with bisphosphonates and other agents. In: Sarel, S., Mechoulam, R., Agranat, I. (Editors), Trends in medicinal chemistry '90. Blackwell Scientific Publications, Oxford, 1992, pp. 293–298.
3. Francis, M.D., Martordam, R.R., Chemical, biochemical and medicinal properties of diphosphonates. In: Hilderbrand, R.L. (Editor), The role of phosphonates in living systems. CRC Press, Boca Raton, 1983, pp. 55–96.
4. Sunberg, R.J., Ebetino, F.H., Mosher, C.T., Roof, C.F., Designing drugs for stronger bones. Chemtech 1991; 21: 304–309.
5. Blackburn, G.M., England, D.A., Kolkman, F., Phosphonates and bisphosphonates as analogues in biological chemistry: principals and practice. J. Chem. Soc. Chem. Commun. 1981; 17: 930–932.
6. Rowe, D.J., Hayes, S.J., Inhibition of bone resorption by difluoromethylene diphosphonate in organ culture. Metab. Bone Dis. Rel. Res. 1983; 5: 13–16.
7. Storm, T., Thamsborg, G., Steiniche, T., Genant, H.K., Sørensen, O.H., Effect of intermittent cyclical etidronate therapy on bone mass and fracture rate in women with postmenopausal osteoporosis. N. Engl. J. Med. 1990; 322(18): 1265–1271.

8. Watts, N.B., Harris, S.T., Genant, H.K., et al., Intermittent cyclical etidronate treatment of post-menopausal osteoporosis. N. Engl. J. Med. 1990; 323(2); 73–79.
9a. Sietsema, W.K., Ebetino, F.H., Bisphosonates in development for metabolic bone disease. Exp. Opin. Invest. Drugs 1994; 3(12): 1255–1276.
9b. Sietsema, W.K., Ebetino, F.H., Salvagno, A.M., Bevan, J.A., Antiresorptive dose response relationship across three generations of bisphosphonates. Drugs Exp. Clin. Res. 1989; XV(9): 389–396.
10. Bauss, F., BM 21.0955, monosodium salt, monohydrate. Drugs of the Future 1994; 19(1): 13–16.
11. Benedict, J.J., Perkins, C.M., inventors. The Procter and Gamble Company, assignee. Methods of treating diseases with certain geminal diphosphonates. US 4902679. 1990, Feb 20.
12. Fleisch, H., Russell, R.G., Francis, M.D., Disphosphonates inhibit formation of calcium phosphate crystals in vitro and pathological calcification in vivo. Science 1969; 165: 1264–1266.
13. Francis, M.D., Hovancik, K., Boyce, R.W., NE-58095: A diphosphonate which prevents bone erosion and preserves joint architecture in experimental arthritis. Int. J. Tissue React. 1989; XI(5): 239–252.
14. Boises, E., Gall, R., inventors. Boehringer Mannheim GmbH, assignee. Diphosphonic acid derivatives, processes for the preparation thereof and pharmaceutical compositions containing them. US 4719203. 1988, 1 12.
15. Boises, E., Gall, R., inventors. Boehringer Mannheim GmbH, assignee. Certain 1-hydroxy ethane-1,1-diphosphonic acid derivatives useful in treating calcium metabolic disturbances. US 4687767. 1987, 8 18.
16. Isomura, Y., Takeuchi, M., Abe, T., inventors. Yamanouchi Pharmaceutical Company Ltd, assignee. Heterocycle-substituted bis(phosphonic acid) derivatives and bone absorption inhibitors containing them. JP 02048587. 1990, Feb 19.
17. Abe, T., Kawamuki, K., Kudo, M., Ouchi, N., Isomura, Y., Takeuchi, M., Sakamoto, S., Murase, K., Kawashima, H., Biological activity of a new bisphosphonate, YM084, in animals [Abstract]. J. Bone Miner. Res. 1989; 4 (suppl. 1): S358.
18. Ebetino, F.H., Benedict, J.J., inventors. Norwich Eaton Pharmaceuticals Inc, assignee. Novel heterocycle-substituted diphosphonate compounds, pharmaceutical compositions, and methods of treating abnormal calcium and phosphate metabolism. EP 274158. 1987, 7 13.
19. Green, J.R., Jaeggi, K.A., Mueller, K., A new highly potent, anti-osteolytic bisphosphonate: CGP 42446 [Abstract]. J. Bone Miner. Res. 1990; 5 (suppl. 2): S79.
20. Isomura, Y., Takeuchi, M., Abe, T., inventors. Yamanouchi Pharmaceutical Company Ltd, assignee. Heterocyclic bisphosphonic acid derivatives as bone resorption inhibitors. EP 354806. 1990, Feb 14.
21. Hümpel, M., Günzel, P., Biere, H., Junginger, B., ZK 90695: A new antiarthritic drug with tissue targeting properties. Agents Actions 1991; 32(1/2): 22–23.
22. Isomura, Y., Takeuchi, M., Sakemoto, S., Abe, T., inventors. Yamanouchi Pharmaceutical Company Ltd, assignee. Preparation and testing of (cycloalkylamino)methylenebisphosphonic acids for use as bone resorption inhibitors, antiinflammatories, and antirheumatics. EP 325482. 1989, Jul 26.
23. Isomura, Y., Takeuchi, M., Kawamuki, K., Kudo, M., Abe, T., Fujita, S., Murase, K., The rational design of new bisphosphonates [Abstract]. J. Bone Miner. Res. 1990; 5 (suppl.2): S234.
24. Benedict, J.J., Johnson, K.Y., inventors. The Procter and Gamble Company, assignee. New cyclic diphosphonic acid compounds-useful for treating calcium and phosphate metabolism disorders. EP 189662. 1986, Aug 6.
25. Benedict, J.J., Degenhardt, C.R., Perkins, C.M., Johnson, K.Y., Bevan, J.A., Olson, H.M., Cyclic-geminal bis(phosphonates) as inhibitors of bone resorption [Abstract]. Calcif. Tissue Int. 1985; 38 (suppl.): S31.
26. Ebetino, F.H., Degenardt, C.R., Jamieson, L.A., Burdsall, D.C., Recent work on the synthesis of phosphonate-containing, bone-active heterocycles. Heterocycles 1990; 30(2): 855–862.
27. Ploger, W., Schmidt-Dunker, M., Gloxhuber, C., inventors. Henkel and Co. GmbH, assignee. Azacycloalkane-2,2-diphosphonic acids. US 3988443. 1976, 10 26.
28a. Dunn, C.J., Nugent, R.A., inventors. The Upjohn Company, assignee. Geminal bisphosphonic acids and derivatives as antiarthritic agents. WO 90/12017. 1990, Oct 18.
28b. Nugent, R.A., Murphy, M., Schlachter, S.T., et al., Pyrazoline bisphosphonate esters as novel antiinflammatory and antiarthritic agents. J. Med. Chem. 1993; 36: 134–139.
29. Ebetino, F.H., Jamieson, L.A., The design and synthesis of bone-active phosphinic acid analogues: I. The pyridylaminomethane phosphonoalkylphosphinates. Phosphorus Sulfur Silicon 1990; 51/52: 23–26.
30. Ebetino, F.H., inventor. Norwich Eaton Pharmaceuticals Inc, assignee. Methylene phosphonoalkylphosphinates, pharmaceutical compositions, and methods for treating abnormal calcium and phosphate

metabolism. EP 298553. 1989, 1 11.

31. Ebetino, F.H., McOsker, J.E., The design and discovery of a novel class of bone active agents: The aminomethane phosphonoalkylphosphinates [Abstract]. J. Bone Miner. Res. 1989; 4(suppl. 1): S165.

32. Ebetino, F.H., McOsker, J.E., Borah, B., Emge, T.J., Crawford, R.J., Berk, J.D., Studies on a potent new antiresorptive bisphosphonate class: cis-octahydro-1-pyrindine-6,6-bisphosphonic acid, NE-58025 and its analogues. In: Christiansen, C., Overgaard, K. (Editors), Proceedings of the Third International Symposium on Osteoporosis, Copenhagen, 1990; 3: 14–18.

33. Ebetino, F.H., Kaas, S.M., Crawford, R.J., Bisphosphonates: molecular modelling, structure-activity relationships and the rational design of new analogues. Phosphorus Sulfur Silicon 1993; 76: 151–154.

34. Takeuchi, M., Sakamoto, S., Yosida, M., Abe, T., Isomura, Y., Studies on novel bone resorption inhibitors. I. Synthesis and pharmacological activities of aminomethylene bisphosphonate derivatives. Chem. Pharm. Bull. 1993; 41(4): 688–693.

35. Benedict, J.J., Degenhardt, C.R., Poser, J.W., inventors. The Procter and Gamble Company, assignee. Diphosphonate-derivatized macromolecules. US 5011913. 1991, 4 30.

36. Boises, E., inventor. Boerhinger Mannheim GmbH, assignee. New N-peptidyl-amino-alkane-1,1-diphosphonic aid derivatives useful for treating disorders of calcium metabolism. US 4666895. 1985, 5 19.

Bisphosphonate on bones
O. Bijvoet, H.A. Fleisch, R.E. Canfield and G. Russell (eds.)
© 1995 Elsevier Science B.V. All rights reserved.

CHAPTER 10

Mechanisms of action of bisphosphonates: Studies with bone culture systems

Clemens Löwik and Gabri van der Pluijm

Department of Endocrinology and Metabolic Diseases, University Hospital, Leiden, The Netherlands

I. Introduction

Bone resorption can be increased by stimulation of the activity of existing mature osteoclasts and/or by increasing osteoclast number through enhanced recruitment from hemopoietic precursors (osteoclastogenesis). The latter involves a multistep process of osteoclast development including proliferation, chemotaxis and differentiation of early osteoclast progenitors into tartrate-sensitive acid phosphatase (TSAcP) postmitotic osteoclast precursors, further differentiation of these post-mitotic TSAcP cells into tartrate-resistant acid phosphatase (TRAcP) osteoclast precursors (terminal differentiation), and fusion of these TRAcP mononuclear cells with other precursors or existing osteoclasts into multinuclear, resorbing osteoclasts (see also Fig. 1). Furthermore, there is much evidence that all these processes are regulated by osteoblasts and/or bone marrow-derived stromal cells with osteogenic potential. Through the production of various cytokines and extracellular matrix

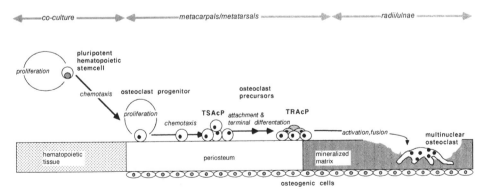

Fig. 1.

molecules, they provide the essential microenvironment for osteoclast formation and activity. In addition, osteogenic cells can also produce (and activate) several proteolytic enzymes (i.e. collagenase and plasminogen activators) which are not only involved in activation of certain locally acting cytokines (i.e. TGFβ and IGFs) but which can also regulate the initiation of resorption through mineral exposure by removing the unmineralized layer of organic material (osteoid). The fact that osteoclasts are only found in bony tissue, and are specialized in bone resorption, strongly suggests that their attachment, final differentiation and activation must be regulated by some 'bone specific signals' or 'solid phase cytokines' [1]. It seems most likely that these 'signals' are bound to the surface of the mineralized bone matrix which also forms the actual substrate of the osteoclast. These 'signals' might indeed be cytokines bound to extracellular matrix components like proteoglycans, although it is hard to imagine how this might create specificity towards the formation of an osteoclast phenotype since most cytokines have a pleiotropic action. It is more likely that this kind of signaling mechanism is involved in the regulation of early proliferation and differentiation steps in osteoclastogenesis. More conceivable candidates for the induction of the osteoclast phenotype are the extracellular bone matrix components themselves. One of the most abundant non-collagenous proteins is osteocalcin, which until now is the only real bone-specific protein known. It has been reported that osteocalcin (and its γ-Gla residues) can act as chemoattractant for possible osteoclast precursors and stimulate osteoclast attachment, differentiation and activation [2]. Several Arg-Gly-Asp (RGD)-containing proteins have been identified: fibronectin (FN), osteopontin (OP), bone sialoprotein (BSP), thrombospondin (TSP), and vitronectin (VN) [3, 4]. Their RGD sequence is recognized by specific cell surface receptors called integrins [5–7]. RGD-containing extracellular matrix molecules and their cellular receptors, the integrins, are needed for cellular attachment, spreading, migration, and terminal differentiation of cells. They are also involved in the homing of certain myeloid cells towards specific organs. Integrins might also be involved in the homing of osteoclasts or their precursors to bone. Studies with isolated osteoclasts and immunocytochemical evaluation in vivo have shown that a vitronectin-like receptor ($\alpha v \beta 3$) [8, 9] can be a mediator of osteoclast attachment to RGD-containing extracellular bone matrix molecules like osteopontin or bone sialoprotein [10]. In addition, recent evidence suggests that the RGD-containing proteins osteopontin and bone sialoprotein can also evoke immediate cell signals through the ($\alpha v \beta 3$) vitronectin receptor on osteoclasts which can activate the osteoclast [11]. With respect to these findings, it is interesting to note that osteopontin and osteocalcin can form specific complexes in vitro, which may be responsible for a bone-specific adhesion and differentiation of osteoclasts or their precursors [12]. After recognition and adhesion to the substrate, subsequent activation of the osteoclasts occurs. This is associated with polarization, formation of podosomes, a clear zone, and a ruffled border with proton pumps, followed by the start of the resorption process itself. The latter involves the release of protons and proteolytic enzymes, leading to a demineralization and digestion of the mineralized bone matrix [13].

II. In vitro studies of the mechanism of action of bisphosphonates

As described above, osteoclastic resorption is the final result of a series of complex sequential events. Therefore, in order to study the mechanism of action of bisphosphonates using in vitro assays, it is important to understand the characteristics of each assay system used. In the next paragraphs the most frequently used in vitro assays to study osteoclast formation and osteoclast activity will be discussed including their advantages and restrictions. We will also describe their application to study the mechanism of action of bisphosphonates. Moreover, in order to understand the relevance of the in vitro findings they should be compared with in vivo findings.

1. Monitoring of osteoclast activity

First, in vitro systems are described in which predominantly osteoclast activity is monitored and their application to study the effects of bisphosphonates.

(a) Macrophage- and osteoclast-mediated resorption of devitalized bone particles

Although macrophages are closely related to osteoclasts, it is now clear that mature macrophages, in contrast to mature osteoclasts, are unable to form resorption pits in thin slices of bone or dentine [14]. However, macrophages are able to demineralize ^{45}Ca-labeled bone particles (most probably by phagocytosis) and have therefore been used as a model system for osteoclastic resorption [15]. From studies using this system to test the potency of various bisphosphonates, it can be concluded that the activity of macrophages which ingest the bisphosphonate coated bone particles is inhibited. This inhibition is most probably caused by inhibiting cellular metabolism or through a cytotoxic effect since high doses are required and little specificity was found. Cl_2MDP was the most potent bisphosphonate, and there is accumulating evidence that Cl_2MDP acts predominantly through a cytotoxic mechanism [16, 17]. This property has now been applied by using liposomes containing Cl_2MDP to selectively eliminate all macrophages in vivo in order to study macrophage repopulation [18, 19]. The ability of liposome-encapsulated APD to decrease macrophages is far less potent than Cl_2MDP which is in line with findings of Reitsma who found that Cl_2MDP is more cytotoxic when ingested by macrophages [17].

When techniques became available to isolate enriched populations of osteoclasts, experiments investigating the effects of bisphosphonates on resorption of labeled devitalized bone particles were also performed. Carano et al. [20] showed that inhibition of chicken osteoclast activity was most effective when the bisphosphonates were bound to bone. In addition, they found that osteoclastic bone-binding capacity decreased by 30–40% after 72 h of bisphosphonate treatment, whereas resorption was inhibited > 90%. This led them to conclude that most of the inhibitory effects could not be due to their impact on cell-matrix attachment. They further showed that inhibition of bone resorption was only seen after 24–72 h of treatment and could be due to a reduction of proton accumulation in the resorption cavity.

They found, however, that relatively high concentrations of bisphosphonates in solution did not affect the ATP-dependent proton transport in inside-out plasma membrane vesicles. These observations and the finding that bisphosphonates inhibit protein synthesis in osteoclasts as well as in fibroblasts led them to conclude that bisphosphonates act predominantly as metabolic inhibitors with selectivity for osteoclasts resulting from high affinity binding of bisphosphonates to bone mineral. However, since the inhibition of resorption took at least > 24 h and was most prominent after 72 h, an effect on osteoclast formation contributing to the resorption cannot be excluded in these experiments. Although these studies show that bone-bound bisphosphonate can directly affect mature resorbing osteoclasts, the relative potency of different bisphosphonates to inhibit resorption in these systems was not similar to that found in vivo.

(b) The bone slice assay or pit formation assay

This assay [14, 21–26] is particularly suitable for the study of the activity and morphology of isolated mature osteoclasts and thus the resorption process itself. It comprises cell populations, enriched in osteoclasts, that are seeded on thin slices of dentine or bone. Osteoclasts can be isolated from various mammalian and avian sources [27]. Resorbing activity of individual osteoclasts is monitored microscopically by measuring pit formation (volume or area) or release of label from prelabelled bone slices [25]. Although much progress has been made, the main problem with the use of this system is related to the purity of the cell preparation, the viability of the isolated osteoclasts and the integrity of the cells at the end of the purification procedure (see for review [28]). The bone slice assay can be used to examine the effects of a variety of substances on the behavior of mature osteoclasts regarding attachment and resorption, but provides limited information on regulation of osteoclast differentiation and formation. From a practical point of view, for the qualification of pit volume or area, the bone slice assay requires expensive technical equipment and is fairly laborious.

Using the pit assay, Flanagan and Chambers [29, 30] have also shown that bisphosphonates are more effective inhibitors of osteoclastic resorption when bone slices are pretreated with bisphosphonate. They furthermore showed that bone-bound Cl_2MDP reduced the number of osteoclasts and their viability as shown by morphological features of cell injury and degeneration (retracted lamellipodia). This confirms that Cl_2MDP acts predominantly through cytotoxicity when ingested by osteoclasts.

Sato and Grasser [31] showed that APD, EHDP, and ABP inhibit the excavation of bone slices by isolated rat osteoclasts. A clear discrepancy was found between concentrations needed to obtain effective inhibition of resorption and toxic effects on mature osteoclasts. It was concluded that osteoclast elimination was not the mechanism of bisphosphonate action in the bone slice assay, but that bisphosphonates affect the cytoskeleton of osteoclasts. Osteoclast motility and 'ruffled' border formation and, thus, bone degradation were impaired. The fact that inhibition of osteoclastic resorption in this assay was already observed for one day led them to suggest that inhibition of osteoclast differentiation did not significantly contribute to their mechanism of action. Interestingly, they found that bisphosphonates, especially APD, at low concentrations (10^{-9} M) could even stimulate formation of resorption pits. Again, in these studies there was no clear correlation between relative in vitro and in vivo potency of the bisphosphonates to inhibit bone resorption.

In a more recent study it was shown in vivo that ^{3}H-alendronate (ABP) was not uniformly distributed in bone of newborn rats after 24 h after administration, but concentrated primarily under osteoclasts [32]. This is in contrast to earlier findings with Tc-labeled bisphosphonates, used as scintigraphic agents, which localize especially in areas of high bone formation [33]. An explanation for this discrepancy might be that these young rats have a very high bone turnover, which makes it possible that within 24 h a cycle of formation (when the bisphosphonate is bound) is already followed by resorption (when the analysis was performed). From their in vivo findings and studies with the pit formation assay, the authors hypothesize that alendronate binds to exposed hydroxyapatite of the bone matrix and is locally released in the resorption lacuna during acidification. Subsequently, the rise in bisphosphonate concentration (calculated to be around 1 mM) stops membrane ruffling and resorption, without destroying the osteoclasts. The local rise in bisphosphonate concentration causes, according to the authors, increased leakiness to calcium and probably other ions due to enhanced permeability of the osteoclast membrane. The increase in intracellular calcium concentrations is thought to be protective against irreversible damage to the osteoclasts since it is known that high Ca_i^{2+} concentrations can stop osteoclast activity [34].

Interestingly, another possible mechanism of action was recently described by Sahni and co-workers also using the pit assay [35]. They confirmed that bisphosphonates added to the mineral before addition of osteoclasts could very effectively inhibit resorption, but there was no correlation with the relative potency in vivo of the various bisphosphonates. When, however, the inhomogeneous osteoclast-enriched cell population (which also contains relatively large numbers of osteoblasts) was pretreated for only 5 min with bisphosphonates before allowing them to adhere onto the bone slice, the inhibitory effect was obtained at very low concentrations (as low as 10^{-11} M), but more importantly, the relative efficacies of the tested bisphosphonates closely paralleled their relative in vivo potencies. Furthermore, by using an osteoblastic cell line, which is a powerful promoter of osteoclastic resorption in vitro, they obtained evidence that this inhibitory effect of bisphosphonates was most probably mediated through an effect on osteoblasts rather than osteoclasts. They suggested that bisphosphonates somehow inhibit the production of an osteoblast-derived osteoclastic resorption-stimulating activity since the inhibition of resorption also occurred using conditioned medium of pretreated osteoblastic cells. Although the osteoclast/osteoblast cell preparation was only cultured for 24 h, after a 25-min settlement period on the bone slices, an effect on osteoclast formation cannot be excluded since the number of multinuclear osteoclasts was significantly increased in control cultures after 24 h, whereas the number of mononuclear TRAcP-positive cells was strongly reduced, suggesting that new osteoclast formation has taken place. In keeping with this are the recent findings of Fenton and co-workers [72] showing that indeed osteoclast differentiation and proliferation occur during the first 24 h of culture. They reported a 50–60% increase in the number of multin-ucleated TRAcP-positive cells between 2 and 24 h. Since Sahni et al. found that only Cl_2MDP significantly reduced the number of multinuclear osteoclasts without affecting the number of mononuclear TRAcP-positive cells, they suggested that the inhibition was independent of osteoclast formation. Unfortunately, no information on the number of osteoclast nuclei during culture was given, which is a much better indicator of osteoclast formation. The fact that the maximal obtainable inhibition was only around 65%, irrespective of which bisphosphonate was used, and could be further inhibited by calcitonin (which is a direct inhibitor of osteoclast activity!) to 96% strongly suggests that not only osteoclastic activity is inhibited. It therefore cannot be excluded that the pretreatment of the osteoblasts with bisphosphonates leads to inhibition of the production of an osteoclast-differentiation factor, which in fact would be in line with findings of Hughes et al. [62] and Löwik et al.[1] using different in vitro systems (described below).

(c) Bone organ cultures

Another method to study osteoclast biology in vitro is the bone organ culture system [36]. Pregnant mice or rats are injected with ^{45}Ca, and the prelabelled fetal long bones or fetal/neonatal calvaria are dissected and cultured in chemically defined medium. Osteoclastic resorption, measured as $\%^{45}Ca$-release combined with histological examination, can be studied in the presence of various factors. The bone explants used consist of various cell types, and during culture multiple sequential events take place. Many of the bone organ assays are, however, often poorly characterized. For a better understanding of the effects of factors and phar-macological compounds on the processes of osteoclast development and resorption (especially when ^{45}Ca-release is used as an endpoint), one should be aware of the characteristics of the system used. A very important question is, what is the stage of development of the osteoclast at the start of the experiment? What is the relative contribution of precursors and/or progenitors, which during culture develop into mature osteoclasts, to resorption (measured as ^{45}Ca-release), or is ^{45}Ca-release for the greatest part dependent on already present mature osteoclasts?

(d) Fetal radii or neonatal calvaria

The most widely used systems to study bone resorption are 19-day-old fetal rat radii and 2- or 5-day-old neonatal mouse calvaria [36]. In our laboratory, 17-day-old fetal mouse radii (see Fig. 2) are used, which are exactly at the same developmental stage as 19-day-old rat radii. In these systems, mature osteoclasts are already present at time of explantation, and ^{45}Ca-release is for the greatest part due to the activity of these resorbing mature osteoclasts and to some degree due to fusion and differentiation of late direct precursors. In line with this are the findings of Boonekamp and co-workers who have shown that removal of the periosteum of fetal rat radii, which is a source of osteoclast progenitors and precursors, had no significant effect on ^{45}Ca release [35]. Apart from this similarity between radii and neonatal calvaria, an important difference is that resorption in calvaria is largely dependent on endogenous prostaglandin synthesis, since resorption can be

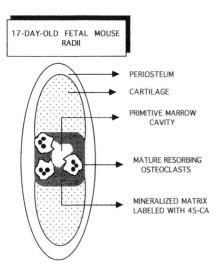

17-DAY-OLD FETAL MOUSE RADII

→ PERIOSTEUM

→ CARTILAGE

→ PRIMITIVE MARROW CAVITY

→ MATURE RESORBING OSTEOCLASTS

→ MINERALIZED MATRIX LABELED WITH 45-CA

RESORPTION IS ALMOST TOTALLY DEPENDENT ON:

MATURE FUNCTIONING OSTEOCLASTS.

Fig. 2.

inhibited by indomethacin [38]. This difference explains the contradictory findings of the effects of certain cytokines (i.e. TGFβ and LIF) on bone resorption.

In fetal rat radii [37] and neonatal mouse calvaria [39, 40], in which osteoclasts were already present at time of explantation, all tested bisphosphonates (EHDP, Cl$_2$MDP and APD) were found to inhibit the osteoclastic resorption at relatively high concentrations. Boonekamp found, using 19-day-old fetal rat radii, that Cl$_2$MDP was about 10 times more potent in this assay than the other two bisphosphonates, which did not reflect the relative differences in potencies in vivo. It was suggested that the inhibitory effect of bisphosphonates in this system, which only occurred at high concentrations, was predominantly due to impairment of cellular metabolism or cytotoxicity for mature resorbing osteoclasts ingesting bisphosphonate-bound bone. This was later confirmed by other studies described above.

2. Monitoring of osteoclast development

Now we will discuss systems in which osteoclast development can be studied and their application to study the effects of bisphosphonates.

(a) Fetal mouse metacarpals or metatarsals

One can take advantage of the fact that during embryonic development the degree of differentiation of tissues, including bones, not only proceeds in time but that there is also a gradual decrease in the degree of differentiation going from

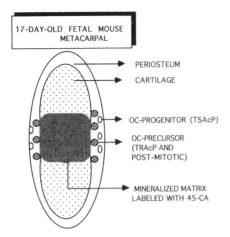

RESORPTION IS TOTALLY DEPENDENT ON:

DIFFERENTIATION, INVASION AND FUSION
OF OC-PRECURSORS INTO MATURE OCs.

Fig. 3.

proximal towards distal. For example, at day 17 of fetal development of the mouse, the radii and ulnae already contain mature resorbing osteoclasts which have already formed a primitive marrow cavity. In contrast, in metatarsals or metacarpals of the same animal, no mature osteoclasts are present in the mineralized matrix but only osteoclast precursors and progenitors which, however, are still confined to the periosteum (see Fig. 3). Bone resorption under basal conditions, measured as ^{45}Ca-release, in this system is totally dependent on the formation of mature osteoclasts from precursors present in the periosteum. These precursors still have to invade the mineralized matrix, differentiate, and fuse into mature, multinucleated, resorbing osteoclasts. We have shown that irradiation of these explants with a dose of 5 Gray totally abolished proliferation but had no effect on basal and PTH-stimulated resorption, indicating that only postmitotic events are involved [41]. This is in line with the findings of Scheven and co-workers [42]. However, TNFα-stimulated resorption could be totally abolished by irradiation, indicating that there are also resting osteoclast progenitors present in the periosteum which do not contribute to basal resorption but can be stimulated to proliferate by certain cytokines [41].

When bisphosphonates are applied in this system (see Table 1), resorption and multinuclear osteoclast formation can be blocked at much lower concentrations than those needed to block resorption in radii derived from the same animals. By applying irradiation (5 Gray) to block possible osteoclast progenitor proliferation, we showed that the inhibition of resorption by APD and Me$_2$-APD was independent of proliferation. Furthermore, the inhibitory effect of both bisphosphonates could be restored after addition of PTH, which also acts at a postmitotic level. These results show that the nitrogen-containing bisphosphonates tested and PTH have opposite actions that are both exerted at a postmitotic level in osteoclast formation.

Table 1.

Bisphosphonate	Mature OC Radii	OC-precursors/progenitors		$(= IC_{50radii/coculture})$
		Metacarpals	Coculture	
APD (pamidronate)	2×10^{-5}	5×10^{-6}	2.5×10^{-6}	8
Dimethyl-APD	5×10^{-5}	5×10^{-7}	5×10^{-7}	80
EB-1053	8×10^{-6}	5×10^{-7}	2.5×10^{-7}	32
NE-58025	10^{-5}	2×10^{-6}	7.5×10^{-7}	13
NE-58095 (risedronate)	8×10^{-6}	2×10^{-7}	8×10^{-8}	100
MK-217 (alendronate)	2×10^{-4}	2×10^{-7}	4×10^{-8}	5000
BM 21.09555	$> 10^{-5}$	n.d.	10^{-8}	> 1000

The reversibility of bisphosphonate-inhibited resorption by PTH also indicates that the inhibitory effect is not due to cytotoxicity [43,50]. A potential problem with the metacarpal/metatarsal system is the variability between experiments which is due to the exact time of mating and thus the exact stage of development of the explant (i.e day 17 early or late), which leads to differences in the proportion of osteoclast progenitors and precursors (own unpublished observation). This can be critical especially for factors which act only on the proliferation of osteoclast progenitors, leading to differences in responsiveness from experiment to experiment. However, apart from this drawback the use of 17-day-old fetal mouse radii/ulnae together with metacarpals/metatarsals of the same animals offers the opportunity to compare effects of compounds at different levels of osteoclast development [41, 44–48].

(b) Co-culture system

The co-culture system, originally developed by Burger et al. [49], is an extension of the metacarpal/metatarsal system, in that 17-day-old metacarpals or metatarsals can be made free of osteoclast progenitors and precursors by removing ('stripping') the periosteum with collagenase. These osteoclast-free explants can then be co-cultured together with hemopoietic tissue (fetal liver or bone marrow clots), which can serve as source of osteoclast progenitors or precursors (Fig. 4). Resorption in this system is totally dependent on osteoclast formation from pluripotent hemopoietic stem cells or very early progenitors. This system represents all sequential steps that lead to osteoclastic resorption and is therefore very suitable to study the process of osteoclastogenesis in more detail. Another advantage of the co-culture system is that the bone explant and/or the osteoclast precursor source can be separately pretreated before co-culture.

Boonekamp et al. [37] showed that 24-h pretreatment of 'stripped' bone explants with bisphosphonates could entirely prevent osteoclastic resorption of the mineralized matrix. When, however, treatment of the explant is postponed until after the development of mature osteoclasts, the bisphosphonate dose required for an inhibitory effect is increased 100-fold for the amino bisphosphonate APD, but not for Cl_2MDP and EHDP. It was concluded that high concentrations of all bisphosphonates inhibit the resorbing osteoclast but that low doses of the amino-bisphosphonate can specifically inhibit osteoclast formation. Pretreatment of the

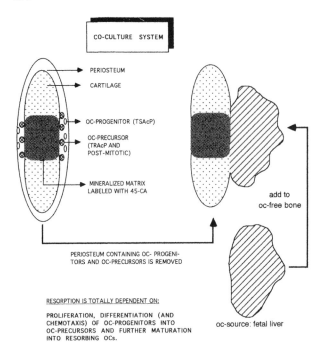

Fig. 4.

precursor source for 24 h had no effect on resorption after subsequent co-culture with untreated osteoclast-free bone explants. It was therefore not likely that bone resorption was inhibited by a direct cellular effect of bisphosphonates present in the medium. The observation that APD pretreatment of the osteoclast-free bone rudiments does not inhibit the resorption of that part of the cartilaginous matrix that is calcified after the start of the co-culture suggests that mineral-bound APD interferes with a signal from the calcified matrix that directs the accession of these osteoclasts. When the osteoclast-free bone explants were cultured together with a source of osteoclast progenitors/precursors but separated from each other by a filter with a pore size of 8 mm, cells migrated through the filter towards the calcified matrix and only acquired the characteristics of mature, TRAcP-positive osteoclasts upon direct contact with the bone explant [1]. This acquisition of TRAcP activity and subsequent resorption of the explant could be prevented by exposure of the system to the amino-bisphosphonate dimethyl-APD (Me$_2$-APD), whereas migration of cells through the filter was not affected. These findings suggest that the bisphosphonate does not affect migration of precursors but interferes with a matrix factor that is essential for the attachment and/or subsequent transformation of the osteoclast precursors into the mature phenotype (terminal differentiation and activation) [1].

Apart from differences in inhibitory action between amino-bisphosphonates and first-generation bisphosphonates (EHDP and Cl$_2$MDP), we have found that low doses ($< 5.10^{-7}$ M) amino-bisphosphonates, in contrast to Cl_2MDP and EHDP, can act synergistically with PTH and enhance osteoclastic resorption in the co-culture system [50]. We have recently found that this enhancement at low doses is associated with a strong increase in IL-6 production [51,73], which we have shown stimulates osteoclastogenesis [48]. This increase in IL-6 production was also found in osteoclast-free bone explants, indicating that this effect is mediated by osteogenic cells. This stimulatory action of amino-bisphosphonates at low doses in association with increased IL-6 levels might explain the in vivo observations in patients that only amino-bisphosphonates can induce a transient and small increase in temperature and acute-phase proteins, together with lymphopenia and a transient increase in urinary hydroxyproline [52, 53, 73]. The latter is indicative for increased resorption, whereas the others are indicative for increased IL-6 levels [54]. These phenomena occur in patients only during the first 24–48 h of treatment, probably when the concentration of the bisphosphonate on bone is still low, and disappear when higher concentrations and equilibrium have been reached. It would be interesting to study whether the effects are more pronounced in patients which receive the amino-bisphosphonate by a daily (2 h) infusion than in patients receiving just one high-dose bolus injection.

It is important to note that the co-culture system was the first system in which the relative potency of the tested bisphosphonates corresponded to their relative potencies in vivo. The predictive power of the co-culture system for its in vivo antiresorptive efficacy was also shown in a clinical protocol in patients with Paget's disease [55] as well as in a rat model [56]. In another study of our group, it was found that the amino group in the bisphosphonate structure is essential for its inhibitory action and that certain modifications, e.g. dimethylation (Me_2-APD), not only leads to increased potency but also to a decrease in (metabolic) side effects [57]. This finding has been the basic foundation of the development of new, more potent amino-bisphosphonates like EB1053, NE 58095, BM 21.0955, CGP42.446 and YM 175.

(c) The bone marrow culture system

For examination of osteoclast differentiation in vitro, the bone marrow culture system is widely used. Marrow cells, derived predominantly from mammalian sources, are currently used for studies of the effects of bone-resorbing or -inhibiting agents on the process of osteoclast differentiation. Marrow-derived multinucleated cells share many characteristics with real osteoclasts, including TRAcP activity, calcitonin receptors [58], and vitronectin receptors [59]. Besides the ability to study osteoclast-like cell formation, another advantage of the assay is its relative simplicity. However, there are also clear restrictions. One major problem is the fact that the natural substrate, bone or mineralized cartilage, is absent, and as a result osteoclast activation (resorption) cannot be determined. To overcome this problem, bone marrow can of course be seeded on bone slices and pit formation can be assayed, but this, however, is very tedious and time consuming. Secondly, the complex mixture of various cell populations hinders the identification of osteoclast precursors and progenitors. Culturing monoclonal subpopulations with their natural substrate (i.e. on bone slices or together with bone rudiments) may contribute to a better understanding of osteoclast biology, as was shown by Scheven et al. [60] and Hagenaars et al. [61].

The effects of bisphosphonates in solution on the formation of osteoclast-like cells from their mononuclear hemopoietic progenitors have been investigated by several investigators in long-term bone marrow cultures or bone-marrow-derived macrophages. In long-term cultures of human bone marrow, several bisphosphonates did not inhibit proliferation of progenitors of osteoclast-like cells, but strongly inhibited the $1,25(OH)_2D_3$-stimulated formation of osteoclast-like cells with the same relative potencies as in vivo [62]. These confirmed our findings using the co-culture system.

Cecchini et al. have studied the effects of bisphosphonates on the proliferation and viability of mouse bone-marrow-derived macrophages or nucleated bone marrow cells [63]. They postulated that mononuclear phagocytes, like bone-marrow-derived macrophages or their immediate precursors, can either act as a local pool of osteoclast precursors or act as accessory cells by the release of local factors and cytokines. These bone-marrow-derived macrophages were found to be very sensitive to bisphosphonates with respect to their (M-CSF-induced) proliferation. Since osteoclasts and macrophages might share a common early progenitor, the authors suggested that bisphosphonates may impair the replication of osteoclast progenitors. In a later report, they showed that bisphosphonates caused a dose-dependent and specific disappearance of macrophage colonies among the hemopoietic series, whereas polymorphonuclear phagocyte colony formation remained unaffected [64]. In these studies of Cecchini on macrophage proliferation, the relative potency of the various bisphosphonates tested also reflected their relative potency in vivo.

III. Interpretation and conclusion

For a meaningful interpretation of all the different in vitro findings, it is important to recognize the in vivo effects of bisphosphonates in time. When any bisphosphonate is given at an effective dose, inhibition of osteoclastic resorption (decrease in serum calcium and urinary hydroxyproline) can be measured 24–48 h after administration and decreases for a certain time until a new equilibrium is reached [53, 65, 66]. Establishment of this equilibrium is strongly dependent on the dose given [65]. Histological evaluation shows that initially (3–7 days) there is an increase in osteoclast numbers and an even larger increase in the number of nuclei per osteoclast, but these osteoclast are inactive and not attached to bone [67–69]. This direct inhibition of osteoclast activity is followed by a gradual decrease in osteoclast numbers [53, 69, 70]. The paradoxical initial increase in osteoclasts and their nuclei might be simply explained by a secondary transient increase in PTH levels in the serum leading to increased recruitment. Since the osteoclast precursors are not able to acquire TRAcP activity due to the matrix-bound bisphosphonate but are still able to fuse, this will lead to an increased number of inactive (less TRAcP-positive) osteoclasts. Since this increase in inactive osteoclasts seems to be due to a systemic counter-mechanism, this effect is not found in vitro. Another explanation for the initial increase in osteoclasts might be the transient increase in osteocalcin, found in APD-treated patients with Paget's disease, which has been shown to increase osteoclast recruitment [71]. Since the osteocalcin content in fetal bones is very low or even absent, this might explain why the effect is not found in vitro. A third explanation for the initial increase in multinuclear cells not attached to bone might be that per definition these cells are not osteoclast but multinuclear giant cells recruited, directly or indirectly, in response to a foreign agent, that is, bisphosphonate. This would be in line with the findings of Cecchini that APD or ABP treatment in mice leads to a strong increase in F4/80-positive macrophages, some of which are TRAcP-positive (personal communication). When this transient 'compensatory' response to inhibition of mature osteoclasts is over, the continued inhibition of new osteoclast formation will lead to a further decrease in osteoclast numbers. Concerning the structure-activity relation of bisphosphonates, as yet, it seems that there is no big difference between the various mineral-bound bisphosphonates in their capacity to inhibit osteoclast activity directly, whereas there is a great difference in their capacity to inhibit osteoclast formation, in that the N-containing bisphosphonates are the most potent.

In conclusion, all these various findings in vitro and in vivo appear very different when looked at separately, and suggest totally different mechanisms of action. When, however, studied in more detail and put into perspective, we can conclude that bisphosphonates, depending on their structure, dose, and way of application can inhibit bone resorption by a direct effect on the activity of osteoclasts and by an effect on osteoclast formation. As discussed, inhibition of these processes can be mediated either by osteoblasts or through the mineralized matrix.

References

1. Löwik, C.W.G.M., van der Pluijm, G., van der Wee-Pals, B., van Treslong-de Groot, H. and Bijvoet, O.L.M., Migration and phenotypic transformation of osteoclast precursors into mature osteoclasts: the effect of a bisphosphonate. J. Bone Miner. Res. 1988; 185: 185–192.
2. Lian, J.B., Osteocalcin: Functional studies and postulated role in bone resorption. In: Suttie, J.W. (Editor), Current advances in vitamin K research. Elsevier Science Publishers, Amsterdam, 1988, pp. 245–257.
3. Heinegård, D., Jirskog-Hed, B., Oldberg, Å., Reinholt, F.P. and Wendel, M., Bone macromolecules. In: Cohn, D.V., Glorieux, F.H. and Martin, T.J. (Editors), Calcium regulation and bone metabolism — basic and clinical aspects. Elsevier Science Publishers, Amsterdam, 1989, pp. 181–187.
4. Gehron-Robey, P., The biochemistry of bone. Endocrinol. Metab. North Am. 1989; 18: 859–902.
5. Albeda, S.M. and Buck, C.A., Integrins and other cell adhesion molecules. FASEB J. 1990; 4: 2868–2880.
6. Ruoslahti, E. and Pierschbacher, M.D., New perspectives in cell adhesion: RGD and integrins. Science 1987; 238: 491–497.
7. Ruoslahti, E., Integrins. J. Clin. Invest. 1991; 87: 1–5.
8. Davies, J., Warwick, J., Totty, N., Philip, R., Helfrich, M. and Horton, M., The osteoclast functional antigen, implicated in the regulation of bone resorption, is biochemically related to the vitronectin receptor. J. Cell. Biol. 1989; 109: 1817–1826.
9. Horton, M.A. and Davies, J., Perspectives: adhesion receptors in bone. J. Bone Miner. Res. 1989; 4: 803–809.
10. Reinholt, F.P., Hultenby, K., Oldberg, Å. and Heinegård, D., Osteopontin: a possible anchor of

osteoclasts to bone. Proc. Natl. Acad. Sci. USA 1990; 87: 4473–4475.

11. Miyauchi, A., Alvarez, J., Greenfield, E.M., Teti, A., Grano, M., Colucci, S., Zambonin-Zallone, A., Ross, F.P., Teitelbaum, S.L., Cheresh, D. and Hruska, K.A., Recognition of osteopontin and related peptides by an $\alpha_v\beta_3$ integrin stimulates immediate cell signals in osteoclasts. J. Biol. Chem. 1991; 266: 20369–20374.

12. Ritter, N.M., Farah-Carson, M.C. and Butler, W.T., Evidence for the formation of a complex between osteopontin and osteocalcin. J. Bone Miner. Res. 1992; 7: 877–885.

13. Vaes, G., Cellular biology and biochemical mechanism of bone resorption. A review of recent developments on the formation, activation and mode of action of osteoclasts. Clin. Orthop. Rel. Res. 1988; 231: 239–271.

14. Boyde, A., Ali, N.N. and Jones, S., Resorption of dentine by isolted osteoclasts in vitro. Br. Dent. J. 1984; 156: 216–220.

15. Teitelbaum, S., Stewart, C.C. and Kahn, A.J., Rodent peritoneal macrophages as bone resorbing cells. Calcif. Tissue Int. 1979; 27: 255–261.

16. Chambers, T.J., Diphosphonates inhibit bone resorption by macrophages in vitro. J. Pathol. 1980; 132: 255–262.

17. Reitsma, P.H., Teitelbaum, S.T., Bijvoet, O.L.M. and Kahn, A.J., Differential action of the bisphosphonates (3-amino-1-hydroxy propylidene)-1,1-bisphosphonate (APD) and disodium dichloromethylene bisphosphonate (Cl_2MDP) on rat macrophage-mediated bone resorption in vitro. J. Clin. Invest. 1982; 70: 927–933.

18. van Rooijen, N. and Nieuwmegen, R.V., Elimination of phagocytic cells in the spleen after intravenous injection of liposome-encapsulated dichloromethylene diphosphonate. Cell. Tissue Res. 1984; 238: 355–358.

19. van Rooijen, N. and Kors, N., Effects of intracellular diphosphonates on cells of the mononuclear phagocyte system: in vivo effects of liposome-encapsulated diphosphonates on different macrophage subpopulations in the spleen. Calcif. Tissue Int. 1989; 45: 153–156.

20. Carano, A., Teitelbaum, S.L., Konsek, J.D., Schlesinger, P.H. and Blair, H.C., Bisphosphonates directly inhibit the bone resorption activity of isolated avian osteoclasts in vitro. J. Clin. Invest. 1990; 85: 456–461.

21. Chambers, T.J., Revell, R.A., Fuller, K. and Athanasou, N.A., Resorption of bone by isolated rabbit osteoclasts. J. Cell. Sci. 1984; 66: 383–399.

22. Boyde, A., Dillon, C.E. and Jones, S.J., Measurement of osteoclastic pits with a tandem scanning electron microscope. J. Micros. 1989; 158: 261–265.

23. Arnett, T.R. and Dempster, D.W., A comparative study of disaggregated chick and rat osteoclasts in vivo; effects of calcitonin and prostaglandins. Endocrinology 1987; 120: 602–608.

24. Kanehisa, T.R. and Heersche, J.N.M., Osteoclastic bone resorption; in vitro analysis of the rate of resorption and migration of individual osteoclasts. Bone 1988; 9: 73–79.

25. de Vernejoul, M.C., Horowitz, M., Demignon, J., Neff, L. and Baron, R., Bone resorption by isolated chick osteoclasts in culture is stimulated by murine spleen cell supernatant fluids (osteoclast-activating factor) and inhibited by calcitonin and prostaglandin E_2. J. Bone Miner. Res. 1988; 3: 69–80.

26. Walsh, C.A., Beresford, J.N., Birch, M.A., Boothroyd, B. and Gallagher, J.A., Application of reflected light microscopy to identify and quantitate resorption by isolated osteoclasts. J. Bone Miner. Res. 1991; 7: 661–671.

27. Teti, A. and Zambonin Zallone, A., Osteoclasts isolation and culture. Workshop A of the 13th annual meeting of the American Society of Bone and Mineral Research 'Osteoclast Biology: Methods and Pitfalls', 1991, pp. 11–24.

28. Baron, R. and Chatterjee, D., Isolation and purification of osteoclasts for biochemical and molecular biological studies. Workshop A of the 13th annual meeting of the American Society of Bone and Research 'Osteoclast Biology: Methods and Pitfalls', 1991, pp. 1–10.

29. Flanagan, A.M. and Chambers, T.J., Dichloromethylenebisphosphonate (Cl_2MBP) inhibits bone resorption through injury to osteoclasts that resorb Cl_2MBP-coated bone. Bone Miner. 1989; 6: 33–43.

30. Flanagan, A.M. and Chambers, T.J., Inhibition of bone resorption by bisphosphonates: interactions between bisphosphonates, osteoclasts and bone. Calcif. Tissue Int. 1991; 49: 407–415.

31. Sato, M. and Grasser, W., Effects of bisphosphonates on isolated rat osteoclasts as examined by reflected light microscopy. J. Bone Miner. Res. 1990; 5; 31–40.

32. Sato, M., Grasser, W., Endo, N., Akins, R., Simmons, H., Thompson, D.D., Golub, E. and Rodan, G.A., Bisphosphonate action: Alendronate localization in rat bone and effects on osteoclast

ultrastructure. J. Clin. Invest. 1991; 88: 2095–2105.

33. Bisaz, S., Jung, A. and Fleish, H., Uptake by bone of pyrophosphate, diphosphate and their technetium derivates. Clin. Sci. Mol. Med. 1978; 54: 265–268.

34. Zaidi, M., Datta, H.K., Patchell, B., Moonga, B. and MacIntyre, I. Calcium-activated intracellular calcium elevation: A novel mechanism of osteoclast regulation. Biochem. Biophys. Res. Commun. 1989; 159: 68–71.

35. Sahni, M., Guenther, H.L., Fleish, H., Collin, P. and Martin, T.J., Bisphosphonate act on rat bone resorption through the mediation of osteoblasts J. Clin. Invest. 1993; 91: 2004–2011.

36. Stern, P.A. and Raisz, L.G., Organ culture of bone. In: Simmons, D.J. and Kunin, A.S. (Editors), Skeletal research and experimental approaches. Academic Press, New York, 1979, pp. 21–59.

37. Boonekamp, P.M., Van der Wee-Pals, L.J.A., van Wyk-van Lennep, M., Thesingh, C.W. and Bijvoet, O.L.M., Two modes of action of bisphosphonates on osteoclastic resorption of mineralized matrix. Bone Miner. 1986; 1: 27–40.

38. Lerner, U.H., Modifications of the mouse calvarial technique improve the responsiveness to stimulators of bone resorption. J. Bone Miner. Res. 1987; 2: 375–383.

39. Shinoda, H., Adamek, G., Felix, R., Fleisch, H., Schenk, R. and Hagan, P., Structure-activity relationships of various bisphosphonates. Calcif. Tissue Int. 1983; 35: 87–99.

40. Lerner, U.H. and Larsson, Å., Effects of four bisphosphonates on bone resorption, lysosomal enzyme release, protein synthesis and mitotic activities in mouse calvarial bones in vitro. Bone 187; 8: 179–189.

41. van der Pluijm, G., Most, W., van der Wee-Pals, L., de Groot, H., Papapoulos, S. and Löwik, C., Two distinct effects of recombinant human tumor necrosis factor-α on osteoclast development and subsequent resorption of mineralized matrix. Endocrinology 1991; 129: 1596–1604.

42. Scheven, B.A.A., Burger, E.H., Kawilarang-de Haas, E.W.M., Wassenaar, A.M. and Nijweide, P.J., Effects of ionizing irradiation on formation and resorbing activity of osteoclasts in vitro. Lab. Invest. 1985; 53: 72–79.

43. van der Pluijm, G., Modulation of osteoclastic resorption by bisphosphonates and cytokines. Thesis, Leiden, 1992.

44. Hoekman, K., Löwik, C.W.G.M., van der Ruit, M., Bijvoet, O.L.M., Verheijen, J.H. and Papapoulos, S.E., The effect of tissue type plasminogenactivator (tPA) on osteoclastic resorption in embryonic mouse long bone explants; a possible role for the growth factor domain of tPA. Bone Miner. 1992; 17: 1–13.

45. Slootweg, M.C., Most, W.W., van Beek, E., Schot, L.P.C., Papapoulos, S.E. and Löwik, C.W.G.M., Osteoclast formation together with IL-6 production in mouse long bones is increased by insulin-like growth factor I. J. Endocrinol. 1992; 132: 433–438.

46. Antonioli Corboz, V., Cecchini, M., Felix, R., Fleisch, H., van der Pluijm, G. and Löwik, C., Effect of macrophage colony stimulating factor (M-CSF) on in vitro osteoclast formation and bone resorption. Endocrinology 1992; 130: 437–442.

47. van Beek, E., van der Wee-Pals, L., van de Ruit, M., Nijweide, P., Papapoulos, S. and Löwik, C., Leukemia inhibitory factor inhibits osteoclastic resorption, growth, mineralization and alkaline phosphatase activity in fetal mouse metacarpal bones in culture. J. Bone Miner. Res. 1993; 8: 191–198.

48. Löwik, C.W.G.M., van der Pluijm, G., Bloys, H., Hoekman, K., Aarden, L.A., Bijvoet, O.L.M. and Papapoulos, S.E., Parathyroid hormone (PTH) and PTH-like protein (PLP) stimulate interleukin-6 production by osteogenic cells: a possible role of interleukin-6 in osteoclastogenesis. Biochem. Biophys. Res. Commun. 1989; 162: 1546–1552.

49. Burger, E.H., van der Meer, J.W.M., van de Gevel, J.S., Gribnau, G.C., Thesingh, C.W. and van Furth, R., In vitro formation of osteoclasts from long-term cultures of bone marrow phagocytes. J. Exp. Med. 1982; 156; 1604–1614.

50. van der Pluijm, G., Löwik, C.W.G.M., de Groot, H., Alblas, M.J., van der Wee-Pals, L.J.A., Bijvoet, O.L.M. and Papapoulos, S.E., Modulation of PTH-stimulated osteoclastic resorption by bisphosphonates in fetal mouse bone explants. J. Bone Miner. Res. 1991; 6: 1203–1210.

51. van der Pluijm, G., van Beek, E., Löwik, C. and Papapoulos, S., Involvement of IL-6 in modulation of osteoclastic resorption by bisphosphonates. J. Bone Miner. Res. 1990; 5 (suppl.2): abstr. 642, S234.

52. Bijvoet, O.L.M., Frijlink, W.B., Jie, K., van der Linden, H., Meyer, C.J.L.N., Mulder, H., van Paassen, H.C., Reitsma, P.H., te Velde, J., de Vries, E. and van der Wey, J.P., APD in Paget's disease of bone. Role of the mononuclear phagocyte system? Arthritis Rheum. 1980; 23: 1193–1204.

53. Harinck, H.I.J., Bijvoet, O.L.M., Blanksma, H.J. and Dahlinghaus-Nienhuys, P.J., Efficacious man-

agement with aminobisphosphonate (APD) in Paget's disease of bone. Clin. Orthop. Rel. Res. 1987; 217: 79–98.

54. Nijsten, N.W.M., de Groot, E.R., Ten Duis, H.J., Klasen, H.J., Hack, C.E. and Aarden, L.A., Serum levels of IL-6 and acute phase responses. Lancet 1987; 17: 921–923.

55. Papapoulos, S.E., Hoekman, K., Löwik, C.W.G.M., Vermeij, P. and Bijvoet, O.L.M., Application of an in vitro model and a clinical protocol in the assessment of the potency of a new bisphosphonate. J. Bone Miner. Res. 1988; 4: 775–781.

56. van der Pluijm, G., Binderup, L., Bramm, E., van der Wee-Pals, L., de Groot, H., Binderup, E., Löwik, C. and Papapoulos, S., Disodium 1-hydroxy-3-(1-pyrroliddinyl)-propylidene-1,1bisphosphonate (EB 1053) is a potent inhibitor of bone resorption in vitro and in vivo. J. Bone Miner. Res. 1992; 7: 981–986.

57. Boonekamp, P.M., Löwik, C.W.G.M., van der Wee-Pals, L.J.A., van Wyk-van Lennep, M. and Bijvoet, O.L.M., Enhancement of the inhibitory action of APD on the transformation of osteoclasts precursors into resorbing cells after dimethylation of the amino group. Bone Miner. 1987; 2: 29–42.

58. Mundy, G.R. and Roodman, G.D., Osteoclast ontogeny and function. In: Peck, W.A. (Editor), Bone and mineral research. Elsevier Science Publishers, Amsterdam, 1987, pp. 209–279.

59. Horton, M.A., Osteoclast-specific antigens. In: ISI Atlas of Science: Immunology. 1988; 1: 35–43.

60. Scheven, B.A.A., Visser, J.W.M. and Nijweide, P.J., In vitro osteoclast generation from different bone marrow fractions including a highly enriched haemopoietic stem cell population. Nature 1986; 321; 79–81.

61. Hagenaars, C.E., van der Kraan, A.A.M., Kawilarang-Haas, E.W.M., Visser, J.W.M. and Nijweide, P.J., Osteoclasts formation from cloned pluripotent hemopoietic stem cells. Bone Miner. 1989; 6: 179–189.

62. Hughes, D.E., MacDonald, B.R., Russell, R.G.G. and Gowen, M., Inhibition of osteoclast-like cell formation by bisphosphonates in long-term cultures of human bone marrow. J. Clin. Invest. 1989; 83: 1930–1935.

63. Cecchini, M.G., Felix, R., Fleisch, H. and Cooper, P.H., Effect of bisphosphonates on proliferation and viability of mouse bone marrow-derived macrophages. J. Bone Miner. Res. 1987; 2: 135–142.

64. Cecchini, M.G. and Fleisch, H., Bisphosphonates in vitro specifically inhibit, among the hematopoietic series, the development of the mouse mononuclear phagocyte lineage. J. Bone Miner. Res. 1990; 5: 1019–1027.

65. Reitsma, P.H., Bijvoet, O.L.M., Potokar, M., van der Wee-Pals, L.J.A., van Wijk-van Lennep, M., Apposition and resorption of bone during oral treatment with (3-amino-1-hydroxypropylidene)-1,1-bisphosphonate (APD). Calcif. Tissue Int. 1983; 35: 357–361.

66. Bijvoet, O.L.M., Vellenga, C.J.L.R. and Harinck, H.I.J., Paget's disease of bones: Assessment, therapy and secondary prevention. In: Kleerekoper, M. and Krane, S.M. (Editors), Clinical disorders of bone and mineral metabolism. Mary Ann Liebert Publishers, New York, 1989, pp. 525–542.

67. Miller, S.C. and Jee, W.S.S., The effect of dicloromethylene diphosphonate, a pyrophosphate analog on bone and cell structure in the growing rat. Anat. Rec. 1979; 193: 439–462.

68. Marie, P.J.H., Hott, M. and Garba, M.T., Inhibition of bone matrix apposition by (3-amino-1-hydroxypropylidene)-1,1-bisphosphonate (AHPrBP) in the mouse. Bone 1985; 6: 193–200.

69. Marshall, M.J., Wilson, A.S. and Davie, M.W., Effects of (3-amino-1-hydroxypropylydene)-1-bisphosphonate on mouse osteoclasts. J. Bone Miner. Res. 1990; 5: 955–962.

70. Chappard, D., Petitjean, M., Alexandre, C., Vico, L., Minaire, P. and Riffat, G., Cortical osteoclasts are less sensitive to etidronate than trabecular osteoclasts. J. Bone Miner. Res. 1991; 6: 673–680.

71. Papapoulos, S.E., Frolich, M., Mudde, A.H., Harinck, H.I.J., van de Berg, H. and Bijvoet, O.L.M. Serum osteocalcin in Paget's disease of bone: basal concentrations and response to bisphosphonate treatment. J. Clin. Endocrinol. Metab. 1987; 65: 89–94.

72. Fenton, A.J., Nicholson, G.C. and King, K., Osteoclast differentiation and proliferation occur during the first 24 hours of the isolated rat osteoclast assay. J. Bone Miner. Res. 1993; 8 (suppl.1): S383, abstr. 1064.

73 Schweitzer, D.H., Oostendorp-van de Ruit, M., van der Pluijm, G., Löwik, C.W.G.M., and Papapoulos, S.E. Interleukin-6 and the acute phase response during treatment of patients with Paget's disease with the nitrogen-containing bisphosphonate dimethylaminohydroxypropylidene bisphoshonate. J. Bone Miner. Res. 1995; (in press).

Bisphosphonate on bones
O. Bijvoet, H.A. Fleisch, R.E. Canfield and G. Russell (eds.)
© 1995 Elsevier Science B.V. All rights reserved.

CHAPTER 11

Mechanisms of action of bisphosphonates: Information from animal models

Roman C. Mühlbauer

Department of Pathophysiology, University of Berne, Murtenstrasse 35, CH-3010 Berne, Switzerland

I. Introduction

A great variety of animal models have helped the development of the bisphosphonates which are now used successfully in humans. In this chapter, the main in vivo techniques which were used to accomplish this task will be described. The discussion of the results will focus on the information obtained from in vivo models only. However, for a more detailed understanding of the mechanism of action of bisphosphonates, it is also necessary to consider other techniques, such as 'ex vivo in vitro' or 'in vitro', which are discussed elsewhere in this book. Since special chapters are devoted to the action of bisphosphonates on 'in vivo' mineralization and calcification, these topics have been excluded from this chapter. This also applies to the effect of bisphosphonates in tumour models and models of arthritis as well as to the topic quality of bone, i.e. bone strength.

The great majority of studies cited in this chapter were performed in the rat. This animal lacks Haversian bone remodelling, and for this reason, studies using the rat have been criticized for many years for generating results which are possibly irrelevant to man. According to our experience and that of many other investigators in the field, this is not the case. For example, clodronate efficiently inhibits 'immobilization osteoporosis' in rats [1]. This effect was confirmed in paraplegic patients [2]. Quantitative morphometric evaluation of the rat metaphysis has allowed the determination of differences in potency of various amino-bisphosphonates to inhibit bone resorption [3]. Similar differences were found in man [4]. Also as shown in Fig. 1, the range of effective doses as well as the relative potency of various bisphosphonates to inhibit arotinoid-induced hypercalcaemia in the rat (see below) and tumoural hypercalcaemia in patients was similar. These similarities in response between the rat and man are possibly due to the fact that a large part of human bone loss occurs through the thinning of trabeculae and compact bone, which is not a 'Haversian disease' [5]. Therefore, the rat is an adequate model to study

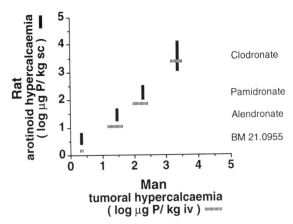

Fig. 1. Comparison of the range of effective doses of various bisphosphonates to inhibit hypercalcaemia in rats and man. The results for rats were obtained with the arotinoid test [14]. For the sake of comparison with human data, the total dose given during the whole assay period (3 days) was used. Fifty per cent inhibition of arotinoid-induced increase of plasma calcium was considered the lowest effective dose. For man the total dose of bisphosphonates necessary (single as well as multiple infusions) to lower calcaemia in tumour-induced bone disease, as summarized in [4], were used. The range of doses given as mg compound were transformed into µg P (phosphorus)/kg body weight, assuming a mean body weight of 70 kg. (Copyright R.C. Mühlbaner 1993, used with permission.)

modalities of prevention or treatment of bone loss, provided that an appropriate model is chosen and the limitations of the model realized.

II. Effect of bisphosphonates in intact animals with normal or stimulated bone resorption by the administration of low calcium diet

1. Effects assessed by histological techniques and microradiography

(a) Effect at the tissue level

In growing rats, treatment with bisphosphonates leads to a marked impairment of normal metaphyseal remodelling [3, 6–15]. In this condition, the resorption of columns of calcified cartilage as well as periosteal bone resorption are inhibited. This leads to a club-shaped, radiologically more dense appearance of the metaphysis. In growing rats, this effect can easily be visualized by microradiography after short-term treatment [6–11, 14].

Using quantitative morphometric evaluation of longitudinal sections of proximal rat tibiae, an increase in bone volume was found after treatment with etidronate [16]. In this system pamidronate was about 20 times more potent and alendronate 100 times more potent than clodronate in increasing trabecular bone volume [3].

The effects of bisphosphonates have also been investigated in a model of tooth (molar) drifting. A very high alveolar bone turnover occurs in this model, as molars drift physiologically at a rate of 6.7 μm per day. Bone resorption as well as bone formation occur at spatially well-defined sites, so that remodelling cycles can also be assessed [17]. Using this method, a strong inhibition of bone resorption was observed with clodronate and pamidronate. Clodronate inhibited alveolar bone resorption [18] and reduced the molar drift rate [19]. Interestingly, this effect was observed at a dose which did not inhibit resorption in vertebrae from the same animals [18].

When the longitudinal growth or the trabecular thickness was measured, it became evident that bisphosphonates may also inhibit bone formation [3, 16]. This effect varied according to the compound and dose investigated. Indeed, at low doses the inhibition of bone formation was absent or low, while it increased with increasing doses. The effect of bisphosphonates on bone resorption is, however, considerably larger than on bone formation, leading to a net gain in bone mass under these conditions.

The rat models reported so far were useful to describe the main effects of bisphosphonates. The advantage of these models is that the effects can be visualized already after 1 week of treatment, since they are amplified by the inhibition of growth-dependent metaphyseal remodelling. It should, however, be kept in mind that in rats at the age used and at the site investigated in these experiments, the remodelling by bone multicellular units (BMU, see Chapter 1) is not yet appreciable, and therefore the situation is different from that in adult man.

In the adult dog and sheep a significant amount of BMU-based bone remodelling occurs. Therefore, the effects of bisphosphonates on the trabecular bone remodelling dynamics can be investigated in these models.

In iliac crest biopsies from old sheep, 3 months of treatment with tiludronate leads to a marked decrease in osteoclast perimeter and activation frequency, indicating an inhibition of bone resorption [20]. In this model the treatment also induced a very large decrease in the tetracycline-based bone formation rate. Therefore, bone turnover was dramatically depressed, and it is not sure whether in these conditions a net gain in bone mass can be expected.

In adult dogs, risedronate also leads to a decrease in bone resorption as evidenced by reduced resorption depth and a large decrease in activation frequency [21]. Net bone formation, as shown by trabecular wall thickness, did not decrease but, on the contrary, increased somewhat. This effect was explained by the increase in the formation period observed. These results were obtained after 84 days of cyclic intermittent treatment. This is a relatively short period of treatment for adult dogs. Therefore, it is conceivable that the increased wall thickness may not reflect a permanent gain in trabecular bone mass but rather a transient phenomenon. Indeed, the coupling between bone resorption and bone formation does not occur immediately. If the eroded spots, at any individual BMU, fill up normally with new bone under bisphosphonate treatment but fewer new BMUs are created, a transient increase of trabecular bone mass may be observed. To provide conclusive evidence that bisphosphonates are also able to increase trabecular bone mass in intact adult dogs, it is essential that these results are further substantiated by those from a much longer treatment period.

(b) Effect at the cellular (osteoclast) level

In spite of a strong inhibition of bone resorption, large numbers of osteoclasts have been observed in rats treated with bisphosphonates for short periods of time [6, 8, 14, 19, 22–24]. Therefore, there is an apparent paradox between the inhibition of bone resorption by bisphosphonates and the number of osteoclasts found.

In growing rats osteoclasts remain physiologically associated with the same trabecular region during the whole short life-span of the tissue, i.e. for about 5 days [25]. Osteoclasts have been found all along and in close contact with the primary trabeculae in rats treated for 7 days with BM 21.0955 [14]. Thus, it is reasonable to assume that osteoclasts from these bisphosphonate-treated animals survived for 7 days and that they were distributed over the whole trabecular surface — the trabeculae growing in length — since they could not be resorbed due to a functional inhibition of the osteoclasts. Consequently, as a general rule, osteoclast counts per total area may not be a relevant parameter, but should be given as a function of the boundary length of the trabecular surfaces which might increase conspicuously under bisphosphonate treatment. The fact that usually the osteoclasts of bisphosphonate-treated animals are also larger than normal should be taken into account, too. Nevertheless, using these corrections, a significant increase in the trabecular surface covered by osteoclasts was still found with BM 21.0955 [14].

Osteoclasts from treated animals appeared morphologically abnormal and with more nuclei [6, 8, 9, 14, 22–24, 26, 27]. An increased rate of incorporation and accumulation of [^{3}H]-thymidine-labelled nuclei was found in treated animals [23]. Ultrastructurally, the osteoclasts in animals treated with etidronate and clodronate appeared functionally inhibited, as defined by smaller ruffled borders and a reduced number of cytoplasmatic vacuoles [8, 28]. Treatment with alendronate led to similar changes even in rats in which bone resorption was stimulated by infusion of PTHrP [29]. The osteoclast membranes were in close apposition to the bone surface, indicating that adhesion, as a partial indicator of viability, was not affected in these cells.

It was also found, at least in mice given pamidronate, that despite an increased number of osteoclasts and nuclei per cell, the number of acid phosphatase-stained osteoclasts was markedly reduced, suggesting a functional inhibition [26]. However, in rats given BM 21.0955, an important increase in tartrate-resistant, acid phosphatase-positive osteoclasts was found [14]. Thus, no general conclusion can be drawn. The result may depend not only on the type and dose of bisphosphonates, the age and species of the experimental animals used, and on the fact that no reliable histochemical marker of osteoclast activity is available yet, but also on the period of treatment chosen. Indeed, there is little doubt that bisphosphonates, when administered for a short period of time in vivo, increase the number of osteoclasts. However, long-term administration has led to conflicting results in that, after 140 days of treatment with etidronate and clodronate, osteoclast counts had not increased, and the bone surface covered with osteoclasts had markedly decreased [28]. This contrasts with the observation that after 13 weeks of treatment with YM 175, large numbers of osteoclasts were still found [30]. As shown in mice subjected to prolonged low-dose irradiation which destroys osteoclast precursor cells, osteoclast numbers are markedly decreased beyond 10 weeks of irradiation [31]. If extrapolated to the rat, this result does not support an inhibitory effect of YM 175 on osteoclast recruitment in vivo.

Osteoclast recruitment in vivo has also been investigated in a model using the early post-natal mouse caudal vertebrae. In the most distal vertebrae, primary ossification centres still develop after birth, and they are subsequently invaded by osteoclasts which have been generated by the proliferation and differentiation of progenitors. In this model, treatment with alendronate did not impair osteoclast generation but inhibited their activity after invasion of the calcified cartilage rudiment [32].

This body of evidence suggests that short-term treatment with submaximal doses of bisphosphonates does not seem to inhibit either osteoclast recruitment or their attachment to the bone surface in vivo. Osteoclast survival seems also not to be influenced. Therefore, the bisphosphonates investigated do appear to inhibit exclusively the activity of mature osteoclasts. Although the results from long-term treatment may indicate fundamental differences between compounds, the data need to be substantiated further to allow definitive conclusions to be drawn.

2. Effects of bisphosphonates on calcium metabolism as assessed by biochemical measurements

(a) Calcium balance studies

Balance studies are a valuable tool to assess whether bisphosphonate treatment leads to an increased retention of calcium in the whole animal. Such an increased daily retention of calcium has been observed for clodronate [33], for a low-dose [1 mg P (phosphorus)/kg body weight] of etidronate [33], for pamidronate [9] and very recently for BM 21.0955 (H. Fleisch, personal communication). With this technique, however, it is not possible to find out whether an effect is due to a change of resorption or formation of bone or both.

(b) ^{45}Ca kinetics

From a calcium balance study and the disappearance curve of intravenously injected ^{45}Ca in the same animal, many variables of calcium metabolism can be obtained by analysing the data according to a two-compartment model [33]. Among these, the rate of calcium flux into bone (bone formation) and out of bone (bone resorption) are the most relevant. ^{45}Ca kinetic studies represent one of the most complete methods of investigation of calcium metabolism in the rat.

Using this method, it has been found that a low dose (1 mg P/kg) of etidronate inhibits bone resorption significantly, with little effect on bone formation [33]. At a ten-fold higher dose, however, bone resorption as well as the flux of calcium into bone decrease dramatically. This decrease is associated with an increased urinary output as well as a reduced intestinal absorption of calcium, leading to a marked decrement in calcium retention. This high dose of etidronate inhibits mineralization [34] and decreases $1,25(OH)_2D_3$ synthesis. Treatment with this vitamin D metabolite prevents the fall in intestinal calcium absorption but fails to restore the defect in mineralization [35, 36], indicating that etidronate has a direct effect on this process.

Clodronate leads to a marked dose-dependent decrease in bone resorption and, to a lesser extent, of bone formation. This is associated with an increase of net intestinal calcium absorption and little change in urinary output [33]. Therefore, calcium retention increases by about 20% in rats treated with doses of 1 or 10 mg P/kg of clodronate.

Very recently, a similar increase of calcium retention (25%) has been observed with BM 21.0955, but at a 1000 times lower dose (H. Fleisch, personal communication).

(c) Time course to reach the maximal bisphosphonate effect

Based on the urinary excretion of hydroxyproline, it has been shown for pamidronate that the maximal effect is reached, depending on the dose, within 3–8 days after starting treatment. Thereafter the excretion remains constant [9].

Using the urinary excretion of [^{3}H]-tetracycline from chronically prelabelled rats as index of bone resorption, the maximal effect of daily administered clodronate is reached 4 days after starting treatment [37]. In the same system, but with a single injection of alendronate or BM 21.0955, the maximal effect also occurs after 4 or 3 days respectively [14, 37]. In the latter experiment the maximal effect persisted for the time of observation (4 and 5 days), indicating that a single administration of bisphosphonate is able to suppress bone resorption for a longer period than expected from its presence in blood. However, this is not surprising since, due to their bone-seeking properties, bisphosphonates are deposited in/on bone.

(d) Plasma calcium and calcium homeostasis

(i) In rats with sufficient dietary calcium supply The question arises whether bisphosphonates can adversely affect the homeostasis of plasma calcium by inhibiting bone resorption more than bone formation. Under conditions of normal dietary calcium supply, only a minor and insignificant decrease in plasma calcium at high doses of clodronate [33] and pamidronate [9] has been observed. When one of the bisphosphonates with prevailing inhibitory activity on bone resorption (1-hydroxypentane-1,1-bisphosphonate) was administered, a marked stimulation of the calcium balance, a rise in plasma $1,25(OH)^2D^3$ and intestinal calcium absorption were observed. Interestingly, this homeostatic response was not attenuated in thyroparathyroidectomized rats, indicating that PTH is not an essential mediating factor for stimulating $1,25(OH)^2D^3$ production as a response to an increase in skeletal mineral retention [38]. A similar response of serum $1,25(OH)^2D^3$ has also been found with clodronate and YM-175 [39] as well as BM 21.0955 (H. Fleisch, personal communication), indicating that most probably this homeostatic response applies for all bisphosphonates at doses which increase calcium balance.

Bisphosphonates which inhibit mineralization may lead to hypercalcaemia. This is a prominent finding at high doses of etidronate [33] and to a much lesser degree for other bisphosphonates known to inhibit crystallization in vitro [40, 41]. Since a close correlation has been found between the inhibition of mineralization and decreased intestinal calcium absorption with only a small increase in plasma calcium [40], this suggests that the decreased calcium absorption may also represent a homeostatic response to impaired mineralization.

There is also some evidence that the hour-to-hour calcium homeostasis may not be adversely affected in bisphosphonate-treated animals. A diurnal rhythm of bone resorption has been found in the rat by following the urinary excretion of [^{3}H]-tetracycline. Food intake was followed by a marked increase in bone resorption. Although bone resorption was considerably depressed by treatment with alendronate, the postprandial peak of bone resorption expressed as percent of the daily resorption was unchanged [37]. This suggests that an adequate modulation of bone resorption for calcium homeostasis still persists under bisphosphonate treatment.

(ii) In rats on reduced dietary calcium supply The issue of adequate plasma calcium homeostasis during treatment with bisphosphonates may be even more relevant in a situation of reduced calcium intake. Using ^{45}Ca kinetics, it has become evident that a progressive decrease in dietary calcium supply does not affect bone formation, but that bone resorption increases accordingly [42]. Animals treated with clodronate also respond to the lowering of calcium intake with an increase in bone resorption, but according to their reduced needs (bone formation), the response starts at a lower calcium intake. These results indicate that in this model, the powerful stimulation of bone resorption by low calcium diet can overcome the inhibition of bone resorption by clodronate, thus allowing adequate calcium homeostasis. In contrast, during lactation in rats on a slightly subnormal calcium intake, clodronate leads to a marked hypocalcaemia in spite of an important increase in serum 1,25(OH)^{2}D^3 [43]. However, although lactation produces a large drain of calcium into milk, calcium intake may still have been too large to challenge the clodronate-inhibited bone resorption. This view is supported by the finding that clodronate also completely prevents the bone loss associated with this condition. In another study, again using a low calcium diet but for 6 months, low doses of etidronate only partially prevented the bone loss, presumably indicating an adequate contribution of bone to the calcium homeostasis [44]. These discrepancies may indicate fundamental differences between the various models used.

Very recently, the issue of adequate calcium homeostasis under bisphosphonate treatment has also been investigated with the [^{3}H]-tetracycline technique. The response of bone resorption to a low calcium diet has been investigated in rats treated with clodronate and BM 21.0955 [45]. Although under basal conditions there was a strong inhibition of bone resorption by the bisphosphonate treatment, normal stimulation at low bisphosphonate doses and a small response at high bisphosphonate doses were induced by a low calcium intake. Presumably, the latter response is homeostatically adequate if the reduced bone formation at high bisphosphonate doses is taken into account. When the bisphosphonate treatment was discontinued, the low calcium diet induces a strong rise in bone resorption also in the rats which had previously received the high dose of clodronate but not those with BM 21.0955, indicating a difference in the persistence of the effect between the two compounds in this model.

III. Effect of bisphosphonates in models of pharmacologically and pathologically stimulated bone resorption

Bisphosphonates are effective in inhibiting bone resorption in models with locally induced resorption such as in paralysis induced by nerve severance, experimental periodontal bone loss [46, 47], post-extraction alveolar ridge resorption [48], and air pressure application to the middle ear [49]. Administration of PTH, PTHrP, $1,25(OH)^2D^3$, arotinoid, corticosteroids [50, 51] and heparin [52] as well as female and male castration led to the development of model systems suitable for studying bisphosphonate effects on systemically increased resorption. For tumour models see elsewhere in this book.

Since no clear cut structure-activity relationship for bisphosphonates has been found [41], a rational drug design is not yet possible. Therefore, reliable, rapid and potentially simple methods are needed, to allow a large number of compounds to be screened.

The remainder of this chapter will therefore be focussed on the information derived from 'screening' methods and from some animal models of osteopenia.

1. Stimulation of bone resorption in thyroparathyroidectomized rats by pharmacological means

In animal models in which pharmacological means are used to stimulate bone resorption, calcaemia has been used as an index of bone resorption. However, the measurement of calcaemia can be considered reliable only if PTH and calcitonin are excluded, i.e. the animals are thyroparathyroidectomized, and the flux of calcium from the intestine is negligible. This is achieved either by feeding the rats a low calcium diet or by overnight fasting before a blood sample is taken.

(a) PTH and PTHrP stimulated bone resorption

Early in the development of the bisphosphonates, it was found that clodronate could inhibit the hypercalcaemia induced by injections of parathyroid extract [53]. With this model, a large number of active compounds were identified [54–56]. By using modifications of this protocol, namely infusing either human or bovine PTH 1-34, the efficacy of clodronate was confirmed [57] and the potency of alendronate and YM 529 shown [58, 59]. Recently, the efficacy of pamidronate was further verified in the rat in a more sophisticated 'gene transfer' model of hyperparathyroidism [60]. Fibroblasts transfected with the human PTH gene were injected intraperitoneally and served as a continuous PTH release source. Hypercalcaemia and bone loss became evident 20 days after the injection. In this system a significantly higher bone mineral density was observed after treatment with pamidronate.

However, in animals treated with PTH, calcaemia may not be reliable as an index of bone resorption. Indeed, plasma calcium will be influenced by the stimulatory effect of PTH on the renal reabsorption of calcium. Although the known bisphos-phonates do not influence the renal handling of calcium directly, interference with this mechanism cannot be excluded for newly developed analogues. Furthermore, the fear exists that due to the renal effects of PTH, false-negative results may be generated.

How important the renal contribution can be has recently been shown in a study using PTHrP [61]. Bovine PTH as well as PTHrP shifted the relationship between urinary calcium excretion and plasma calcium, indicating an increased renal reabsorption. The correction of the PTHrP-induced hypercalcaemia by pamidronate was only partial, while a large effect was seen on urinary calcium excretion. This indicated that under these conditions, the renal reabsorption is an important determinant in the increase of plasma calcium. In a second study using this system, the potent effect of BM 21.0955 on bone resorption, as shown with fasting urinary calcium, was demonstrated, while only a slight effect on plasma calcium resulted. Also, this bisphosphonate did not affect the renal reabsorption of calcium enhanced with PTHrP [62].

(b) Arotinoid-stimulated bone resorption

Pharmacological means to stimulate bone resorption without the concomitant calcaemic effects of PTH have been investigated. A vitamin A analogue (ethyl *p*-[(E)-2-(5,6,7,8-tetrahydro-5,5,8,8-tetramethyl-2-naphthyl)- 1-propenyl]benzoate) efficiently stimulated bone resorption but was devoid of a stimulatory effect on renal calcium reabsorption [63]. Its action seems to be mediated by an increased osteoclast number, secondary to an increased proliferation of precursor cells, since irradiation of the rats prevented the hypercalcaemia. Bone formation was unchanged as assessed with ^{45}Ca kinetics. Due to these properties a screening method was developed in which this arotinoid replaced PTH. Because of its high sensitivity and reproducibility, the effect of bisphosphonates on bone resorption could be investigated with a much smaller number of animals than previously needed.

A large number of compounds have been screened [13, 14] and BM 21.0955 selected for further development. Dose-response curves indicate that BM 21.0955 is 10 times more potent than alendronate, 50 times more potent than pamidronate and about 500 times more potent than clodronate in inhibiting arotinoid-stimulated hypercalcaemia. Tiludronate was also found to be effective in this model [64].

The duration of the inhibitory effect of bisphosphonates was also investigated using this model. While alendronate remains effective 6 days after a single administration [65], about 50% of the initial effect is lost for clodronate and BM 21.0955 [14, 65]. This partial inhibition is, however, maintained for the following 13 days with clodronate and 10 days with BM 21.0955.

This screening method has proved to be very powerful in the detection of inhibitors of bone resorption. However, the question remains of whether the results can be extrapolated to man. Figure 1 shows a comparison of the range of effective doses of four bisphosphonates which inhibit hypercalcaemia in the rat and in man. The correlation found is excellent, indicating the usefulness of the arotinoid model. This good predictive value for doses effective in man, based on kg body weight, may exquisitely depend on the fact that bisphosphonates are not known to be metabolized in vivo. Thus, differences in metabolic rate between rats and man are probably not relevant.

(c) 1,25(OH)$_2$D$_3$ stimulated bone resorption

Very recently, CGP 42'446 was found to be the most active bisphosphonate so far investigated in a rat model, similar to the one described above, but in which hypercalcaemia was induced with 1,25(OH)$_2$D$_3$ [66].

Finally, pamidronate suppresses 1,25-(OH)$_2$D$_3$-induced hypercalcaemia in a long-term model. These experiments were performed in intact rats given very large doses of 1,25(OH)$_2$D$_3$. Hypercalcaemia was reduced 2 days after a single intravenous administration. This effect was still significant after 19 days [67].

2. Effect of bisphosphonates in models of osteopenia

(a) Effect of bisphosphonates in models of immobilization

Bone loss in one leg was induced in rats by nerve severance [1, 44, 59, 68–74], cutting ligaments of one hind limb [50], spinal cord section [75], and by maintaining animals in restrictive cages [76]. The effect of bisphosphonates on inhibiting bone loss was also investigated in a denervation model of the cat tail [77].

The mechanism by which immobilization leads to increased bone resorption and bone loss is still poorly understood. Many different mechanisms have been proposed. Recently, a strong increase in bone plasma flow was observed in paraplegic rats. This effect was progressive and was associated with an increase in vascular buds in the metaphysis. It has therefore been suggested that the increased blood flow is secondary to the change of vascular architecture at this site [75]. However, in spite of treatment with pamidronate, which prevented the resorption of trabecular bone, blood flow was still significantly higher, indicating that this was not secondary to increased bone resorption.

In the rat models described above, etidronate, clodronate, dimethylaminomethylene bisphosphonate, pamidronate, alendronate, YM 084 and YM 529 efficiently inhibited the loss of bone induced by immobilization, as assessed by ash weight, calcium or morphometric measurements. In some of these studies, the amount of bone found in the immobilized limb of bisphosphonate-treated animals even exceeded the bone mass of unimmobilized limbs of control animals, indicating that in growing rats, the effect of bisphosphonates stems partially from the impairment of normal metaphyseal remodelling. Indeed, when the bone loss as well as the bisphosphonate effect were compared in young (130–140 g) and old (400 g) rats, much smaller effects were observed in the latter [72].

In the denervated cat tail model, etidronate failed to inhibit the loss of bone [77]. Since also in another study, etidronate as well as clodronate were unable to inhibit the development of dietary-induced osteoporosis [78], cats are perhaps not suitable for this type of investigation.

(b) Effect of bisphosphonates on simulated weightlessness

As assessed with single photon absorptiometry on dissected bones, tail suspension of rats significantly decreased bone density at sites containing pure cortical as well as a mixture of cortical and trabecular bone in the unloaded hind limbs [79]. Treatment with alendronate led to an increased bone density even above control (unsuspended) levels. This finding was most prominent at the site where trabecular bone was also measured, but less at the cortical site. Again, this result is compatible with the view that these effects of bisphosphonate were partially due to the impairment of normal metaphyseal remodelling.

(c) Effect of bisphosphonates in models of female and male castration

Until now, ovariectomy has been most widely used. The great majority of studies were performed or started in growing rats [21, 44, 64, 80–85], fewer in 'adult' [86] or in 'aged', i.e. 1-year-old rats [21, 59, 87], in adult baboons [88–90] or dogs [91, 92].

As assessed by quantitative histomorphometry, ovariectomy induces increased bone turnover both with a concomitant loss in bone mass [80, 83, 84] or without net loss [81]. While etidronate provides only partial protection against bone loss [80], risedronate, alendronate and 2-(2-pyridinyl)ethylidene-1,1 bisphosphonate increase bone volume above that observed in non-ovariectomized rats [80, 81, 83]. Therefore, the same limitations apply to results from growing animals, as discussed previously in this chapter. It would be preferable if such experiments would be started at an age of about half a year, since physiologically growth in rats ceases at 29 weeks of age [93].

In a 1 week on, 3 weeks off treatment regimen, bands with dense cancellous bone alternating with poorly preserved trabeculae were observed. This indicates that the effect of risedronate was not maintained during the whole period without treatment and that only the trabeculae formed during treatment are protected from resorption during the treatment interval [80]. When the same total dose of alendronate is given in two or eight injections per month, the maximal effect for high doses appears to depend on the total dose given. On the contrary, for smaller doses the effect on trabecular bone volume is greater when the compound is given more frequently [83]. Similarly, for tiludronate the effect on bone mineral density is slightly higher with the continuous compared with cyclical treatment [86].

In an extensive study performed in adult ovariectomized baboons, alendronate prevented the decrease in trabecular bone volume and bone density at a low dose. At the high dose an increase in lumbar density was found at 6 and 12 months of treatment. At the latter time point the lumbar bone density of treated animals even exceeded that of non-ovariectomized baboons which had conspicuously risen during this time [88]. It is not clear whether this increase in bone density indicates accumulation of bone mass by still some growth or increased mineralization by reduced turnover. Indeed, theoretically if bone turnover decreases with ageing or with the effect of the bisphosphonate, the bone as a whole will become older and consequently more heavily mineralized.

In dogs, ovariohysterectomy leads to a marked increase in bone resorption as shown by an increase in erosion depth and loss of trabecular volume. This loss of bone was prevented by BM 21.0955 [92].

Castration of 1-year-old male rats leads within 4 months to a significant bone loss of trabecular and cortical bone in femurs, as assessed by microradiography. Since growth has ceased at this age, effects of bisphosphonates on the growth-dependent metaphyseal remodelling are not to be expected. Clodronate prevented the loss of bone at the proximal and distal end of femurs as well as in the diaphysis. The effect on ash weight was, however, only partial [94]. Tiludronate, given for 2 or 3 months, starting 1 month after castration, has been reported to be also effective in this model [65].

IV. Conclusion

A great variety of animal models assisted in the development of several bisphosphonates which are now successfully used in man as inhibitors of bone resorption. The overwhelming body of knowledge about the effects of bisphosphonates has been obtained from growing rats. It is feared that in young rats, the growth-dependent modelling drift and the lack of an appreciable amount of BMU-based turnover at this age may limit the relevance of the findings obtained from them. However, as discussed in this chapter, the information on the effects of bisphosphonates obtained from growing rats were not misleading. On the contrary, it appears that in growing rats, the effects of bisphosphonates are amplified by the inhibition of growth-dependent modelling. Therefore, these models may represent animal systems with an optimal cost/benefit ratio.

However, if the aim is the investigation of the effect of bisphosphonates on net bone gain, rats older than 6 months, adult dogs, baboons or sheep are the animals of choice.

Efficient animal models together with other techniques such as 'ex vivo in vitro' or 'in vitro' which allow particular mechanisms to be understood represent a promising strategy for future research on bisphosphonates.

Acknowledgements. I wish to thank Dr. M.G. Cecchini and Prof. H. Fleisch for critical review. Many thanks also go to G. Mühlbauer for typing the manuscript and retrieving the literature, to Dr. C.M. Lim-Taylor for correcting the English typescript, and to O. Aeby for the help with the illustration.

Received for publication, 15 January 1993.

References

1. Fleisch, H., Russell, R.G.G., Simpson, B. and Mühlbauer, R.C., Prevention by a diphosphonate of immobilization 'osteoporosis' in rats. Nature 1969; 223: 211–212.
2. Minaire, P., Bérard, E., Meunier, P.J., Edouard, C., Goedert, G. and Pilonchéry, G., Effects of disodium dichloromethylene diphosphonate on bone loss in paraplegic patients. J. Clin. Invest. 1981; 68: 1086–1092.
3. Schenk, R., Eggli, P., Fleisch, H. and Rosini, S., Quantitative morphometric evaluation of the inhibitory activity of new aminobisphosphonates on bone resorption in the rat. Calcif. Tissue Int. 1986; 38: 342–349.
4. Fleisch, H., Bisphosphonates: Pharmacology and use in the treatment of tumour-induced hypercalcaemic and metastatic bone disease. Drugs 1991; 42: 919–944.
5. Frost, H.M., Jaworski, Z.F.G. and Jee, W.S.S., On the rat model of human osteopenias and osteoporoses. Abstracts of the Second Workshop on Using the Live Rat in Skeletal Studies, 25th Annual Scanning Microscopy Meeting, Chicago, Illinois, USA, 11–14 May 1992, pp. 64–67.

6. Schenk, R., Merz, W.A., Mühlbauer, R., Russell, R.G.G. and Fleisch, H., Effect of ethane-1-hydroxy-1,1-diphosphonate (EHDP) and dichloromethylene diphosphonate (Cl_2 MDP) on the calcification and resorption of cartilage and bone in the tibial epiphysis and metaphysis of rats. Calcif. Tissue Res. 1973; 11: 196–214.

7. Miller, S.C. and Jee, W.S., The comparative effects of dichloromethylene diphosphonate (Cl_2MDP) and ethane-1-hydroxy-1,1-diphosphonate (EHDP) on growth and modeling of the rat tibia. Calcif. Tissue Res. 1977; 23: 207–214.

8. Miller, S.C. and Jee, W.S., The effect of dichloromethylene diphosphonate, a pyrophosphate analog, on bone and bone cell structure in the growing rat. Anat. Rec. 1979; 193: 439–462.

9. Reitsma, P.H., Bijvoet, O.L.M., Verlinden-Ooms, H. and van der Wee-Pals, L.J.A., Kinetic studies of bone and mineral metabolism during treatment with (3-amino-1-hydroxypropylidene)-1,1-bisphosphonate (APD) in rats. Calcif. Tissue Int, 1980; 32: 145–157.

10. Rowe, D.J., Effects of a fluorinated bisphosphonate on bone remodeling in vivo. Bone 1985; 6: 433–437.

11. Felix, R., Fleisch, H. and Schenk, R., Effect of halogenmethylenebisphosphonates on bone cells in culture and on bone resorption in vivo. Experientia 1986; 42: 302–304.

12. Benedict, J.J., Degenhardt, C.R., Perkins, C.M., Johnson, K.Y., Bevan, J.A. and Olson, H.M., Cyclic germinal bis(phosphonates) as inhibitors of bone resorption (Abstract 113). Calcif. Tissue Int. 1986; 38 (Suppl): S31.

13. Sietsema, W.K., Ebetino, F.H., Salvagno, A.M. and Bevan, J.A., Antiresorptive dose-response relationships across three generations of bisphosphonates. Drugs Exp. Clin. Res. 1989; 15: 389–396.

14. Mühlbauer, R.C., Bauss, F., Schenk, R. et al., BM 21.0955, a potent new bisphosphonate to inhibit bone resorption. J. Bone Miner. Res. 1991; 6: 1003–1011.

15. Pataki, A., Heizmann, H., Müller, K. et al., A histomorphometric study on the effects of the bisphosphonate compound CGP 42446 on rat bone (Abstract 11). Satellite Workshop of the XIth ICCRH Conference. Bisphosphonates — From the Laboratory to the Patient, Siena, Italy, April 29 and 30, 1992. Bone Miner. 1992; 17 (Suppl 1): S13.

16. Miller, S.C. and Jee, W.S., Ethane-1-hydroxy-1,1-diphosphonate (EHDP). Effects on growth and modeling of the rat tibia. Calcif. Tissue Res. 1975; 18: 215–231.

17. Vignery, A. and Baron, R., Dynamic histomorphometry of alveolar bone remodeling in the adult rat. Anat. Rec. 1980; 196: 191–200.

18. Vignery, A. and Baron, R., Comparative effects of APD and Cl2MDP on bone in the rat: In vivo and in vitro studies. Metab. Bone Dis. Rel. Res. 1980; 2 S: 381–387.

19. Hardt, A.B., Bisphosphonate effects on alveolar bone during rat molar drifting. J. Dent. Res. 1988; 67: 1430–1433.

20. Delmas, P.D., Vergnaud, P., Arlot, M.E., Pastoureau, P. and Meunier, J., The in vivo anabolic effect of hPTH-(1-34) is blunted when bone resorption is blocked by a bisphosphonate (Abstract 214). Thirteenth Annual Meeting of the American Society for Bone and Mineral Research, San Diego, California, August 24-28, 1991. J. Bone Miner. Res. 1991; 6 (Suppl 1): S136.

21. McOsker, J.E. and Sietsema, W.K., Preclinical pharmacology of risedronate, a novel bisphosphonate. In: Christiansen, C. and Overgaard, K. (Editors), Osteoporosis 1990, Third International Symposium on Osteoporosis, Copenhagen 1990. Osteopress ApS, Copenhagen, 1990, pp. 1079–1081.

22. Gotcher, J., Kimmel, D. and Jee, W.S.S., A dose response study of Cl2MDP in a growing rat. J. Dent. Res. 1976; 55B: B303.

23. Miller, S.C., Jee, W.S., Kimmel, D.B. and Woodbury, L., Ethane-1-hydroxy- 1,1-diphosphonate (EHDP) effects on incorporation and accumulation of osteoclast nuclei. Calcif. Tissue Res. 1977; 22: 243–252.

24. Evans, R.A., Baylink, D.J. and Wergedal, J., The effects of two diphosphonates on bone metabolism in the rat. Metab. Bone Dis. Rel. Res. 1979; 2: 39–48.

25. Kimmel, D.B. and Jee, W.S.S., Bone cell kinetics during longitudinal bone growth in the rat. Calcif. Tissue Int. 1980; 32: 123–133.

26. Marie, P.J., Hott, M. and Garba, M.T., Inhibition of bone matrix apposition by (3-amino-1-hydroxypropylidene)-1,1- bisphosphonate (AHPrBP) in the mouse. Bone 1985; 6: 193–200.

27. Marshall, M.J., Wilson, A.S. and Davie, M.W.J., Effects of (3-amino-1- hydroxypropylidene)-1,1-bisphosphonate on mouse osteoclasts. J. Bone Miner. Res. 1990; 5: 955–962.

28. Evans, R.A., Howlett, C.R., Dunstan, C.R. and Hills, E., The effect of long-term low-dose diphosphonate treatment on rat bone. Clin. Orthop. 1982; 165: 290–299.

29. Sato, M., Grasser, W., Endo, N. et al., Bisphosphonate action. Alendronate localization in rat bone and effects on osteoclast ultrastructure. J. Clin. Invest. 1991; 88: 2095–2105.

30. Fujimoto, R., Nii, A., Okazaki, A., Miki, H. and Kawashima, H., Effect of disodium dihydrogen (cycloheptylamino) methylene bisphosphonate monohydrate (YM 175) on the bone formation and resorption in rats and dogs. Histological examination (Abstract 335). Twelfth Annual Meeting of the American Society for Bone and Mineral Research, Atlanta, Georgia, August 28–31, 1990. J. Bone Miner. Res. 1990; 5 (Suppl 2): S157.

31. Anderson, N.D., Colyer, R.A. and Riley, L.H.Jr., Skeletal changes during prolonged external irradiation: Alterations in marrow, growth plate and osteoclast populations. Johns Hopkins Med. J. 1979; 145: 73–83.

32. Cecchini, M.G., Castagna, M., Schenk, R. and Fleisch, H., A new 'in vivo' model for studying 'de novo' osteoclastogenesis: The post-natal mouse caudal vertebrae (Abstract 595). Twelfth Annual Meeting of the American Society for Bone and Mineral Research, Atlanta, Georgia, August 28–31, 1990. J. Bone Miner. Res. 1990; 5 (Suppl 2): S223.

33. Gasser, A.B., Morgan, D.B., Fleisch, H.A. and Richelle, L.J., The influence of two diphosphonates on calcium metabolism in the rat. Clin. Sci. 1972; 43: 31–45.

34. Fleisch, H., Bisaz, S., Schenk, R. and Russell, R.G.G., Pyrophosphate, pyrophosphatases, diphosphonates and mineralisation. XIII International Congress of Pediatrics, Vienna, August 29–September 4, 1971, pp. 265–270.

35. Bonjour, J.P., DeLuca, H.F., Fleisch, H. et al., Reversal of the EHDP inhibition of calcium absorption by 1,25- dihydroxycholecalciferol. Eur. J. Clin. Invest. 1973; 3: 44–48.

36. Bonjour, J.P., Trechsel, U., Fleisch, H., Schenk, R., DeLuca, H.F. and Baxter, L.A., Action of 1,25-dihydroxyvitamin D_3 and a diphosphonate on calcium metabolism in rats. Am. J. Physiol. 1975; 229: 402–408.

37. Mühlbauer, R.C. and Fleisch, H., A method for continual monitoring of bone resorption in rats: evidence for a diurnal rhythm. Am. J. Physiol. 1990; 259: R679–R689.

38. Bonjour, J.P., Trechsel, U., Taylor, C.M. and Fleisch, H., Parathyroid hormone-independent regulation of $1,25(OH)_2D$ in response to inhibition of bone resorption. Am. J. Physiol. 1988; 254: E260–E264.

39. Kawashima, H., Nagao, Y., Ishitobi, Y., Kinoshita, H. and Fukushima, S., Bisphosphonates increase serum 1,25-dihydroxyvitamin D in rats via stimulating renal production of the hormone. Contrib. Nephrol. 1991; 91: 140–145.

40. Trechsel, U., Schenk, R., Bonjour, J.P., Russell, R.G.G. and Fleisch, H., Relation between bone mineralization, Ca absorption, and plasma Ca in phosphonate-treated rats. Am. J. Physiol. 1977; 232: E298–E305.

41. Shinoda, H., Adamek, G., Felix, R., Fleisch, H., Schenk, R. and Hagan, P., Structure-activity relationships of various bisphosphonates. Calcif. Tissue Int, 1983; 35: 87–99.

42. Morgan, D.B., Gasser, A., Largiadèr, U., Jung, A. and Fleisch, H., Effects of a diphosphonate on calcium metabolism in calcium-deprived rats. Am. J. Physiol. 1975; 228: 1750–1756.

43. Brommage, R. and Baxter, D.C., Inhibition of bone mineral loss during lactation by Cl2MBP. Calcif. Tissue Int. 1990; 47: 169–172.

44. Shiota, E., Effects of diphosphonate on osteoporosis induced in rats. Roentgenological, histological and biomechanical studies. Fukuoka Igaku Zasshi 1985; 76: 317–342.

45. Antic, V.N., Mühlbauer, R.C. and Fleisch, H., Effect of low calcium diet on bone resorption in bisphosphonate (BP) treated rats (Abstract 2). Satellite Workshop of the XIth ICCRH Conference. Bisphosphonates — From the Laboratory to the Patient, Siena, Italy, April 29 and 30, 1992. Bone Miner. 1992; 17 (Suppl 1): S11.

46. Leonard, E.P., Reese, W.V. and Mandel, E.J., Comparison of the effects of ethane-1-hydroxy-1,1-diphosphonate and dichloromethylene diphosphonate upon periodontal bone resorption in rice rats (*Oryzomys palustris*). Arch. Oral Biol. 1979; 24: 707–708.

47. Gotcher, J.E. and Jee, W.S.S., The progress of the periodontal syndrome in the rice rat. II. The effects of a diphosphonate on the periodontium. J. Periodont. Res. 1981; 16: 441–455.

48. Olson, H.M. and Hagen, A., Inhibition of post-extraction alveolar ridge resorption in rats by dichloromethane diphosphonate. J. Periodont. Res. 1982; 17: 669–674.

49. Adachi, K. and Chole, R.A., Inhibition of osteoclast recruitment at a local site by 1-hydroxyethylidene-1,1-bisphosphonate (HEBP). Ann. Otol. Rhinol. Laryngol. 1990; 99: 738–741.

50. Cabanela, M.E. and Jowsey, J., The effects of phosphonates on experimental osteoporosis. Calcif. Tissue Res. 1971; 8: 114–120.

51. Jee, W.S.S., Black, H.E. and Gotcher, J.E., Effect of dichloromethane diphosphonate on cortisol-induced bone loss in young adult rabbits. Clin. Orthop. 1981; 156: 39–51.

52. Hähnel, H., Mühlbach, R., Lindenhayn, K., Schaetz, P. and Schmidt, U.J., Zum Einfluss von Diphosphonat auf die experimentelle Heparinosteopathie. Z. Alternsforsch. 1973; 27: 289–292.

53. Fleisch, H., Russell, R.G. and Francis, M.D., Diphosphonates inhibit hydroxyapatite dissolution in vitro and bone resorption in tissue culture and in vivo. Science 1969; 165: 1262–1264.

54. Russell, R.G.G., Mühlbauer, R.C., Bisaz, S., Williams, D.A. and Fleisch, H., The influence of pyrophosphate, condensed phosphates, phosphonates and other phosphate compounds on the dissolution of hydroxyapatite in vitro and on bone resorption induced by parathyroid hormone in tissue culture and in thyroparathyroidectomised rats. Calcif. Tissue Res. 1970; 6: 183–196.

55. Mühlbauer, R.C. and Fleisch, H., Effect of various polyphosphates on ectopic calcification and bone resorption in rats. Miner. Electrolyte Metab. 1981; 5: 296–303.

56. Benedict, J.J., Johnson, K.Y., Bevan, J.A. and Perkins, C.M., A structure/activity study of nitrogen heterocycle containing bis(phosphonates) as bone resorption inhibiting agents (Abstract 114). Calcif. Tissue Int. 1986; 38 (Suppl): S31.

57. Doppelt, S.H., Neer, R.M. and Potts, J.T.Jr., Human parathyroid hormone 1-34-mediated hypercalcemia in a rat model, and its inhibition by dichloromethane diphosphonate. Calcif. Tissue Int. 1981; 33: 649–654.

58. Thompson, D.D., Seedor, J.G., Grasser, W., Rosenblatt, M. and Rodan, G.A., Effect of alendronate (bisphosphonate) in animal models of hyperparathyroidism. Contrib. Nephrol. 1991; 91: 134–139.

59. Kudo, M., Abe, T., Motoie, H. et al., Pharmacological profile of new bisphosphonate, 1-hydroyy-2-(imidazo[1,2-a]pyridin-3- yl)ethane-1,1-bis(phosphonic acid) (Abstract 11). Satellite Workshop of the XIth ICCRH Conference. Bisphosphonates — From the Laboratory to the Patient, Siena, Italy, April 29 and 30, 1992. Bone Miner. 1992; 17 (Suppl 1): S13.

60. Mitlak, B.H., Rodda, C.P., Von Deck, M.D., Dobrolet, N.C., Neer, R.M. and Nussbaum, S.R., Pamidronate reduces PTH-mediated bone loss in a gene transfer model of hyperparathyroidism in rats. J. Bone Miner. Res. 1991; 6: 1317–1321.

61. Rizzoli, R., Caverzasio, J., Chapuy, M.C., Martin, T.J. and Bonjour, J.P., Role of bone and kidney in parathyroid hormone-related peptide-induced hypercalcemia in rats. J. Bone Miner. Res. 1989; 4: 759–765.

62. Rizzoli, R., Caverzasio, J., Bauss, F. and Bonjour, J.P., Inhibition of bone resorption by the bisphosphonate BM 21.0955 is not associated with an alteration of the renal handling of calcium in rats infused with parathyroid hormone-related protein. Bone 1992; 13: 321–325.

63. Trechsel, U., Stutzer, A. and Fleisch, H., Hypercalcemia induced with an arotinoid in thyroparathyroidectomized rats. A new model to study bone resorption in vivo. J. Clin. Invest. 1987; 80: 1679–1686.

64. Barbier, A., Emonds-Alt, X., Brelière, J.C. and Ethgen, D., In vitro and in vivo osseous pharmacological profile of tiludronate. Implication for osteoporosis treatment. In: Christiansen, C. and Overgaard, K. (Editors), Osteoporosis 1990, Third International Symposium on Osteoporosis, Copenhagen 1990. Osteopress ApS, Copenhagen, 1990, pp. 1127–1130.

65. Stutzer, A., Fleisch, H. and Trechsel, U., Short- and longterm effects of a single dose of bisphosphonates on retinoid-induced bone resorption in thyroparathyroidectomized rats. Calcif. Tissue Int. 1988; 43: 294–299.

66. Green, J.R., Müller, K. and Jaeggi, K.A., Pharmacological characterization of bisphosphonate compounds containing a basic nitrogen substituent (Abstract 6). Satellite Workshop of the XIth ICCRH Conference. Bisphosphonates — From the Laboratory to the Patient, Siena, Italy, April 29 and 30, 1992. Bone Miner. 1992; 17 (Suppl 1): S12.

67. Okada, M., Noguchi, S., Hasegawa, Y. and Inukai, T., Effect of pamidronate in a rat hypercalcemia model induced by cholecalciferol. Arzneim. Forsch. Drug Res. 1992; 42: 543–546.

68. Mühlbauer, R.C., Russell, R.G., Williams, D.A. and Fleisch, H., The effects of diphosphonates, polyphosphates, and calcitonin on 'immobilisation osteoporosis' in rats. Eur. J. Clin. Invest. 1971; 1: 336–344.

69. Michael, W.R., King, W.R. and Francis, M.D., Effectiveness of diphosphonates in preventing 'osteoporosis' of disuse in the rat. Clin. Orthop. 1971; 78: 271–276.

70. Cates, J., Sheets, D.D. and Johnston, C.C.Jr., Prevention of disuse osteoporosis in the rat. Clin. Res. 1971; 19: 473.

71. Lane, J.M. and Steinberg, M.E., The role of diphosphonates in osteoporosis of disuse. J. Trauma 1973; 13: 863–869.

72. Lindenhayn, K., Hähnel, H., Schmidt, U.J. and Kalbe, I., Effekt von Dimethylaminomethylendiphosphonat auf die Immobilisationsosteoporose der Ratte. Dtsch. Gesundh-Wesen 1975; 30: 2291–2293.
73. Kawashima, H., Nagao, Y., Abe, T. et al., Immobilization causes a decrease in serum 1,25-dihydroxyvitamin D in rats, which is prevented by bisphosphonates (Abstract 713). Eleventh Annual Meeting of the American Society for Bone and Mineral Research, Montreal, Quebec, Canada, September 9–14, 1989. J. Bone Miner. Res. 1989; 4 (Suppl): S296.
74. Thompson, D.D., Seedor, J.G., Weinreb, M., Rosini, S., Rodan, G.A., Aminohydroxybutane bisphosphonate inhibits bone loss due to immobilization in rats. J. Bone Miner. Res. 1990; 5: 279–286.
75. Schoutens, A., Verhas, M., Dourov, N. et al., Bone loss and bone blood flow in paraplegic rats treated with calcitonin, diphosphonate, and indomethacin. Calcif. Tissue Int. 1988; 42: 136–143.
76. Goldovskaya, M.D., Vnukova, Z.E., Shvets, V.N., Rodionova, S.S., Orlov, O.I. and Kabitskaya, O.E., Reactions of bone and osteoclasts to bisphosphonates and vitamin D_3 in hypokinetic rats. Kosm. Biol. Aviakosm. Med. 1989; 23: 47–51.
77. Ellsasser, J.C., Moyer, C.F., Lesker, P.A. and Simmons, D.J., Effect of low doses of disodium ethane-1-hydroxy-1,1-diphosphonate on disuse osteoporosis in the denervated cat tail. Clin. Orthop. 1973; 91: 235–242.
78. Jowsey, J. and Holley, K.E., Influence of diphosphonates on progress of experimentally induced osteoporosis. J. Lab. Clin. Med. 1973; 82: 567–575.
79. Apseloff, G., Girten, B., Walker, M. et al., Aminohydroxybutane bisphosphonate prevents bone loss in a rat model of simulated weightlessness. Curr. Ther. Res. Clin. Exp. 1991; 50: 794–803.
80. Wronski, T.J., Dann, L.M., Scott, K.S. and Crooke, L.R., Endocrine and pharmacological suppressors of bone turnover protect against osteopenia in ovariectomized rats. Endocrinology 1989; 125: 810–816.
81. Movsowitz, C., Epstein, S., Fallon, M., Ismail, F. and Thomas, S., Hyperostosis induced by the bisphosphonate (2-PEBP) in the oophorectomized rat. Calcif. Tissue Int. 1990; 46: 195–199.
82. Togari, A., Arai, M., Hironaka, M., Matsumoto, S. and Shinoda, H., Effect of HEBP (1-hydroxyethylidene-1,1-bisphosphonate) on experimental osteoporosis induced by ovariectomy in rats. Jpn. J. Pharmacol. 1991; 56: 177–185.
83. Seedor, J.G., Quartuccio, H.A. and Thompson, D.D., The bisphosphonate alendronate (MK-217) inhibits bone loss due to ovariectomy in rats. J. Bone Miner. Res. 1991; 6: 339–346.
84. Wronski, T.J., Yen, C.F. and Scott, K.S., Estrogen and diphosphonate treatment provide long-term protection against osteopenia in ovariectomized rats. J. Bone Miner. Res. 1991; 6: 387–394.
85. Hannuniemi, R. and Virtamo, T., Clodronate has an inhibitory effect on bone loss in ovariectomized rats (Abstract 7). Satellite Workshop of the XIth ICCRH Conference. Bisphosphonates — From the Laboratory to the Patient, Siena, Italy, April 29 and 30, 1992. Bone Miner. 1992; 17 (Suppl 1): S12.
86. Ammann, P., Rizzoli, R., Slosman, D.O. and Bonjour, J.P., Effects of intermittent cyclical versus continuous treatment with the bisphosphonate tiludronate on bone mineral density sequentially evaluated by dual energy x-ray (Abstract 1). Satellite Workshop of the XIth ICCRH Conference. Bisphosphonates — From the Laboratory to the Patient, Siena, Italy, April 29 and 30, 1992. Bone Miner. 1992; 17 (Suppl 1): S11.
87. McOsker, J.E., Li, X.J., Smith, J.A. and Stevens, M.L., Skeletal effects of combined estrogen and risedronate treatment in ovariectomized rats (Abstract 731). Fourteenth Annual Meeting of the American Society for Bone and Mineral Research, Minneapolis, Minnesota, September 30–October 4, 1992. J. Bone Miner. Res. 1992; 7 (Suppl 1): S275.
88. Thompson, D.D., Seedor, J.G., Solomon, H. et al., Alendronate prevents bone loss in estrogen deficient baboons. In: Christiansen, C. and Overgaard, K. (Editors), Osteoporosis 1990, Third International Symposium on Osteoporosis, Copenhagen 1990. Osteopress ApS, Copenhagen, 1990, pp. 1015–1017.
89. Balena, R., Markatos, A., Lafage, M.H., Masarachia, P., Gentile, M. and Rodan, G.A., The long term effects of alendronate on bone remodeling in the spine of ovariectomized baboons (Abstract 82). Fourteenth Annual Meeting of the American Society for Bone and Mineral Research, Minneapolis, Minnesota, September 30–October 4, 1992. J. Bone Miner. Res. 1992; 7 (Suppl 1): S113.
90. Balena, R., Lafage, M.H., Markatos, A., Seedor, J.G. and Rodan, G.A., The effect of two years alendronate treatment on cortical bone remodeling (Abstract 942). Fourteenth Annual Meeting of the American Society for Bone and Mineral Research, Minneapolis, Minnesota, September 30–October 4, 1992. J. Bone Miner. Res. 1992; 7 (Suppl 1): S328.
91. de Vernejoul, M.C., Jiang, Y., Lacheretz, F. et al., Prevention of bone loss following tiludronate

administration to ovariectomized beagle dogs. In: Christiansen, C. and Overgaard, K. (Editors), Osteoporosis 1990, Third International Symposium on Osteoporosis, Copenhagen 1990. Osteopress ApS, Copenhagen, 1990, pp. 1119–1122.

92. Monier-Faugere, M.C., Friedler, R.M., Bauss, F. and Malluche, H.H., A new bisphosphonate, BM21.0955, prevents bone loss occurring after cessation of ovarian function in experimental dogs (Abstract 739). Fourteenth Annual Meeting of the American Society for Bone and Mineral Research, Minneapolis, Minnesota, September 30–October 4, 1992. J. Bone Miner. Res. 1992; 7 (Suppl 1): S277.

93. Casez, J.P., del Pozo, E., Modrowski, D., Ruch, W. and Jaeger, P., Biological and biochemical correlates of skeletal growth in female rats from birth to senescence (Abstract 739). Thirteenth Annual Meeting of the American Society for Bone and Mineral Research, San Diego, California, August 24–28, 1991. J. Bone Miner. Res. 1991; 6 (Suppl 1): S269.

94. Wink, C.S., Onge, M.S. and Parker, B., The effects of dichloromethylene biphosphonate on osteoporotic femora of adult castrate male rats. Acta Anat. (Basel) 1985; 124: 117–121.

Bisphosphonate on bones
O. Bijvoet, H.A. Fleisch, R.E. Canfield and G. Russell (eds.)
© 1995 Elsevier Science B.V. All rights reserved.

CHAPTER 12

Studies with isolated cells and cell systems

Rolf Felix

Pathophysiologisches Institut, Universität Bern, Murtenstraße 35, CH-3010 Bern, Schweiz

I. Introduction

Bisphosphonates inhibit bone resorption in vitro and in vivo. They bind with high affinity to calcium phosphate crystals, inhibiting their growth and dissolution (see Chapter 5). This high affinity for hydroxyapatite explains why bisphosphonates, when given in vivo, accumulate in bone.

It was originally thought that these compounds decrease bone resorption by inhibiting the dissolution of the crystals. It was, however, soon realized that there is no good correlation between the effect of different bisphosphonates on crystal dissolution and on bone resorption. Clodronate diminishes bone resorption more than etidronate, whereas the reverse relationship is observed with the dissolution of the mineral [1]. This has led to the suggestion that bisphosphonates inhibit bone resorption by acting directly on cells. The osteoclasts, which dissolve mineral, are probably the target cells. Until recently, no osteoclasts in culture were available to study the above hypothesis. Therefore, the effect of bisphosphonates on calvaria cells has been studied. Later, macrophages were also used. Finally, today osteoclasts can be isolated from bone [2], or they can be grown in culture starting from bone marrow or spleen cells [3].

II. The effect of bisphosphonates, mainly etidronate and clodronate, on connective tissue cells in culture

1. Uptake of etidronate and clodronate by calvaria cells and fibroblasts

Calvaria cells and fibroblasts in culture take up etidronate and clodronate slowly and linearly with time for at least 48 h [4]. The intracellular concentration reaches a value up to three times that of the medium. After subcellular fractionation into nuclei, lysosomes, mitochondria, microsomes and cytosol, 70% to 80% of labelled bisphosphonates have been found in the supernatant [5]. This is the only fraction having a relative specific radioactivity (percentage of radioactivity divided by the percentage of protein for each fraction) higher than 1. This indicates that bisphosphonates accumulate in the cytosol and not in cell organelles. The absolute concentration cannot be determined with this method, so it cannot be excluded that in organelles such as e.g. mitochondria, bisphosphonates reach concentrations high enough to affect cellular metabolism. Such a possibility is also supported by the observation that bisphosphonates delay the release of calcium from kidney mitochondria [6, 7].

2. Effect on cell proliferation

Etidronate does not have any effect on the proliferation of calvaria cells and fibroblasts, whereas clodronate inhibits growth when cells are confluent but has no influence during rapid proliferation (log phase) [4]. The reason for the absence of an effect in the log phase may be that in rapidly dividing cells the compound never reaches a concentration high enough to induce inhibition of growth. When clodronate is removed from the culture, cells slowly recover after 1 week of treatment, 2 weeks being needed for full recovery. Whether this long period is needed for regeneration of inactivated enzymes, of new cells or for the release of the compound is not known. Different effects on the growth of cartilage cells have been found, namely slight inhibition [4, 8] and stimulation [9]. The reason for this difference is not known.

Whether or not bisphosphonates act directly on DNA synthesis is not known. Large concentrations, higher than 500 μM, of methylenebisphosphonate and hydroxymethylenebisphosphonate inhibit α-DNA polymerase [10]. Phosphonocompounds are more potent, and they act more strongly on viral DNA polymerase than on the cellular enzyme [11, 12].

3. Effect on glycolysis

The effect on cell growth might be due indirectly to an effect on cell metabolism. Glycolysis, studied by measuring lactate production, is inhibited by etidronate and clodronate [4], but when the oxidative metabolism is blocked by incubating the cells under nitrogen, this inhibition is lost [4, 13]. It appears to be influenced by extreme conditions such as lack of oxygen. On the other hand, this inhibition prevails after lysis of the cells, as lactate production measured in homogenates of bisphosphonate-treated cells is decreased by the same degree as in the culture. Addition of bisphosphonates to the homogenate of control cells has no effect, thus excluding an immediate direct effect on the enzymes catalysing glycolysis [13]. In the homogenate, the cellular content is highly diluted, so the possibility that a soluble cellular factor is responsible for the inhibition is unlikely. The amount or activity of glycolytic enzyme(s) seems to be diminished in cultured cells treated with bisphosphonate. A small decrease in lactate dehydrogenase activity has been observed in cells treated with clodronate, but not in ones treated with etidronate [14]. This enzyme is, however, not involved in the regulation of the glycolytic flux and therefore appears not to be the main site where bisphosphonates act.

The main regulatory enzyme is known to be phosphofructokinase. It has been reported that PPi inhibits phosphofructokinase of rabbit muscle [15], although it is not known whether bisphosphonate might have a similar effect. Bisphosphonate have been found to inhibit phosphofructokinase of *Entamoeba histolytica*, resulting in a diminished growth of the parasite [16]. This finding is not, however, valid for mammalian cells, as they possess a phosphofructokinase which uses ATP as substrate and not PPi as the parasitic enzyme [17, 18].

In conditions quite different from the ones described above, clodronate and etidronate added to calvaria cells cultured in suspension for 24 h increase lactate production at low concentrations (10^{-6} to 10^{-5} M) and decrease it at higher ones [19]. Clodronate also decreases glycolysis in cultured calvaria [20–22].

Clodronate inhibits lactate production more strongly than etidronate. This correlates with the stronger inhibition of bone resorption by clodronate [1]. At the time when these observations were made, it was postulated that lactic acid is needed to dissolve the mineral in bone resorption. The inhibition of bone resorption has, therefore, been explained by such a decreased acid production [4]. Today it is known that osteoclasts do not produce lactic acid but H_2CO_3 to dissolve mineral [3]. The postulated mechanism is, therefore, not valid.

About 15 years ago, new bisphosphonate were synthesized and investigated. Some of them contain a long aliphatic side-chain (R1) with up to 11 C-atoms (Fig. 1; [22]). These compounds, having a lipophilic part and two negatively charged phosphonate groups, are by definition detergents. Not surprisingly, they destroy calvaria cells when added to the culture at the usual concentration of 250 μM [22]. At lower concentrations they increase lactate production. The reason for this effect is probably that the cell membrane gets damaged by these bisphosphonate and therefore permeable to ions and small molecules. This may force the cell to augment its pumping activity in order to transport these intracellular constituents back into the cell. More energy may be needed, leading to an augmentation in glycolysis.

Interestingly, amino-bisphosphonates have properties similar to those of long-chain bisphosphonates towards cells [22]. They also increase lactate production. Pamidronate with only 3 C-atoms is the most active compound (Fig. 2). The potency decreases as the number of C-atoms in the side-chain containing the amino group increases, 6-amino-1-hydroxyhexylidene-1,1-bisphosphonate having only a slight effect. These data suggest that amino-bisphosphonates might also interact with the cell membrane, leading finally to increased ATP consumption.

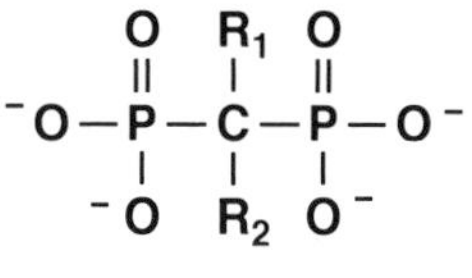

$$
\begin{array}{ccccc}
 & O & R_1 & O & \\
 & \| & | & \| & \\
^-O & -P & -C & -P & -O^- \\
 & | & | & | & \\
 & ^-O & R_2 & O^- &
\end{array}
$$

Fig. 1. General formula of geminal bisphosphonate.

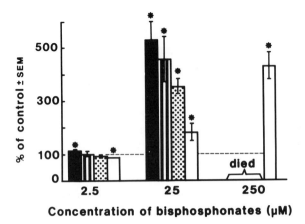

Fig. 2. Effect of amino-bisphosphonates on lactate production by rat calvaria cells. Cells were cultured for 8 days in the presence or absence of bisphosphonates. Lactate production was measured from day 7 to 8 (16 h), calculated per 10^6 cells and expressed as percentage of control (mean±SEM for 8 dishes). Pamidronate: black; alendronate: filled with lines; 5-amino-1-hydroxypentylidene-1,1-bisphosphonate: dashed; 6-amino-1-hydroxyhexylidene-1,1-bisphosphonate: open. * significantly different from control; $P < 0.05$.

Table 1.

The effect of bisphosphonates on the metabolism of glucose. Cells were cultured from days 1–7 in the presence or absence of bisphosphonate in Erlenmeyer flasks. On day 7 fresh medium containing [U–^{14}C]-glucose ±bisphosphonates was added and the cells were incubated for 15 h. The mean ±S.E.M. of n flasks is given as percentage of the control value (absence of bisphosphonate). The oxidation of glucose in the control flasks was 12.9 ± 0.47 (8) nmol/μg DNA, and the lactate production 0.84 ± 0.02 (8) μmol/μg DNA.

Treatment	Concentration (mM)	Oxidation of glucose (%)	Production of lactate (%)
No bisphosphonate	0	100 ± 1.5 (8)	100 ± 1.5 (8)
Etidronate	0.25	65.2 ± 8.2[a] (7)	68.5 ± 9.8[a] (8)
Clodronate	0.25	42.4 ± 1.4[a] (7)	34.6 ± 2.7[a] (8)

[a] Significantly different from control $p < 0.05$.

4. Effect on oxidative glucose metabolism

Beside glycolysis, etidronate and clodronate also diminished the oxidative glucose metabolism of cultured calvaria cells ([19]; Table I; Felix and Fleisch, unpublished). Impaired activity of glucose-6-phosphate dehydrogenase, 6-phospho-gluconate dehydrogenase and lactate dehydrogenase has also been observed in homogenates of mouse calvaria cultured for 48 h in the presence of clodronate [14]. Etidronate has no effect on any of the enzymes studied.

A diminished glucose metabolism might result in a smaller amount of ATP available for the cell and impair its activity. Indeed, clodronate at a concentration of 250 μM decreases ATP content by about 20%, whereas lower concentrations and also etidronate have no effect [23]. Energy-dependent transport systems maintaining the intracellular concentration of small molecules and ions might be one of the activities injured by a shortage of available ATP. Cellular potassium content has been found to be decreased in cultured connective tissue cells treated with clodronate, but not with etidronate [4].

5. Effect on fatty acid oxidation and tricarboxylic acid cycle

Diminution of glucose metabolism might turn on another pathway. The oxidation of fatty acids is indeed increased by clodronate, but not by etidronate [24]. This effect seems to be a special property of methylenebisphosphonates possessing halogen substituents, because all these compounds are active in the following order of potency: $Cl_2 > Br_2 > F_2 > Cl$ [25]. The oxidation of palmitate is more influenced than that of octonate. Since the oxidation of long-chain fatty acids, but not that of octonate, is dependent on the transport of these acids as carnitine esters into the mitochondria [26, 27], it is possible that clodronate may interact with this transport system. Another possibility might be that this bisphosphonate interacts with the fatty acid-binding protein, which seems to participate in the cellular transport of hydrophobic long-chain fatty acids, but has low affinity for medium-chain fatty acids [28]. Although the inhibition of glycolysis and the increase in β-oxidation appear at the same time, namely 2 days after the addition of clodronate to the culture, it is unlikely that the two effects are connected with each other. Several facts exclude such a possibility [24].

The rate of the tricarboxylic cycle also seems to be augmented. In mouse calvaria treated with etidronate and clodronate, an increase in CO_2 production from [6-^{14}C]citrate, [U-^{14}C]leucine and [1-^{14}C]acetate has been observed [14, 21]. We ourselves have found no effect on CO_2 release from [2-^{14}C]pyruvate and [U-^{14}C]glutamine in cultured calvaria cells (Felix and Fleisch, unpublished). Furthermore, a competitive inhibition of succinate dehydrogenase by PPi and methylenebisphosphonate has been reported [29].

6. Effect on glycogen content

Clodronate and to a certain degree also etidronate increase the glycogen content of rabbit ear cartilage cells in culture [30]. Whether this observation is related to the inhibition of the glycolytic pathway is not known. Another possibility could be that bisphosphonates inhibit protein phosphatases. Since glycogen synthesis and phosphorylase are regulated by phosphorylation and dephosphorylation [31], such an impairment would lead to increased glycogen formation and a diminished breakdown.

7. Effect on alkaline phosphatase, and osteocalcin synthesis

Clodronate increases strongly, etidronate only very weakly, the activity of alkaline phosphatase in cultured calvaria cells [32]. This effect is comparable to the one on fatty acid oxidation described above, since only halogenated methylene bisphosphonates possess this property in the order $Cl_2 > Br_2 > F_2 > Cl$, whereas hydroxymethylenebisphosphonate and methylenebisphosphonate are not active or only weakly [25]. None of the other bisphosphonates tested increased alkaline phosphatase in cultured calvaria cells [22, 33]. It has been found that many compounds are able to increase the alkaline phosphatase activity of cultured cells (for references see [32]). Such an effect has also been observed for substrates of the enzyme [34]. Since bisphosphonates are analogues of PPi and since PPi is a substrate of alkaline phosphatase, this might be a possible mechanism. Cortisol also increased alkaline phosphatase activity in HeLa cells [35]. This effect is dependent on protein synthesis, although the increase in enzyme activity is not due to the formation of more enzyme molecules. In this particular case it was found that the enzyme is a phosphoprotein and that the induced form has only half of a phosphate group associated with the control enzyme [36]. This alteration in phosphate content may be due to a cortisol-mediated inhibition of a protein kinase or the induction of a specific protein phosphatase [36]. Halogenmethylenebisphosphonates might interact with a protein kinase. Thus, by inhibiting such an enzyme, the bisphosphonates could generate an alkaline phosphatase with fewer phosphate groups.

The effect on alkaline phosphatase is not restricted to conditions in vitro, but can also be seen in vivo, this having been observed in the epiphyseal growth plate [37] and in bone [38, 39]. In vivo, however, etidronate is more active than clodronate.

Clodronate decreases the release of osteocalcin from calvaria in culture [40], confirming the in vivo observations. In rats, clodronate and alendronate strongly inhibit the increase of plasma osteocalcin induced by 1,25-dihydroxycholecalciferol [40]. The data suggest a direct effect of bisphosphonates on osteoblasts which is independent of bone resorption.

8. Effect on synthesis of collagen and proteoglycans

Clodronate also increases collagen synthesis in rabbit articular chondrocytes and rat calvaria cells and bone explants in culture. Etidronate has no effect on chondrocytes but decreases collagen formation in bone tissue [41], although the type of collagen is not affected. Clodronate increases the hydroxylation of lysine which leads to a higher number of crosslinks between hydroxylysine residues [42]. It has been observed in fibroblasts that up to 40% of newly synthesized collagen is degraded intracellularly prior to secretion [43]. Clodronate inhibits this effect in calvaria cells [44]. The net increase of collagen synthesis mediated by this bisphosphonate is therefore due in part to a decreased intracellular degradation. Extracellular breakdown is not influenced.

Clodronate, but not etidronate, increases the formation of proteoglycans in rabbit articular chondrocytes in culture [8]. The degradation does not seem to be affected. These results are different from those found in vivo where, at least in the case of etidronate, the synthesis and degradation of proteoglycans are inhibited in the epiphysis of animals treated with etidronate [45–47]. Lysozyme, which is responsible for proteoglycan disaggregation, disappears upon etidronate treatment, and large aggregations of proteoglycans which inhibit mineralisation, are formed

[48]. It has been suggested that the latter effect is at least partially responsible for the inhibition of cartilage mineralization induced by this bisphosphonate.

9. Effect on the production of prostaglandins and of proteases

Since prostaglandins are known to stimulate bone resorption [49], studies on whether bisphosphonates may act by inhibiting their synthesis have been carried out. Indeed, in calvaria cells labelled with ^{14}C-arachidonic acid, clodronate and etidronate strongly diminish the formation of ^{14}C-prostaglandin E_2 [50, 51]. The incorporation of arachidonic acid into the different lipid fractions is not changed. Pamidronate and bisphosphonates with an aliphatic side-chain increase prostaglandin synthesis at high concentrations and inhibit it at low ones [50, 51]. This increase is probably due to a higher incorporation into and release of arachidonic acid from the lipids. Finally, the effect of bisphosphonates on prostaglandin synthesis and on bone resorption has been compared in cultured calvaria [51]. Clodronate, etidronate, pamidronate and alendronate have been given in vivo for 3 days and the bone then explanted in culture. A good correlation between inhibition of prostaglandin synthesis and bone resorption has been observed for etidronate and clodronate. On the other hand, high concentrations of amino-bisphosphonates increase prostaglandin synthesis and strongly inhibit bone resorption. At lower concentrations, both events are inhibited. In conclusion, the effect of etidronate and clodronate on prostaglandin synthesis might be a mechanism by which they inhibit bone resorption in certain situations. It is less likely that amino-bisphosphonates act in a similar way, at least at high concentrations.

With a possible effect on rheumatoid arthritis in mind, the effect of bisphosphonates on the release of prostaglandins and proteases by chondrocytes in vitro has been investigated. In one study they have been found to increase the secretion of prostaglandin E_2 and collagenase by rabbit articular chondrocytes stimulated with interleukin-1 [9], but to inhibit in another using human articular chondrocytes [52]. In agreement with the latter, tiludronate and etidronate decrease the production of collagenase, neutral casein- and proteoglycan-degrading proteases in rabbit articular chondrocytes and synovial cells stimulated with conditioned medium from peripheral blood mononuclear cells [53]. In contrast to this observation, in bone in vitro clodronate and pamidronate have no effect on collagenase release and activity at concentrations at which they inhibit bone resorption [54].

III. Effect of bisphosphonates on macrophages

Mononuclear phagocytes have been found in close association with active resorption sites [55, 56]. Here they may act indirectly as accessory cells by releasing cytokines, such as interleukin 1 (IL-1), interleukin 6 (IL-6) and tumour necrosis factor alpha (TNFα) [57]. Alternatively, they may provide a local pool of osteoclast precursors [55]. Consequently, the possibility arises that bisphosphonates might, besides a direct action on osteoclasts, also inhibit bone resorption by acting on macrophages. The effect of bisphosphonates on these cells in vitro has been studied in different ways.

Macrophages and monocytes resorb bone particles [58], but this process is different from bone resorption performed by an osteoclast. No ruffled border and no clear zone are observed on the macrophage attached to bone surfaces [59]. Resorption of bone particles is inhibited by clodronate and pamidronate, whereas the cell attachment to such particles treated with bisphosphonate is not influenced [60]. Interestingly, when clodronate is added 8 h after the bone particles have been brought into contact with the macrophages, no inhibition of resorption is observed during the next 88 h. This indicates that the compound acts on these cells only when bound to the bone mineral prior to cell attachment. The amino-bisphosphonate pamidronate acts either when preincubated for 24 h with macrophages in the absence of mineral or when bound to the crystals. Furthermore, it has been observed that etidronate and clodronate are more potent when added to macrophages bound to apatite crystals than when added in solution [61]. The compounds seem to be taken up by the cells during resorption, probably by phagocytosis of coated mineral. It has also been observed that bisphosphonates inhibit migration of macrophages [62].

Bisphosphonates at low concentrations of 10^{-7} to 10^{-6} M inhibit the growth and differentiation of bone marrow cells to macrophages [63]. The proliferation of bone marrow derived macrophages is similarly diminished, whereas about 40 to 100 times higher concentration is needed to affect the viability of these mature cells in the absence of a growth stimulant. The order of relative potency of the various bisphosphonates inhibiting proliferation (alendronate > pamidronate > clodronate > etidronate) coincides with the sequence of potency of inhibiting bone resorption in vivo [64]. Furthermore, the effect of the bisphosphonates on the growth of cells of the mononuclear phagocytic lineage is specific among the haematopoietic series, as shown by the following experiments. Bone marrow cells have been grown in the presence of different growth factors. Macrophages are the only cells the growth and survival of which is impaired by bisphosphonates [65]. Since they are known to be highly pinocytic, it is possible that they concentrate bisphosphonates intracellularly, leading to toxic concentrations [66]. The inhibition of proliferation by amino-bisphosphonates, but not by clodronate, disappears when iron-saturated transferrin is added to the culture (M. Cecchini et al., unpublished). The mechanism is not known. PPi participates in intracellular iron metabolism. Iron is, at least partially, taken up by the cell as iron-transferrin. Intracellularly, it is released and distributed to different organelles and proteins. Thus, transfer seems to be mediated by PPi [67–69]. Whether bisphosphonates interfere by competing with PPi is not known. Binding of phosphonates, but not of geminal bisphosphonates, to transferrin has been described [70].

Recently, it has been found that bisphosphonates inhibit squalene and cholesterol biosynthesis [71] and that there appears to be a relationship between this inhibitory activity and the effectiveness for inhibition of bone resorption. As complete inhibition of sterol biosynthesis results in cell death, phagocytic accumulation of bisphosphonates in macrophages and osteoclasts may lead to a complete inhibition of sterol biosynthesis and may contribute to cytotoxicity.

A specific effect of bisphosphonates on the function of mononuclear phagocytes has been observed in lymphocyte proliferation [72]. Pamidronate indirectly inhibits the growth of lymphocytes by acting on the macrophages, probably by damaging and even destroying them. Measurement of ^{3}H-thymidine incorporation into unstimulated peripheral mononuclear cells has indicated a stimulation of proliferation at 10^{-6} M alendronate and an inhibition at higher concentrations [73]. The bisphosphonates probably influence production of IL-1, a growth factor for lymphocytes [74].

The fact that cytokines like IL-1, IL-6 and TNFα stimulate bone resorption [75–77] and induce inflammation [74, 78, 79] is a further reason to investigate whether bisphosphonates inhibit their production. The release of IL-1, measured with the thymocyte comitogenic assay, is inhibited by etidronate at high concentrations [80]. When etidronate was given in vivo to ovariectomized rats, diminished IL-1 production by peritoneal macrophages, stimulated in vitro with lipopolysaccharides, was observed [81]. No effect on the release of IL-1 by peritoneal macrophages and by the macrophage cell line P388D1, treated with several different BPs, has been found [9]. Bone particles and collagen stimulate the release of IL-1 from human blood mononuclear cells [82]. Pretreatment of the bone particles with etidronate decreases the ability to stimulate. Finally, it has been shown that pamidronate induces TNFα production in human blood in vitro [83]. This suggests that amino-bisphosphonates activate monocytes and macrophages to release cytokines. Such a release seems also to occur in vivo and to induce the acute phase reaction, observed when an amino-bisphosphonate is given to a patient for the first time [84]. Bisphosphonates seem also to influence the release of fibronectin from mononuclear phagocytes [85]. This effect might not be specific and may be related to the general toxic effect on these cells.

IV. The effect on osteoclasts

Bisphosphonates affect disaggregated osteoclasts resorbing bone, dentin or ivory slices in vitro. One unresolved question resulting from such experiments is the following: in vivo the relative potency of bisphosphonates covers a large range. One of the most powerful compounds, *N,N*-methylpentyl-1-3-amino-1-hydroxypropylidenebisphosphonate, is about 10,000 times more active than etidronate, the weakest of all [64]. In contrast, in vitro all the bisphosphonates inhibit bone-resorbing osteoclasts with a similar potency. Recently, the experimental protocol to study the effect of bisphosphonates on osteoclasts has been modified [86]. Osteoclasts in suspension have been preincubated with bisphosphonates in the absence of any mineral for only 5 min, washed and then incubated on ivory without adding bisphosphonates. These treatments, using very low concentrations down to 10^{-11} M, affected the osteoclasts. A similar order of relative potency in inhibiting bone resorption has been found as observed in vivo. Furthermore, these data indicate that the inhibition of the osteoclast activity in this in vitro system is indirectly mediated by the osteoblastic cells. Bisphosphonates seem to interact, in addition to a direct effect on osteoclasts, specifically and with high affinity with certain components of the osteoblast.

The site and concentration of bisphosphonates in bone has been investigated by injected ^{3}H-alendronate into young rats at an amount necessary to inhibit bone resorption [87]. Autoradiography of cut bone slices indicates that the bisphosphonate accumulates mainly on the bone surface below the osteoclast. Its concentration in the resorbing space has been estimated at the range of 0.1 to 1.0 mM, an unexpectedly high concentration. Experiments in vitro indicate that under such conditions the membrane of osteoclasts become permeable for K^+, H^+ and Ca^+ and that the cell loses its activity to resorb bone [88].

The osteoclast possesses a powerful H^+-ATPase which pumps protons through the membrane of the ruffled border towards the bone, in order to dissolve the mineral [89]. This enzyme, a very important tool for this cell, has been investigated to see whether it is inhibited by bisphosphonates [90]. Such a direct effect could not observed. As a result and as inhibition of bone resorption by bisphosphonates appears slowly, with a delay similar to that of the inhibition of protein synthesis, it has been suggested that these compounds disturb the energy balance in the osteoclast. The deficiency in ATP might result in impairment of energy-utilizing processes, such as H^+-ATPase and synthesis of macromolecules [90].

The effect of bisphosphonates on osteoclastogenesis has been studied in long-term culture of human bone marrow cells [91]. They inhibit the formation of multinuclear cells with the same relative potency with which they inhibit bone resorption in vivo. The effect seems to be on the differentiation, but not on the proliferation of their precursor cells, contradicting results obtained with growing murine bone marrow-derived macrophages [63]. Since there is some doubt whether multinuclear cells formed in human marrow culture are osteoclast-like cells, it might be worth repeating the experiment with murine cells [3].

V. Effect on other cells and systems

Clodronate stimulates neutrophil peroxidase activity, measured either spectrophotometrically or by chemiluminescence in whole cells [92, 93]. On the other hand, an inhibition of hydrogen peroxide production in monocytes has been observed [94]. An activation of glutaminase in calvaria with high concentrations of etidronate and clodronate has been reported [95]. Experiments have been described in which bisphosphonates act by binding calcium, resulting in an effect on the membrane, thus altering the deformability of sickled erythrocytes [96], changing the osmotic permeability of the frog bladder wall [97] and protecting lymphocytes against damage by antilymphocytic serum [98]. No effect on ATP-driven calcium transport has been found in short-term experiments of 15 min in erythrocytes by etidronate and clodronate at a concentration of 0.5 mM [99].

Recently, it has been shown that clodronate inhibits contraction of vascular smooth muscle in vitro [100]. The results indicate an action firstly on intracellular mobilization of Ca^{2+} and secondly on L-type Ca^{2+} channels. This effect is probably not related to the interaction of 1,3-diphosphonates, a new class of calcium entry blockers, with receptors for calcium channel ligands [101], since these compounds are, in contrast to geminal bisphosphonates, completely esterified with buthanol and, therefore, highly lipophilic.

Bisphosphonates influence adenylate cyclase, alkaline phosphatase, inorganic pyrophosphatase and lysomal enzymes (for details see review [102]). Acid phosphatase and aryl sulphatase are competitively inhibited by clodronate [103], and in cultured calvaria this bisphosphonate decreases acid phosphatase [20]. These effects on lysosomal enzymes might be one way in which certain bisphosphonates inhibit bone resorption.

VI. Conclusion

The data described here show that bisphosphonates act on cells in vitro in a variety of ways. The question arises whether these results provide any information about the action of the drugs in vivo, mainly on bone resorption.

There is constant discussion as to whether the concentrations of bisphosphonates used in vitro are comparable to the ones present in vivo. Data have been published [87] indicating that in vivo the osteoclast seems to be exposed to an unexpectedly high concentration of bisphosphonates. This implies that the concentrations used in vitro are in no way too high; they might rather be too low. Most experiments in vitro have, however, been done with calvaria cells and not with osteoclasts. As bisphosphonates act in vitro on several cell types, and because there appears not to be one type which is especially sensitive to bisphosphonates, the findings with calvaria and other cells are probably also valid for analogous reactions in osteoclasts. The effect of bisphosphonates probably also depends on the amount taken up — this could explain why macrophages, a cell with a high pinocytic rate, are more sensitive than other cells [65]. In vivo they probably induce the acute phase reaction when given for the first time. So far, however, no mechanism of this phenomenon has been elucidated from in vitro experiments. The in vitro data show that cellular effects of bisphosphonates depend strongly on the structure of the side chains R1 and R2 (Fig. 1). This is also the reason why all bisphosphonates do not have the same potency in inhibiting bone resorption in vivo and why there are differences in side effects. The gastrointestinal disturbances appearing after oral administration of bisphosphonates could originate from the action of the compounds on the cell membrane of the intestinal mucosa.

Bisphosphonates influence many biochemical reactions and pathways in cultured cells. This suggests that they may act at many sites in the cell and probably in a quite unspecific fashion. Are some of these effects relevant to find the mechanism of how bisphosphonates inhibit bone resorption? The inhibition of the glucose metabolism by etidronate and clodronate, which may result in energy shortage in the cells, could be relevant. Important for the amino-bisphosphonates is their interaction with the cell membrane. The possible leakage of ions and small molecules forces the cell to pump these components back, thus requiring additional ATP. This might lead to an energy deficiency which finally impairs the activity of the cell. This hypothesis is supported by the observation that osteoclasts treated with bisphosphonates in vitro slowly lose their activity [90].

Finally, there is the observation that bisphosphonates act in vitro on osteoblasts with a very high affinity. They inhibit osteoclastic bone resorption indirectly mediated by osteoblasts [86]. Such a mechanism could operate in addition to a direct effect of bisphosphonates on osteoclasts. These findings open a new approach to investigate the molecular pharmacology of bisphosphonate action.

References

1. Reynolds, J.J., Minkin, C., Morgan, D.B., Spycher, D. and Fleisch, H., The effect of two diphosphonates on the resorption of mouse calvaria in vitro. Calcif. Tissue Res. 1972; 10: 302–313.
2. McSheehy, P.M.J. and Chambers, T.J., Osteoblastic cells mediate osteoclastic responsiveness to parathyroid hormone. Endocrinology 1986; 118: 824–828.
3. Suda, T., Takahashi, N. and Martin, T.J., Modulation of osteoclast differentiation. Endocrine Rev. 1992; 13: 66–80.
4. Fast, D.K., Felix, R., Dowse, C., Neuman, W.F. and Fleisch, H., The effects of diphosphonates on the growth and glycolysis of connective-tissue cells in culture. Biochem. J. 1978; 172: 97–107.
5. Felix, R., Guenther, H.L. and Fleisch, H., The subcellular distribution of [^{14}C]dichloromethylene-bisphosphonate and [^{14}C]1-hydroxyethylidene-1,1-bisphosphonate in cultured calvaria cells. Calcif. Tissue Int. 1984; 36: 108–113.
6. Guilland, D.F. and Fleisch, H., The effect of in vivo treatment with EHDP and/or 1,25-DHCC on calcium uptake and release in isolated kidney mitochondria. Biochem. Biophys. Res. Commun. 1974; 61: 906–911.
7. Guilland, D.F., Sallis, J.D. and Fleisch, H., The effect of two diphosphonates on the handling of calcium by rat kidney mitochondria in vitro. Calcif. Tissue Res. 1974; 15: 303–314.
8. Guenther, H.L., Guenther, H.E. and Fleisch, H., Effects of 1-hydroxyethane-1,1-diphosphonate and dichloromethane-diphosphonate on rabbit articular chondrocytes in culture. Biochem. J. 1979; 184: 203–214.
9. Evéquoz, V., Trechsel, U. and Fleisch, H., Effect of bisphosphonates on production of interleukin 1-like activity by macrophages and its effect on rabbit chondrocytes. Bone 1985; 6: 439–444.
10. Eriksson, B., Oeberg, B. and Wahren, B., Pyrophosphate analogues as inhibitors of DNA polymerases of cytomegalovirus, herpes simplex virus and cellular origin. Biochim. Biophys. Acta 1982; 696: 115–123.
11. Eriksson, B., Larsson, A., Helgstrand, E., Johansson, N.G. and Oeberg, B., Pyrophosphate analogues as inhibitors of herpes simplex virus type 1 DNA polymerase. Biochim. Biophys. Acta 1980; 607: 53–64.
12. Nordenfelth, E., Oeberg, B., Helgstrand, E. and Miller, E., Inhibition of hepatitis B dane particle DNA polymerase activity by pyrophosphate analogs. Acta Pathol. Microbiol. 1980; 88: 169–175.
13. Felix, R. and Fleisch, H., The effect of bisphosphonates on glycolysis in cultured calvaria cells and their homogenate. Experientia 1983; 39: 1293–1295.
14. Ende, J.J. and van Rooijen, H.J.M., Some effects of EHDP and Cl$_2$MDP on enzyme activity and substrate utilization by mouse calvaria in tissue culture. Proc. Kon. Ned. Akad. Wet. 1979; 82: 55–63.
15. Bar-Tana, J. and Cleland, W.W., Rabbit muscle phosphofructokinase. II. Product and dead end inhibition. J. Biol. Chem. 1974; 249: 1271–1276.
16. Eubank, W.B. and Reeves, R.E., Analog inhibitors for the pyrophosphate-dependent phosphofructokinase of *Entamoeba histolytica* and their effect on culture growth. J. Parasitol. 1982; 68: 599–602.
17. Reeves, R.E., South, D.J., Blytt, H.J. and Warren, L.G., Pyrophosphate: D-fructose 6-phosphate 1-phosphotransferase: A new enzyme with the glycolytic function of 6-phosphofructokinase. J. Biol. Chem. 1974; 249: 7737–7741.

18. Reeves, R.E., Serrano, R. and South, D.J., 6-Phosphofructokinase (pyrophosphate): Properties of the enzyme from Entamoeba histolytica and its reaction mechanism. J. Biol. Chem. 1976; 251: 2958–2962.

19. Ende, J.J., Some effects of EHDP and Cl$_2$MDP on the metabolism of isolated bone cells. Proc. Kon. Ned. Akad. Wet. 1978; C-81: 252–264.

20. Morgan, D.B., Monod, A., Russell, R.G.G. and Fleisch, H., Influence of dichloromethylene diphosphonate (Cl$_2$MDP) and calcitonin on bone resorption, lactate production and phosphatase and pyrophosphatase content of mouse calvaria treated with parathyroid hormone in vitro. Calcif. Tissue Res. 1973; 13: 287–294.

21. Ende, J.J. and van Rooijen, H.J.M., Some effects of EHDP and Cl$_2$MDP on the metabolism of mouse calvaria in tissue culture. Proc. Kon. Ned. Akad. Wet. 1979; 82: 43–54.

22. Shinoda, H., Adamek, G., Felix, R., Fleisch, H., Schenk, R. and Hagan, P., Structure-activity relationships of various bisphosphonates. Calcif. Tissue Int. 1983; 35: 87–99.

23. Felix, R., and Fleisch, H., Effect of diphosphonates on ATP and Pi content, Pi uptake and energy charge of cultured calvaria cells. Experientia 1982; 38: 644–646.

24. Felix, R. and Fleisch, H., Increase in fatty acid oxidation in calvaria cells cultured with diphosphonates. Biochem. J. 1981; 196: 237–245.

25. Felix, R., Fleisch, H. and Schenk, R., Effect of halogenmethylene-bisphosphonates on bone cells in culture and on bone resorption in vivo. Experientia 1986; 42: 302–304.

26. Bremer, J., Carnitine and its role in fatty acid metabolism. Trends Biochem. Sci. 1977; 2: 207–209.

27. McGarry, J.D. and Foster, D.W., Regulation of hepatic fatty acid oxidation and ketone body production. Annu. Rev. Biochem. 1980; 49: 395–420.

28. Ockner, R.K. and Manning, J.A., Fatty acid binding protein: Role in esterification of absorbed long chain fatty acid in rat intestine. J. Clin. Invest. 1976; 58: 632–641.

29. Rosen, S.W. and Klotz, I.M., Phosphorus analogs as inhibitors of the beef heart succinic dehydrogenase system. Arch. Biochem. Biophys. 1957; 67: 161–168.

30. Felix, R., Fast, D.K., Sallis, J.D. and Fleisch, H., Effect of diphosphonates on glycogen content of rabbit ear cartilage cells in culture. Calcif. Tissue Int. 1980; 30: 163–166.

31. Cohen, P., Protein phosphorylation and the control of glycogen metabolism in skeletal muscle. Phil. Trans. R. Soc. Lond. B. 1983; 302: 13–25.

32. Felix, R. and Fleisch, H., Increase in alkaline phosphatase activity in calvaria cells cultured with diphosphonates. Biochem. J. 1979; 183: 73–81.

33. Moore, N.C. and Chipman, J.K., Direct modulatory effect of hexasodium N,N,N',N'-ethylenediamine-tetramethylene-phosphonate on bone cell function in vitro. Bone Miner. 1990; 8: 157–168.

34. Cox, R.P. and Pontecorvo, G., Induction of alkaline phosphatase by substrates in established cultures of cells from individual human donors. Proc. Natl. Acad. Sci. USA 1961; 47: 839–845.

35. Cox, R.P. and MacLeod, C.M., Hormonal induction of alkaline phosphatase in human cells of tissue culture. Nature 1961; 190: 85–87.

36. Bazzell, K.L., Price, G., Tu, S., Griffin, M., Cox, R. and Ghosh, N., Cortisol modification of HeLa 65 alkaline phosphatase: Decreased phosphate content of the induced enzyme. Eur. J. Biochem. 1976; 61: 493–499.

37. Felix, R., Herrmann, W. and Fleisch, H., Stimulation of precipitation of calcium phosphate by matrix vesicles. Biochem. J. 1978; 170: 681–691.

38. Ende, J.J., Some effects of EHDP and Cl$_2$MDP on the activity of alkaline and acid phosphatase in rat bone. Proc. Kon. Ned. Akad. Wet. 1978; C-81: 150–161.

39. Weisbrode, S.E., Capen, C.C. and Pendley, C.B., II. Effect of dichloromethylene diphosphonate on morphology, enzyme activity, and ash content of bones of thyroparathyroidectomized rats. Calcif. Tissue Res. 1978; 25: 119–126.

40. Stronski, S.A., Bettschen-Camin, L., Wetterwald, A., Felix, R., Trechsel, U. and Fleisch, H., Bisphosphonates inhibit 1,25-dihydroxyvitamin D3-induced increase of osteocalcin in plasma of rats in vivo and culture medium of rat calvaria in vitro. Calcif. Tissue Int. 1988; 42: 248–254.

41. Guenther, H.L., Guenther, H.E. and Fleisch, H., The effects of 1-hydroxyethane-1,1-diphosphonate and dichloromethanediphosphonate on collagen synthesis by rabbit articular chondrocytes and rat bone cells. Biochem. J. 1981; 196: 293–301.

42. Guenther, H.L., Guenther, H.E. and Fleisch, H., The influence of 1-hydroxyethane-1,1-diphosphonate and dichloromethanediphosphonate on lysine hydroxylation and cross-link formation in rat bone, cartilage and skin collagen. Biochem. J. 1981; 196: 303–310.

43. Bienkowski, R.S., Baum, B.J. and Crystal, R.G., Fibroblasts degrade newly synthesised collagen within the cell before secretion. Nature 1978; 276: 413–416.
44. Gallagher, J.A., Guenther, H. and Fleisch, H.A., Rapid intracellular degradation of newly synthesized collagen by bone cells: Effect of dichloromethylenebisphosphonate. Biochim. Biophys. Acta 1982; 719: 349–355.
45. Larsson, S.E., The metabolic heterogeneity of glycosaminoglycans of the different zones of the epiphyseal growth plate and the effect of ethane-1-hydroxy-1,1-diphosphonate (EHDP) upon glycosaminoglycan synthesis in vivo. Calcif. Tissue Res. 1976; 21: 67–82.
46. Larsson, A. and Larsson, S.E., Light microscopic and ultrastructural observations on the short-term effects of ethylene-1-hydroxy-1,1-diphosphonate (EHDP) on rat tibia epiphysis. Acta Path. Microbiol. Scand. Sect. A 1976; 84: 17–27.
47. Larsson, A. and Larsson, S.E., The effects of ethylene-1-hydroxy-1,1-diphosphonate on cellular transformation and organic matrix of the epiphyseal growth plate of the rat — a light microscopic and ultrastructural study. Acta Path. Microbiol. Scand. Sect. A 1978; 86: 211–223.
48. Howell, D.S., Muniz, O.E., Blanco, L.N. and Pita, J.C., A micropuncture study of growth cartilage in phosphonate (EHDP) induced rickets. Calcif. Tissue Int. 1980; 30: 35–42.
49. Dietrich, J.W., Goodson, J.M. and Raisz, L.S., Stimulation of bone resorption by various prostaglandins in organ culture. Prostaglandins 1975; 10: 231–240.
50. Felix, R., Bettex, J.D. and Fleisch, H., Effect of diphosphonates on the synthesis of prostaglandins in cultured calvaria cells. Calcif. Tissue Int. 1981; 33: 549–552.
51. Ohya, K., Yamada, S., Felix, R. and Fleisch, H., Effect of bisphosphonates on prostaglandin synthesis by rat bone cells and mouse calvaria in culture. Clin. Sci. 1985; 69: 403–411.
52. McGuire, M.K.B., Russell, R.G.G., Murphy, G. and Reynolds, J.J., Effects of diphosphonates on human cells in vitro. Inhibition of production of prostaglandins and collagenase. In: Donat, A. and Courvoisier, B. (Editors), Diphosphonates and bone. Imprimerie Médecine et Hygiène, Geneva, 1982, p. 399–403.
53. Emonds-Alt, X., Brelière, J.C. and Roncucci, R., Effects of 1-hydroxyethylidene-1,1-bisphosphonate and (chloro-4 phenyl)thiomethylene bisphosphonic acid (SR 41319) on the mononuclear cell factor-mediated release of neutral proteinases by articular chondrocytes and synovial cells. Biochem. Pharmacol. 1985; 34: 4043–4049.
54. Delaissé, J.M., Eeckhout, Y. and Vaes, G., Bisphosphonates and bone resorption: Effects on collagenase and lysosomal enzyme excretion. Life Sci. 1985; 37: 2291–2296.
55. Baron, R., Neff, L., Tran Van, P., Nefussi, J.R. and Vignery, A., Kinetic and cytochemical identification of osteoclast precursors and their differentiation into multinucleated osteoclasts. Am. J. Pathol. 1986; 122: 363–378.
56. Hume, D.A., Loutit, J.F. and Gordon, S., The mononuclear phagocyte system of the mouse defined by immunohistochemical localization of antigen F4/80: Macrophages of bone and associated connective tissue. J. Cell. Sci. 1984; 66: 189–194.
57. Mundy, G.R. and Roodman, G.D., Osteoclast ontogeny and function. In: Peck, W.A. (Editor), Bone and mineral research annual 5. Elsevier, Amsterdam, 1987, pp. 209–279.
58. Teitelbaum, S.L., Stewart, C.C. and Kahn, A.J., Rodent peritoneal macrophages as bone resorbing cells. Calcif. Tissue Int. 1979; 27: 255–261.
59. Kahn, A.J., Stewart, C.C. and Teitelbaum, S.L., Contact-mediated bone resorption by human monocytes in vitro. Science 1978; 199: 988–989.
60. Reitsma, P.H., Teitelbaum, S.L., Bijvoet, O.L.M. and Kahn, A.J., Differential action of the bisphosphonates (3-amino-1-hydroxypropylidene)-1,1-bisphosphonate (APD) and disodium dichloromethylidene bisphosphonate (Cl_2MDP) on rat macrophage-mediated bone resorption in vitro. J. Clin. Invest. 1982; 70: 927–933.
61. Chambers, T.J., Diphosphonates inhibit bone resorption by macrophages in vitro. J. Pathol. 1980; 132: 255–266.
62. Stevenson, P.H. and Stevenson, J.R., Cytotoxic and migration inhibitory effects of bisphosphonates on macrophages. Calcif. Tissue Int. 1986; 38: 227–233.
63. Cecchini, M.G., Felix, R., Fleisch, H. and Cooper, P.H., Effect of bisphosphonates on proliferation and viability of mouse bone marrow-derived macrophages. J. Bone Miner. Res. 1987; 2: 135–142.
64. Mühlbauer, R.C., Bauss, F., Schenk, R., Janner, M., Bosis, E., Strein, K. and Fleisch, H., BM 21.0955, a potent new bisphosphonate to inhibit bone resorption. J. Bone Miner. Res. 1991; 6: 1003–1011.
65. Cecchini, M.G. and Fleisch, H., Bisphosphonates in vitro specifically inhibit, among the hematopoietic series, the development of the mouse mononuclear phagocyte lineage. J. Bone Min. Res. 1990;

5: 1019–1027.

66. Mönkkönen, J., Urtti, A., Paronen, P., Elo, H.A. and Ylitalo, P., The uptake of clodronate (dichloromethylenebisphosphonate) by macrophage in vivo and in vitro. Drug Metab. Dispos. 1989; 17: 690–693.

67. Cowart, R.E., Swope, S., Loh, T.T., Chasteen, N.D. and Bates, G.W., The exchange of Fe^{3+} between pyrophosphate and trasferrin: Probing the nature of an intermediate complex with stopped flow kinetics, rapid multimixing, and electron paramagnetic resonance spectroscopy. J. Biol. Chem. 1986; 261: 4607–4614.

68. Konopka, K., Mareschal, J.C. and Crichton, R.R., Iron transfer from transferrin to ferritin mediated by pyrophosphate. Biochem. Biophys. Res. Commun. 1980; 96: 1408–1413.

69. Nilsen, T. and Romslo, I., Iron uptake and heme synthesis by isolated rat liver mitochondria. Diferric transferrin as iron donor and the effect of pyrophosphate. Biochim. Biophys. Acta 1985; 842: 162–169.

70. Harris, W.R. and Nesset-Tollefson, D., Binding of phosphonate chelating agents and pyrophosphate to apotransferrin. Biochemistry 1991; 30: 6930–6936.

71. Amin, D., Cornell, S.A. and Gustafson, S.K., Needle, S.J. Ullrich, J.W., Bilder, G.E. and Perrone, M.H., Bisphosphonates used for the treatment of bone disorders inhibit squalene synthase and cholesterol biosynthesis. J. Lipid Res. 1992; 33: 1657–1663.

72. De Vries, E., Van der Weij, J.P. and Veen, C.J.P., van Paassen, H.C., Jager, M.J., Sleeboom, H.P., Bijvoet, O.L.M. and Cats, A., In vitro effect of (3-amino-1-hydroxypropyl idene)-1,1-bisphosphonic acid (APD) on the function of mononuclear phagocytes in lymphocyte proliferation. Immunology 1982; 47: 157–163.

73. Cappelli, R., Adami, S., Tartarotti, D., Rosini, S. and Lo Cascio, V., 4-Amino-1-hydroxybuthylidene-1,1-bisphosphonate stimulates proliferation of peripheral mononuclear cells. Calcif. Tissue Int. 1987; 41 (Suppl): S21.

74. Durum, S.K., Schmidt, J.A. and Oppenheim, J.J., Interleukin 1: An immunological perspective. Ann. Res. Immunol. 1985; 3: 263–287.

75. Gowen, M. and Mundy, G.R., Actions of recombinant interleukin 1, interleukin 2, and interferon-γ on bone resorption in vitro. J. Immunol. 1986; 136: 2478–2482.

76. Löwik, C.W.G.M., van der Pluijm, G., Bloys, H., Hoekman, K., Bijvoet, O.L.M., Arden, L.A. and Papapoulos, S.E., Parathyroid hormone (PTH) and PTH-like protein (PLP) stimulate interleukin-6 production by osteogenic cells: a possible role of interleukin-6 in osteoclastogenesis. Biochem. Biophys. Res. Commun. 1989; 162: 1546–1552.

77. Bertolini, D.R., Nedwin, G.E., Bringman, T.S., Smith, D.D. and Mundy, G.R., Stimulation of bone resorption and inhibition of bone formation in vitro by human tumor necrosis factors. Nature 1986; 319: 516–518.

78. Kishimoto, T., The biology of interleukin-6. Blood 1989; 74: 1–10.

79. Vilcek, J. and Lee, T.H., Tumor necrosis factor: New insights into the molecular mechanisms of its multiple actions. J. Biol. Chem. 1991; 266: 7313–7316.

80. Aida, Y., Toda, Y., Shimakoshi, Y., Yamada, K. and Aono, M., Effects of disodium ethane-1-hydroxy-1,1-diphosphonate (EHDP) on interleukin 1 production by macrophages. Microbiol. Immunol. 1986; 30: 1199–1206.

81. Matsuda, T., Matsui, K., Shimakoshi, Y., Aida, Y. and Hukuda, S., 1-Hydroxyethylidene-1,1-bisphosphonate decreases the postovariectomy enhanced interleukin 1 secretion from peritoneal macrophages in adult rats. Calcif. Tissue Int. 1991; 49: 403–406.

82. Pacifici, R., Carano, A., Santoro, S.A., Rifas, L., Jeffrey, J.J., Malone, J.D., McCracken, R. and Avioli, L.V., Bone matrix constituents stimulate interleukin-1 release from human blood mononuclear cells. J. Clin. Invest. 1991; 87: 221–228.

83. Sauty, A., Pecherstorfer, M., Juillerat, L., Leuenberger, Ph., Burckhardt, P. and Thiébaud, D., IL-1β, IL-6 and TNFα levels in serum of patients treated with pamidronate (APD). Calcif. Tissue Int. 1993; 52 (Suppl. 1): S76 (abstract 301).

84. Bijvoet, O.L.M., Frijlink, W.B., Jie, K., van der Linden, H., Meijer, C.J.L.M., Mulder, H., van Paassen, H.C., Reitsma, P.H., te Velde, J., de Vries, E. and van der Wey, J.P., APD in Paget's disease of bone: Role of the mononuclear phagocyte system? Arthritis Rheum. 1980; 23: 1193–1204.

85. Mian, M., Adami, S., Rigo, A., Bonazzi, L., Braga, V. and Lo Cascio, V., Effects of vitamin D metabolites and bisphosphonates in fibronectin release from monocyte-derived macrophages. Int. J. Tissue Reac. 1991; 18: 139–143.

86. Sahni, M., Guenther, H.L. Collin, P., Martin, T.J. and Fleisch, H., Bisphosphonates act on rat bone

resorption through the mediation of osteoblasts. J. Clin. Invest. 1993; 91: 2004–2011.

87. Sato, M., Grasser, W., Endo, N., Akins, R., Simmons, H., Thompson, D.D., Golub, E. and Rodan, G.A., Bisphosphonate action: Alendronate localization in rat bone and effects on osteoclast ultrastructure. J. Clin. Invest. 1991; 88: 2095–2105.

88. Zimolo, Z., Wesolowski, G. and Rodan, G.A., Alendronate effects on ammonium permeability in mammalian osteoclastic cells. Calcif. Tissue Int. 1993; 52 (Suppl. 1): S38 (abstract 151).

89. Chatterjee, D., Chakraborty, M., Leit, M., Neff, L., Jamsa-Kellokumpu, S., Fuchs, R. and Baron, R., Sensitivity to vanadate and isoforms of subunits A and B distinguish the osteoclast proton pump from other vacuolar H^+-ATPases. Proc. Natl. Acad. Sci. 1992; 89: 6257–6261.

90. Carano, A., Teitelbaum, S.L., Konsek, J.D., Schlesinger, P.H. and Blair, H.C., Bisphosphonates directly inhibit the bone resorption activity of isolated avian osteoclasts in vitro. J. Clin. Invest. 1990; 85: 456–461.

91. Hughes, D.E., MacDonald, B.R., Russell, R.G.G. and Gowen, M., Inhibition of osteoclast-like cell formation by bisphosphonates in longterm cultures of human bone marrow. J. Clin. Invest. 1989; 83: 1930–1935.

92. Kowolik, M.J. and Hyvönen, P.M., The effect of dichloromethylene bisphosphonates on human gingival crevicular neutrophil myeloperoxidase activity. Arch. Oral Biol. 1990; 35 (Suppl.): 201S–203S.

93. Kowolik, M.J., Hyvönen, P.M., Sutherland, R. and Raeburn, J.A., The effect of two bisphosphonates on human neutrophil chemiluminescence and myeloperoxidase activity. J. Bioluminescence. Chemilumines. 1991; 6: 223–226.

94. Stock, J.L., Coderre, J.A. and Levine, P.H., Effects of calcium-regulating hormones and drugs on human monocyte chemiluminescence. J. Clin. Endocrinol. Metab. 1982; 55: 956–960.

95. Biltz, R.M., Pellegrino, E.D., Letteri, J.M. and Pinkus, L.M., Inorganic phosphate, pyrophosphate and the diphosphonates activate bone (calvaria) glutaminase. Adv. Exp. Med. Biol. 1984; 178: 217–221.

96. Van Duzzee, B.F., Sunberg, R.J. and Benedict, J.J., Effect of etidronate disodium on filterability of sickle cell erythrocytes. J. Pharm. Sci. 1980; 69: 599–600.

97. Shakhmatova, E.I., Kabachnik, M.I., Medved, T.Y.A. and Natochin, Y.U.V., Ability of diphosphonates to bind calcium and their effect on osmotic permeability of the frog bladder wall. Byull. Eksp. Biol. Med. 1982; 93: 71–74.

98. Zernov, I.N., Stefani, D.V. and Vel'tishchev, Y.U.E., Assessment of the protective action of diphosphonate compounds against damage to T-lymphocytes and antilymphocytic serum. Bull. Exp. Biol. Med. 1979; 78: 253–254.

99. Felix, R. and Fleisch, H., The effect of pyrophosphate and diphosphonates on calcium transport in red cells. Experientia 1977; 33: 1003–1005.

100. Paspaliaris, V. and Leaver, D.D., Clodronate inhibits contraction and prevents the action of L-type calcium channel antagonists in vascular smooth muscle. J. Bone Min. Res. 1991; 6: 835–841.

101. Rossier, J.R., Cox, J.A., Niesor, E.J. and Bentzen, C.L., A new class of calcium entry blockers defined by 1,3-diphosphonates: Interactions of SR-7037 (Belfosdil) with receptors for calcium channel ligands. J. Biol. Chem. 1989; 264: 16598–16607.

102. Felix, R., Shinoda, H. and Fleisch, H., Biochemical effects of bisphosphonates. In: Donath, A. and Courvoisier, B. (Editors), Diphosphonate and bone. Proc. IV Symp. CEMO, Nyon, 1981. Imprimerie Médecine et Hygiène, Geneva, 1982, pp. 20–45.

103. Felix, R., Russell, R.G.G. and Fleisch, H., The effect of several diphosphonates on acid phosphohydrolases and other lysosomal enzymes. Biochim. Biophys. Acta 1976; 429: 429–238.

Bisphosphonate on bones
O. Bijvoet, H.A. Fleisch, R.E. Canfield and G. Russell (eds.)
© 1995 Elsevier Science B.V. All rights reserved.

CHAPTER 13

Alendronate: The bone surface and bisphosphonate action on bone resorption

Gideon A. Rodan

Department of Bone Biology and Osteoporosis Research, Merck Research Laboratories, West Point,
PA 19486, USA

This chapter will consider the action of bisphosphonates in the context of the discussion on 'the osteoclast bone interface and bone resorption' (see Chapter 3).

I. Bisphosphonate uptake in bone

A dominant feature of all bisphosphonates is their uptake in bone as a result of the binding of the P-C-P backbone to hydroxyapatite. This binding can be demonstrated in vitro and is probably similar for all bisphosphonates, especially the 1-hydroxy derivatives, regardless of their pharmacological activity. By incubating radioactive alendronate (ALN, 4-amino-1-hydroxybutylidene-1,1-bisphosphonate sodium) with bone particles (mesh size 180), we found that under equilibrium conditions the capacity for ALN was about 100 nmoles/mg and the apparent dissociation constant about 1 mM. The binding of etidronate (ethane-1-hydroxy-1,1-bisphosphonate) was very similar, suggesting that this property does not account for the differences in the pharmacological potency of the two compounds [1]. Other bisphosphonates are likely to bind to apatite surfaces with similar affinity, with only minor differences imposed by the carbon side-chains on the pKa's of the two phosphonate groups. The OH side-chain of C in P-C-P, which is shared by alendronate, etidronate and many other compounds in this group, also contributes to the binding affinity. Since binding occurs primarily through the interaction of the phosphonate moieties with calcium on the surface of hydroxyapatite, it is strongly influenced by pH, which determines the ionization of the phosphonate groups. In vitro studies have shown that 50% of the ALN bound at pH 7.2 to bone particles was released at pH 3.5 [1]. This is of significant pharmacological importance in view of the acidification of the bone surface associated with osteoclastic activity, as discussed below.

In vivo, bisphosphonate binding to bone should occur on surfaces where hydroxyapatite is most exposed and closest to the circulation. This probably includes surfaces immediately before or after resorption and newly formed crystals at bone formation sites. These are the classical hot spots, visualized by bone-seeking tracers and by the technetium-tagged bisphosphonates used in bone scans. Indeed, administration of pharmacologically effective doses of high specific activity tritiated alendronate to rat pups [1] and adult animals (unpublished data) showed preferential localization to sites of bone resorption, identified by the presence of osteoclasts. There was also a substantial presence of grains on surfaces which were not covered by cells and looked either like pre- (resting) or post- (scalloped) resorption surfaces.

The tremendously high capacity of hydroxyapatite for bisphosphonate predicts the pharmacokinetics observed for these compounds. Bone will extract bisphosphonate, like a hydroxyapatite column, from the blood capillaries which perfuse bone, possibly during a single passage. About 5% of the cardiac output flows through bone. In younger animals or other conditions characterized by active bone turnover, such as in hyperparathyroidism and the early postmenopausal period, a larger fraction of bisphosphonate should be extracted from blood more rapidly. Since bisphosphonates, due to the bulky phosphonate charged groups, do not penetrate cells easily, this is the major route for bisphosphonate disappearance from the bloodstream into a body compartment. The other route is its excretion by the kidney. The uptake of bisphosphonate in bone, as described in detail in other sections of this volume, peaks between 2 and 4 h.

The second consequence of the large capacity of bone for bisphosphonate is that it will stay in bone for the duration of the lifetime of that segment of tissue, which is again consistent with the pharmacokinetic observations.

These pharmacokinetic properties and the adsorption of bisphosphonate to hydroxyapatite on the bone surface have strong implications regarding the mode of action of these compounds. They suggest that, unlike most other drugs where the circulating concentration determines the pharmacological activity, in this case the determinant concentration will be the presence of this drug on the bone surface [1, 2]. This is supported by the fact that the same total dose of alendronate has similar effects if given as a bolus or as multiple divided doses [3].

The second consequence of these pharmacokinetics is that the drug can be active for some time after its administration, since its half-life on the bone surface is very long. Indeed, the earliest pharmacological activity is seen about 24 h after administration, and the duration of action from a single dose extends for at least 2–3 weeks and for multiple doses (continuous treatment) for as long as 3–4 months. We really do not know for sure the dynamics of the generation of resorption surfaces and how long they persist prior to being repopulated by bone-forming cells. Bisphosphonates, administered as radioactive markers to animals, could help address these questions.

To summarize this section, the uptake of bisphosphonates by hydroxyapatite in bone is a dominant feature of these compounds; the first site of uptake, at low concentrations, is the resorption surface where hydroxyapatite is most exposed and most accessible. This feature, along with the excretion in the urine, accounts for the rapid clearance from the plasma, for the preferential localization in bone, for the duration of action, which exceeds the presence of the drug in the circulation, and for the general safety of these compounds.

II. Fate of bisphosphonate on the bone surface

The amount of bisphosphonate on the mineral surface, at least for alendronate, is minute compared with the saturating capacity. Since saturation of bone particles in vitro is seen only around 10 mM and full inhibition of bone resorption in vitro is seen after preincubation with 0.1–1 μM [4], the amount of bisphosphonate on the apatite surface is only 1/1000 to 1/10,000 of its saturating capacity. These small amounts of bisphosphonate probably do not have a significant effect on crystal dissolution or on the structural properties of the bone, unlike the larger amounts of fluoride in fluorosis, which affect both crystal growth and dissolution.

It is also unlikely that the small amount of bisphosphonate forms a protective layer, which interferes with osteoclast attachment. Indeed, in vitro studies showed no interference with osteoclast attachment [4], and there are both in vitro and in vivo indications that osteoclasts may start resorbing bisphosphonate- covered bone and stop early, producing smaller pits in vitro and shallower resorption depths in vivo [5].

However, if osteoclast resorption is initiated, the early steps of acidification of the resorption space would release the bisphosphonate found there and increase its concentration locally in the resorption space, which is sealed by the clear zone. The local elevated bisphosphonate concentration could interfere with processes essential for bone resorption, such as the activity of hydrolytic enzymes. We have also repeatedly found on autoradiography ^{3}H-alendronate silver grains on osteoclasts, which suggested that ALN has penetrated these cells [1]. The local elevated concentration, produced by bisphosphonate released from the bone surface due to acidification, may lead to the penetration of bisphosphonate into osteoclasts. Alternatively, it could penetrate into the cells via pinocytosis or phagocytosis through the very active ruffled border.

This sequence of events may explain the selective action of bisphosphonates on osteoclasts, which may be the only cells capable of producing, via acidification, the local elevation in bisphosphonate concentration. The relatively higher circulating concentration produced by i.v. administration may reach 'threshold' levels for monocytes/macrophages and cause the acute phase response observed in some cases for potent aminobisphosphonates [6].

After cessation of resorption, bone formation takes place on the ^{3}H-ALN covered surfaces, and ALN becomes buried in the bone. This was observed both 1 week [1] and 7 weeks after ^{3}H-ALN administration (manuscript in preparation). The ALN buried in the bone would have no pharmacological activity, since it is not on the bone surface, accessible to osteoclasts, and would stay there until this bone is turned over.

III. Cellular effects of the bisphosphonate alendronate

Forty-eight hours after administration of alendronate, there was a total absence of ruffled border in osteoclasts [1] as previously reported by Plasmans et al. [7]. Twenty-four hours after administration of alendronate, one could see in cells which showed a distinct clear zone on EM that the ruffled border appeared disorganized [1]. The convolutions of the membrane were not distinctly visible. We do not know yet the molecular mechanism for producing these effects and whether or not effects on osteoclasts are similar to those responsible for the acute phase response (APR) produced by amino-bisphosphonates injected intravenously [6]. The APR is most likely due to effects on macrophages/monocytes and is mediated by IL-1 and/or IL-6. These effects are usually produced after intravenous injections of relatively high doses of amino-bisphosphonates, which could produce transiently micromolar concentrations in the circulation. The developmental relationship of osteoclasts to macrophages makes this relationship interesting. In vitro studies have detected direct effects on macrophages at micromolar concentrations [8].

In a recent report, Sahni et al. [9] showed that preincubation of freshly isolated osteoclasts, or osteoblasts prior to their addition to osteoclasts, with low concentrations of bisphosphonates (10^{-10}–10^{-6} M) inhibited in vitro osteoclast pit formation. The potency of several bisphosphates in this assay paralleled their potency in vivo.

Alendronate effects on membrane function were observed in isolated osteoclasts in vitro. After 10–30 min exposure, intracellular calcium increased, and following exposure to ammonium chloride or low pH, there were changes in membrane permeability to $NH4^+$ or H^+ [10]. It is not known if these effects are direct or indirect, and so far they could not be attributed to specific K^+ or Ca^{++} channels, using known inhibitors. Moreover, osteoclasts seeded on bone slices preincubated in alendronate lose the ability to extrude H^+ in the absence of extracellular Na^+ [11], interpreted as a lack of H^+ pumping ability. Electrophysiological measurements showed no membrane 'leakiness' and no effects on K^+ currents [12]. It is possible that by virtue of its P-C-P structure, ALN interferes with phosphorylation by competing with ATP or may inhibit phosphatases and block dephosphorylation. Both reactions are very important in the regulation of cellular function, including vesicular traffic and membrane function. Further studies are needed to explore these possibilities. The src-dependent tyrosine phosphorylation seems to be essential to osteoclast function, since the genetic knock-out of c-src in mice produced osteopetrosis [13], and the major defect was the lack of ruffled border in osteoclasts, similar to that produced by ALN [14]. However, if this is a general manifestation of osteoclast inactivation, its relationship to the mechanism of src or bisphosphonate action remains to be established.

IV. Conclusions

In considering the mode of action of alendronate, the following facts have to be taken into account: (a) Alendronate (ALN) localizes on the bone surface, and its pharmacological activity is determined by the uptake in bone rather than its concentration in the circulation; and (b) the capacity of bone hydroxyapatite for bisphosphonate is very large, and the bisphosphonate would not come off in any significant amounts, unless some local changes are produced, such as acidification by osteoclasts. Thus, given these features, the bisphosphonate activity on osteoclasts has to act at the bone-osteoclast interface, albeit other actions are not excluded. At that interface, our studies favor the hypothesis that alendronate is released as a result of osteoclastic acidification; the rise in local concentration causes direct effects on osteoclasts, manifested as disappearance of the ruffled border. The molecular events seem to include changes in ion transfer across the osteoclast membrane, but the molecular basis for these changes remains to be elucidated. Osteoclast activity ceases, the cells move away, ALN diffuses or readsorbs to the apatite surface, which is colonized by bone-forming cells. Bone formation follows the aborted resorption, and the small amount of ALN on the bone surface becomes incorporated into the mineralized bone where it is pharmacologically inactive. The result is a positive bone balance.

V. Summary

Autoradiography following in vivo administration of radioactive alendronate shows the highest uptake on bone resorption surfaces. Studies show that when the mineral is covered with bisphosphonate following the injection of a pharmaco- logically active dose, the sealing of osteoclasts to bone surfaces still occurs as in control bones, but the cells lack a ruffled border. It can be calculated that following acidification of the interface, the release of alendronate on the bone surface would locally increase its concentration to 0.1–1 mM, which inhibits resorption and causes disappearance of the ruffled border by mechanisms which remain to be elucidated. Following inactivation, the osteoclasts move away, and the surface is covered by bone formation, which incorporates the bisphosphonate into the matrix and renders it pharmacologically inactive.

References

1. Sato, M., Grasser, W., Endo, N., Akins, R., Simmons, H., Thompson, D.D., Golub, E. and Ro- dan, G.A., Bisphosphonate action: alendronate localization in rat bone and effects on osteoclast ultrastructure. J. Clin. Invest. 1991; 88: 2095–2105.

2. Flanagan, A.M. and Chambers, T.J., Inhibition of bone resorption by bisphosphonates: interactions between bisphosphonates, osteoclasts, and bone. Calcif. Tissue Int. 1991; 49: 407–415.

3. Seedor, J.G., Quartuccio, H.A. and Thompson, D.D., The bisphosphonate alendronate (MK-217) inhibits bone loss due to ovariectomy in rats. J. Bone Miner. Res. 1991; 6(4): 339–346.

4. Sato, M. and Grasser, W., Effects of bisphosphonates on isolated rat osteoclasts as examined by reflected light microscopy. J. Bone Miner. Res. 1990; 5: 31–40.

5. Steiniche, T., Hasling, C., Charles, P., Eriksen, E.F., Melsen, F. and Mosekilde, L., The effects of etidronate on trabecular bone remodeling in postmenopausal spinal osteoporosis: a randomized study comparing intermittent treatment and an ADFR regime. Bone 1991; 12: 155–163.

6. Adami, S., Bhalla, A.K., Dorizzi, R., Montesanti, F., Rosini, S., Salvagno, G. and Lo Cascio, V., The acute-phase response after bisphosphonate administration. Calcif. Tissue Int. 1987; 41: 326–331.
7. Plasmans, C.M.T., Jap, P.H.K., Kuypers, W. and Slooff, T.J.J., Influence of a diphosphonate on the cellular aspect of young bone tissue. Calcif. Tissue Int. 1980; 32: 247–256.
8. Mian, M., Adami, S., Rigo, A., Bonazzi, L., Braga, V. and Lo Cascio, V., Effects of vitamin D metabolites and bisphosphonates on fibronectin release from onocyte-derived macrophages. Int. J. Tissue React. 1991; XVIII(3): 139–143.
9. Sahni, M., Guenther, H.L., Fleisch, H., Collin, P. and Martin, T.J., Bisphosphonates act on rat bone resorption through the mediation of osteoblasts. J. Clin. Invest. 1993; 91: 2004–2011.
10. Zimolo, Z., Tanaka, H. and Rodan, G.A., Alendronate (ALN) increases the membrane permeability of multinucleated osteoclast-like cells to NH_4^+, H^+ and Ca^{++}. Bone Miner. 1992; 17: S146.
11. Zimolo, Z., Wesolowski, G. and Rodan, G.A., Alendronate effects on NH_4^+ permeability and intracellular pH regulation in mammalian osteoclastic cells. Bone Miner. 1994; 25: S70.
12. Ypey, D.L., Weidema, A.F., Boxman, I.L.A., Nijweide, P.J.J. and Rodan, G.A., Aminobisphosphonates produce no short term gross effects on membrane integrity and K^+ conductance of rat and chick osteoclasts at neutral pH. J. Bone Miner. Res. 1993; 8: S391.
13. Soriano, P., Montgomery, C., Geske, R. and Bradley, A., Targeted disruption of the c-src proto-oncogene leads to osteopetrosis in mice. Cell 1991; 64: 693–702.
14. Boyce, B.F., Yoneda, T., Lowe, C., Soriano, P. and Mundy, G.R., Requirement of $pp60^{c-src}$ expression for osteoclasts to form ruffled borders and resorb bone in mice. J. Clin. Invest. 1992; 90: 1622–1627.

Bisphosphonate on bones
O. Bijvoet, H.A. Fleisch, R.E. Canfield and G. Russell (eds.)
© 1995 Elsevier Science B.V. All rights reserved.

CHAPTER 14

Effects of bisphosphonates on bone biomechanics

José Luis Ferretti

Consejo de Investigaciones de la Universidad Nacional de Rosario (CIUNR); Centro de Estudios de Metabolismo Fosfocálcico (CEMFoC), Universidad Nacional de Rosario; Instituto de Investigaciones Metabólicas (IDIM), Libertad 836, 1er. Piso, 1012 Buenos Aires, Argentina

I. Introduction

Biomechanical properties of bones are obviously in closer relation to the determination of the fracture risk than any other bone quality indicator. However, they have been investigated barely, especially concerning the repercussion of effects of hormones and drugs on bone composition and/or structure. Bisphosphonates (BPs) represent a paradigmatic example within this context [12].

This lack of information derives from the low reliability of non-invasive determinations of bone strength which has restricted experimental designs almost exclusively to animal models. Furthermore, only bones from some of the higher mammals show both modelling and remodelling activities as they grow into adult human bones. Nevertheless, some studies involving 'static' (low-strain rate) mechanical testing of bones from either only-modelling or modelling-remodelling species have brought some insight on BP effects on bone biomechanics.

The interpretation of results from those experiments is based on the following assumptions [13, 23]:

1. A deforming force acting on a bone induces some degree of strain, inversely related to bone stiffness. As a result of that strain, a corresponding amount of stress (force per unit area) is induced on bone structure.
2. Each bone is able to stand a certain amount of stress under linearly elastic conditions (i.e. linear relationship between stress and strain and complete reversibility of deformation) up to a critical, 'yielding' load. If the load is increased further, bone structure begins to fail because of the production of microcracks (non-elastic or plastic behaviour) and may suffer a fracture.
3. The mechanical quality of a bone integrated as an organ is defined by its resistance to deformation and fracture and by its ability to absorb energy under elastic conditions (the so-called 'structural' properties).

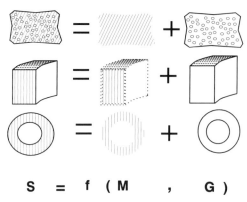

$$S = f(M, G)$$

Fig. 1. Schematic representation of bone structural properties (S) as functions of material (M) and geometric properties (G).

4. Bone structural properties should be regarded as functions of both bone tissue quality (expressed by intrinsic or 'material' properties) and bone macroarchitecture (described by extensive or 'geometric' properties, Fig. 1).
5. Bone material properties (e.g. material stiffness or Young's modulus of elasticity, limit elastic stress, energy absorption per unit volume, etc.) depend on bone composition and microarchitecture.
6. Bone geometric properties (e.g. volume, section area) are given by the amount and/or spatial distribution of bone tissue resulting from modelling-remodelling activities.
7. Bone modelling-remodelling is mechanically oriented by bone strain history. As bone strain is locally modulated by material stiffness, it could be accepted that, up to some extent, bone geometry depends on bone material properties.
8. A feedback mechanism governing bone geometry as dependent on bone strain, this being modulated by material quality, can therefore be proposed (Fig. 2) in agreement with the 'mechanostat' concept [27, 63]. The setpoint for this mechanism could be influenced by genetic and nutritional factors, as well as by the weight of the biomass bones have to bear [23].

The effects of BPs, as well as of any other agent, on bone biomechanics must be understood as a consequence of an interference with the referred interrelationships between material, geometric and structural properties.

Bones behave mechanically as anisotropic structures, i.e. showing a high dependence on the direction or mode of action of the deforming forces. Therefore, structural and material properties of a given bone may differ according to the way it is tested (compression, tension, bending, torsion, etc.). Four different tests were used to investigate BP effects on mechanical properties of normal or osteopenic bones: bending, torsion or compression of long bones (effects on cortical tissue) and torsion or compression of vertebral bodies (effects on trabecular tissue). Some reports referred also to the use of non-invasive, resonance frequency or ultrasound velocity measurements to assess bone material properties.

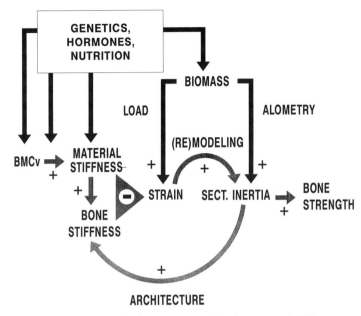

Fig. 2. Proposed feedback mechanism controlling bone strength [19].

Data are available on the effects of the following BPs on bone biomechanics.

1. Disodium etidronate (EHDP, EHBP)

Effects of EHBP on normal bone may be negative, especially at high doses: 10 (but not 5) mg/kg/day of P as EHBP given i.p. for 10 days reduced the torsional torque of femur diaphyses from normal chicks in conjunction with an inhibition of bone mineralization, regardless of a diet supplementation with 50–800 ppm of sodium fluoride and of changes in growth gain [11].

A beneficial EHBP action was demonstrated, however, on osteopenic models: treatment with 0.1–2.0 mg/kg/day for 6 months prevented the deleterious repercussion of immobilization or of ovariectomy (OvX) and/or Ca restriction on rat tibial mass, mineral content and resistance to fracture, though no changes on bone material properties could be shown [54]. A partial prevention of OvX-induced impairment in compressive strength of rat femoral neck and vertebral bodies was also achieved with 3–25 mg/kg/day s.c. for 3 months [35]. Doses up to 10 mg/kg/day given s.c. for 2 weeks failed, however, to prevent immobilization-derived depression of humeral compressive strength in growing rats, while 30 mg/kg/day depressed this even more with respect to non-immobilized controls with the same model [34]. These results were attributed to inhibition of bone mineralization at high doses [34, 60]. Doses of 10 (but not 1) mg/kg/day given i.p. for 20 days to growing rats in our laboratory [22] partially prevented the reduction in bending stiffness and the abnormal increment in energy absorption (but not the impairment in strength)

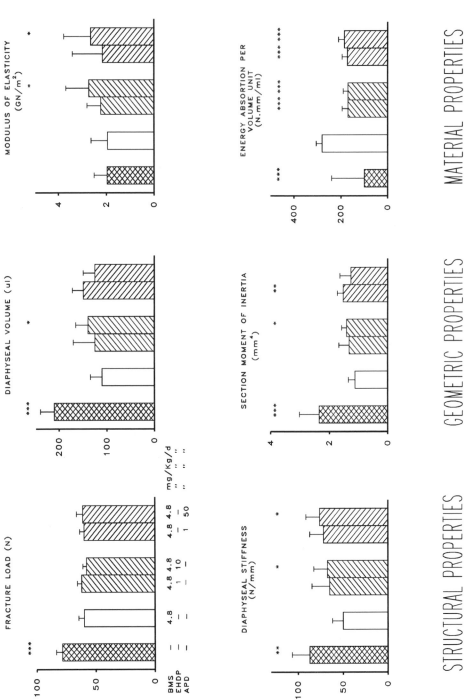

Fig. 3. Effects of EHDP and APD on betamethasone (BMS)-afected bones. 0.05 (*), 0.01 (**) and 0.001 (***) levels of statistical significance of differences with untreated (left bars) animals are indicated [18].

of femur diaphyses provoked by simultaneous s.c. injections of 4.8 mg/kg/day of betamethasone (Fig. 3). These effects were associated with a partial protection against the corticoid-induced reduction in diaphyseal volume and sectional moment of inertia and to a striking, abnormal increase in the material modulus of elasticity, the etiopathogeny of which remained undetermined.

The protective EHBP effects referred to parallel the reduction of vertebral fracture rate observed in osteoporotic postmenopausal women after a long-term, intermittent cyclic treatment, in which an increase of vertebral mineral content, a decrease in the risk of trabecular plate perforation and a reduction of activation frequency and resorption depth of bone modelling units were demonstrated [41, 55–58, 60, 65, 66].

2. Clodronate (Cl$_2$BP)

Only weak effects of Cl$_2$BP were reported in normal rats. An enhancement of tibial ash and vertebral compressive strength was observed with 4 mg/kg/wk for 25 weeks. No effects were demonstrated, however, with 12 or 50 mg/kg/wk in bone mass or strength in vertebra, tibia (torsion), femur diaphysis (bending) or femoral neck (compression) [40]. Shorter treatments (10 mg/kg/day for 21 days) enhanced femoral bone mass but not strength [39].

Preliminary reports on the protective effect of Cl$_2$BP in osteopenic models were more consistent. The immobilization-induced impairment in bone mass and torsional strength and stiffness of rat femur diaphyses was prevented by doses of 10 mg/kg/day for 21 days [39] or 12.5 mg/kg/day for 6 weeks followed by 6.25 mg/kg/day for a further 6 weeks [15]. Also, the OvX-induced reduction in bone mass and ultimate compressive load in rat vertebrae and femoral neck were prevented by 3 or 25 (not 1) mg/kg/wk for 12 weeks, a comparatively stronger effect than that obtained with the same doses of EHBP [35].

3. Pamidronate (APD)

The response of small-rodent cortical bone to pamidronate has been shown to be biphasic. Doses of 0.1 or 1.0 mg/kg/week s.c. from the 13th to the 65th week of age in normal mice improved the ultimate strength of femur diaphyses in bending [30]. The same was observed when giving 0.0045–0.45 mg/day i.p. for 25 days to growing rats, but doses from 4.5 to 45 mg/kg/day reduced bone strength [17]. Effects on diaphyseal stiffness (load-to-deformation ratio) were absent up to 0.045 mg/kg/day and negative from 0.45 mg/kg/day onwards with this model, indicating a dissociation between APD actions on bone strength and deformability at low to medium doses (Fig. 4). Changes in cortical bone strength correlated well with those produced in geometric properties in the long-term treated mice. In the 25-day-treated rats, however, high doses evoked an impairment of diaphyseal strength and stiffness despite an improvement of geometric properties (Fig. 5). This can be explained as (1) the architecturally meaningful moment of inertia of diaphyseal cross-sections was not enhanced despite the increased bone mass, suggesting an uncoupling of

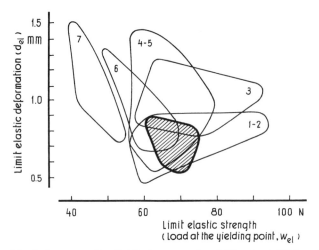

Fig. 4. Representative distribution zones for yielding load (Wel) and deformation (del) pairs of values of femur diaphyses from control (pointed area) and APD-treated rats with doses of 0.0045–0.045 (1-2), 0.45 (3), 1.4–4.5 (4-5), 14 (6), and 45 mg/kg/day (7) for 25 days [13].

osteoclast-osteoblast modelling activities, and (2) there was a significant decrease in bone mineralization (DEXA-assessed). The dose-related increase in bone mass seemed therefore to have been mechanically irrelevant [17]. This interpretation is in agreement with current concepts on BP effects at the bone cell level, especially concerning modelling activities [7, 9, 48] and with data on bone metabolism and composition obtained with a similar model and identical dose-time design [47]. In the long-term mice model, however, bone mineralization remained unchanged up to 40 weeks of treatment and increased thereafter [30].

Different results were obtained studying cortical bone from larger, remodelling mammals. No effects of oral doses of 0.5 mg/kg/day or s.c. doses of 0.45 μmol/kg of APD with an 1 week on/3 week off scheme repeated 3 times were observed on cortical bone from beagle dams studied through both torsion and bending tests [1, 32].

These reports point out a species dependency of BP action on cortical bone biomechanics related to the only-modelling or modelling-remodelling condition of bones. Important differences between treatments may also reflect dose/time-dependence of mineralization changes [14].

Positive effects of APD were particularly clear on cancellous bone from highly remodelling species when studied after long-term treatments. Ultrasound determination of material properties of cancellous bone from dogs orally treated with 2.5–25.0 mg/kg/day of APD for one year confirmed the correlation between dose-related variations of bone modulus of elasticity (material stiffness) and tissue mineralization [31]. Evidence was afforded that APD enhanced both trabecular thickness and the packing density of bone crystals (increase in lattice parameters and decrease in crystal size) and reduced the solubility of bone mineral without altering the bone chem-

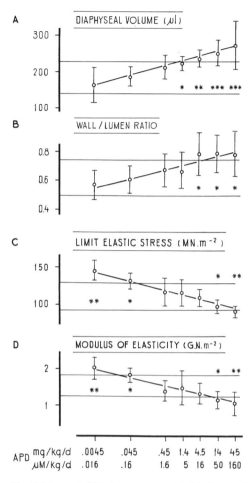

Fig. 5. Means ± SD of some geometric (A, B, adjusted to body weight) and material properties (C, D) of rats treated with APD for 25 days. 0.05 (*), 0.01 (**) and 0.001 (***) levels of statistical significance of differences with controls (zone between horizontal lines) are indicated [13].

istry of Ca, Mg and P. The repercussion of these changes on the structural properties of cancellous bone was also demonstrated. Administration of 0.5 mg/kg/day orally or 0.45 μmol/kg s.c. of APD with that on-off scheme increased the torsional and compressive strength and the ultrasound-assessed material properties (modulus of elasticity and maximum shear stress) of spongy bone samples from beagle dogs [1, 32].

A protective activity of APD on osteopenic rat models was also described. Doses of 50 (but not 1) mg/kg/day i.p. for 20 days partially prevented the biomechanical repercussion of a simultaneous treatment with 4.8 mg/kg/day s.c. of betamethasone on rat femur diaphyses [22]. Effects were similar to those observed with EHBP (Fig. 3) and consonant with some clinical observations [46]. The abnormal increase in modulus of elasticity induced by APD in this model, homologous to that observed with EHBP, resembled the referred APD actions on normal cancellous bone after longer treatments [31].

Also, the OvX-induced decrease in vertebral (but not tibial) strength was prevented in rats treated with 1 mg/kg APD for 8 weeks [1a]. Positive effects of 2–8 mg/kg/day APD p.o. for 6 months were also shown on femurs from both immobilized (IM) and overcharged (OC) limbs of OvX, hemi-sciaticectomized rats [20], in consonance with non-mechanical observations made with a similar model [50]. Diaphyseal strength was enhanced because of an improvement of stress resistance of bone material associated with an increase of BMD, without any change in geometric properties with respect to OvX controls (Fig. 6). Diaphyseal stiffness was depressed, however, because of a reduction in the modulus of elasticity of bone material (Fig. 7). The naturally positive relationship between material quality and bone mineral content was maintained in both APD-treated and -untreated rats. This suggested the participation of additional, undetermined factors in the APD-induced increase in bone deformability. Nevertheless, the resulting abnormal flexibility of APD-treated bones induced them to undergo a greater strain for a given body weight, thus enhancing tissue ability to absorb energy above that of weight-paired controls. This effect may have led to an adaptive maintenance of modelling-dependent bone geometric properties that prevented BP-treated bones from any reduction in cross-sectional moment of inertia with respect to untreated, OvX animals. The correlation between this geometric parameter and material modulus of elasticity for all the bones studied showed, in fact, the usual negative, hyperbolic pattern (Fig. 8). The OC bone values plotted higher than IM ones from the same animals, showing the significant influence of in vivo mechanical stimulation on the pathogenesis of APD effects. The potentiation of APD protection from OvX-induced biomechanical changes by pre-treatment with a bone formation stimulator as IGF-1 [1a] is in consonance with this thinking.

4. Dimethyl-pamidronate (Me$_2$-APD, mildronate, olpadronate)

Long-term oral treatment of normally growing rats with Me$_2$-APD on femur biomechanics in bending showed positive effects on bone structural properties. These effects were evident even at very high doses (8–200 mg/kg/day for 6 months, or 45–90 mg/kg/day for 3 months) [18, 19, 24]. Diaphyseal ultimate strength, stiffness and energy absorption ability increased in relation to dose, body weight and bone deformability (indicating an effect on mechanostatic responsiveness). These changes were linearly associated to improvements in cross-sectional properties at the midshaft (more marked in moment of inertia than in area) and in the DEXA-determined BMD, with no negative effects on volumetric (pQCT-assessed) cortical BMD and bone material properties. Effects were more evident in males than in age-paired females because of the naturally greater biomass (Fig. 9) and lower bone material stiffness of the former [23, 24].

These results point out that, at variance with that found after a 25-day parenteral treatment with APD, a long-term oral administration of Me$_2$-APD to normal rats

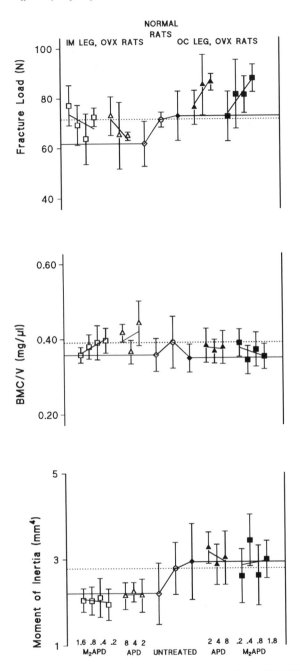

Fig. 6. Fracture load, mineral content per unit volume (BMC/V) and section moment of inertia of femur diaphyses from control rats and from immobilized (IM) and overcharged (OC) limbs of ovariectomized (OvX), hemi-sciaticectomized rats untreated or treated with APD or Me_2-APD (oral doses in mg/kg/ day) for 6 months [16].

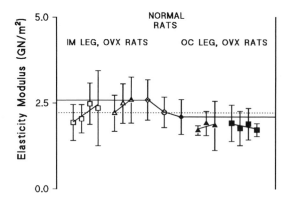

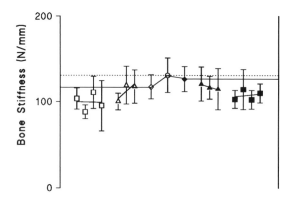

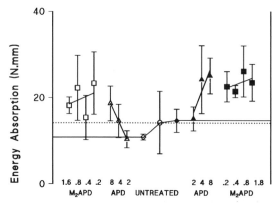

Fig. 7. Elastic modulus (material stiffness), bone stiffness and energy absorption of femur diaphyses from control rats and from immobilized (IM) and overcharged (OC) limbs of ovariectomized (OvX)-hemisciaticectomized rats untreated or treated with APD or Me$_2$-APD (oral doses in mg/kg/day) for 6 months [16].

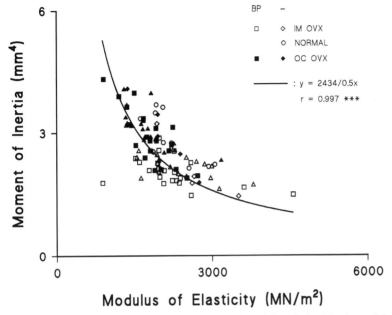

Fig. 8. Correlation between moment of inertia and modulus of elasticity (material stiffness) of femur diaphyses from normal rats and from immobilized (IM) and overcharged (OC) limbs of ovariectomized (OvX), hemisciaticectomized rats untreated (−) or treated (BP) with APD or Me$_2$-APD at the doses indicated in Figs. 6 and 7 [16].

(1) improved, rather than impaired, bone stiffness, showing no dissociation with effects on bone strength; (2) enhanced cross-sectional moment of inertia with no interference upon osteoclast-osteoblast modelling coordination; (3) improved bone structural and geometric properties and DEXA-assessed BMD altogether (yet not bone material properties) even at very high doses without any biphasism of effects; and (4) showed a high dependency upon in vivo mechanical stimulation of weight-bearing bones. The more important participation of bone geometric properties in the determination of effects of Me$_2$-APD with respect to those of APD may be related to the enhancement of the anti-resorbing activity with no negative effects on mineralization, resulting from methylation of the amino group [10, 43].

A protective action of oral doses of 0.2–1.6 mg/kg/day of Me$_2$-APD given for 6 months on both immobilized (osteopenic) and overcharged femurs from OvX rats was also shown [20]. Analogously to those evoked by APD at equivalent (10-fold higher) doses (Figs. 6 and 7), these changes derived mainly from an improvement of bone ability to withstand stress and to elastically absorb energy and were highly dependent on the mechanical stimulation history. Lack of variation of cross-sectional moment of inertia and the unexpected decrease of bone stiffness in these conditions contrasted with Me$_2$-APD effects on normal rat femurs (Fig. 9). This suggested that oestrogens may play a role in the determination of the nature of BP-induced changes on those crucial properties in intact rats.

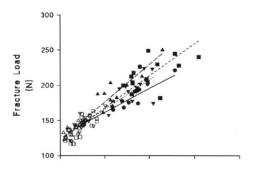

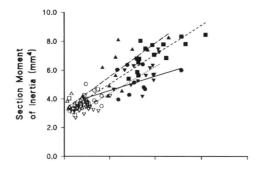

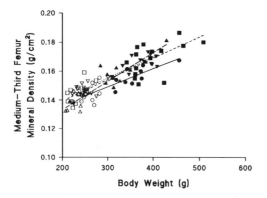

Fig. 9. Effects of oral doses of 8 (down-pointing triangles), 40 (squares: short dashed line) and 200 (up-pointing triangles; long-dashed line) mg/kg/day of Me_2-APD given during 6 months to growing rats on fracture load (a), section moment of inertia (b) and mineral density (c) of femur diaphyses. Covariance analysis indicated significant differences between treated groups in (a) and (b), and with control animals (circles; continuous line) in every case.

5. Alendronate (AHBP)

Alendronate effects on bone biomechanics were widely investigated. Results in normal animals were not conclusive, however, perhaps because of their dependency on sex and time of administration. Oral doses of 0.5–5.0 mg/kg/day given to young rats and beagles, or of 2–8 mg/kg/day administered to adult beagles for 6 months, failed to improve torsional stiffness, angle of deformation, torque (strength) and energy absorption of their femurs [16]. Also s.c. injections of 0.03–0.3 mg/kg/day for 2 weeks were ineffective on bending strength and stiffness of humeri, tibiae or femurs in normal rats [3]. Even a 33% reduction in torque was observed in a rat group receiving 2.5 mg/kg/day, though careful studies with wide dose ranges in rats, pigs, dogs and baboons showed no deleterious changes in bone quality [49]. These results are similar to those obtained with APD in beagles [1, 32]. Long-term treatment (105 weeks) of rats with oral doses of 1.0 or 3.7 mg/kg/day, however, increased bone mass and strength (and less evidently stiffness) in vertebrae (compression) and femur shafts (bending) with respect to aging controls, preserving bone structure and showing a dose-dependency [33]. These positive effects were attributed to a strong inhibition of bone resorption during growth and to an attenuation of BMU-based bone resorption in the age-related bone loss period. They were much more evident in males than in females as a weight-related phenomenon, as previously observed with Me_2APD [17, 19, 24]. Enhancement of bone formation by prostaglandin E_2 administration potentiated these effects in the short term (25 days) [38].

On the other hand, protective effects of AHBP on osteopenic models were reported by many investigators. Positive AHBP changes were reported after testing this BP as a protective drug against weightlessness repercussion on bone. The reduction in male rat humeral, femoral and tibial strength and stiffness after 14-day tail suspension was prevented by the s.c. injection of 0.03–0.3 mg/kg/day of AHBP [3, 3a] or 1 mg/kg/day of P as AHBP [2]. These effects were consistent with the AHBP-induced prevention of the impairment of bone mineral density shown under those and comparable conditions [59]. No changes were detected in bone geometric properties. This protective AHBP property contrasted with the lack of effects of maximal doses of gallium nitrate on a similar model [2].

Also, protective effects of s.c. doses of at least 18–28 μg/kg of AHBP twice weekly for 6–12 months were demonstrated against the chronic repercussion of an OvX-induced impairment in BMD, apparent density, geometric properties and histomorphometric parameters on rat bone strength and stiffness as tested in vertebral bodies during compression (showing a positive correlation between bone strength and bone volume fraction) and in femoral midshafts and necks in bending [51, 52, 62]. Similar results were obtained testing vertebral (but not femoral) strength in AHBP-protected (0.05–0.25 mg/2 weeks i.v. for 2 years) OvX baboons [4, 61]. Concomitant administration of prostaglandin E_2 as a bone formation enhancer potentiated the effects shown in OvX rats [38], in consonance with that observed with APD [1].

This promising compound [49] is now being tested in a large fracture intervention trial in order to demonstrate its effectiveness in reducing fracture rate in women aged 55–80 years [8].

6. Tiludronate

Positive effects of tiludronate on normal bone biomechanics were invasively demonstrated at a higher phylogenetic level than those of any other BP. Doses of 10–126 mg/kg/day given for one year with the drinking water to young baboons enhanced radial transversal stiffness and bending strength (calculated from resonance frequency analysis) in a dose-related fashion. This change was correlated with an increment in bone mineral, though no variation was detected on bone ability to absorb energy [5, 6, 28, 29]. The calculated buckling strength was also found increased at the highest doses one year after withdrawal of treatment. The directly assessed torsional strength was unaffected at the end of treatment, but torsional stiffness was increased in proportion to the dose. One year later, however, no differences in invasively determined biomechanical properties were detected with respect to untreated controls.

Protective properties of doses of 8–32 mg/kg/day given on a 3 month on/3 month off scheme for one year were also demonstrated on impact force of the femoral neck and fast-torsional strength of femur shafts from OvX beagles [6]. No positive changes were reported on femoral head biomechanics with lower doses. The OvX-induced impairment of rat vertebral bone mass and compressive strength was prevented by 50 mg/kg/day after one 3 month on/3 month off cycle, yet lesser effectiveness was observed at lower doses [42].

The positive effects of tiludronate on some aspects of long bone biomechanics resemble those of APD in rodents [17] rather than those in remodelling species [31, 32, 32a]. They seem to be less consistent, however, than Me_2-APD actions on normal rat femurs [18, 19].

7. Cyclic derivatives

Dose-dependent, protective effects of 1-hydroxy-2-(imidazo(1,2-A)-pyridin-3-yl)-ethane-1,1-bisphosph onate (YM175) on mineral content and compressive strength (but not stiffness) of humeri from immobilized limbs were shown in either intact or OvX rats [34, 37]. Effects started at doses as low as 0.003 mg/kg/day s.c. or 0.1 mg/kg p.o. 5/wk for 3 months and were also found in shorter treatments (1–10 mg/kg/day p.o. for 2 weeks). Potency was found to be, respectively, 100 and 10,000 times greater than those of APD and EHDP on this model. In consonance, doses of 0.1 (partially) or 1 mg/kg (completely) given 5 weeks p.o. during 18 months prevented spongy bone from OvX-induced trabecular perforations and preserved vertebral strength in beagles [42]. A preventive activity of an 8-day treatment with YM175 on the biomechanical repercussion of experimental tumoral osteolysis in rats was also shown [36]. In every case results were correlative with effects on bone mineral content.

As shown, BP effects on bone biomechanics are dependent on (1) type of compound (newly developed drugs as AHBP or Me$_2$APD were shown to be more effective and to affect less negatively or even positively bone mineralization than first-generation derivatives); (2) dose-time scheme of administration (chronic, intermittent plans as well as parenteral administration give better results); (3) species (better responses of cancellous bone in remodelling mammals and of cortical bone in only-modelling rodents than vice versa); (4) type of bone (cancellous bone reacts more sensitively than cortical tissue); (5) intensity of modelling/remodelling (more noticeable results obtained in young, immobilized or castrated subjects); (6) mechanical stimulation history (coadjutant action of biomass and exercise to beneficial effects); (7) responsiveness of bone mechanostatic mechanisms (proportionality between effects and bone deformability); (8) endocrine status (absence of gonadal function may interfere with favourable results on bone geometry and induce a negative influence of BPs on bone stiffness); and (9) interaction with simultaneous treatments (glucocorticoid therapy, bone formation inducers, immobilization, weightlessness, OvX, etc. may potentiate, reduce or even change the sign of some BP effects).

Nevertheless, bone strength (at variance with bone stiffness, that shows large variations under different conditions) is positively affected in most of cases unless very high, demineralization-inducing doses are given. This effect seems to depend on improvements in both bone mineralization (including crystal package) and geometric properties, in variable proportion according to the type of compound or dosage assayed. Among geometric changes, those evoked on cross-sectional moment of inertia of long bones and bone fraction volume in vertebral bodies (highly dependent on mechanical stimulation history and bone ability to absorb energy) seem to be crucial for the determination of bone structural properties under most of the reviewed experimental conditions unless a lack of mineralization has taken place.

Taking into account the above comments (Fig. 2), the induction of bone strengthening by BPs as a result of improvements in both material and geometric parameters in many cases (a curious, distinctive property of BPs among current bone-seeking agents) should be regarded as derived from an 'anti-natural' behaviour of bone tissue [21, 23]. This effect could indeed be interpreted as a departure from the normal functioning rules of the mechanostat. Such a condition may emerge from BP-induced threshold effects on the activation-resorption phase of bone modelling [26] and/or on the activation frequency and resorption depth of bone remodelling units [45, 57] besides eventual changes induced in bone stiffness. This hypothesis could explain the experimentally shown dependency of the BP-induced improvement in mechanical properties of both normal and osteopenic bones upon mechanical stimulation under treatment [53] (Fig. 10) and bone deformability. Through this mechanism BP therapy could in fact counteract the biomechanical repercussion of bone-losing conditions.

Therefore, and as far as the earlier evaluations of their effects on fracture risk in osteoporotic humans seem to indicate [41, 45, 58, 65, 66], current and newly developed BPs should be regarded as useful, promising drugs [25, 44, 64] for treatment of bone-weakening diseases.

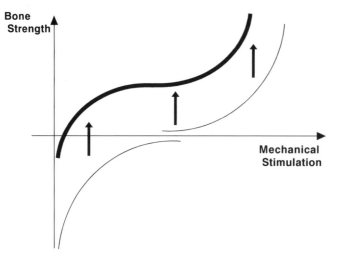

Fig. 10. Diagrammatic representation of BP-induced threshold effects (arrows, thick curve) on the postulated influence [21] of mechanical stimulation history on bone strength through modulation of bone modeling (thin curve, right) and remodeling (thin curve, left).

Acknowledgements. Drs. J.R. Zanchetta, R. Capozza, G. Cointry (CEMFoC-IDIM), E. Montuori, N. Mondelo and E. Roldán (Department of Experimental Pharmacology, Gador S.A., Buenos Aires) actively collaborated in the experiments discussed in this paper. Etidronate, pamidronate and dimethyl-pamidronate were in every instance kindly provided by Gador S.A.

References

1. Acito, A.J., Kasra, M., Lee, J.M. and Grynpas, M.D., Effects of intermittent administration of pamidronate on the mechanical properties of canine cortical and trabecular bone. J. Orthop. Res. 1994; 12: 742–746.

1a. Amman, P., Rizzoli, R., Meyer, J.M., Slosman, D. and Bonjour, J.P., Pamidronate improves trabecular bone mass/strength and, in association with IGF-1, cortical bone quality in ovariectomized rats. Bone Miner. 1994; 25(S1): S59.

2. Apseloff, G., Girten, B., Walker, M. et al., Aminohydroxybutane bisphosphonate prevents bone loss in a rat model of simulated weightlessness. Curr. Ther. Res. 1991; 5: 794–803.

3. Apseloff, G., Girten, B., Walker, M. et al. Aminohydroxybutane bisphosphonate and clenbuterol prevent bone changes and retard muscle atrophy respectively in tail-suspended rats. J. Pharmacol. Exp. Ther. 1993; 264: 1071–1078.

3a. Apseloff, G., Girten, B., Weisbrode, S.E. et al. Effects of aminohydroxybutane bisphosphonate on bone growth when administered after hind-limb bone loss in tail-suspended rats. J. Pharmacol. Exp. Ther. 1993; 267: 515–521.

4. Balena, R., Toolan, B.C., Shea, M. et al. The effects of 2-year treatment with the aminobisphosphonate alendronate on bone metabolism, bone histomorphometry, and bone strength in ovariectomized nonhuman primates. J. Clin. Invest. 1993; 92: 2577–2586.

5. Barbier, A., Bonjour, J.P., Geusens, P., de Vernejoul, M.C. and Lacheretz, F., Tiludronate: a bisphosphonate with a positive effect on bone quality in experimental models. J. Bone Miner. Res. 1990; 5(S1): S217.

6. Barbier, A., Geusens, P., Lacheretz, F. et al. Interest in biomechanical analysis in the experimental bone quality evaluation: the study of tiludronate as an example. Bone Miner. 1992; 17(S1): S12.

7. Bijvoet, O.L.M., Papapoulos, S.E., Loewik, C.W.G.M., Harinck, H.I.T., Manipulation of cell-cell interaction in bone with bisphosphonate in the interpretation of bone and calcium homeostasis in man. In: Cohn, D.V., Martin, T.J. and Meunier, P.J., eds. Calcium regulation and bone metabolism. Basic and clinical aspects 9. Amsterdam: Elsevier, 1987; 93–104.

8. Black, D.M., Reiss, T.F., Nevitt, M.C. et al. Design of the fracture intervention trial. Osteoporosis Int. 1993; 3(S3): S29–S39.

9. Boonekamp, P.M., Bijvoet, O.L.M., van der Wee-Pals, L.J.A. and van Wijk-van Lennep, M.L.L., Effect of bisphosphonates on bone resorption need not imply altered osteoclast function. In: Ornoy, A., Harell, A. and Sela, J., eds. Current advances in skeletogenesis. Amsterdam: Excerpta Medica, 1985; 59–64.

10. Boonekamp, P.M., Loewik, C.W.G.M., van der Wee-Pals, L.J.A., van Wijk-van Lennep, M.L.L. and Bijvoet, O.L.M., Enhancement of the inhibitory action of APD on the transformation of osteoclast precursors into resorbing cells after dimethylation of the amino group. Bone Miner. 1987; 2: 29–42.

11. Chan, M.M., Riggins, R.S. and Rucker, R.B., Effect of ethane-1-hydroxy-1,1-diphosphonate (EHDP) and dietary fluoride on biomechanical and biochemical changes in chick bone. J. Nutr. 1977; 107: 1747–1754.

12. Cooper, C., Fogelman, I. and Melton, L.J., Bisphosphonates and vertebral fracture: an epidemiological perspective. Osteoporosis Int. 1991; 2: 1–4.

13. Currey, J.D., The mechanical properties of materials and the structure of bone. In: Currey, J.D., ed. The mechanical adaptation of bones. New Jersey: Princeton University Press, 1984; 3–37.

14. De Vernejoul, M.C., Pointillart, A., Bergot, C. et al. Different schedules of administration of (3-amino-1-hydroxypropylidene)-1,1-bisphosphonate induce different changes in pig bone remodeling. Calcif. Tissue Int. 1987; 40: 160–165.

15. Dziedric-Goclawska, A., Kaminski, A., Kusy, R.P. and Yamuchi, M., The effect of Cl2MBP on mechanical properties, mineral content and bone volume in immobilized rats. Bone Miner. 1994; 25(S1): S59.

16. Einhorn, T., Peter, C.P., Clair, J., Rodan, G.A. and Thompson, D.D., Effect of alendronate on mechanical properties of bone in rats and dogs. J. Bone Miner. Res. 1990; 5(S1): S97.

17. Ferretti, J.L., Cointry, G., Capozza, R., Montuori, E., Roldán, E. and Pérez Lloret, A., Biomechanical effects of the full range of useful doses of (3-amino-1-hydroxypropylidene)-1,1-bisphosphonate (APD) on femur diaphyses and cortical bone tissue in rats. Bone Miner. 1990; 11: 101–109.

18. Ferretti, J.L., Mondelo, N., Capozza, R.F., Cointry, G.R., Zanchetta, J.R., and Montuori, E., Effects of large doses of olpadronate (dimethyl-pamidronate) on mineral density, cross-sectional architecture, and mechanical properties of rat femurs. Bone 1995; 16: in press.

19. Ferretti, J.L., Mondelo, N., Vázquez, S., Bogado, C.E., Montuori, E. and Zanchetta, J.R., Mineral density and structural properties of male and female rat femora as affected by dimethyl-pamidronate. J. Bone Miner. Res. 1991; 6(S1): S128.

20. Ferretti, J.L., Mondelo, N., Capozza, R., Vázquez, S., Montuori, E. and Zanchetta, J.R., Pamidronate and dimethyl-pamidronate effects on femur biomechanics in ovariectomized-hemisciaticectomized rats. Bone Miner. 1992; 17(S1): S12.

21. Ferretti, J.L., Scheinsohn, V., Macchi, M. and Zanchetta, J.R., Biological determination of diaphyseal thickness according to mechanical quality of bone material in several vertebrate species. J. Bone Miner. Res. 1992; 7(S2): S243–S245.

22. Ferretti, J.L., Delgado, C.J., Capozza, R. et al. Protective effects of disodium etidronate and pamidronate against the biomechanical repercussion of betamethasone-induced osteopenia in growing rat femurs. Bone Miner. 1993; 20: 265–276.

23. Ferretti, J.L., Capozza, R.F., Mondelo, N. and Zanchetta, J.R., Interrelationships between densitometric, geometric and mechanical properties of rat femurs. Inferences concerning mechanical regulation of bone modeling. J. Bone Miner. Res. 1993; 8: 1389–1396.

24. Ferretti, J.L., Mondelo, N., Peluffo, V. et al. Sub-chronic effects of high doses of mildronate on femur densitometric (DEXA), tomographic (pQCT) and mechanical properties in young rats. Bone Miner. 1994; 25(S2): S12.

25. Fleisch, H., The possible uses of bisphosphonates in osteoporosis. In: De Luca, H.F. and Mazess, R. eds. Osteoporosis: physiological basis, assessment, and treatment. Amsterdam: Elsevier, 1990; 323–329.

26. Frost, H.M., Intermediary organization of the skeleton. Boca Raton: CRC Press, 1986.

27. Frost, H.M., The mechanostat: a proposed pathogenic mechanism of osteoporoses and the bone mass effects of mechanical and nonmechanical agents. Bone Miner. 1987; 2: 73–86.

28. Geusens, P., Nijs, J., van der Perre, G. et al. Longitudinal skeletal effect of tiludronate on bone density and strength in monkeys. In: Christiansen, C. and Overgaard, K., eds. Osteoporosis 1990 1. Copenhagen: Osteopress, 1990; 366–367.

29. Geusens, P., Nijs, J., Van der Perre, G. et al. Longitudinal effect of tiludronate on bone mineral density, resonant frequency, and strength in monkeys. J. Bone Miner. Res. 1992; 7: 599–609.

30. Glatt, M., Pataki, A., Blaettler, A. and Reife, R., APD long-term treatment increases bone mass and mechanical strength of femora of adult mice. Calcif. Tissue Int. 1986; 39: A72.

31. Grynpas, M.D., Acito, A., Dimitru, M., Mertz, B.P. and Very, J.M., Changes in bone mineralization, architecture and mechanical properties due to long-term (1 year) administration of pamidronate (APD) to adult dogs. Osteoporosis Int. 1992; 2: 74–81.

32. Grynpas, M.D., Acito, A., Kasra, M., Renlund, R. and Pritzker, K.P.H., The effect of pamidronate (APD) administration on canine bone. Bone Miner. 1992; 17(S1): S15.

33. Guy, J.A., Shea, N., Peter, C.P., Morrissey, R. and Hayes, W.C., Continuous alendronate treatment throughout growth, maturation, and aging in the rat results in increases in bone mass and mechanical properties. Calcif. Tissue Int. 1993; 53: 283–288.

34. Kawamuki, K., Abe, T., Kudo, M. et al. Effect of YM175 on bone positively correlates with its concentration in bone. J. Bone Miner. Res. 1990; 5(S1): S245.

35. Kippo, K., Lepola, V., Hannuniemi, R. et al. Bone effects of two bisphosphonates (clodronate and etidronate) in ovariectomized rats. Bone Miner. 1994; 25(S1): S60.

36. Kudo, M., Abe, T., Kawamuki, K. et al. Effect of YM175 on experimental hypercalcemia and tumor-induced osteolysis in rats. J. Bone Miner. Res. 1990; 5(S1): S166.

37. Kudo, M., Abe, T., Motoie, H. et al. Pharmacological profile of new bisphosphonate 1-hydroxy-2-(imidazo(1,2-a)pyridin-3-yl)-ethane-1,1-bis(phosph onic acid). Bone Miner. 1992; 17(S1): S13.

38. Lauritzen, D.B., Balena, R., Shea, M. et al. Effects of combined prostaglandin and alendronate treatment on the histomorphometry and biomechanical properties of bone in ovariectomized rats. J. Bone Miner. Res. 1993; 8: 871–879.

39. Lepola, V., Jalovaara, P. and Väänänen, K., The influence of clodronate on the torsional strength of the growing rat tibia in immobilization osteoporosis. Bone 1994; 15: 367–371.

40. Lepola, V., Hannuniemi, R., Kippo, K., Jalovaara, P. and Väänänen, K., Long-term effects of clodronate on bone strength. Bone Miner. 1994; 25(S1): S60.

41. Miller, P.D., Watts, N.B., Genant, H.K. et al. Intermittent cyclical etidronate therapy in postmenopausal osteoporosis: analysis of fracture risk factors and one-year follow-up of bone mass changes. In: Christiansen, C. and Overgaard, K., eds. Osteoporosis 1990 3. Copenhagen: Osteopress, 1990; 1403–1405.

42. Ohnishi, H., Nakamura, T., Tsurukami, H., Murakami, H., Abe, M. and Barbier, A., Tiludronate increases the mechanical competence of lumbar vertebral body reduced after ovariectomy in rats. Bone Miner. 1994; 25(S1): S61.

43. Papapoulos, S.E., Hoekman, K., Löwik, W.G.M., Vermeij, P. and Bijvoet, O.L.M., Application of an in vivo model and a clinical protocol in the assessment of the potency of a new bisphosphonate. J. Bone Miner. Res. 1989; 4: 775–781.

44. Papapoulos, S.E., Bijvoet, O.L.M., Valkema, R. et al. New bisphosphonates in the treatment of osteoporosis. In: Christiansen, C., ed. Osteoporosis 1990 3. Copenhagen: Osteopress, 1990; 1294–1300.

45. Parfitt, A.M., Use of bisphosphonates in the prevention of bone loss and fractures. Am. J. Med. 1991; 91(5B): 42S–46S.

46. Reid, I.R., King, A.R., Alexander, C.J. and Ibbertson, H.K., Prevention of steroid-induced osteoporosis with (3-amino-1-hydroxypropylidene)-1,1-bisphosphonate (APD). Lancet 1988; 8578: 143–146.

47. Reitsma, P.H., Bijvoet, O.L.M., Veerlinden-Ooms, H. and van der Wee-Pals, L.J.A., Kinetic studies of bone and mineral metabolism during treatment with (3-amino-1-hydroxypropylidene)-1,1-bisphosphonate (APD) in rats. Calcif. Tissue Int. 1980; 32: 145–157.

48. Reitsma, P.H., Bijvoet, O.L.M., Potokar, M., van der Wee-Pals, L.J.A. and van Wijk-van Lennep, M.M.L., Apposition and resorption of bone during oral treatment with (3-amino-1-hydroxypropylidene)-1,1-bisphosphonate (APD). Calcif. Tissue Int. 1983; 35: 357–361.

49. Rodan, G.A., Seedor, J.G. and Balena, R., Preclinical pharmacology of alendronate. Osteoporosis Int. 1993; 3(S3): S7–S12

50. Schoutens, A., Verhas, M., Dourov, N. et al. Bone loss and bone blood flow in paraplegic rats treated with calcitonin, diphosphonate, and indomethacin. Calcif. Tissue Int. 1988; 42: 136–143.

51. Shea, M., Guy, J.A., Seedor, G.J., Rodan, G.A. and Hayes, W.C., Alendronate preserves geometric and tissue properties in the femora of aging estrogen-deficient rats. Bone Miner. 1994; 25(S1): S62.
52. Shea, M., Balena, R., Guy, J.A. et al. Alendronate preserves the mechanical and histomorphometrical properties in vertebrae of aging estrogen-deficient rats. Bone Miner. 1994; 25(S1): S62.
53. Shellhart, W.C., Hardt, A.B., Moore, R.N. and Erickson, L.C., Effects of bisphosphonate treatment and mechanical loading on bone modeling in the rat tibia. Clin. Orthop. Rel. Res. 1992; 278: 253–259.
54. Shiota, E., Eguchi, M., Kawamura, H. and Shimauchi, T., Effects of bisphosphonate on osteoporosis induced in rats. In: Christiansen, C. and Overgaard, K., eds. Osteoporosis 1990 2. Copenhagen: Osteopress, 1990; 1147–1149.
55. Steiniche, T., Hasling, C., Charles, P., Eriksen, E.F., Melsen, F. and Mosekilde, L., The effects of etidronate on trabecular bone remodeling in postmenopausal osteoporosis: a randomized study comparing intermittent treatment and an ADFR regime. Bone 1991; 12: 155–164.
56. Storm, T., Thamsborg, G., Steiniche, T., Genant, H.K. and Sorensen, O.H., Effect of intermittent cyclical etidronate therapy on bone mass and fracture rate in women with postmenopausal osteoporosis. N. Engl. J. Med. 1990; 322: 1265–1271.
57. Storm, T., Thamsborg, G., Kollerup, G. et al. Five years of intermittent, cyclical etidronate therapy increases bone mass and reduces vertebral fracture rate in postmenopausal osteoporosis. Bone Miner. 1992; 17(S1): S24.
58. Storm, T., Steiniche, T., Thamsborg, G. and Melsen, F., Changes in bone histomorphometry after long-term treatment with intermittent, cyclic etidronate for postmenopausal osteoporosis. J. Bone Miner. Res. 1993; 8: 199–208.
59. Thompson, D.D., Seedor, J.G., Weinreb, M., Rosini, S. and Rodan, G.A., Aminohydroxybutane bisphosphonate inhibits bone loss due to immobilization in rats. J. Bone Miner. Res. 1990; 5: 279–286.
60. Togari, A., Arai, M., Hironaka, M., Matsumoto, S. and Shinoda, H., Effect of EHBP (1-hydroxy-ethylidene-1,1-bisphosphonate) on experimental osteoporosis induced by ovariectomy in rats. Jpn. J. Pharmacol. 1991; 56: 177–185.
61. Toolan, B.C., Shea, M., Myers, E.R. et al. The effect of long term alendronate treatment on vertebral strength in ovariectomized baboons and rats. J. Bone Miner. Res. 1991; 6(S1): S248.
62. Toolan, B.C., Shea, M., Myers, E.R. et al. Effects of 4-amino-1-hydroxybutylidene bisphosphonate on bone biomechanics in rats. J. Bone Miner. Res. 1992; 7: 1399–1406.
63. Turner, C.H., Homeostatic control of bone structure: an application of feedback theory. Bone 1991; 12: 203–218.
64. Turner, C.H., Toward a cure for osteoporosis: reversal of excessive bone fragility. Osteoporosis Int. 1991; 2: 12–19.
65. Wasnich, R.D., Ross, P.D., Genant, H.K. et al. Cyclical etidronate therapy increases bone mass and reduces fracture incidence: a 4-year, prospective study. In: Christiansen, C. (ed), IV International Symposium on Osteoporosis and Consensus Development Conference, Hong Kong 1993; 134.
66. Watts, N.B., Harris, S.T., Genant, H.K. et al. Intermittent cyclical etidronate treatment of postmenopausal osteoporosis. N. Engl. J. Med. 1992; 323: 73–79.

Bisphosphonate on bones
O. Bijvoet, H.A. Fleisch, R.E. Canfield and G. Russell (eds.)
© 1995 Elsevier Science B.V. All rights reserved.

CHAPTER 15

Pharmacodynamics of bisphosphonates in man; implications for treatment

Socrates E. Papapoulos

Department of Endocrinology and Metabolic Diseases, University Hospital, Leiden, The Netherlands

I. Introduction

Bisphosphonates are taken up preferentially by the skeleton and affect bone surface-related processes. They accumulate on active bone surfaces, they can be taken up by bone cells, they may be locally released by desorption from the surface, or they can be embedded in bone. Detailed analysis of this sequence of events in vivo is impossible with current pharmacokinetic techniques. There are additional limitations in the assessment of the pharmacokinetics of bisphosphonates. For example, measurement of bisphosphonate concentrations in biological fluids has been until recently difficult, and information had to be obtained from experiments with radiolabelled compounds precluding, thus, studies in humans. Even in animal studies with radiolabelled bisphosphonates, however, classical pharmacokinetic concepts and analyses are not applicable due to the long retention time of the drugs in bone, which makes a pharmacokinetic steady state very difficult to obtain. Moreover, bisphosphonates affect a bone surface-related process, while the drug which is embedded in bone during bone remodelling is biologically inert; there are presently no valid models which can distinguish between these two bone compartments in vivo even with the use of sensitive and specific assays for measuring bisphosphonate concentrations. Understanding, therefore, the pharmacological properties of these drugs and designing appropriate therapeutic regimens depend to a large extent on the interpretation of pharmacodynamic data. Such information can more or less accurately be derived in vivo due to the properties of bisphosphonates to concentrate specifically in bone and to suppress bone resorption, a biological response which can readily be quantitated. In this chapter the pharmacodynamic background of bisphosphonate treatment will be reviewed and the use of this information in designing therapeutic strategies will be discussed.

II. Assessment of the antiresorptive potency of bisphosphonates in man

As discussed earlier in this volume, there have been considerable difficulties in the accurate assessment of the relative antiresorptive potencies of bisphosphonates in vitro and hence of the appropriate ranking of the various compounds and of the choice of relevant therapeutic doses. Even with the availability of suitable in vitro resorption assays and in vivo animal models, the problem of directly extrapolating these results to human studies remained. Harinck et al. [1], while studying the short-term effects of bisphosphonate treatment (pamidronate) in patients with Paget's disease, observed that the rate of decrease of bone resorption, assessed by measuring urinary hydroxyproline excretion, was exponential and independent of initial disease activity (Figure 1). This allowed these investigators to express the response to bisphosphonate as a fractional decrease of the excess of bone resorption. In this way, results from patients with variable disease activity could be uniformly analysed, and only small groups of patients treated for short periods (up to 10 days) were needed to obtain information about the magnitude of the anti-resorptive action of the drug. This analysis was applied to data of patients treated with various doses of pamidronate, and a linear log dose-response relationship between dose and time taken for hydroxyproline excess to decrease by 50% was

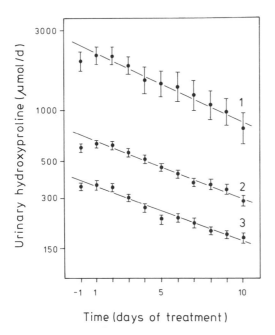

Time (days of treatment)

Fig. 1. Decrease of urinary hydroxyproline excretion during treatment with oral pamidronate 600 mg/ day in 83 patients with Paget's disease of bone without prior bisphosphonate therapy. Patients are grouped according to pretreatment hydroxyproline excretion; 3: <500 μmol/day, n=44; 2: 500–1000 μmol/day, n=27; 1: >1000 μmol/day, n=12. Means and SE of log values are given. From Harinck et al. [1].

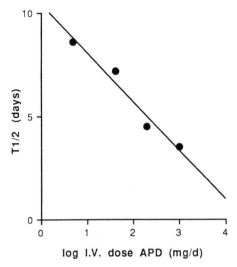

Fig. 2. Relation between different doses (log values) of i.v. pamidronate (2, 5, 10 and 20 mg) and time to decrease the initial excess of urinary hydroxyproline excretion by 50% in 4 groups of patients with Paget's disease, without prior bisphosphonate therapy, treated for 10 days. Adapted from Harinck et al. [1].

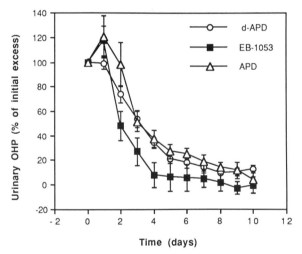

Fig. 3. Urinary hydroxyproline excretion (OHP) expressed as percentage of initial excess in three groups of patients with Paget's disease treated for 10 days with i.v. pamidronate 20 mg/day (triangles), dimethyl-APD 4 mg/day (open circles) or EB-1053 4 mg/day (closed squares). Means ± SE are shown.

obtained (Figure 2). The approach was tested prospectively in studies with other bisphosphonates such as dimethyl-APD [2] and EB-1053. The former is about 5 times more potent than pamidronate, while the latter bisphosphonate is about 10 times more potent than pamidronate in vitro [3]. As shown in Figure 3, when three groups of patients with Paget's disease were given pamidronate (20 mg/

day), dimethyl-APD (4 mg/day) or EB-1053 (4 mg/day) for 10 days, the first two bisphosphonates induced a very similar suppression of resorption, while the third was slightly more potent. Harinck et al. [1] also analysed data obtained with intravenous clodronate and calculated that the time required for 50% reduction in urinary hydroxyproline excretion with 300 mg/day i.v. clodronate was about 3 days; this makes clodronate about 10 to 20 times less potent than pamidronate, as already predicted by the in vitro resorption assay [4]. Thus, with the use of appropriate in vitro resorption assays and small groups of patients with Paget's disease, rapid and accurate information about the relative potencies of bisphosphonates to suppress bone resorption can be obtained. Caution is needed, however, in the way the drug is given. Although oral administration provides similar information to intravenous administration [5, 6], the former is not recommended for such studies because of the low and variable intestinal absorption (1–5%) which is characteristic of all bisphosphonates and cannot be adequately controlled in pharmacodynamic studies requiring precise knowledge of the concentration of the bisphosphonate delivered in the circulation.

III. Bisphosphonates in the study of bone cell-cell interaction in man

The pharmacodynamic information obtained with the use of Paget's disease as a clinical model have also led to the in vivo evaluation of forced changes in bone cellular dynamics in addition to their validity in assessing the anti-resorptive potency of bisphosphonates. In Paget's disease bone resorption is tightly coupled to bone formation [7]. During the early phase of treatment of patients with Paget's disease with bisphosphonates, there is a rapid suppression of bone resorption. In this initial phase bone formation is not affected and decreases later as a result of the coupling between bone resorption and bone formation [1, 8–13]. It has now been unequivocally demonstrated that a short course of bisphosphonate which suppresses bone resorption effectively will lead in the long run to a secondary suppression of bone formation even if the treatment is given for only a few days. This was shown by following the sequential changes in serum alkaline phosphatase activity and in urinary excretion of hydroxyproline as indices of bone formation and resorption, respectively. The short initial half-life of urinary hydroxyproline corresponds to the short turnover of osteoclasts. On the other hand, the delayed decrease in serum alkaline phosphatase activity corresponds to estimates of osteoblast turnover time. The induced uncoupling of bone resorption and bone formation with bisphosphonate treatment and the resulting positive bone balance are associated with marked changes in calcium metabolism. There is a fall in serum calcium which stimulates PTH secretion and 1,25-dihydroxyvitamin D production. These in turn increase the renal tubular reabsorption of calcium (PTH) and its intestinal absorption (1,25-DHH). During the period of uncoupling there is, thus, a great increase in external calcium balance, the magnitude of which is limited only by the capacity of the intestine to absorb calcium. As the equilibrium between bone resorption and bone formation is slowly restored, these transient changes in calcium homeostasis revert to normal, and a new steady state is obtained at a lower level of bone turnover. Despite the often marked reductions in bone resorption, the adaptive changes of calcium metabolism prevent the development of symptomatic hypocalcaemia. Appreciation of the transient changes not only simplified the treatment of patients with Paget's disease and emphasised the importance of dose and duration of treatment for long-term responses but demonstrated also the magnitude of the adaptation of calcium metabolism to the needs of skeletal homeostasis [14].

IV. The acute-phase response

In some patients treated for the first time with nitrogen-containing bisphosphonates, there is an increase in body temperature within the first 3 days of treatment associated with flu-like symptoms (e.g. malaise and myalgias). This effect is transient and reverses without any specific treatment within a few days. It has been reported with the use of pamidronate, alendronate, aminohexane, dimethyl-APD [5, 6, 12, 15–17]. In a detailed analysis of a large group of patients with Paget's disease treated with pamidronate and followed daily in a metabolic ward, Harinck et al. [5] reported that 54% of patients treated with pamidronate orally (600 mg/day) and 63% of those treated intravenously (20 mg/day) had an increase in body temperature of more than 0.5°C. The rise in temperature was not related to the activity of the disease, to the mode of the drug administration or to dose/kg body weight. The incidence of a similar rise in temperature in patients with Paget's disease treated with either oral or intravenous dimethyl-APD was 18.6% [6]. In studies with different nitrogen-containing bisphosphonates, Adami et al. [16] reported that this is a dose-related effect, and in a recent study in postmenopausal women treated orally with low doses of alendronate, no febrile reactions were recorded [18]. It should be noted that in most of the studies reporting such a reaction the exact level of temperature is not mentioned — it is described rather as a febrile reaction — and it is, therefore, impossible to estimate its true incidence according to bisphosphonate and dose. Such reactions have not been reported with the use of etidronate or clodronate and are independent of the specific bone pathology. The mechanism underlying this response is unclear. The clinical and biochemical picture, however, strongly resemble an acute phase reaction. Apart from the rise in temperature there is also a transient decrease in lymphocyte count and transient changes in acute phase reactants in serum (e.g. C-reactive protein in serum; Figure 4). Of considerable interest is the observation that patients exposed to a nitrogen-containing bisphosphonate once do not show this reaction when they are re-treated with the same or another nitrogen-containing bisphosphonate even if the interval between the two treatments is years apart [6, 16]. On the other hand, previous treatment with etidronate does not preclude the acute-phase response to subsequently administered nitrogen-containing bisphosphonates, but it has been reported that clodronate does [16]. An acute-phase reaction is generally thought to be mediated by cytokines such as Interleukin-6 and TNF-α. Studies of circulating levels of these cytokines in patients treated with nitrogen-containing

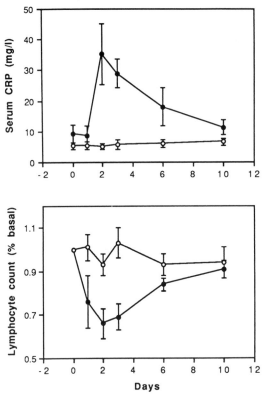

Fig. 4. Sequential changes in serum C-reactive protein and in percent lymphocyte count in two groups of patients with Paget's disease (8 patients per group) during treatment with pamidronate 20 mg/day for 10 days. Closed circles: patients treated for the first time with a nitrogen-containing bisphosphonate. Open circles: patients who had been treated in the past with pamidronate and were studied during a recurrence of their disease.

bisphosphonates are equivocal, and although there is some evidence in support of an involvement of these cytokines in the bisphosphonate-induced acute-phase reaction, hard proof is still lacking. With the available data we can only hypothesise about the nature of this effect. The primary question is whether this is a side effect of treatment or a phenomenon related to the biological response and/or to the mechanism of action of the drugs. A side effect of treatment seems highly unlikely as it does not occur upon re-treatment. It appears, therefore, to be related to the action of the bisphosphonate at the bone-bone marrow interface. Interleukin-6, for example, is produced by osteoblasts and stromal cells of the bone marrow in response to various factors and stimulates osteoclastogenesis and bone resorption [19]. This cytokine is also increased in the bone marrow of patients with Paget's disease [20]. In addition, fetal bones from rodents produce Il-6 in culture, and this production can be stimulated by treatment with other cytokines such as Il-1, growth factors or hormones such as PTH and PTHrP [21–23]. Some nitrogen-containing bisphosphonates given at low doses increase the production of Il-6 from these bone explants, while clodronate, which does not elicit an acute-phase response, has no such effect [24]. With higher doses Il-6 production is suppressed. It may, therefore, be that during the initial exposure of bone to nitrogen-containing bisphosphonates, Il-6 is locally released, and if this release is high, the cytokine enters the systemic circulation at a level sufficient to induce an acute-phase response. In this respect, it is interesting to note that patients with Paget's disease who showed transient temperature rises and haematological changes with pamidronate treatment also had an increase in urinary hydroxyproline excretion during the first day of treatment [5]. It is tempting to speculate that this initial increase in bone resorption is mediated by the above-mentioned cytokine-modulated mechanism. It should also be noted that the magnitude of the acute-phase response to nitrogen-containing bisphosphonates, even when severe, is much less than that observed in response to an infectious agent. How may this potential sequence of events explain the lack of any response upon re-treatment? Bisphosphonates have a very long residence time in the skeleton, and small amounts are probably locally released from bone constantly. Such low concentrations may stimulate local release of the cytokines in concentrations which are inadequate for a systemic response but at the same time adequate to preclude a general response to new bisphosphonate treatment. This hypothesis needs, however, to be tested in practice.

V. Factors affecting the response to bisphosphonates

As mentioned earlier, bisphosphonates are taken up at active bone surfaces, and the rate of bone turnover will, therefore, be a major determinant of the uptake of the drug by the skeleton. The higher the bone turnover, the higher the retention of bisphosphonate in the skeleton. The dose of the drug and in particular the way this is delivered will further determine the biological response. Although the total dose, if given within a short period of time, is important for the effect on bone resorption, the concentration which is presented to bone at any particular time appears to be the major determinant of the anti-resorptive effect. These statements are elaborated in the following paragraphs with the help of data obtained in three different states of bone turnover. First, normal bone turnover, second, unopposed bone resorption and third, increased bone turnover.

1. Normal bone turnover

When a bisphosphonate is given as a single i.v. infusion to healthy subjects with normal bone turnover, bone resorption is quickly suppressed. Netelenbos et al. [25] showed that a single infusion of pamidronate (20 mg) to healthy volunteers decreased urinary hydroxyproline excretion to 43% of basal values after 3 days. While during the follow-up period there was a tendency for the values to return to the basal level, they were still 55% of basal after one month and 77% of basal after two months. Passeri et al. [26] treated patients with osteoporosis with the more potent bisphosphonate alendronate 5 mg/day i.v. for two consecutive days. The mean rate of bone resorption in these patients was normal. Three months later urinary hydroxyproline excretion was still 75% of basal. Therefore, one or two infusions with bisphosphonate doses which suppress bone resorption effectively can have long-term effects on bone metabolism when bone turnover is normal. If bone turnover is low, as in some patients with osteoporosis, this effect may be amplified.

2. Unopposed bone resorption

The situation is different in conditions with unopposed bone resorption, the typical example being malignancy-associated hypercalcaemia. After a short i.v. course with a bisphosphonate, bone resorption is suppressed to values which depend on the dose and the compound used [13, 27–33]. This suppression of bone resorption is associated with a decrease in serum calcium concentrations. The response is, however, short-lived, and if the malignancy is left untreated, the rate of resorption returns to basal within two to four weeks, and hypercalcaemia recurs. It has been shown, for example, that in patients with malignancy-associated hypercalcaemia following successful treatment with pamidronate, hypercalcaemia recurred within 3 weeks in 50% of patients who received no additional anti-tumour treatment [34]. Thus, in the presence of unopposed increased bone resorption induced by local and/or systemic factors, the effect of bisphosphonate treatment is quickly reversed. It should be noted that in practice the study of bisphosphonate pharmacodynamics in tumour patients has certain limitations due to the gravity of the condition as well as to the possible contribution of the tumour turnover to the levels of urinary hydroxyproline. With the recently developed methods for the measurement of specific bone collagen degradation products, more accurate information may be obtained regarding the exact level of suppression of bone resorption. It is unlikely, however, that such information will add anything new to the general concept of the quick reversal of the effect.

3. Increased bone turnover

In conditions with increased bone turnover, the picture is more complex, and the response to bisphosphonate appears to depend on the driving force of the abnormality. For example, hyperparathyroidism is characterized by increased bone turnover due to increased secretion of PTH. It is generally believed that PTH affects bone metabolism through an effect on the osteogenic cells rather than on the osteoclasts which do not have receptors for the peptide [35]. In response to PTH osteogenic cells release factors which in turn affect the formation and/or the activity of the osteoclasts [36]. In this way in hyperparathyroidism the rate of bone remodelling increases. Short-term bisphosphonate administration to patients with primary hyperparathyroidism suppresses bone resorption, as expected. The effect is, however, quickly reversed due to the continuing secretion of PTH which probably generates new active bone remodelling sites. Whether PTH can also reverse the effect of bisphosphonates which have already been taken up by bone surfaces is unclear at present. In vitro studies have shown that the effects of bisphosphonates on osteoclastic resorption can be reversed by PTH depending on the class of the compound. For example, addition of PTH to cultures of fetal bone explants of rodents can reverse the anti-resorptive effect of the newer potent bisphosphonates dimethyl-APD and EB-1053 but not that of clodronate and pamidronate [37]. No human studies have addressed this particular issue yet, but some indications that this may also be the case in vivo are discussed further.

Carcinoma of the prostate metastasises frequently to the skeleton, and up to 62% of patients have bone metastases at the time of diagnosis [38]. Metastases are typically osteosclerotic rather than osteolytic. Biochemical and histological studies have, however, shown that bone resorption is also increased and that in such patients there is a close relation between bone formation and bone resorption, with an overall increase in bone turnover [39–41]. It appears that factors which are produced by the carcinoma cells and have a mitogenic effect on osteoblasts may also stimulate osteogenic cells to release substances which can in turn stimulate osteoclast formation and/or activity leading to increased bone resorption. Alternatively, carcinoma cells may release factors which can directly stimulate bone resorption, as is the case with other malignancies. A short course of bisphosphonates induces a predictable suppression of bone resorption [42, 43]. This is, however, again short-lived, and within 6 weeks the rate of resorption has returned to pre-treatment levels (own unpublished observations), a response similar to that seen during increased parathyroid activity independently of the extent of the disease.

In contrast to the above-mentioned two conditions, in Paget's disease of bone the primary abnormality lies in the osteoclast, and suppression of bone resorption with a short course of bisphosphonates can be sustained for a long period. The possibility that this is due to higher local concentrations of bisphosphonate in Paget's disease because of the focal nature of the defect and because of targeting a higher concentration in a smaller area seems unlikely as similar results have been obtained in patients with limited as well as with extensive involvement of the skeleton, provided that an adequate dose is given. In addition, when Paget's disease is accompanied by increased parathyroid activity, suppression of resorption is not sustained for long.

This information about the effect of the rate of bone turnover on the response to bisphosphonates is summarised in Figure 5.

4. Implications for treatment

It is clear that a short course of bisphosphonate will suppress bone resorption rapidly independently of its initial rate. The duration, however, of this effect will mainly depend on the initial rate as well as on its driving force. The question which arises is whether the total dose of bisphosphonate or the peak concentration presented to bone is more important. In other words, will the same effect be obtained by dividing the dose and giving it over a longer period of time? Animal data have already provided evidence that this is generally not the case. For example, Reitsma et al. [44] treated young growing rats with different parenteral

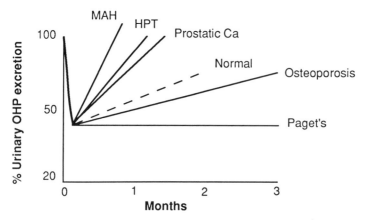

Fig. 5. Schematic representation of the induction and duration of the effect of short courses with intravenous bisphosphonates on bone resorption in conditions with different rates of bone turnover (and different mechanisms for increased bone turnover when this is abnormal). MAH: malignancy-associated hypercalcaemia; HPT: hyperparathyroidism; Prostatic Ca: carcinoma of the prostate.

doses of pamidronate and followed the changes in bone resorption by measuring urinary hydroxyproline excretion. With a dose of 1.6 μmol/kg/day, there was a suppression of bone resorption of about 50% within two days of treatment. In contrast, with a dose of 0.16 μmol/kg/day, suppression of resorption did not exceed 40% even after 15 days of treatment. Comparable data in humans are not available, but analysis of published results leads to the same conclusions. For example, Thiebaud et al. [45] recently showed that single infusions of 30 mg pamidronate given to patients with osteoporosis every 3 months led to a decrease in urinary hydroxyproline excretion by about 43% after one year. We found that oral pamidronate (150 mg) given daily suppressed urinary hydroxyproline excretion by about 25% after one year in patients with osteoporosis [46]. Assuming an absorption of the bisphosphonate of 1%, this means that the total dose of bisphosphonate delivered over a year orally was about 550 mg or roughly four times higher than the total dose delivered intravenously (120 mg). Yet the suppression of resorption obtained with the intravenous administration was considerably higher. The situation is more complex in conditions with excessive bone resorption as there appear to be threshold doses above which similar effects can be obtained with either short or divided administration of the bisphosphonate as long as this is given within a certain period of time. For example, in malignancy-associated hypercalcaemia we found similar effects on bone resorption with dimethyl-APD given by single infusion (10 mg) or orally (200 mg/day) for a maximum of 7 days (equivalent to about 14 mg). The exact duration of this period needs, however, still to be defined, but it appears to be a few weeks.

The above-mentioned studies coupled with an increasing understanding of bone biology have led to the formulation of the following therapeutic concepts. Firstly, in conditions with increased bone resorption short courses with high doses of bisphosphonate should be administered; the limiting factor of the level of the dose being the toxicological profile of the compound. Continuous administration of low doses will induce incomplete responses even if the total dose is the same. Secondly, when bone resorption is not excessive and bone turnover is low or normal, caution is needed when giving short courses with high doses as these may induce marked and sustained suppression of bone resorption, leading in the long term to an overall excessive suppression of bone turnover due to the coupling between the processes of bone resorption and formation. This may impair the ability of bone to remodel with all its consequences especially in patients with osteoporosis.

VI. Side effects to bisphosphonate treatment

Detailed discussion of the side effects to treatment lies outside the scope of this chapter. However, as some of the potential toxic effects of bisphosphonates may occur at the bone tissue level and are related to the individual pharmacological profile of the drug, relevant issues will be briefly discussed here for completeness. There is remarkably little toxicity associated with bisphosphonate treatment as long as the general as well as the individual properties of the compounds are taken into consideration. Toxicity can be distinguished into local and generalized and to toxicity at the target level.

1. Local toxicity

Mild gastrointestinal complaints have been reported with variable but rather low frequency with the oral use of all bisphosphonates. Aminobisphosphonates, however, given orally can induce more severe gastrointestinal side effects such as heartburn, nausea or vomiting. In patients treated with enteric-coated pellets of pamidronate, some cases of serious oesophagitis have been documented. This side effect is dose- and formulation-dependent. For example, pamidronate doses higher than 300 mg/day induce gastrointestinal side effects of varying severity in up to 50% of patients and doses above 600 mg/day are hardly tolerated by the majority of patients [5]. These are more frequent if the drug is given in solution. On the other hand, with the use of doses lower than 300 mg/day and of formulations such as enteric-coated tablets or soft gelatin capsules, the incidence of these complaints decreases considerably. In a preliminary report of the use of very low oral doses of alendronate, no such effects were encountered [18]. This side effect limits the use of the full potential of oral aminobisphosphonates in the treatment of patients with increased bone resorption in whom high, suppressive doses are needed. This problem may be overcome by improved oral formulations, and various industries are exploring this possibility. As a general rule, bisphosphonates should be administered on an empty stomach with adequate water (about two glasses). They should never be given together with food and calcium-containing preparations or before going to bed. Another side effect is the local irritation at the site of bisphosphonate infusion, and mild thrombophlebitis has been observed in a few patients. This is again a problem of aminobisphosphonates and has not been described with clodronate. Aminobisphosphonates should never be administered intramuscularly or directly into the vein but should be given by infusion. There is not enough information about these side effects with other new nitrogen-containing bisphosphonates, but in our studies with dimethyl-APD no such effects were encountered with the use of suppressive oral or intravenous doses [6].

2. General toxicity

Bisphosphonates when infused in high concentrations may rapidly chelate calcium in the circulation. Calcium-bisphosphonate complexes may be formed which can be nephrotoxic. As the primary aim of treatment is not the achievement of high peak blood concentrations, bolus intravenous injections should be avoided, and the drugs should be administered by slow infusion. This might be possible in the future with some new extremely potent bisphosphonates, but evidence for that is currently lacking. It has been further shown that the duration of infusion does not have any effect on the therapeutic response and infusing the same amount of bisphosphonate over 2 or 24 hours had the same effect on bone resorption [46, 47]. The minimal duration of the infusion should, however, be determined separately for every individual compound. Some cases of conjunctivitis or uveitis have been encountered during treatment with intravenous pamidronate. There is no clear cause and effect relationship, and data with other new bisphosphonates are not yet available to determine whether this effect is structure-related. Earlier fears that clodronate may predispose to leukaemia were not substantiated by long-term studies and careful analysis of the data.

With the earlier developed bisphosphonates (etidronate, clodronate, pamidronate) no evidence of renal or liver toxicity has been found with a wide range of doses. Occasional reported cases of renal toxicity are probably related to dose or mode of administration of the bisphosphonate [49]. Information about the newer compounds currently in phases 2 and 3 of clinical development are not generally available.

3. Toxicity at the target tissue

All bisphosphonates when given at very high doses may impair the mineralisation of newly formed osteoid. The induction of osteomalacia depends on the therapeutic window of every individual compound or its activity to toxicity ratio. With etidronate the difference between the dose required for effective suppression of increased bone resorption and that for inhibiting mineralisation is small, and histological osteomalacia has been documented in patients with Paget's disease treated with high but also with low doses of oral etidronate [50–52]. This is not the case with clodronate and pamidronate, which do not affect the mineralisation of newly formed osteoid. Data with other bisphosphonates in humans are scarce, but in animal studies alendronate and risedronate have been reported to have a very large activity to toxicity ratio.

Acknowledgements. I thank all the physicians and the nursing staff of the Clinical Investigation Unit of the University Hospital in Leiden for their contribution to the studies performed in our Unit. Our studies were supported in part by a programme grant from the Dutch Organization for Scientific Research (NWO 900-541-191).

References

1. Harinck, H.I.J., Bijvoet, O.L.M., Blanksma, H.J. and Dalinghaus-Nienhuys, P.J., Efficacious management with aminobisphosphonate (APD) in Paget's disease of bone. Clin. Orthop. 1987; 217: 79–98.
2. Papapoulos, S.E., Hoekman, K., Löwik, C.W.G.M., Vermeij, P. and Bijvoet, O.L.M., Application of an in vitro model and a clinical protocol in the assessment of the potency of a new bisphosphonate. J. Bone Miner. Res. 1989; 4: 775–781.
3. van der Pluijm, G., Binderup, L., Bramm, E. et al. Disodium 1-hydroxy-3-(1-pyrrolidinyl)-propylidene-1,1-bisphosphonate (EB-1053) is a potent inhibitor of bone resorption in vitro and in vivo. J. Bone Miner. Res. 1992; 7: 775–781.
4. Boonekamp, P.M., van der Wee-Pals, L.J.A., van Wijk-van Lennep, M.M.L., Thesingh, C.W. and Bijvoet, O.L.M., Two modes of action of bisphosphonates on osteoclastic resorption of mineralized matrix. Bone Miner. 1986; 1: 27–39.
5. Harinck, H.I.J., Papapoulos, S.E., Blanksma, H.J., Moolenaar, A.J., Vermeij, P. and Bijvoet, O.L.M., Paget's disease of bone: early and late responses to three different modes of treatment with aminohydroxypropylidene bisphosphonate (APD). Br. Med. J. 1987; 295: 1301–1305.
6. Schweitzer, D.H., Zwinderman, A.H., Vermeij, P., Bijvoet, O.L.M. and Papapoulos, S.E., Improved treatment of Paget's disease with dimethylaminohydroxypropylidene bisphosphonate. J. Bone Miner. Res. 1993; 8: 175–182.
7. Harinck, H.I.J., Bijvoet, O.L.M., Vellenga, C.J.L.R., Blanksma, H.J. and Frijlink, W.B., Relation between signs and symptoms in Paget's disease of bone. Q. J. Med. 1986; 58: 133–151.
8. Yates, A.J.P., Gray, R.E.S., Urwin, G.H. et al. Intravenous clodronate in the treatment and retreatment of Paget's disease of bone. Lancet 1985; i: 1474–1477.
9. Frijlink, W.B., te Velde, J., Bijvoet, O.L.M. and Heynen, G., Treatment of Paget's disease of bone with (3-amino-1-hydroxypropylidene)-1,1-bisphosphonate (APD). Lancet 1979; i: 799–803.
10. Thiebaud, D., Jaeger, P., Gobelet, C., Jacquet, A.F. and Burckhardt, P., A single infusion of the bisphosphonate AHPrBP (APD) as treatment of Paget's disease of bone. Am. J. Med. 1988; 85: 207–212.
11. Atkins, R.M., Yates, A.J.P., Gray, R.E.S. et al. Aminohexane diphosphonate in the treatment of Paget's disease of bone. J. Bone Miner. Res. 1987; 2: 273–279.
12. O'Doherty, D.P., Bickerstaff, D.R., McCloskey, E.V. et al., Treatment of Paget's disease of bone with aminohydroxybutylidene bisphosphonate. J. Bone Miner. Res. 1990; 5: 483–491.
13. Kanis, J.A. and McCloskey, E.V., The use of clodronate in disorders of calcium and skeletal metabolism. In: Kanis, J.A., ed., Calcium Metabolism. Prog. Basic Clin. Pharmacol. 1990; 4: 89–136.
14. Bijvoet, O.L.M., Papapoulos, S.E., Lowik, C.W.G.M. and Harinck, H.I.J., Manipulation of cell-cell interaction in bone with bisphosphonate in the interpretation of bone and calcium homeostasis in man. In: Cohn, D.V. et al., eds., Calcium Regulation and Bone Metabolism — Basic and Clinical Aspects, vol 9. Amsterdam: Excerpta Medica 1987: 93–104.
15. Bijvoet, O.L.M., Frijlink, W.D., Jie, K. et al., APD in Paget's disease of bone. Role of the mononuclear phagocyte system. Arthritis Rheum. 1980; 23: 1193–1204.
16. Adami, S., Bhalla, A.K., Dorizzi, R. et al., The acute phase response after bisphosphonate administration. Calcif. Tissue Int. 1987; 41: 326–331.
17. Adami, S., Salvagno, G., Guarrera, G. et al., Treatment of Paget's disease of bone with intravenous 4-amino-1-hydroxybutylidene-1,1-bisphosphonate. Calcif. Tissue Int. 1986; 39: 226–229.
18. Harris, S.T., Gertz, B.J., Genant, H.K. et al., The effect of short term treatment with alendronate on vertebral density and biochemical markers of bone remodeling in early postmenopausal women. J. Clin. Endocrinol. Metab. 1993; 76: 1399–1406.
19. Löwik, C.W.G.M., Differentiation inducing factors: Leukemia inhibitory factor and interleukin 6. In: Gowen, M., ed., Cytokines and Bone Metabolism, chapter 11. Boca Raton: CRC Press 1991:

300–324.
20. Roodman, G.D., Kurihara, N., Ohsaki, Y., Kukita, T., Hosking, D., Demulder, A. and Singer, F.S., Interleukin-6: a potential autocrine/paracrine factor in Paget's disease of bone. J. Clin. Invest. 1992; 89: 46–52.
21. Löwik, C.W.G.M., van der Pluijm, G., Bloys, H. et al., Parathyroid hormone (PTH) and PTH-like protein (PLP) stimulate Interleukin-6 production by osteogenic cells: a possible role of Interleukin-6 in osteoclastogenesis. Biochem. Biophys. Res. Commun. 1989; 162: 1546–1552.
22. Feyen, J.H.M., Elford, P., Dipadova, R.E. and Trechsel, U., Interleukin-6 is produced by bone and modulated by parathyroid hormone. J. Bone Miner. Res. 1989; 4: 633–638.
23. Slootweg, R., Most, W.W., van Beek, E., Schot, L.P.C., Papapoulos, S.E. and Lowik, C.W.G.M., Osteoclast formation together with interleukin-6 production in mouse long bones is increased by insulin growth factor I. J. Endocrinol. 1992; 132: 434–438.
24. van der Pluijm, G., van Beek, E., Löwik, C. and Papapoulos, S., Involvement of Il-6 in modulation of osteoclastic resorption by bisphosphonates. J. Bone Miner. Res. 1990; 5 (suppl 2): S234.
25. Netelenbos, J.C., van Ginkel, F.C., Lips, P. et al., Effect of single infusion aminohydroxypropylidene on calcium and bone metabolism in healthy volunteers monitored during 2 months. J. Clin. Endocrinol. Metab. 1991; 72: 223–228.
26. Passeri, M., Baroni, M.C., Pedrazzoni, M. et al., Intermittent treatment with intravenous 4-amino-1-hydroxybutylidene-1, 1-bisphosphonate (AHBuBP) in the therapy of postmenopausal osteoporosis. Bone Miner. 1991; 15: 237–248.
27. Bickerstaff, D.R., O'Doherty, D.P., McCloskey, E.V., Hamdy, N.A.T. and Kanis, J.A., Effects of aminobutylidene diphosphonate in hypercalcemia due to malignancy. Bone 1991; 12: 17–20.
28. Thiebaud, D., Jaeger, P. and Burckhardt, P., Response to retreatment of malignant hypercalcemia with the bisphosphonate AHPrBP (APD): respective role of kidney and bone. J. Bone Miner. Res. 1990; 5: 221–226.
29. Harinck, H.I.J., Bijvoet, O.L.M., Plantingh, A.S.T. et al., Role of bone and kidney in tumor-induced hypercalcemia and its treatment with bisphosphonate and sodium chloride. Am. J. Med. 1987; 82: 1133–1142.
30. Dumon, J.C., Magritte, A. and Body, J.J., Efficacy and safety of the bisphosphonate tiludronate for the treatment of tumor-associated hypercalcemia. Bone Miner. 1991; 15: 257–266.
31. Fleisch, H., Bisphosphonates: pharmacology and use in the treatment of tumour-induced hypercalcaemic and metastatic bone disease. Drugs 1991; 42: 919–944.
32. Fitton, A. and McTavish, D., Pamidronate, a review of its pharmacological properties and therapeutic efficacy in resorptive bone diseases. Drugs 1991; 41: 289–318.
33. Papapoulos, S.E. and van Holten-Verzandvoort, A.T.M., Modulation of tumour-induced bone resorption by bisphosphonates. J. Steroid Biochem. Mol. Biol. 1992; 43: 131–136.
34. Harinck, H.I.J. and Bijvoet, O.L.M., Clinical aspects of the treatment of tumor-induced hypercalcemia with APD. In: Burckhardt, P., ed., Disodium pamidronate (APD) in the treatment of malignancy-related disorders. Bern: Hans Huber Publishers 1989: 64–71.
35. Nijweide, P.J., Burger, E.H. and Feyen, J.H., Cells of bone: proliferation, differentiation and hormonal regulation. Phys. Rev. 1986; 66: 855–886.
36. Rodan, G.A. and Martin, T.J., Role of osteoblasts in hormonal control of bone resorption — a new hypothesis. Calcif. Tissue Int. 1981; 33: 191–200.
37. van der Pluijm, G., Löwik, C.W.G.M., de Groot, H. et al., Modulation of PTH-stimulated osteoclastic resorption by bisphosphonates in fetal mouse bone explants. J. Bone Miner. Res. 1991; 6: 1203–1210.
38. Tofe, A.J., Francis, M.D. and Harvey, W.J., Correlation of neoplasms with incidence and localization of skeletal metastases: an analysis of 1,355 diphosphonate bone scans. J. Nucl. Med. 1975; 16: 986–989.
39. Charhon, S.A., Chapuy, M.C., Delvin, E.E., Valentin-Opran, A., Edouard, C.M. and Meunier, P.J., Histomorphometric analysis of sclerotic bone metastases from prostatic carcinoma with special reference to osteomalacia. Cancer 1983; 51: 918–924.
40. Percival, R.C., Urwin, G.H., Harris, S. et al., Biochemical and histological evidence that carcinoma of the prostate is associated with increased bone resorption. Eur. J. Surg. Oncol. 1987; 13: 41–49.
41. Urwin, G.H., Percival, R.C., Harris, S., Beneton, M.N.C., Williams, J.L. and Kanis, J.A., Generalized increase in bone resorption in carcinoma of the prostate. Br. J. Urol. 1985; 57: 721–723.
42. Adami, S., Salvagno, G., Guarrera, G. et al., Dichloromethylene diphosphonate in patients with prostatic carcinoma metastatic to the skeleton. J. Urol. 1985; 134: 1152–1154.

43. Pelger, R.C.M., Lycklama, A., Nijeholt, A.A.B. and Papapoulos, S.E., Short-term metabolic effects of pamidronate in patients with prostatic cacrinoma and bone metastases. Lancet 1989; ii: 865.
44. Reitsma, P.H., Bijvoet, O.L.M., Verlinden-Ooms, H. and van der Wee Plas, L.J.A., Kinetic studies of bone and mineral metabolism during treatment with (3-amino-1-hydroxypropylidene)-1, 1-bisphosphonate (APD) in rats. Calcif. Tissue Int. 1980; 32: 145–157.
45. Thiebaud, D., Burckhardt, P., Melchior, J. et al., Two years' effectiveness of intravenous pamidronate (APD) versus oral fluoride for osteoporosis occurring in the postmenopause. Osteoporosis Int. 1994; 4: 76–83.
46. Papapoulos, S.E., Landman, J.O., Bijvoet, O.L.M. et al., The use of bisphosphonates in the treatment of osteoporosis. Bone 1992; 13 (suppl 1): S41–S49.
47. Zysset, E., Ammann, P., Jenzer, A. et al., Comparison of a rapid (2h) versus a slow (24h) infusion of alendronate in the treatment of hypercalcemia of malignancy. Bone Miner. 1992; 18: 237–249.
48. Ralston, S.H., Alzaid, A.A., Gallaher, S.J., Gardner, M.D., Cowan, R.A. and Boyle, I.T., Clinical experience with aminohydroxypropylidene bisphosphonate (APD) in the management of cancer-associated hypercalcaemia. Q. J. Med. 1988; 69; 258: 825–834.
49. Bounameaux, H.M., Sheifferli, J., Montani, J.-P., Jung, A. and Chatelanat, F., Renal failure associated with intravenous disphosphonates. Lancet 1983; i: 471.
50. Boyce, B.F., Fogelman, I., Ralston, S., Smith, L., Johnston, E. and Boyle, I.T., Focal osteomalacia due to low-dose diphosphonate therapy in Paget's disease. Lancet 1984; i: 821–824.
51. Russell, R.G.G., Smith, R., Preston, C.J., Walton, C.J. and Woods, C.G., Diphosphonates in Paget's disease. Lancet 1974; i: 894–898.
52. Evans, R.A., Dunstan, C.R., Holls, E. and Wong, S.Y.P., Pathological fracture due to severe osteomalacia following low-dose diphosphonate treatment of Paget's disease of bone. Aust. NZ. J. Med. 1983; 13: 277–279.

Bisphosphonate on bones
O. Bijvoet, H.A. Fleisch, R.E. Canfield and G. Russell (eds.)
© 1995 Elsevier Science B.V. All rights reserved.

CHAPTER 16

Determination of bisphosphonates in biological fluids

Bogdan K. Matuszewski

Merck Research Laboratories, West Point, PA 19486, USA

I. Introduction

The development of analytical methods for the determination of geminal bis-phosphonates in biological fluids presents a great challenge to analytical chemists. The majority of these compounds (Fig. 1) do not possess any chromophores for direct ultraviolet (UV), fluorescence and electrochemical (EC) detection. They are all highly polar and are not amenable to direct gas chromatographic (GC) analyses.

In addition, because of the presence of four acidic hydrogens in the molecule and, in the case of amino bisphosphonates, an amino group, these compounds have up to five pK_a values covering the entire pH range, which makes the development of adequate conditions for high-pressure liquid chromatographic (HPLC) determination difficult. This high polarity of the molecule also prevents the utilization of the common liquid-liquid or solid-phase extraction (SPE) methods for the isolation of the compound from biological fluids. The successful development of the analytical procedures for bisphosphonates in biological fluids at ng/ml levels requires three key steps: the efficient isolation of this highly polar and water-soluble material from the sample matrix, derivatization to convert this non-chromophoric molecule into a highly absorbing, fluorescing or volatile (for GC analysis) analogue, and utilization of some non-conventional chromatography to quantify and separate the highly polar and potentially unstable derivative from the impurities extracted from urine and plasma. These three steps will be described in some detail for all the assays covered in this review.

The assays described in the literature are almost exclusively concerned with compounds listed in Fig. 1, and these methods will be reviewed here. All these bisphosphonates were administered to both animal species and humans [1]. Since the selection of the detection technique and assay method depends on the presence of a derivatizable functional group in the molecule (for example, a primary amino group), all bisphosphonates listed in Fig. 1 were divided into three categories: those

1

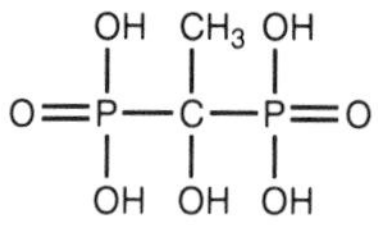

1-Hydroxyethylidene-
bisphosphonic acid (etidronate)

2

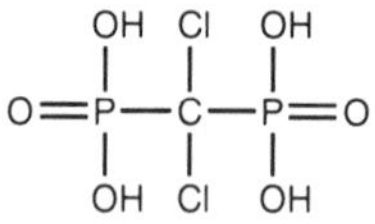

Dichloromethylene-
bisphosphonic acid (clodronate)

3

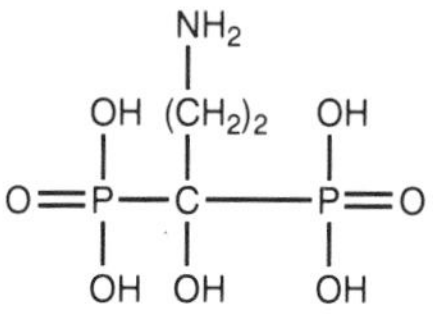

3-Amino-1-hydroxypropylidene-
bisphosphonic acid (pamidronate)

4

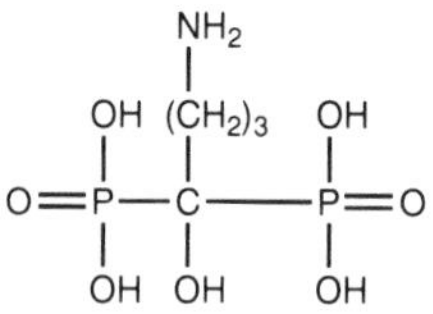

4-Amino-1-hydroxybutylidene-
bisphosphonic acid (alendronate)

5

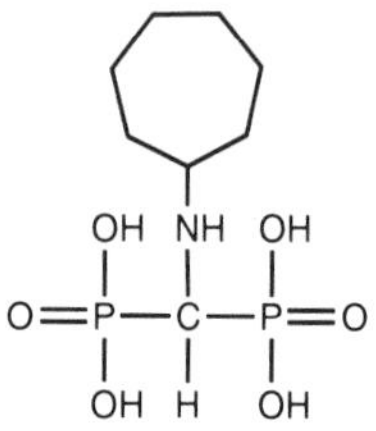

Cycloheptylamino-
methylenebisphosphonic
acid (YM 175)

6

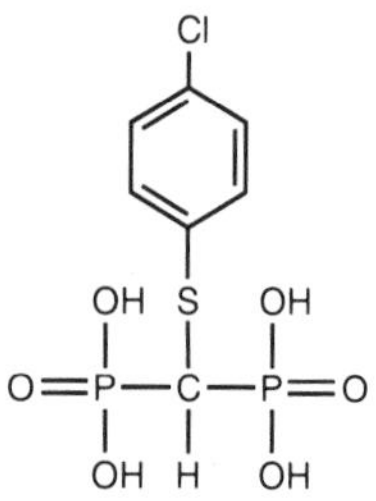

Chloro-4-phenylthiomethylidene-
bisphosphonic acid (tiludronate)

Fig. 1. Chemical structures of selected bisphosphonates

containing a primary or secondary amino group, compounds with no amino group present, and bisphosphonates possessing an UV-absorbing chromophore for direct detection without the need of derivatization.

The sensitivity of an analytical procedure in biological matrices is usually characterized by the lowest limit of quantitation (LOQ) per unit volume (ml) of the biological fluid used for the analysis. Various criteria are being used to define this LOQ. In order to make comparisons between different methods described in this review, the LOQ will be defined as the lowest concentration that can be assayed with adequate accuracy ($\leq 15\%$) and a relative standard deviation (precision, % RSD) of $\pm 10\%$.

A variety of methods have been described for the determination of bisphosphonates in pharmaceutical dosage forms [2–7], where isolation of the drug from the matrix and high sensitivity of detection are usually not required. These methods will not be reviewed here.

II. Assays of bisphosphonates not containing a primary amino group in the molecule

1. Etidronate (**1**)

Two older methods for the determination of etidronate (**1**) in urine and plasma are available [8, 9]. Both were based on potentially non-specific, spectrophotometric determination of products of either a competitive formation of a complex with **1**, which changes the absorption properties of an indicator (xylenol orange, XO) [8], or photochemical decomposition of **1** with UV radiation [9].

The first method [8] was based on the removal of **1** from urine using hydroxylapatite or calcium hydroxide, solubilization of the recovered residues of **1** and adsorption by cation exchange on a strong acid type resin, and titration of the effluent with a binary complex of thorium-diaminocyclohexanetetracetate (Th-DCTA) to form a ternary species (Th-DCTA)$_2$-**1**. As a colorimetric indicator XO was used and formed a similar, but weaker, ternary species (Th-DCTA-XO). Deprotonation of XO (H_3I^{2-} to H_2I^{3-}) occurred during formation of the latter species and caused a yellow to blue-violet colour change which was monitored spectrophotometrically. Analyses required 500 ml of urine, and the limit of detection (undefined) was reported as 0.1 ppm (about 100 ng/ml). The accuracy and precision of the method varied with the concentration, and in the samples containing 5–23 ppm of **1**, a standard deviation of 0.7 ppm (3–14%) was obtained.

The method of Bisaz et al. [9] was based on co-precipitation of **1** with calcium phosphate, elimination of inorganic phosphate as an insoluble triethylamine-phosphomolybdate complex, decomposition of the P-C-P bond with a polychromatic UV light, and spectrophotometric determination of the inorganic phosphate released. The method has been utilized for determination of **1** both in urine (5 ml) and plasma (2 ml). The isolation of **1** from biological fluids was based on the observation that calcium phosphate binds **1** very strongly, and a small precipitate of calcium phosphate is sufficient to coprecipitate **1** [10] (step 1). In step 2, the sediment was redissolved in 2 M HCl and heated for 30 min at 100°C in order to hydrolyse pyrophosphate and other acid-labile phosphate compounds into inorganic phosphate. The latter was then removed from the solution through formation of an insoluble triethylamine-phosphomolybdate complex (step 3) by the addition of ammonium molybdate and triethylamine. In order to oxidize any blue molybdate complexes formed, a solution of bromine in water was added before the addition of reagents. After removal of the inorganic phosphates, **1** was co-precipitated from the filtrate using calcium chloride and 10 M solution of sodium hydroxide. The solid extract after dissolution in 1 M HCl was then decomposed to an inorganic phosphate by UV photolysis for 2 hours using a quartz high pressure mercury-vapour lamp (120 W). The irradiation was performed in quartz tubes (internal diameter 12–14 mm) placed at 10 cm from the light source. Samples were prepared in duplicate: one was subjected to photolysis, the other was kept in the dark and used as blank to measure the trace amounts of inorganic phosphate not precipitated in the complex. After irradiation inorganic phosphate generated was determined spectrophotometrically, following addition of ammonium molybdate and ascorbic acid and heating for 10 min at 100°C. The absorbance was measured at 820 nm (in 1 cm cell), and the difference in the absorbance between the irradiated sample and blank corresponded to the amount of **1**.

The assay in plasma required initial protein precipitation with trifluoroacetic acid (TFA), followed by the addition of 10 M sodium hydroxide to form the precipitate. After dissolving the precipitate in 1 M HCl, a second precipitation with 10 M NaOH was performed, followed by hydrolysis in 1 M HCl as in step 2 for urine. The remaining steps were similar to those in urine, except a 5-cm cell was used for the absorbance measurements.

The LOQ of the method was estimated at 2000 ng/ml of urine and 100 ng/ml of plasma, with better than 90% recovery in both matrices. Similarly, as with the method of Ligget [8], Bisaz's assay [9] was very time consuming; only 6–8 samples could have been processed by an analyst in a single day.

Both methods for etidronate were developed in the early 1970s before the HPLC technique was fully available. Because of the large volumes of biological fluids required for analysis, a very long and time consuming multi-step sample preparation procedure, lack of sensitivity, and potential for poor specificity, these methods were not useful for supporting pharmacokinetic studies with **1**. However, these early studies contributed greatly to the design of isolation procedures from urine and plasma which were in later methods based almost exclusively on co-precipitation with calcium phosphate developed in these early studies.

2. Clodronate (**2**)

Determination of **2** was performed in serum and urine using ion-exchange HPLC with a flame photometric detector [11], and in urine by HPLC with the post-column addition of a thorium (Th)-ethylenediaminetetracetic acid (EDTA)-xylenol (XO) mixed ligand complex and absorbance detection [12], or by capillary GC with mass spectrometric (MS) detection [13].

In the HPLC method with flame photometric detection [11], a flame phosphorous detector (FPD) built from commercially available components was utilized.

After co-precipitation of **2** with calcium phosphate and hydrolysis of any pyrophosphate present into orthophosphate, in a similar manner to that described by Bisaz et al. [9], the organic phosphate was separated, precipitated again with NaOH and then dissolved in a 9:1 (v/v) mixture of water and saturated solution of EDTA in water. An aliquot of this solution was injected directly for HPLC analysis. As an HPLC mobile phase hydrochloric acid (0.025 M solution A, and 1.0 M solution B) and a column packed with an anion-exchange resin (100 mm, AG 1-XB resin) were utilized. After injection, sample was introduced onto the column using solution B, and after 10 min, solution A was used to elute **2** from the column. The total effluent from the HPLC column was introduced into a FPD consisting of a nebulizer and a burner assembly with a hydrogen-argon-air flame. An interference filter with the maximum wavelength of emission at 525 nm was applied to isolate the phosphorous emission, which was detected by a photomultiplier tube. The linear response of the FPD was reported to be in the range of 0.025 to about 800 μg/ml of injected standards. Detector performance was severely degraded when chromatographic eluents other than deionized water or hydrochloric acid were used. The LOQ in serum using this method was about 500 ng/ml when 5 ml of serum was processed. This LOQ was adequate for determination of serum profiles (0–10 h) following single oral doses of 1600 mg of **2**. The method has been also used for the determination of **2** in urine, but the LOQ was higher than 30 μg/ml.

The HPLC/FPD method was used for determination of **2** in more than 3000 serum and urine specimens of animal and human origin, and allowed determination of up to 15 samples per day, assuming samples were prepared the day prior to the chromatographic analysis. The method suffers from poor precision and accuracy at lower concentrations due to the high flame background light, the necessity to separate large amounts of calcium phosphate salts and EDTA from small amounts of **2** by the chromatographic procedure, and the dependence of the response factor on small changes in the chromatographic variables.

Another recently described HPLC method for the determination of **2** in urine was based on post-column addition of a Th-EDTA-XO mixed ligand complex and monitoring the changes in the absorbance at 550 nm of the post-column reagent [12]. These changes in absorbance were due to the ligand-exchange reaction in which XO was replaced with **2**. This method was similar to the spectrophotometric method for determination of etidronate in urine [8] described earlier, but was more specific due to the HPLC separation of **2** from endogenous urine impurities on an anion-exchange column using nitric acid (30 mM) as a mobile phase followed by post-column addition of the reagent. Urine samples were injected into the column without any pretreatment or dilution, but the LOQ of the method was only about 2 μg/ml.

Because of their low volatility and highly polar nature, phosphonic acids cannot be analysed readily with GC, and derivatization procedures to convert them to relatively volatile analogues are required. Several derivatization reactions for phosphonic acids have been described in the literature, including trimethylsilylation [3, 14, 15], diazoalkylation [16], and dimethyl-*tert*-butylsilylation [17]. GC and electron impact (EI) MS of silylated phosphonates has been extensively studied by Harvey and Horning [14].

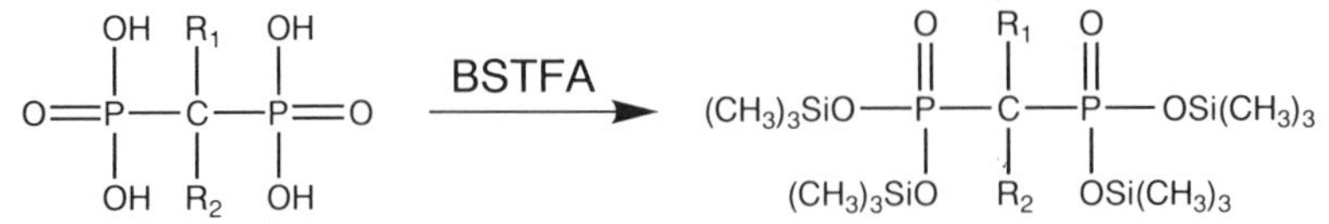

$$\begin{array}{ccc} \text{OH} & \text{R}_1 & \text{OH} \\ | & | & | \\ \text{O}=\text{P}-\text{C}-\text{P}=\text{O} \\ | & | & | \\ \text{OH} & \text{R}_2 & \text{OH} \end{array} \quad \xrightarrow{\text{BSTFA}} \quad \begin{array}{ccc} \text{O} & \text{R}_1 & \text{O} \\ \| & | & \| \\ (\text{CH}_3)_3\text{SiO}-\text{P}-\text{C}-\text{P}-\text{OSi}(\text{CH}_3)_3 \\ | & | & | \\ (\text{CH}_3)_3\text{SiO} & \text{R}_2 & \text{OSi}(\text{CH}_3)_3 \end{array}$$

2, R_1=Cl; R_2=Cl   **8**, R_1=Cl; R_2=Cl
7, R_1=CH₃; R_2=Br   **9**, R_1=CH₃; R_2=Br

Fig. 2. Derivatization of **2** and internal standard (**7**) for GC/NCI/SIM/MS determination of **2**.

A sensitive and highly selective method for the determination of **2** in urine, based on capillary GC/MS, has been recently described [13]. It was based on trimethylsilylation of **2** (Fig. 2) with BSTFA [N,O-bis(trimethylsilyl)trifluoroacetamide] and detection of the derivatives **8** and **9** in methane-negative chemical ionization (NCI)/ selective ion monitoring (SIM) mode. (C-methyl monobromomethylene) bisphosphonic acid (**7**) was used as an internal standard (IS).

EI and ammonia CI of the derivatives **8** and **9** produced intense ions at high m/ z values (Fig. 3A and B). However, SIM using these ionization methods was not suitable for the analysis of **2** in urine because of inadequate sensitivity and selectivity.

Ammonia CI/MS/MS detection technique was also utilized, but sensitivity of the method was poor. Therefore, methane NCI/MS and quantitation in the SIM mode of a fragment ion at m/z 424 (Fig. 3D) was utilized in the quantitative work. This fragment ion was generated by the loss of a neutral fragment, Me₃SiCl, from the molecular ion. The capillary column used in the GC was an OV-1, 25 m, i.d. 0.31 mm, and film thickness 0.1 μm. The injection port temperature was 250°C, and the oven was programmed from 120°C to 230°C at 10°C per min. The quantitative studies were carried out by adding known quantities of **2** and 500 ng of an IS (**7**) in blank urine samples (1 ml) and extraction of bisphosphonates on a Dowex anion exchange resin (150 mg). The resin was first washed with water (2 ml), the sample was added, and after washing the resin again with 10 ml water, the bisphosphonates were eluted with 0.5 ml 2 M HCl. An aliquot (0.2 ml) of the eluent in a separate vial was evaporated to dryness with a stream of air at 80°C, followed by the addition of acetonitrile (0.1 ml) and BSTFA (0.1 ml). After heating the mixture at 80°C for 2 hr, an aliquot (1 μl) was injected into the GC.

The precision of the assay in urine at 500 ng/ml was 13.2%, and the recoveries of the extraction at 5 and 10 μg/ml were better than 90%.

III. Assays of amino bisphosphonates

1. Bisphosphonates containing a primary amino group

(a) Pamidronate (**3**)

The presence of the primary amino group in aminobisphosphonates creates the possibility of derivatization to form fluorescent or UV-absorbing derivatives.

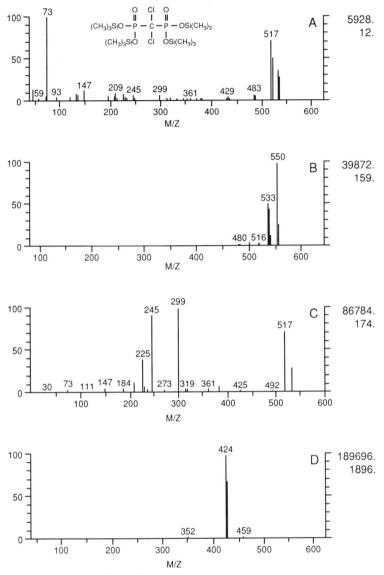

Fig. 3. Mass spectra of the trimethylsilylated **2**. (A) Electron ionization mass spectrum; (B) positive ammonia chemical ionization spectrum; (C) collision-induced daughters of the protonated molecular ion (m/z 533); (D) negative chemical ionization spectrum (reprinted from [13] with permission).

This provided a basis for the development of several assays for **3** in plasma and urine [18–20]. In addition, a method based on post-column oxidation of **3** to orthophosphate and post-column reaction with molybdenum-ascorbate to yield a chromophore detected at 820 nm was developed [21, 22]. The details of some of these methods are provided below.

(i) Assays based on derivatization of the amino group. Flesch and Hauffe's method for determination of **3** in urine was based on derivatization of the primary amino group with fluorescamine and HPLC with fluorescence detection [18].

The co-precipitation procedure of pamidronate in urine was similar to that described by Bisaz et al. [9]. Urine samples (2 ml) were treated with 1.5 M trichloroacetic acid (TCA, 0.5 ml), and after addition of calcium chloride (20 μl, 2.5 M) and sodium dihydrogen phosphate (40 μl, 0.5 M), the pH was adjusted to 12.0 using first NaOH (6.25 M) and finally NaOH (0.5 M). After isolation of the precipitate and dissolution in HCl (1 ml, 0.1 M), a second precipitation was performed using 0.5 M NaOH. After centrifugation, the precipitate was dissolved in EDTA solution (0.13 M, pH 9, 0.2 ml), and 0.1 ml fluorescamine dissolved in acetonitrile (1 mg/ml) was added. The mixture was extracted with dichloromethane (0.2 ml), and a portion of the aqueous phase (10 μl) was injected into the HPLC system. The HPLC column (250 × 4 mm) was packed with Nucleosil C-18 (10 μm particle size), and chromatography was performed at 40°C. The mobile phase consisted of an aqueous solution of 1 mM EDTA (pH 6.5) and methanol (97:3, v/v) pumped at a flow rate of 1 ml/min. A compound similar to **3** but with five instead of two methylene groups present in the molecule was utilized as an internal standard (IS). The fluorescamine derivative of **3** was detected by monitoring the emission at 480 nm after excitation at 395 nm. Using 2 ml of urine, the LOQ was shown to be about 200 ng/ml. The assay has been utilized to measure urine levels after single oral (150 mg) or i.v. (5 mg) doses of **3** to dogs.

An improved method for the determination of **3** in urine and plasma based on fluorescamine derivatization and fluorescence detection has been recently reported [19]. In comparison with the method described in [18], the improved procedure utilizes an IS with four, instead of five, methylene groups in the molecule (Fig. 4), which reduces analysis time and makes integration of the IS peak height easier. In

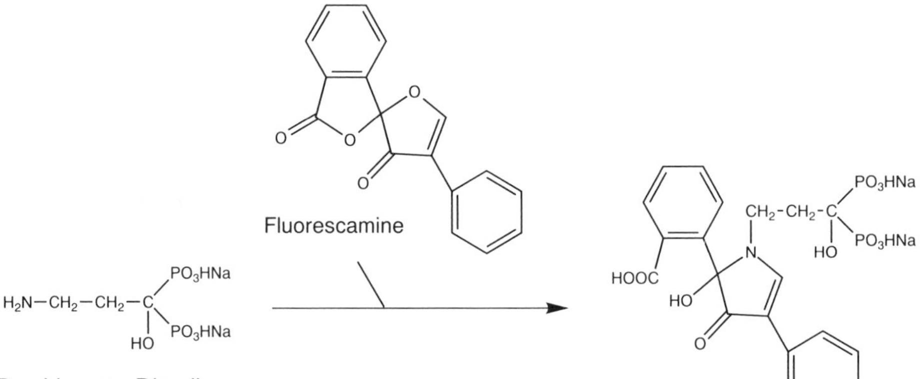

Fig. 4. Derivatization of pamidronate disodium with fluorescamine and structure of the probable reaction product.

addition, the derivatization step was modified, by increasing both the pH (from pH 9 to 10) and the concentration of the fluorescamine solution (from 1 to 3 mg/ml). These changes resulted in increased sensitivity and precision of the method both in plasma and urine. When 2 ml of plasma or urine were processed, the LOQ was about 190 and 165 ng/ml, respectively. This method was sensitive enough to monitor urine concentrations and plasma concentration-time course for **3** in patients after single i.v. infusion of 60 mg in 1 h.

A third method based on derivatization of the primary amino group of **3** has been recently described [20]. This procedure involved derivatization of **3** with phenylisothiocyanate (PITC) and UV detection of the thiourea derivative at 240 nm. Pamidronate was isolated from biological samples by anion-exchange chromatography using quaternary amine extraction cartridges. After sample application and after washing the cartridge several times with water, **3** was eluted with nitric acid (100 mM). The eluate was evaporated under nitrogen at 80°C, and the residue derivatized with PITC at alkaline pH at 80°C for 5 min. After derivatization, samples were evaporated to dryness again and, following reconstitution in the mobile phase, were subjected to HPLC analysis. The thiourea derivatives of **3** were chromatographed on a C-18 reversed phase column using as a mobile phase a mixture of 0.02 M phosphate buffer (pH 7) and acetonitrile containing 0.005 M tetrabutylammonium chloride as an ion-pairing agent.

(ii) Methods based on post-column oxidation and absorbance detection of a complex. All methods for **3** described above were based on pre-column derivatization of the amino group and fluorescence or UV detection of a derivative after HPLC separation. A different approach, based on post-column oxidation of **3** to orthophosphate, formation of a blue phosphomolybdate complex between orthophosphate and molybdenum ascorbate, and detection of this complex at 820 nm, has been employed by Daley-Yates and co-workers for the determination of **3** in plasma and urine [21, 22]. Formation of a similar complex, but without HPLC separation, was the basis of an earlier assay for **1** [9] in urine and plasma. The post-column procedure [21, 22] involved the usual co-precipitation of **3** with calcium chloride, separation of the precipitate by high-performance ion chromatography on a Dionex AS7 anion-exchange column using nitric acid (1 mM) as the mobile phase, and a two-step post-column reaction. In this reaction the HPLC effluent was heated first with persulphate to liberate orthophosphate, followed by simultaneous addition of ascorbic acid and a molybdenum reagent to neutralize excess persulphate and to generate the phosphomolybdate complex. The same IS as used in [19] was employed. The LOQ in urine was established at 450 ng/ml when 1 ml of urine was processed, but was not reported in plasma.

Although, in principle, the post-column procedure [21, 22] seems to be applicable to all bisphosphonates, it is rather complex and has many limitations in terms of sensitivity, specificity, choice of chromatographic conditions, and ruggedness. It requires a complicated HPLC/post-column derivatization system consisting of three pumps, three post-column heating and cooling coils, optimization of ion chromatography and post-column reaction, removal of endogenous orthophosphate

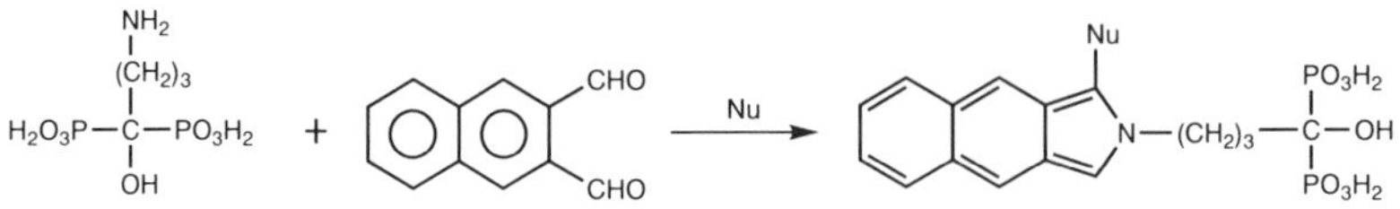

4

11 Nu = CN⁻

12 Nu = ⁻SC(CH₃)₂ CH (COOH) NHCOCH₃

Fig. 5. Chemical derivatization of **4** and formation of fluorescent benzo[f]isoindole derivatives **11** and **12**

from the sample, and the need to dilute urine (1:10) extracts before injection. The method was applied for monitoring the concentration of **3** in urine and plasma of patients during i.v. infusion of 30–120 mg **3** over 2–8 h via a constant-rate infusion pump.

*(b) Alendronate (**4**)*

A series of very sensitive assays for the determination of **4** in urine and plasma (LOQ $\leq$ 5 ng/ml) were recently developed [23, 24]. These assays were based on automated pre-column derivatization of the primary amino group with 2,3-naphthalene dicarboxyaldehyde (NDA) in the presence of either cyanide or thiol nucleophile, followed by fluorescence or electrochemical (EC) detection of the *N*-substituted benz[f]isoindole derivative formed (Fig. 5).

The derivatives **11** and **12** were found to be highly fluorescent, the fluorescence quantum efficiency (Φ_f) for **11**, for example, was 0.82 [23], allowing highly sensitive detection of **4**.

(i) An assay in urine based on HPLC with fluorescence detection.
(1) Detection of Derivative **11**.
Initially, an assay in urine based on the formation of derivative **11** and fluorescence detection was developed [23]. The procedure included (1) the isolation of the drug from urine (5 ml) by co-precipitation of its calcium salt with endogenous phosphates in the presence of alkaline, in a manner similar to that described by Bisaz et al. [9]; (2) a solid-phase anion-exchange sample clean-up; and (3) automated pre-column derivatization followed by fluorescence detection of **11**. In order to make the calcium isolation step compatible with derivatization, which required basic (pH 9) conditions, the calcium ions had to be removed from the acidified mixture to ensure that **4** remained in solution as a free acid and not as an insoluble calcium salt at pH 9. A weak anion exchanger, a diethylamine (DEA) cartridge (step 2), was found to be efficient for removing the calcium ions and other urine impurities from **4** prior to derivatization. Among many reagents commonly used for the determination of primary amines including *o*-phthaldehyde (OPA)-thiol, dansyl chloride and fluorescamine, a newly developed NDA-CN⁻ system was employed [25, 26] because of its superiority over other derivatizing reagents used for this purpose [26, 27]. The derivatization reaction (Fig. 5) was rapid and complete at low concentrations

and at room temperature and produced the desired, highly fluorescent product **11**. The high polarity of **11** and the need for basic HPLC conditions negated the use of conventional reversed-phase columns such as C8 and C18. Instead, a polymeric, non-silica-based HPLC column composed of the co-polymer of styrene and divinyl benzene (150 × 4.6 mm, 5 μm, 100 Å) was utilized. A sodium citrate-dihydrogen phosphate solution, adjusted to pH 8.5 and mixed with methanol (6:4, v/v) was chosen as an HPLC mobile phase to ensure the derivative stability and to control the charge associated with the phosphonate group.

The application of this methodology to the analyses of large numbers of clinical samples made automation of at least some parts of the procedure highly desirable. More important, automation of the derivatization step was necessary to eliminate the need for careful control of the reaction kinetics and to eliminate the problems associated with the potential chemical and photochemical instability of **11**. Instead of a typical pre-column derivatization of many samples and subsequent analyses of these samples over an extended period of time, each sample was derivatized immediately prior to the analysis. This was accomplished using the 'automix' capability of the autosampler (Varian). The samples were processed manually (steps 1 and 2) to the point of placing aliquots of the eluent from the DEA cartridge into sample vials. These solutions were stable for up to five days. The autosampler was then programmed to add the appropriate volumes of solutions containing CN^- and NDA. The sample solution was allowed to react for 15 min and then injected onto the HPLC column. While the chromatographic run was performed on this derivatized sample, the next sample was derivatized exactly in the same manner and injected.

The assay was linear over the concentration range 5–100 ng/ml of urine, and the total recovery (efficiency of extraction and derivatization) within the whole assay range was 94±3% [23]. The LOQ was 5 ng/ml when 5 ml of urine was processed. Urine samples from a pilot bioavailability study, after dosing human subjects with 50 mg of **4**, were analysed using this assay. Derivative **11** was also found to be a good energy acceptor in a typical oxalate ester-hydrogen peroxide chemiluminescent (CL) system. The observation of this emission created the possibility of development of a sensitive assay for the derivatized **4** based on HPLC with CL detection of **11**, but this possibility was not, thus far, explored further.

(2) Detection of Derivative **12**.

Although the LOQ of **4** using the method described in [23] was far superior to all other procedures available for the determination of structurally similar bisphosphonates [18–22], it became evident, after analysis of samples from first clinical study, that the concentration of **4** in many subjects' urine samples after a 50 mg single oral dose was below 5 ng. Since several pharmacokinetic studies with lower oral doses of **4** (20, 10 and 5 mg) were planned, a more sensitive assay in urine (LOQ = 1 ng/ml) was required. In addition, a highly sensitive assay for **4** in plasma was also highly desirable.

In order to achieve these goals, and to replace the CN^- ion, undesirable in the analytical laboratory, with a less toxic nucleophile in the NDA derivatization reaction, several approaches including electrochemical (EC) rather than fluorescence detection (FD) of the derivatives, utilization of a thiol instead of cyanide as a nucleophile (Fig. 5), and several modifications in the sample isolation procedure and in fluorescence detection were pursued [24].

The NDA derivatization reaction of **4** was shown to be effective with *N*-acetyl-D-penicillamine (NAP) to produce the highly fluorescent and EC active derivative **12** (Fig. 5). Therefore, the CN^- ion was eliminated from the original [23] sample preparation procedure and replaced with NAP. In order to increase the LOQ in urine, several changes in the assay were made. These changes included the replacement of a high capacity 500-mg DEA cartridge with a 200-mg cartridge, allowing the decrease in the dilution of the sample before derivatization from 3 to 1 ml, replacement of a borate buffer (250 μl) with bicarbonate buffer (50 μl) in the final mixture before injection on column, and a change in the pH of the derivatization medium from pH 9.1 to 10.7, which was necessary to achieve the maximum conversion of **4** to **12**. Several other changes, including the modification of the mobile phase composition from methanol (40%) to acetonitrile (15%), adjustment of the pH of the mobile phase from 8.5 to 6.3, and gradient elution of late eluting interference peaks, were all needed to achieve the required assay specificity and provided for uninterrupted multi-sample analyses of urine and plasma extracts.

The assay in urine, based on derivative **12**, with the improved LOQ of 1 ng/ml, has been fully validated in the concentration range 1–25 ng/ml (using 5 ml of urine). The chromatograms of blank urine, urine spiked with 2.5 ng/ml of **4** and a subject urine after dosing with **4**, are shown in Fig. 6.

The within-day and inter-day precision of the assay for all concentrations within the standard line was below 8.5%. This assay was used routinely for the analyses of more than 3000 urine samples from various human pharmacokinetic studies with **4**.

(ii) An assay in urine based on electrochemical detection of derivative **11**. Derivatives **11** and **12** were not only highly fluorescent but also EC active, with a half-wave potential of approximately +0.6 to +0.7 V. This low half-wave potential makes these derivatives amenable to highly specific EC detection. Therefore, an HPLC/EC assay for **4** in urine using derivative **11** has been developed [24]. Using the original sample preparation procedure (III)(1)(b)(i)(1), but after replacement of a borate buffer with bicarbonate buffer, which was necessary to eliminate baseline noise and improve assay specificity, the assay in urine was validated in the concentration range of 2.5–50 ng/ml. The within-day precision was less than 9% for all concentrations within the calibration range. The accuracy of the assay was 97–104%, and its specificity was confirmed by the analysis of urine blanks; impurities co-eluting with **11** were not detected.

Since the long-term, day-to-day performance of the fluorescence detectors is usually more reliable than that of the EC detectors and comparable assay sensitivities were achieved using both detectors, the method based on fluorescence detection [(III)(1)(b)(i)(2)] was utilized in support of human pharmacokinetic studies with **4**. Using a modified sample preparation procedure, as described in method

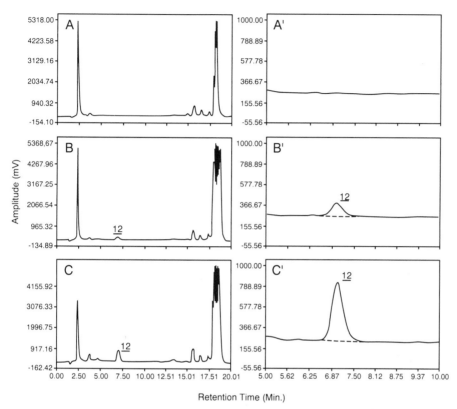

Fig. 6. Representative chromatograms of human urine spiked with **4**, derivatized to **12** with NDA/NAP, and analysed using HPLC with fluorescence detection. (A) Blank control urine, (B) control urine spiked with 2.5 ng/ml **4**, (C) urine sample of a subject (0–36 h collection) participating in a food interaction study after 20 mg dose of **4** (food withheld for 2 h post-dose), the concentration of **4** in the sample analysed was equivalent to 11.0 ng/ml. Chromatograms A', B', and C' show the elution region of **12**.

(III)(1)(b)(i)(2), and EC detection of either **11** or **12**, the development of an assay in urine and plasma with a similar LOQ to FD seems to be feasible [24], but it was not explored further.

*(iii) An assay in plasma based on fluorescence detection of derivative **12**.* The crux of the assay in plasma [24] was the addition of sodium pyrophosphate to the mixture after protein precipitation, to induce the co-precipitation of calcium salts of **4** with other phosphates present in the system. In the presence of pyrophosphate salt, the formation of a characteristic pellet containing **4** was observed. The remaining steps in the assay were the same as in method (III)(1)(b)(i)(2). The LOQ in plasma (5 ng/ml) was higher than in urine (1 ng/ml) since only 1 ml of plasma vs. 5 ml of urine was processed. The assay has been validated in the concentration range of 5–125 ng/ml and was sufficiently sensitive to monitor the concentration of **4** in plasma up to 12 h after i.v. dosing of human subjects with 10 mg of **4** over a period of 2 hours.

2. Bisphosphonates containing a secondary amino group

A highly sensitive method based on HPLC with EC detection and without derivatization has been recently described for a non-chromophoric bisphosphonate **5** (Fig. 1) containing a secondary amino group [28]. The molecule **5**, a cycloheptylaminomethylenebisphosphonic acid, and structurally similar internal standard (a cyclo-octyl analogue), were shown to be electrochemically active and were detected with high specificity at a low electrode potential of +0.55 V operating in the oxidation mode at pH 11. According to the authors [28], this low oxidation was due to an efficient oxidative cleavage of the C-N bond of **5** in an EC detector and formation of cyloheptylamine, a primary amine, which was detected as a fluorescent derivative with fluorescamine having the same retention time as the peak of interest. This low oxidation was limited to **5** and similar bisphosphonates containing a secondary amino group as indicated by the lack of EC activity for pamidronate **3**, a bisphosphonate with primary amino group in the molecule, and **1** and **2**.

Sample preparation was based on co-precipitation of the drug from plasma (1 ml) with calcium phosphate, after deproteination with TFA, followed by the removal of calcium using a cation exchange resin converted from H^+ to K^+ form. The supernatant (200 μl) was basified with 30 μl of 2 M NaOH and 80-μl aliquot was injected into the HPLC system (method A). Solid-phase extraction (SPE) using a Sep-Pak C18 cartridge coupled with method A enabled the extraction of **5** from a large volume (10 ml) of plasma and urine (method B). Compound **5** was retained on this reversed-phase cartridge by a mechanism different from that of many other compounds, probably via specific adsorption of biosphosphonic acid to the silica material, since elution of **5** from the cartridge was easily accomplished using alkaline NaOH solution but was ineffective with acetonitrile. Prior to SPE, compound **5** and IS in 10 ml of plasma were co-precipitated with calcium phosphate, but that in urine with calcium chloride, because urine contained an excess of phosphate ions as compared with calcium ions.

The HPLC system consisted of a polystyrene divinylbenzene-based analytical column (150 × 4.6 mm) operating in the pH range of 1–13, a Coulochem 5100A EC detector (ESA, Bedford, Mass., USA) operating at a potential of +0.55 V, and a mobile phase of acetonitrile-50 mM Na_2HPO_4 buffer containing 1 mM tetrabutylammonium phosphate adjusted to pH 11 with 2 M NaOH (7:93, v/v) at a flow rate of 0.8 ml/min. The LOQ of method A was 5 ng/ml based on 1 ml of plasma used for extraction. The LOQ of method B in both plasma and urine was 1 ng/ml, but required 10 ml of biological fluid for analysis. Using method B, the plasma concentration of **5** in human subjects could be detected up to 6 hours after 5 mg oral dose.

IV. Assay of bisphosphonates containing UV-absorbing chromophore (tiludronet)

Determination of bisphosphonates containing a chromophoric group for direct UV, fluorescence or EC detection does not require, in principle, derivatization.

Assuming adequate assay sensitivity is achieved, the procedure can be greatly simplified in such cases by avoiding pre- or post-column derivatization. In addition to the determination of **5** described above, the assay of **6** (tiludronate) in urine and plasma is an example of such a direct method [29]. The molecule of **6** contains an UV-absorbing (4-chlorophenyl) group and could be detected directly at 280 nm. As in all other procedures for bisphosphonates, the isolation of **6** from biological fluids was accomplished by co-precipitation with calcium phosphate. The solid material after the second precipitation was dissolved in mobile phase containing 0.1 M EDTA, and an aliquot was injected into the HPLC system. The separation was achieved on a polymeric RP column (150 × 4.1 mm, 5 μm), using 0.005 M tetrabutylammonium phosphate/0.05 M sodium hydrogen phosphate (pH 11.8)-acetonitrile (87:13, v/v) as a mobile phase at a flow rate of 1 ml/min. The LOQ of the assay both in plasma and urine was 50 ng/ml using only 0.2 ml of a biological fluid. The assay was used routinely for over a year and was utilized, for example, for the determination of **6** in plasma and urine after a single oral administration of **6** (100 mg) to baboons. In the latter case, assay sensitivity was adequate to monitor the concentrations of **6** in plasma up to 72 h post-dose.

V. Conclusions and future trends

Development of sensitive assays for the determination of bisphosphonates is challenging due to the general lack of chromophores for conventional UV, fluorescence or EC detection, high polarity, and difficulties in designing good chromatographic conditions for their separation from endogenous matrix components.

For bisphosphonates not containing a primary amino group, the most promising and general approach seemed to be based on trimethylsilylation of all four acidic groups of the bisphosphonate and GC separation with MS/negative chemical ionization detection. The same derivatives could be also analysed using either GC/MS/MS technique or liquid chromatography (LC) with MS or MS/MS detection. The LC approach would require development of HPLC conditions compatible with MS detection. Trimethylsilylation was not adequate for the analysis of amino bisphosphonates due to the formation of multiple products and lack of stability of trimethylsilyl derivatives.

The most promising approach for the determination of bisphosphonates containing a primary amino group is based on derivatization with NDA/NAP or NDA/CN⁻, formation of highly fluorescent and EC-active benzo[f]isoindoles, and their detection using fluorescence, chemiluminescence or EC detection. This method seemed to be quite general, and it should be applicable to all bisphosphonates containing primary amino group, including pamidronate **3**.

VI. Summary

The analytical methods for the determination of geminal bisphosphonates in biological fluids were reviewed. The development of these methods is challenging and presents major difficulties due to the lack of a chromophore for direct detection with conventional chromatographic detectors, presence of several functional groups with various pK_a values in the entire pH range, and difficulty in the isolation of these compounds from biological fluids. Although several methods have been described for the analysis of bisphosphonates in pharmaceutical dosage forms, only a few procedures are available for the assay of these compounds in biological fluids. Most of these methods require an elaborate sample preparation procedure, a chemical derivatization for sensitive detection, and very careful selection of chromatographic conditions. The limit of quantitation (LOQ) of these methods varies from 1 to 500 ng/ml depending on the methodology utilized and the chemical structure of the bisphosphonate assayed. The utilization of these methods for pharmacokinetics and toxicology studies was emphasized.

References

1. Fleisch, H., Bisphosphonates; Pharmacology and use in the treatment of tumor-induced hypercalcaemic metastatic bone disease. Drugs 1991; 42: 919–944.
2. Rueppel, N.C., Suba, L.A. and Marvel, J.T., Derivatization of aminoalkylphosphonic acids for characterization by gas chromatography mass spectrometry. Biomed. Mass Spectrom. 1976; 3: 28–31.
3. Ismail, Z., Aldous, S., Triggs, E.J., Smithurst, B.A. and Barry, H.D., Gas chromatographic analysis of didronet tablets. J. Chromatogr. 1987; 404: 372–377.
4. Meek, S.E. and Pietrzyk, J., Liquid chromatographic separation of phosphorous oxo acids and other anions with postcolumn indirect fluorescence detection by aluminium-morin. Anal. Chem. 1988; 60: 1397–1400.
5. DeMarco, J.D., Biffar, S.E., Reed, D.G. and Brooks, M.A., The determination of 4-amino-1-hydroxybutane-1,1-diphosphonic acid monosodium salt trihydrate in pharmaceutical dosage forms by high performance liquid chromatography. J. Pharmacol. Biomed. Anal. 1989; 7: 1719–1727.
6. Kwong, E., Chiu, A.M.Y., McClintock, S.A. and Cotton, M.L., HPLC analysis of an amino bisphosphonate in pharmaceutical formulations using postcolumn derivatization and fluorescence detection. J. Chromatogr. Sci. 1990; 28: 563–566.
7. Tsai, E.W., Ip, D.P. and Brooks, M.A., Determination of alendronate in pharmaceutical dosage formulations by ion chromatography with conductivity detection. J. Chromatogr. 1992; 596: 217–224.
8. Liggett, S.J., Determination of ethane-1-hydroxy-1,1-diphosphonic acid (EHDP) in human feces and urine. Biochem. Med. 1973; 7: 68–77.
9. Bisaz, S., Felix, R. and Fleisch, H., Quantitative determination of ethane-1-hydroxy-1,1-diphosphonate in urine and plasma. Clin. Chim. Acta 1975; 65: 299–307.
10. Jung, A., Bisaz, S. and Fleisch, H., The binding of pyrophosphate and two diphosphonates by hydroxyapatite crystals. Calc. Tissue Res. 1973; 11: 269–280.
11. Chester, T.L., Lewis, E.C., Benedict, J.J., Sunberg, R.J. and Tettenhorst, W.C., Determination of (dichloromethylene)diphosphonate in physiological fluids by ion-exhange chromatography with phosphorous-selective detection. J. Chromatogr. 1981; 225: 17–25.
12. Virtanen, V. and Lajunen, L.H.J., High-performance liquid chromatographic method for simultaneous determination of clodronate and some clodronate esters. J. Chromatogr. (Biomed. Appl.) 1993; 617: 291–298.
13. Auriola, S., Kostiainen, R., Ylinen, M., Monkkonen, J. and Ylitalo, P., Analysis of (dichloromethylene)bisphosphonate in urine by capillary gas chromatography-mass spectrometry. J. Pharm.

Biomed. Anal. 1989; 7: 1623–1629.

14. Harvey, D.J. and Horning, M.G., Derivatives for the characterization of alkyl- and aminoalkylphosphonates by gas chromatography and gas-chromatography-mass spectrometry. J. Chromatogr. 1973; 79: 65–74.

15. Moye, H.A. and Deyrup, C.L., A simple single step derivatization method for the gas chromatographic analysis of the herbicide glyphosate and its metabolite. J. Agric. Food Chem. 1984; 32: 192–195.

16. Rueppel, M.L., Suba, L.A. and Marvel, J.T., Derivatization of aminoalkylphosphonic acids by gas chromatography-mass spectrometry. Biomed. Mass Spectr. 1976; 3: 28–31.

17. Harvey, D.J. and Horning, M.G., The mass spectra of the trimethylsilyl derivatives of some alkyl and aminoalkyl phophonates. Org. Mass Spectrom. 1974; 9: 111–124.

18. Flesch, G. and Hauffe, S.A., Determination of the bisphosphonate pamidronate disodium in urine by pre-column derivatization with fluorescamine, high-performance liquid chromatography and fluorescence detection. J. Chromatogr. 1989; 489: 446–451.

19. Flesch, G., Tominaga, N. and Degen, P., Improved determination of the bisphosphonate pamidronate disodium in plasma and urine by pre-column derivatization with fluorescamine, high-performance liquid chromatography and fluorescence detection. J. Chromatogr. (Biomed. Appl.). 1991; 568: 261–266.

20. Den Hartigh, J., Janssen, M.J. and Vermeij, P., Determination of 3-amino-1-hydroxypropane-1,1-bisphosphonate (APD) in plasma and urine by HPLC. Pharm. Weekbl. Sci. Ed. (No. 3, Suppl.E). 1989; E18. Presented at the 3rd International Symposium on Drug Analysis, Antwerp, May 1989, abstract P 137.

21. Daley-Yates, P.T., Gifford, L.A. and Hoggarth, C.R., Assay of 1-hydroxy-3-aminopropylidene-1,1-bisphosphonate and related bisphosphonates in human urine and plasma by high-performance ion chromatography. J. Chromatogr. (Biomed. Appl.). 1989; 490: 329–338.

22. Hoggarth, C.R., Gifford, L.A. and Daley-Yates, P.T., Chromatographic analysis of bisphosphonates. Anal. Proc. 1990; 27: 18.

23. Kline, W.F., Matuszewski, B.K. and Bayne, W.F., Determination of 4-amino-1-hydroxybutane-1,1-bisphosphonic acid in urine by automated pre-column derivatization with 2,3-naphthalene dicarboxyaldehyde and high-performance liquid chromatography with fluorescence detection. J. Chromatogr. (Biomed. Appl.). 1990; 534: 139–149.

24. Kline, W.F. and Matuszewski, B.K., Improved determination of the bisphosphonate alendronate in human plasma and urine by automated precolumn derivatization and high-performance liquid chromatography with fluorescence and electrochemical detection. J. Chromatogr. (Biomed. Appl.) 1992; 583: 183–193.

25. Carlson, R.G., Srinivasachar, K., Givens, R.S. and Matuszewski, B.K., New derivatizing agents for amino acids and peptides. 1. Facile synthesis of N-substituted 1-cyanobenz[f]isoindoles and their spectroscopic properties. J. Org. Chem. 1986; 51: 3978–3983.

26. de Monitgny, P., Stobaugh, J.F., Givens, R.S., Carlson, R.G., Srinivasachar, K., Sternson, L.A. and Higuchi, T., Naphthalene-2,3-dicarboxyaldehyde/cyanide ion: a rationally designed fluorogenic reagent for primary amines. Anal. Chem. 1987; 59: 1096–1101.

27. Matuszewski, B.K., Givens, R.S., Srinivasachar, K., Carlson, R.G. and Higuchi, T., N-Substituted 1-cyanobenz[f]isoindole: evaluation of fluorescence efficiencies of a new fluorogenic label for primary amines and amino acids. Anal. Chem. 1987; 59: 1102–1105.

28. Usui, T., Watanabe, T. and Higuchi, S., Determination of a new bisphosphonate, YM 175, in plasma, urine and bone by high-performance liquid chromatography with electrochemical detection. J. Chromatogr. (Biomed. Appl.). 1992; 584: 213–220.

29. Fels, J.P., Guyonnet, J., Berger, Y. and Cautreels, W., Determination of (4-chlorophenyl)thiomethylene bisphosphonic acid, a new bisphosphonate, in biological fluids by high-performance liquid chromatography. J. Chromatogr. (Biomed. Appl.). 1988; 430: 73–79.

PART C

THE BISPHOSPHONATES IN THE TREATMENT AND PREVENTION OF BONE PATHOLOGY

Bisphosphonate on bones
O. Bijvoet, H.A. Fleisch, R.E. Canfield and G. Russell (eds.)
© 1995 Elsevier Science B.V. All rights reserved.

CHAPTER 17

Paget's disease of bone: Symptoms, signs and morbidity

Neveen A.T. Hamdy

Department of Endocrinology and Metabolic Diseases, University Hospital, Leiden, The Netherlands

I. Introduction

Paget's disease of bone, named after Sir James Paget, who first accurately observed and described its clinical manifestations in 1877, is a focal disorder of bone remodelling in which bone becomes structurally chaotic, less compact, more vascular and more prone to deformity and fracture. Over the years, light has been shed on the aetiology, pathophysiology, epidemiology and management of Paget's disease of bone [1–12]. Little has been added, however, to the clinical features of the untreated disorder as originally described by Sir James Paget at the turn of the century [13].

> ... It begins in middle age or later, is very slow in progress, may continue many years without influence on the general health, and may give no other trouble than those which are due to changes of shape, size and direction of the diseased bones.
> ... The skull became gradually larger, so that nearly every year, for many years, his hat, and the helmet that he wore as a member of a Yeomanry Corps needed to be enlarged....
> ... The length of the spine seemed lessened, and from a height of six feet one inch, he sank to about 5 feet nine inches.... The arms appeared unnaturally long... the hands hung low down by the thighs and in front of them. Altogether the attitude in standing looked simian, strangely in contrast with the large head....
> ... The left tibia had become larger, and had a well marked anterior curve as if lengthened, while its ends were held in place by their attachments to the unchanged fibula....
>
> *Sir James Paget (1877)*

II. Pathophysiology

Paget's disease of bone is characterised by regional increases in bone turnover. Although geographic, ethnic and genetic factors may play a contributory role to the pathophysiology of the disorder, it is now widely believed that the pathological lesion could be the late manifestation of a slow virus infection resulting in a local, often multifocal abnormality in osteoclast morphology, number and function. The distribution of the lesions and their strict localisation within the boundaries of the part of the skeleton involved tend to support the notion of a possible haematogenous route for the acquisition of the initial insult, analogous to the distribution of bony lesions in haematogenous bacterial osteomyelitis. The demonstration of nuclear inclusion bodies possibly belonging to the paramyxovirus family, in osteoclasts at pathological sites appears to support the hypothesis of a viral aetiology for the abnormalities observed, although the putative organism has not yet been definitely identified. The resulting regional increase in bone resorption is characteristically associated with a proportional increase in bone formation as a result of greatly increased numbers of essentially normal osteoblasts. A ten-fold increase in bone turnover may be observed in involved bones, with up to 100% of the bone surface occupied by active remodelling events. The rapid rates of bone formation result in the 'mosaic pattern' chaotic deposition of woven bone, lacking the structural organisation of lamellar bone, occupying more space, and more prone to distortion by mechanical forces. Excessive fibrous tissue and blood vessels infiltrate the adjacent bone marrow, resulting in highly vascular lesions, particularly in the active stages of the disease. Following treatment, lamellar bone deposition resumes, and the vascularity of the lesions decreases.

III. Clinical features

The disease is most commonly diagnosed after the age of 50 years, and its incidence rises with increasing age. There is a slight male preponderance, and there may be a difference in skeletal distribution between men and women, with the skull and face appearing to be more frequently affected in women compared to a male preponderance for other localisations. Skeletal involvement is heterogeneous, asymmetrical in distribution, and best evaluated by bone scintigraphy. The most common sites affected are the pelvis (in two-thirds of patients), the femur, spine, skull and tibia. The upper extremities are much less frequently affected. The disease may be monostotic (in about 25% of patients) or more commonly polyostotic, involving two or more bones.

The onset of the disease is insidious, and symptoms may vary from minimal to severely disabling, depending on areas of involvement, adjacent structures and activity of the disease. At presentation, 30% of patients will have had symptoms for 10 years or more, but only a third of the lesions is usually symptomatic. A significant percentage of patients is thus asymptomatic at presentation, and the diagnosis is incidentally established clinically (deformity, particularly of a long bone), biochemically (elevated serum alkaline phosphatase activity on biochemical screening for another indication), or radiologically (typical disordered structure of the pagetic bone). Clinical features of the disorder depend on the localisation, activity and extent of the pagetic lesions.

1. Bone pain

Bone pain is the most frequent presenting symptom in Paget's disease of bone. The pain is usually dull, non-specific, but may be boring or nagging in nature. Pain is unrelated to exercise or weight-bearing and bears little relationship to radiographic appearances, although some authors suggest that lesions may be more painful when sclerotic.

Pain is more common in lesions of the long bones. In the presence of microfractures, which may not be necessarily visualised radiographically, it may become sharper and more localised. Headaches or band-like tightness across the forehead are common when Paget's disease is localised to the skull.

Bone pain requires careful evaluation in Paget's disease of bone, as its aetiology is usually multifactorial. Bone pain may be primarily related to the pathological pagetic process, or may arise as a result of complications at the site of a lesion or in adjacent structures. Primarily related to the pagetic process is an increase in bone vascularity in active lesions [14], which may lead to a rise in intramedullary pressure and pain. Pain has indeed been observed to be more common in patients in whom an increase in skin temperature can be demonstrated. Bone pain could also be due to stretching of the periosteum by the increased bone volume due to its disordered deposition during disease activity. Reports of symptomatic relief of pain following decompression by the drilling of holes at the site of the bony lesion possibly substantiate this view. Localised pain may also be due to hyperaemia of the marrow cavity leading to stimulation of adjacent somatic nerve endings, to secondary degenerative changes in adjacent or contralateral joints to a pagetic lesion, or to microfractures in a weight-bearing area.

The pagetic process is often associated with osteoarthritic changes due to unnatural stresses on a weight-bearing joint as a result of deformities [15, 16]. The pelvis is commonly affected in Paget's disease of bone, and the hip joints are thus frequently involved in the disease process, with the degenerative changes occurring on the same side as the pagetic lesion or on the contralateral non-affected side due to altered weight-bearing.

Pain can also occur as a result of neurological compression syndromes, vascular steal syndromes or when the disease is complicated by the development of osteosarcoma.

The vertebrae represent a common site of involvement in Paget's disease of bone, and the lumbar and sacral vertebrae are the ones most frequently affected. The most common presenting symptom is back pain, although the majority of patients with uncomplicated spinal localisation of Paget's disease are asymptomatic. The expanded vertebrae are usually incidentally visualised radiologically or on bone scintigraphy. When present, back pain could be non-specific due to the active pagetic process, or may occur as a result of vertebral compression fractures, spinal stenosis (resulting in radicular pain), a vascular steal syndrome or, commonly, secondary degenerative changes.

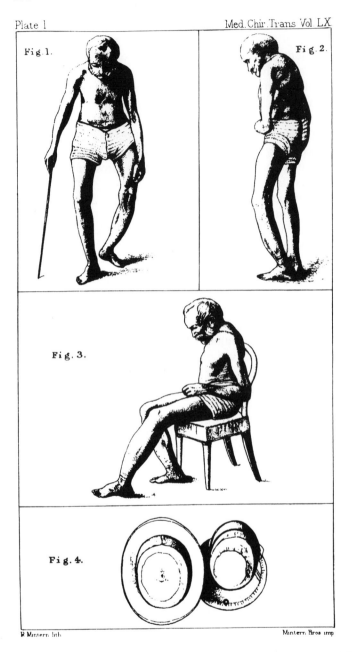

Plate 1   Med.Chir.Trans Vol LX

Fig.1.   Fig.2.

Fig.3.

Fig.4.

R Mintern lith   Mintern. Bros imp

Fig. 1. Reproduction of lithographies, from Sir James Paget's original 1877 publication [13].

2. Deformity

Deformity is the presenting feature in some 20% of patients with Paget's disease of bone and occurs as a result of structural weakness of the pathological bone. The long bones are particularly liable to deformity with resulting anterior (tibia) or lateral (femur and humerus) bowing, depending on mechanical stress and lines of least resistance. Bowing of the femur is often associated with a coxa vara deformity, resulting in external rotation of the lower leg. Lengthening of the affected limb may result in gait abnormalities, and clinically severe secondary arthritis may occur as a result of abnormal mechanical stresses. Fractures may also occur at the sites of maximum bowing.

In the pelvis, involved in about two-thirds of patients, softening of the acetabulum may result in marked deformity, with the femoral head invaginating the pelvic rim, "protrusio acetabuli". Acetabular protrusion may lead to severe hip joint dysfunction and secondary degenerative changes.

Vertebral crush fractures are associated with loss of height and increased curvature of the spine. As a result of spinal bowing, the limbs appear disproportionately long, giving the patient a simian appearance (Figure 1). Occasionally, expanding vertebral bodies may encroach on intervertebral foramina. This may result in interference to the blood supply of the spinal cord and a 'steal syndrome', or in narrowing of the spinal canal and neurological compression features.

The skull is involved in about one-third of patients with Paget's disease of bone, usually associated with more extensive disease elsewhere. Women appear to be more frequently affected than men. Involvement of the vault of the skull results in an increase in the size of the head, which may become triangular in shape. Shortening of the neck due to basilar invagination is observed with involvement of the base of the skull, and the head appears to be sinking onto the shoulders. Radiologically, Paget's disease of the skull may start as a well delineated rarefied area, "osteoporosis circumscripta", involving mostly the frontal or occipital bones, but which may spread to involve the whole of the skull vault. Sclerotic lesions of the skull are, nevertheless, twice as frequent as osteoporotic ones. Involvement of the facial bones is rare but may result in significant cosmetic and dental problems, and marked deformity of the maxillary bones may interfere with speech, mastication and deglutition and may result in loosening of the teeth [17].

3. Local changes

The skin overlying an active pagetic lesion may be warm to palpation, partly due to increased skeletal blood flow [14], but also due to a local increase in metabolic rate and bone turnover with compensatory vasodilatation in the overlying tissues to dissipate the excessive heat generated. The increase in skin temperature is most commonly appreciated in the distal extremities, and the local increase in vascularity is occasionally associated with a bruit, which can be heard on auscultation of the affected site. The increased vascularity of an active pagetic lesion may also compromise the overlying skin blood flow and result in atrophy and the development of slow-healing ulcers.

IV. Biochemical features

The hallmark of active Paget's disease of bone is the balanced increase in bone resorption and formation, traditionally assessed by estimating the urinary excretion of hydroxyproline, the most widely used index of bone collagen degradation, and serum alkaline phosphatase activity, an index of the number of functioning osteoblasts and hence bone formation. Both indices are closely correlated with bone turnover and with the extent and activity of Paget's disease as judged radiologically, scintigraphically and by calcium tracer techniques. These indices may however lie within the normal range in 10–20% of patients with localised monostotic disease, or be inordinately elevated in the case of skull involvement.

Collagen is the major protein of bone, and about 50% of the total urinary hydroxyproline is derived from this source. Dietary collagen is a significant source of hydroxyproline, and dietary restriction of meat and dairy products is required for the accurate interpretation of this index. The need for dietary restriction can, however, be obviated with the use of measurements done on early morning specimens taken after an overnight fast, with values expressed as a ratio of hydroxyproline to creatinine excretion. In Paget's disease of bone, a significant relationship has indeed been demonstrated between fasting hydroxyproline to creatinine ratio and corresponding 24-h urinary excretion of hydroxyproline, and the use of early morning samples has been advocated in the monitoring of response to treatment [18].

A well-characterised biochemical sequence of events is observed in urinary hydroxyproline excretion and serum alkaline phosphatase activity following treatment with inhibitors of osteoclast-mediated bone resorption such as the bisphosphonates. Bone resorption is suppressed early (days), as judged by a decrease in the urinary excretion of hydroxyproline, and a secondary decrease in bone formation follows (weeks), as judged by a decrease in serum alkaline phosphatase activity. The rate and the degree of suppression of bone resorption vary with the potency of the bisphosphonate used, and a complete clinical and biochemical response could be achieved in over 90% of patients with the use of the newer, more potent bisphosphonates. Normalisation of the urinary excretion of hydroxyproline and serum activity of alkaline phosphatase to well within the normal range is a good predictor of a long-lasting remission, whichever the bisphosphonate used and should be aimed at, when devising treatment regimens. These indices should be regularly monitored after remission is achieved (once or twice a year), with an increase in either heralding a relapse in disease activity.

In the event of failure of suppression of alkaline phosphatase activity with the use of adequate suppressive doses of bisphosphonates, or in the case of a rapid relapse after an initial satisfactory response as indicated by an early increase in the enzyme concentrations, malignant transformation of a lesion should be excluded, particularly if associated with persisting symptoms.

Other indices of bone resorption and formation have been examined in the management of Paget's disease of bone. Pyridinoline and deoxypyridinoline are non-reducible intermolecular crosslinks between adjacent mature collagen chains, present only in extracellular collagen fibrils and released in the circulation during the degradation of bone and cartilage. The urinary excretion of these collagen degradation products forms useful and specific indices of bone resorption in Paget's disease of bone. It has been proposed that the urinary excretion of these crosslinks may be a more sensitive index of collagen degradation than hydroxyproline in Paget's disease of bone [19], particularly as they are not affected by dietary gelatin intake. Contrary to the case with the urinary excretion of hydroxyproline, however, data are not yet available on the relationship of these indices to the extent or activity of the disease process. Moreover, recent studies have also demonstrated that these new indices do not appear to offer any advantage over the traditional determination of the urinary excretion of hydroxyproline in the monitoring of response to treatment with inhibitors of bone resorption [20].

Procollagen, the immediate precursor to the α-chain of the final collagen molecule, is a larger protein molecule than collagen, containing additional sequences at both ends. Procollagen is synthesised intracellularly in osteoblasts and is cleaved from the final collagen molecule by specific proteases before it is assembled into fibrils and stabilised by cross-links. The cleaved fragments from the carboxy-terminal pro-peptide of type I procollagen (PICP) are liberated into the circulation where they can be measured by radioimmunoassay. Circulating procollagen peptides are thought to be directly related to the number of collagen molecules formed and are therefore used to quantify type I collagen synthesis and hence bone formation. PICP have indeed been shown to correlate significantly with histologically derived bone formation rates in patients with various disorders of bone metabolism and have been shown to be useful in the clinical monitoring of Paget's disease of bone [21].

Bone formation could also be indirectly assessed by the estimation of serum concentrations of fragments of matrix proteins released in the circulation during the process of bone formation such as osteocalcin. Osteocalcin is the most abundant non-collagenous protein in bone and is synthesised exclusively by osteoblasts. In untreated Paget's disease of bone, osteocalcin concentrations have, however, been found to be normal in about 50% of patients in whom serum alkaline phosphatase activity was increased. In the course of treatment with inhibitors of bone resorption, changes in serum concentrations of osteocalcin do not parallel those of the two traditionally used indices of bone turnover, and an initial increase may be observed after the start of treatment [22]. The use of osteocalcin as an index of bone turnover is thus not advocated in Paget's disease of bone, as it is less sensitive and specific than either urinary excretion of hydroxyproline or serum alkaline phosphatase activity in the assessment of disease activity or in the monitoring of its response to treatment.

Extracellular calcium homeostasis is usually maintained in Paget's disease of bone, although a number of patients may be hypercalciuric and may develop hypercalcaemia on immobilisation, particularly in the presence of extensive skeletal involvement. The risk of urolithiasis is increased in the presence of persistent hypercalciuria. An increase in parathyroid hormone concentrations can also be observed in up to 20% of patients in the presence of normal serum calcium concentrations, particularly in those patients with the greater skeletal involvement.

In the early phase of treatment with inhibitors of bone resorption, the suppression of bone resorption, in the presence of continuing bone formation, results in a decrease in the net efflux of calcium from the skeleton to the extracellular fluid. A fall in serum calcium follows, which stimulates PTH secretion. This in turn increases the renal tubular reabsorption of calcium and enhances intestinal absorption of calcium via stimulation of calcitriol synthesis by the kidney, thus restoring calcium homeostasis. These secondary metabolic effects are not noted with the use of etidronate, as the associated delay in mineralization, particularly with the use of high oral or intravenous doses, inhibits calcium accretion in bone and offsets any hypocalcaemic effect resulting from the inhibition of bone resorption. The unopposed effect of the bisphosphonate on renal tubular reabsorption of phosphate results in hyperphosphataemia, an effect which is dose-dependent in the case of etidronate and only seen very transiently with the use of other bisphosphonates, when it is usually abolished by a secondary increase in PTH secretion [23].

V. Complications

Complications of Paget's disease of bone were also recognised and described by Sir James Paget in his original series of untreated patients whom he observed long-term.

> ... as he was riding and suddenly raised his arms, the bone broke near the shoulder....
> ... cancer appeared late in life, ... possibly not more than might have occurred in accidental coincidences, yet suggesting careful enquiry....

Untreated Paget's disease of bone may remain silent for years, and patients may present with complications including fractures [24], secondary degenerative changes in adjacent or distant joints [15, 16], neurological complications [25] or, more rarely, neoplastic changes [26, 27].

1. Fractures

Pagetic bone is deposited in a disorganised manner, so that the bone is mechanically weak, although increased in volume. Fractures are infrequent, occurring in only about 5% of cases. They represent, however, a serious complication of Paget's disease of bone. They occur most commonly in weight-bearing long bones, at the site of maximal mechanical stresses as a result of bowing, and may be fissure or complete fractures. Long-standing untreated disease resulting in a bowing deformity of a long bone is thus a significant predisposing factor.

Fractures may occur spontaneously or after minimal trauma, may be single or multiple and, in view of the increased vascularity of the lesions, may result in a substantial loss of blood. Fractures may be asymptomatic, but patients may also present with pain and tenderness, often heralding the development of a fissure fracture into a complete one. Fissure fractures may precede the development of a complete fracture by a few weeks.

Some 70–90% of pathological fractures occur in the femur, followed in frequency by fractures of the tibia and forearm. Vertebral compression fractures may also occur when the spine is involved.

Most fractures through pagetic bone heal normally, but union may be delayed, and refracture is common. Fractures of the femoral neck represent a particular management problem, as the bone may be too soft to provide support in the osteolytic phase, or too difficult to penetrate in the sclerotic phase. Deformity may also be so severe that alignment of the shaft may be difficult and internal fixation impossible. Fractures may also be complicated by hypercalcaemia as a result of enforced immobilisation. This may in turn be associated with hypercalciuria and an increased risk of nephrocalcinosis and nephrolithiasis. There is no evidence that fractures are associated with an increased risk of developing osteosarcoma.

2. Osteoarthritis

Osteoarthritis is a very frequent complication of Paget's disease of bone, occurring in joints adjacent to pagetic bone or on the contralateral side as a result of altered lines of mechanical stresses on weight-bearing surfaces. Clinically severe secondary arthritis occurs in a significant proportion of patients with Paget's disease affecting the pelvis. Patients present with pain and limitation of movement in the affected sites. Symptoms may significantly improve by controlling disease activity.

3. Neoplastic change

In Paget's disease of bone, neoplastic changes can occur at the site of any lesion, most commonly in the form of osteosarcoma. It is very difficult to estimate the incidence of this rare but most serious complication of the disorder. Its prevalence increases with age, peaking at the seventh decade, and the most common sites affected are the pelvis, long bones (humerus and femur) and skull. Contrary to primary osteosarcoma which mostly affects the metaphyseal region of bone, Paget's osteosarcoma can occur anywhere along the shaft of a long bone or at any other site affected. A worsening in pain at the site of a known lesion or a change in the pattern of pain may herald osteosarcomatous changes. A fracture may also be the first sign of malignant transformation of a lesion, in which case healing is often delayed. The bony changes may be associated with soft-tissue swelling and tenderness and dilatation of superficial veins. Bone destruction can be demonstrated radiologically in the form of osteolysis with ill-defined boundaries, and bone scintigraphy demonstrates decreased uptake.

The osteosarcomatous lesion is frequently multicentric, and its extreme vascularity increases the risk of haematogenous spread. In over 50% of cases, the anatomical site of the lesion is not amenable to radical amputation. The neoplastic change is also often diagnosed too late, when radical amputation may not alter the prognosis, which is thus very poor. Mean survival has been reported to vary between 7 and 14 months.

4. Neurological complications

Neurological complications may occur in Paget's disease of bone as a result of increased pressure on neurological structures from enlarging bones, or due to interference with the regional neuronal vascular supply.

Cranial nerve compression can occur in Paget's disease of the skull, as a result of narrowing of cranial nerve foramina. The most anatomically susceptible nerves are the optic, auditory and trigeminal nerves, leading, respectively, to progressive loss of vision, deafness and trigeminal neuralgia. Hearing impairment is common in Paget's of the skull and could be conductive, due to fixation of the bone ossicles in the middle ear, or neuronal, due to compression of the VIIIth cranial nerve in the auditory canal. Irreversible hearing loss may occur in 20% of the patients. The lower cranial nerves are less frequently affected. Direct compression of the brain stem in Paget's of the base of the skull may result in progressive confusion.

Paget's disease of the spine can result in nerve root compression, narrowing of the spinal canal or interference with the blood supply to the spinal cord, 'the steal syndrome'. Symptoms may resolve on adequate suppression of disease activity.

5. Cardiovascular complications

In Paget's disease of bone, heart failure is most commonly due to underlying cardiac disease. Rarely, increased vascularity in extensive lesions may result in high output cardiac failure [28]. This complication is seldom, if ever, seen nowadays.

6. Urolithiasis

Renal stones are present in about 5% of patients with Paget's disease of bone. Possible risk factors include hypercalciuria and hypercalcaemia, possibly resulting from immobilisation for concurrent illnesses. Serum uric acid is also often elevated.

References

1. Collins, D.H., Paget's disease of bone — Incidence and subclinical forms. Lancet 1956; ii: 51–57.
2. Nagant de Deuxchaisnes, C. and Krane, S.M., Paget's disease of bone: Clinical and metabolic observations. Medicine 1964; 43: 233–266.
3. Krane, S.M., Paget's disease of bone. Clin. Orthop. Rel. Res. 1977; 127: 24–36.
4. Singer, F.R., Schiller, A.I., Pyle, E.B. and Krane, S.M., Paget's disease of bone. In: Avioli, L. and Krane, S., eds., Metabolic Bone Disease. London: Academic Press, 1978; 489–575.
5. Altman, R.D. and Collins, B., Musculoskeletal manifestations of Paget's disease of bone. Arthritis Rheum. 1980; 23: 1121–1127.
6. Hamdy, R.C., Paget's disease of bone: Assessment and management. New York: Praeger, 1981.
7. Russell, R.G.G., Paget's disease. In: Nordin, B.E.C., ed., Metabolic bone and stone disease. Edinburgh: Churchill Livingstone, 1984; 190–233.
8. Harinck, H.I.J., Bijvoet, O.L.M., Vellenga, C.G.R.L., Blanksma, H.J. and Frijlink, W.B., Relation between signs and symptoms of Paget's disease of bone. Q. J. Med. 1986; 58: 133–151.
9. Meunier, P.J., Salson, C., Mathieu, L., Chapuy, M.C., Delmas, P., Alexandre, C. and Charhon, S., Skeletal distribution of Paget's disease. Clin. Orthop. Rel. Res. 1987; 217: 37–44.

10. Resnick, C.S., Paget's disease of bone: Current status and a look back to 1943 and earlier. Am. J. Radiol. 1988; 150: 249–256.
11. Bijvoet, O.L.M., Vellenga, C.J.L.R. and Harinck, H.I.J., Paget's disease of bones: Assessment, therapy, and secondary prevention. In: Kleerekoper, M. and Krane, S.M., eds., Clinical disorders of bone and mineral metabolism. New York: Liebert, 1989; 525–542.
12. Kanis, J.A., Pathophysiology and treatment of Paget's disease of bone. London: Martin Dunitz, 1991.
13. Paget, J., On a form of chronic inflammation of bones. Medico-Chirurgical Trans. 1877; 60: 37–63.
14. Wootton, R., Reeve, J., Spellacy, E. and Tellez-Yudilevich, M., Skeletal blood flow in Paget's disease of bone and its response to calcitonin therapy. Clin. Sci. Mol. Med. 1978; 54: 69–74.
15. Franck, W., Bress, N., Singer, F. and Krane, S., Rheumatic manifestations of Paget's disease of bone. Am. J. Med. 1974; 56: 592–603.
16. Winfield, J. and Stamp, T.C.B., Bone and joint symptoms in Paget's disease. Ann. Rheum. Dis. 1984; 43: 769–773.
17. Smith, B.J. and Eveson, J.W., Paget's disease of bone with particular reference to dentistry. J. Oral Pathol. 1981; 10: 233–247.
18. Russell, R.G.G., Beard, D.J., Cameron, E.C., Douglas, D.L., Forrest, A.R.W., Guilland-Cumming, D., Paterson, A.D., Poser, J., Preston, C.J., Milford-Ward, A., Woodhead, S. and Kanis, J.A., Biochemical markers of bone turnover in Paget's disease. Metab. Bone Dis. Rel. Res. 1981; 4 and 5: 255–262.
19. Uebelhart, D., Gineyts, E.C., Chapuy, M.C. and Delmas, P.D., Urinary excretion of pyridinium crosslinks: a new marker of bone resorption in metabolic bone disease. Bone Miner. 1990; 8: 87–96.
20. Hamdy, N.A.T., Papapoulos, S.E., Colwell, A., Eastell, R. and Russell, R.G.G., Urinary collagen crosslink excretion: a better index of bone resorption than hydroxyproline in Paget's disease of bone? Bone Miner. 1993; 22: 1–8.
21. Simon, L.S., Krane, S.M., Wortman, P.D., Krane, I.M. and Kovitz, K.L., Serum of Type I and III procollagen fragments in Paget's disease of bone. J. Clin. Endocrinol. Metab. 1984; 58: 110–120.
22. Papapoulos, S.E., Frolich, M., Mudde, A.H., Harinck, H.I.J., VDBerg, H. and Bijvoet, O.L.M., Serum osteocalcin in Paget's disease of bone: basal concentrations and response to bisphosphonate treatment. J. Clin. Endocrinol. Metab. 1987; 65: 89–94.
23. McCloskey, E.V., Yates, A.J.P., Gray, R.E.S., Hamdy, N.A.T., Galloway, J. and Kanis, J.A., Diphosphonates and phosphate homeostasis. Clin. Sci. 1988; 74: 607–612.
24. Stevens, J., Orthopaedic aspects of Paget's disease. Metab. Bone Dis. Rel. Res. 1981; 3: 271–278.
25. Herzberg, L. and Bayliss, E., Spinal cord syndrome due to non-compressive Paget's disease of bone. A spinal artery steal phenomenon reversible with calcitonin. Lancet 1980; 2: 13–15.
26. Smith, J., Botet, J.F. and Yeh, S.D.J., Bone sarcomas in Paget's disease: a study of 85 patients. Radiology 1984; 152: 583–590.
27. Wick, M.R., Siegal, G.P., Unni, K.K., McLeod, R.A. and Greditzer, H.B., Sarcomas of bone complicating osteitis deformans (Paget's disease). Am. J. Surg. Pathol. 1981; 5: 47–59.
28. Howarth, S. Cardiac output in osteitis deformans. Clin. Sci. 1953; 12: 271–275.

Bisphosphonate on bones
O. Bijvoet, H.A. Fleisch, R.E. Canfield and G. Russell (eds.)
© 1995 Elsevier Science B.V. All rights reserved.

CHAPTER 18

Quantitative bone scintigraphy in the evaluation of Paget's disease of bone

C.J.L.R. Vellenga

Twenteborg Ziekenhuis, Zilvermeeuw 1, P.O. Box 7600, 7600 SZ Almelo, The Netherlands

I. Introduction

At present, bone scintigraphy is mostly performed using the radionuclide technetium 99m, linked to a bisphosphonate, either EHDP or MDP. Unlike ^{47}Ca, ^{85}Sr and ^{87m}Sr, which are exchanged with the calcium of the bone pool, and ^{18}F, which is exchanged with the hydroxyl group in hydroxyapatite, the ^{99m}Tc-Sn-EHDP complex travels to the bone as a single entity and probably decomposes at the relevant binding site, thus permitting ^{99m}Tc to become attached to the bone independently of the rest of the complex. ^{99m}Tc has an especially strong affinity to immature osteoid for two reasons: in the first place, for the chemisorption of ^{99m}Tc, the surface provided by the small mineral nuclei exceeds that of the more voluminous mature apatite crystal per unit mass; and in the second place, it exhibits a strong affinity for amorphous Ca-phosphate. Thus, it appears likely that it is not the unmineralized organic portion of bone that is important for the uptake of ^{99m}Tc-Sn-EHDP, but the small nuclei of calcification dispersed throughout the immature bone matrix.

A second factor of importance for the uptake of ^{99m}Tc-Sn-EHDP is the vascularity. The radiopharmaceutical is delivered to the binding site by the bloodstream. However, there is no linear relationship between blood flow and uptake of Tc-compounds. A diffusion-limited saturation effect attributable to the buffer function of the extracellular fluid in bone precludes a further increase in uptake when the blood flow in bone rises above normal levels. On the other hand, a further increase in uptake is seen when the number of vessels supplying the bone is augmented, either by recruitment in experimental models or by pathological processes.

Thus, uptake of ^{99m}Tc-Sn-EHDP is governed mainly by two factors: the first one is the surface area available for adsorption to either hydroxyapatite crystals in mature and immature bone or the nuclei of amorphous calcium salts in immature matrix; the second factor is the number of patent blood vessels in the bone. The rate of local bone metabolism parallels these two factors and is therefore also reflected by the amount of uptake of Tc-compound.

Usually, bone scintigraphy is performed 3 to 4 hours after intravenous injection of 555–740 MBq (15–20 mCi) Tc-MDP or Tc-EHDP. Multiple spot views of the whole skeleton or a whole-body survey are obtained using a large field-of-view gamma-camera. Images are stored digitally on computer disc or tape, and copies of the analogue images are made on transparent film. The digital images can be analysed using a light-pen or track ball, thus quantifying the number of disintegrations of Tc (amount of uptake of radioactivity) in the bony lesion, compared to normal bone and to earlier scintigrams.

Generally, subjective visual assessment of the scintigrams is rather accurate and reliable in respect of changes of uptake during treatment, whereas new lesions or the disappearance of lesions can definitely be identified by non-quantitative viewing. However, it has been demonstrated that visual assessment reflects the logarithm of the actual uptake and that in about 15% of the lesions, changes during treatment for Paget's disease can be missed by the eye [1]. Because scintigraphic changes in Paget's disease during treatment are impressive, it could well be that smaller changes, for example, during treatment of bone metastases, are missed more often by subjective viewing. In these cases quantitative evaluation with the aid of a light-pen and computer can be recommended.

II. Paget's disease

The most and the longest experience with scintigraphic follow-up of treatment effects by bisphosphonates has been obtained in Paget's disease — which was the first bone disease to be treated with bisphosphonates — so this issue will be discussed in detail at first.

1. Radiographic characteristics

Just as the earliest histological event in bone is resorption, the earliest radiological change is a decrease in density of bone. Subsequently, the radiological findings will reflect a local imbalance between bone resorption, causing a decrease in density, and new bone formation, causing either an increase in density or — when mineralization has not yet taken place — a reduced density. These processes co-exist in varying stages of development and alternate from one area to the other. The involved parts of the bone are enlarged and deformed. The spongiosa shows thickened coarse trabeculae which are often separated by large marrow spaces filled with fibrous or fatty bone marrow. The cortex can be dense and thickened or be diffusely demineralized, but can also be lamellar and be dissected by longitudinal osteolytic clefts. The diversity of the roentgenological patterns is great, but they can grossly be distinguished into three categories: osteolytic or osteoporotic phase, mixed or combined phase, and osteosclerotic or osteoplastic phase. These three phases can be encountered everywhere in the skeleton; generally, more than one phase is present in the same patient and frequently in the same bone. There is a large variation in density and structure, and there is considerable overlap among

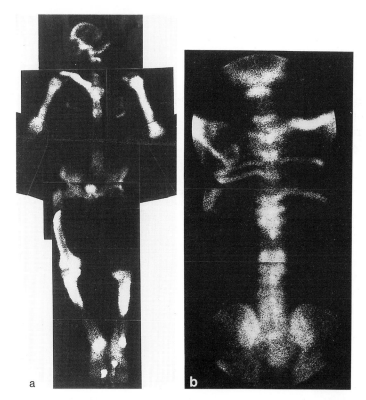

a b

Fig. 1a. Anterior scintigram of polyostotic Paget's disease: homogeneously elevated uptake in multiple bones; some bones are affected partially, others entirely; note the V-shaped demarcation of the lesions in the long bones, the serrated demarcation of the osteoporotic area in the skull, the enhanced visibility of the outlines and anatomical shapes of the bones, the involvement of metatarsal bones and the difference of uptake within lesions. b. Posterior scintigram of Pagets' disease: In the same patient as in a, the increased uptake in some ribs and vertebrae, the left scapula and right clavicle are evident. The normal parts of the skeleton show normal uptake.

the three phases. One may metamorphose into another, but the different types cannot be seen as subsequent stages of evolution. Sometimes a subtle and beginning lesion is osteolytic, sometimes it is sclerotic; some sclerotic lesions become mixed; more commonly, lytic lesions become mixed and subsequently sclerotic, whereas many lesions maintain the same balance of osteolysis and osteoblastosis throughout the years, although architectural changes and deformity of the bone may steadily progress.

2. Scintigraphic survey

The radiological appearance in Paget's disease (described in Chapter 8) always allows a definite and secure diagnosis. Although bone scintigraphy is not considered to be a diagnostic method of high specificity for bone diseases in general, the

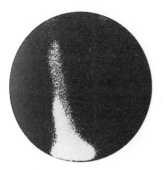

Fig. 2. Primary and secondary front: an area of high uptake in the distal femur is bounded by a typical V-front (secondary front). Proximally, a V-shaped region of lower uptake (primary front) is seen, whereas the normal bone in the most proximal part of the femur is not visible.

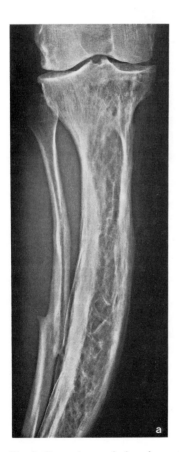

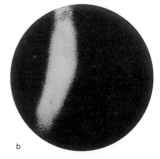

Fig. 3. Gross changes in long bone: (a) severe changes of the tibia, thickening of the cortical bone, coarse and sparse trabeculae and cystic areas; (b) the thickening and bowing of the tibia is clearly visible on the scintigram.

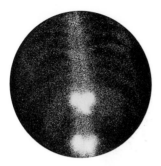

Fig. 4. Vertebral involvement by Paget's disease: The shape of the vertebrae Th12 and L3 is clearly visible due to elevated uptake in Paget's disease. The other vertebrae show a normal pattern.

scintigraphic pattern of Paget's disease is often so characteristic that the diagnosis is unequivocal [2]. The characteristic scintigraphic appearance of Paget's disease is shown in Figure 1. There is a sharply defined area of homogeneous high uptake in the affected bone; the anatomical details are accentuated due to the high uptake, which can be up to 20 times normal. In long bones the area of high activity is always bounded by the articular surface on one side and by a V-shaped front in the diaphysis; despite the sharp boundary between the lesion and the normal bone, not infrequently a band of lower activity is seen along the progression front, reflecting extension of the disease into healthy bone (primary and secondary front) [3] (Fig. 2). Sometimes there is an increased accumulation of radioactivity in the advancing lesion, particularly in the skull. Lesions are encountered more often in the proximal part of a long bone, but an entire bone may be involved from joint to joint. When deformation and expansion are present, this can be seen clearly on the scintigram (Fig. 3a and b; Fig. 7c). In the pelvis the characteristic presentation is a hemipelvic lesion with sharply defined borders at the acetabular and sacro-iliacal joint surfaces. In the spine one or a few vertebrae show uniformly elevated uptake throughout the vertebral body, arch and processi, with normal vertebrae in between (Fig. 4; Fig. 5a and b). Confusion with osteoporotic fracture or metastasis may ensue. In the skull several patterns occur: the lesion can have a sharp undulating margin, corresponding to osteoporosis circumscripta on the X-ray (Fig. 14). Or there is diffuse increase in radioactivity throughout the neurocranium. In this type of lesion, it can sometimes be difficult to decide whether there is pagetic bone or not, if there is only a slight elevation of uptake. In other instances there is high uptake in a grossly deformed skull with obvious basilar invagination (concavity of the base of the skull). The last type of lesion has one or several hot spots, coinciding with osteoporosis on the X-ray and closely mimicking metastatic disease (Fig. 14). The main differential diagnosis on the scintigram comprises fractures, metastatic disease, degenerative osteoarthritis and in some instances hyperparathyroidism.

The scintigram gives a quick and complete survey of all lesions, with the least discomfort and radiation for the patient. Subsequently, X-rays of the affected parts of the skeleton should be taken, in order to visualize the texture and deformation

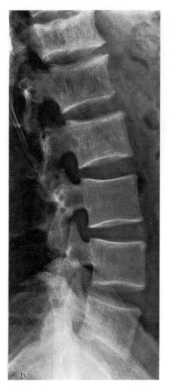
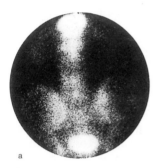

Fig. 5. Correlation of degree of scintigraphic and radiologic involvement of the spine. (a) On the scintigram Th12 shows severe involvement, L1 and L2 show moderate involvement, L3 is normal, L4 and L5 show slight involvement. (b) The radiogram shows also the normal L3 in between the slightly involved L4 and L5, the moderately involved L1 and L2, and the grossly deformed Th12.

of bone and to confirm the diagnosis. One-quarter of the patients has monostotic disease, and one-half has 2–4 lesions. The chance that an additional lesion will be present is always about 70%. The pelvis is the most common site, followed in decreasing order by the tibia, femur, lumbar spine, sacrum and skull. About 15% of the scintigraphically detected lesions are not visible on X-rays. These may be quiescent lesions but generally are areas of early disease and low metabolic activity.

Indeed, a further important aspect of bone scintigraphy is that it not only correlates with metabolism and vascularity, but also with the amount of radiological and macroscopic deformity and with clinical symptoms [5]. So, the higher the uptake in a lesion, the more disturbed the bone texture will be and the higher the occurrence of pain (Figs. 5, 6 and 7).

3. Scintigraphy in the follow-up

Therefore, the bone scintigram is an important monitor of the activity of Paget's disease during treatment. If not treated, natural changes of mean scintigraphic

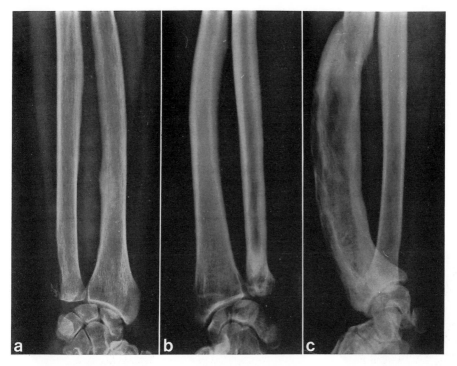

Fig. 6. Different degrees of radiological involvement of the forearm by Paget's disease. (a) minute demineralisation and subtle rarefaction of trabecular structure in the distal radius; (b) moderate involvement with sclerosis of the ulna and thickening of the cortical bone; (c) increased diameter of the cortical bone, gross deformity and bowing of the radius.

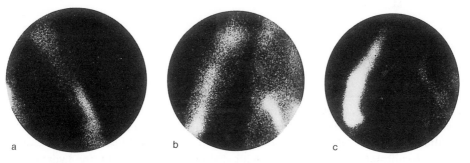

Fig. 7. Scintigrams of same patients as in figure 6: (a) the subtle radiological involvement of Fig. 6a is clearly visible in the scintigram; (b) the distinct radiological involvement of the ulna is reflected as a rather high uptake in the forearm; (c) the very high uptake and deformity of the distal radius are reflected by very high uptake in a grossly deformed bone.

uptake in pagetic lesions are of a minor degree. Patel et al. [4] showed that in individual lesions scan intensity could both decrease or increase over a 2-year period. Even spontaneous normalization can occur. However, scintigraphic changes during

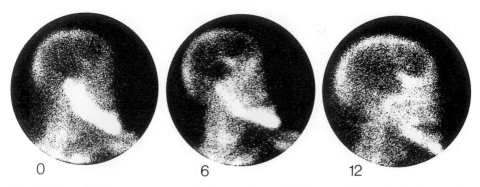

Fig. 8. Scintigraphic improvement during treatment: During APD the very high uptake in the mandible falls to almost normal levels after one year of APD.

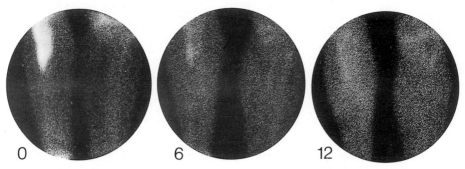

Fig. 9. Scintigraphic normalisation during APD therapy: The ratio in the lesion diminishes from 5.4 times normal to 1.5 after 6 months of APD and to 1.1 after 12 months.

treatment far exceed the natural fluctuations. During treatment with EHDP combined with calcitonin and during treatment with APD, an exponential reduction of radiotracer uptake in all lesions takes place, amounting to an average of about 70% during the first half-year and a further 10% during the second half-year [5, 6]. Even by eye the impressive fall of uptake of radioactivity in the lesions during treatment is unequivocally appreciated (Fig. 8), although especially in lesions with a very high uptake, a reduction in uptake of up to 70% can be interpreted as 'no change' by the eye. In a series of 27 patients with 100 lesions, this occurred 14 times [1].

Despite normalization of the serum alkaline phosphatase and urine hydroxyproline levels, complete normalization of the bone scintigram is not the rule, and only one-third of the individual lesions normalize on the scintigram [5, 6] (Fig. 9), generally those with mild changes on the pre-treatment scintigram, but sometimes lesions with severe scintigraphic involvement may normalize (Fig. 10); in the great majority of patients most individual skeletal lesions retain a residual 20% scintigraphic uptake of the original value [5, 6]. This residual activity does not mean that local metabolism is still elevated but is probably solely caused by persistent abnormality of bone architecture, as is still visible on the radiographs.

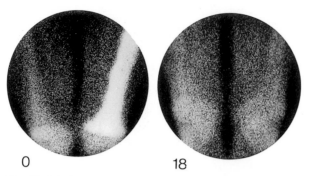

Fig. 10. Scintigraphic normalisation during combination therapy. The initial high uptake in the left femur completely normalizes after 18 months of treatment with calcitonin and EHDP.

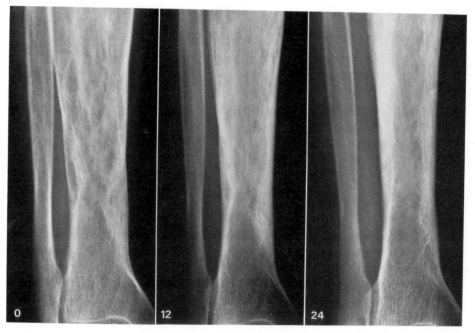

Fig. 11. Radiological improvement during combination therapy: During therapy with calcitonin and EHDP the originally swollen and demineralized tibia becomes slender, the osteolytic spaces fill in with well-mineralized bone, the trabeculae become finer and regain a normal appearance. One year later the pagetic bone has almost normalized, the corticomedullary differentiation is restored, and the V-shaped front between pagetic and normal bone fades away.

Radiological improvement is much slower and more difficult to demonstrate than scintigraphic improvement. It requires careful and exactly reproducible positioning and techniques. In high quality radiography, however, decrease of osteoblastosis, of external bone diameter, of deformation and re-ossification are not a rare occurrence; actually, radiological improvement of pagetic lesions could be demonstrated

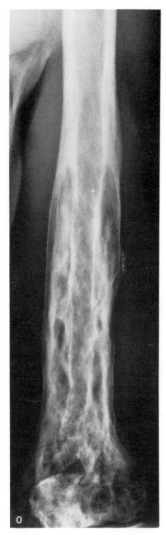 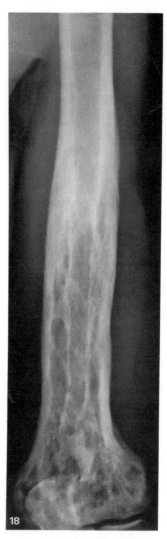

Fig. 12. Radiological improvement during APD therapy: After 18 months, remodelling and remineralization of the humerus are impressive, the broad osteolytic clefts in the cortical bone are filled in with well-mineralized normal bone, and the proximal border of the lesion vanishes.

in 11 of 23 patients, receiving APD; 30% of the individual lesions showed definite improvement (Figure 11 and 12), while in half of the lesions no changes could be demonstrated by radiography [7].

Also during treatment with other bisphosphonates the bone scintigram has been proven to be a useful indicator of the level of metabolism. Ryan et al. [8] demonstrated that Pamidronate has a powerful effect on bone scan appearances in Paget's disease: 65% of 136 lesions in 25 patients improved, 24% remained

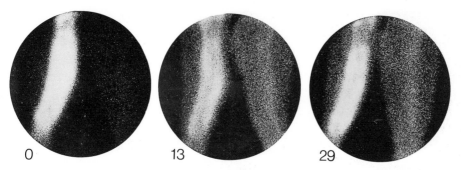

Fig. 13. Diffuse type of scintigraphic recurrence in the tibia: Gross deformation of the tibia is evident. The initially very high uptake improves quite well after 13 months. By 16 months later, however, diffuse increase in uptake is obvious, heralding a relapse of Paget's disease.

unchanged; also in these series complete normalization occurred in only 10% of the lesions. Patel et al. [4] concluded from their study in 29 patients treated with either APD or EHDP that serial bone scans must be used with caution when interpreting the response of Paget's disease to therapy. They found a significant decrease in main lesion intensity in most patients compared to 9 untreated patients. However the summated scintigraphic score did not improve in six patients and even deteriorated in four. Out of 185 lesions 86 improved, but 20 deteriorated. Amelioration and deterioration of individual lesions could occur in the same patient. The large number of 79 unchanged lesions can possibly partly be ascribed to the use of visual assessment and the omission of computerized quantitation. They even identified new lesions in five patients (three in the skull, two in the thoracic spine), although three of these patients showed a satisfactory biochemical response; in six other instances areas of apparently new disease were revealed to be the result of either degenerative disease or bony fracture on repeat bone scanning or radiology.

If, however, a new lesion or deterioration of a known lesion is detected on the bone scintigram during treatment with a bisphosphonate (Figs. 13, 14 and 15), one should seriously consider the possibility of reactivation of Paget's disease, urging a new course of therapy. Of 40 patients on EHDP and/or calcitonin, 21 suffered a clinical and/or biochemical recurrence [9]. One-third was seen first on the scintigram, one-third was first indicated by biochemical determinations, and in one-third the scintigraphic and biochemical relapses coincided. In 2 patients (8%) with a recurrence, the bone scintigram did not deteriorate, and 3 patients (15%) with increasing uptake on the scintigram stayed in biochemical remission.

Scintigraphic deterioration manifested itself as one of four easily detected patterns: most commonly, a diffuse increase of uptake in a lesion could be seen and measured (Fig. 13); not uncommonly, foci of increasing radioactivity originated in a known lesion, especially in the skull (Fig. 14); sometimes, spread of disease beyond the boundaries of the original lesion into adjacent normal bone could be seen (Fig. 15); in six patients new lesions were identified. If deterioration occurs, uptake in one or more lesions rises, whereas other lesions in the same patients remain unaltered.

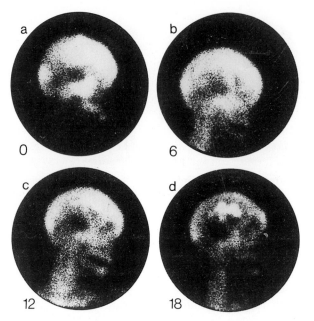

Fig. 14. Focal type of scintigraphic recurrence in the skull: The circumscript area of Paget's disease in the frontal and temporal bone improves to almost normal after 2 years. By 18 months later multiple foci of increased uptake are seen in the same area, coinciding with a clinical recurrence.

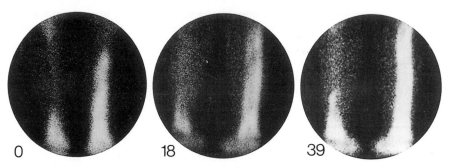

Fig. 15. Progressive type of scintigraphic recurrence in the femora: After 18 months the overall scintigraphic activity has decreased, but the front of activity in the left femur has progressed proximally. After 39 months scintigraphic uptake has increased, and cephalad progression into normal bone of both femora is evident.

III. Conclusion

In conclusion, bone scintigraphy is a reliable parameter for local activity of Paget's disease, although a few pitfalls should be taken into account. Before treatment, the bone scintigram gives a quick and complete survey of the spread of the disease throughout the skeleton and also demonstrates the amount of metabolic activity, of structural changes and of clinical relevance in the individual lesions.

Roentgenography of the affected parts must then be undertaken, to settle the macroscopic bone architecture. During successful treatment with bisphosphonates, a steep fall of uptake of radioactivity in most lesions is compulsory within 6 months, but — due to persistent abnormal bone texture — complete normalization of the scintigram is not mandatory; on the contrary, it is uncommon. According to some investigators, a rise in radionuclide uptake (despite biochemical improvement or normalization) can occur [4].

If carried out with great care, the roentgenogram can also demonstrate improvement of bone texture. However, radiography is painstaking and time-consuming. On the other hand, it should be realized that both methods reflect different processes: whereas radiography uniquely demonstrates pure changes of bone architecture, scintigraphic uptake is mainly governed by metabolism and microscopic qualities (number and size of crystals) of the bone and only to a minor part (15–20%) by structural changes.

References

1. Vellenga, C.J.L.R., Pauwels, E.K.J. and Bijvoet, O.L.M., Comparison between visual assessment and quantitative measurement of radioactivity on the bone scintigram in Paget's disease of bone. Eur. J. Nucl. Med. 1984; 9: 533–537.
2. Vellenga, C.J.L.R., Pauwels, E.K.J., Bijvoet, O.L.M., Frijlink, W.B. and Hermans, J., Untreated Paget's disease of bone studied by scintigraphy. Radiology 1984; 153: 799–805.
3. Vellenga, C.J.L.R., Pauwels, E.K.J. and Bijvoet, O.L.M., Some characteristics of local Paget's and radiologic patterns of Paget's disease of bone. Diagn. Imag. Clin. Med. 1985; 54: 273–281.
4. Patel, U., Callacher, S.J., Boyle, I.T. and McKillop, J.H., Serial bone scans in Paget's disease: development of new lesions, natural variation in lesion intensity and nature of changes seen after treatment. Nucl. Med. Comm. 1990; 11: 747–760.
5. Vellenga, C.J.L.R., Pauwels, E.K.J., Bijvoet, O.L.M., Hosking, D.J. and Frijlink, W.B., Bone scintigraphy in Paget's disease treated with combined calcitonin and diphosphonate (EHDP). Metab. Bone Dis. Rel. Res. 1982; 4: 103–111.
6. Vellenga, C.J.L.R., Pauwels, E.K.J., Bijvoet, O.L.M., Harinck, H.I.J. and Frijlink, W.B., Quantitative bone scintigraphy in Paget's disease treated with APD. Br. J. Radiol. 1985; 58: 1165–1172.
7. Vellenga, C.J.L.R., Mulder, J.D. and Bijvoet, O.L.M., Radiological demonstration of healing in Paget's disease of bone treated with APD. Br. J. Radiol. 1985; 58: 831–837.
8. Ryan, P.J., Gibson, T. and Fogelman, I., Bone scintigraphy following intravenous pamidronate for Paget's disease of bone. J. Nucl. Med. 1992; 33: 1589–1593.
9. Vellenga, C.J.L.R., Pauwels, E.K.J., Bijvoet, O.L.M. and Frijlink, W.B. Scintigraphic aspects of the recurrence of treated Paget's disease of bone. J. Nucl. Med. 1981; 22: 510–517.

Bisphosphonate on bones
O. Bijvoet, H.A. Fleisch, R.E. Canfield and G. Russell (eds.)
© 1995 Elsevier Science B.V. All rights reserved.

CHAPTER 19

The bisphosphonates in treatment and secondary prevention of Paget's disease of bone

Ethel S. Siris and Mary Arden-Cordone

Department of Medicine, Columbia University College of Physicians and Surgeons, 630 West 168 Street, New York, NY 10032, USA

I. Introduction: The nature of Paget's disease

Paget's disease of bone is a localized disorder of bone remodelling, initiated by an abnormality in osteoclast-mediated bone resorption. As described in greater detail in earlier chapters of this volume, increased numbers of larger than normal 'pagetic' osteoclasts promote an increase in bone resorption at affected skeletal sites. Secondarily, there is an increase in the rate of new bone formation, a phenomenon closely coupled to the increase in bone resorption. The newly formed bone is architecturally abnormal, displaying a mosaic pattern of areas of lamellar bone juxtaposed to more primitive woven bone. Pathological sections of such bone, in addition to demonstrating the increased numbers of super-nucleated osteoclasts and normal-appearing osteoblasts during phases of active increased bone turnover, also display the appearance of increased numbers of new blood vessels and, in many cases, a fibrotic bone marrow.

As a consequence of the architectural changes in bone due to the remodelling abnormality just described, pagetic bone may manifest areas of predominantly osteolytic or osteosclerotic character, is typically larger than normal due to the loss of a more compact formation of new bone, and is more vascular than normal bone when the bone remodelling abnormality is active. Not surprisingly, the structurally inferior architecture produces bone that is prone to deformity and, less commonly, fracture. Depending on the number and location of sites of the disorder and on the exuberance of the abnormal remodelling process, there may be no signs or symptoms of the disease — as may be true in the majority of cases of this fairly common disorder — or a variety of clinical findings and problems may occur. It is the purpose of this chapter to discuss the role that bisphosphonate therapy may play (or fail to play) in the alleviation of symptoms and, it is hoped, in the prevention of later complications in patients with Paget's disease.

II. Signs and symptoms

To understand the role of therapy, it is necessary to begin with a review of signs and symptoms of the disorder. Table 1 depicts the sites of Paget's disease determined from an epidemiological study performed by our group that analysed questionnaire responses from over 800 pagetic subjects from throughout the USA [1]. Table 2 shows the signs and symptoms described by these patients — who were clearly a symptomatic group of individuals — both at the time of diagnosis and at the time they were studied, a mean of 13 years after diagnosis was made [1]. A consideration of the potential benefits of treatment requires an attempt to determine which symptoms are most likely to respond to treatment with an agent that decreases the abnormal bone turnover of the pagetic bone.

From Table 2, one can see that bone pain is one of the most common complaints of patients with Paget's disease, and it is a symptom that may be quite difficult to interpret. Pagetic bone pain may be a dull, non-specific ache that appears to reside in the bone itself. Sharper, more localized pain may result from microfractures in the structurally inferior bone, findings that may or may not be readily identifiable

Table 1.

Sites of Paget's disease

Site	Patients (%)
Pelvis/hip	63
Femur	41
Spine	34
Tibia	33
Skull	31
Humerus	23
Forearm	12

Table 2.

Paget's disease symptoms[a]

Symptom	Patients with symptom at diagnosis (%)	Patients with symptom since diagnosis (%) (mean = 13 years)
Bone pain with movement	53	73
Joint pain	44	65
Bone pain at rest	43	68
Heat over bone	29	42
Bowing deformity	22	35
Radicular pain	17	24
Skull enlargement	12	18
Hearing loss	9	18
Headache	9	14
Fracture through pagetic bone	7	12
Asymptomatic	32	25

[a] In 864 patients who completed a questionnaire.

on plain radiographs or even on computed tomography (CT) scans. Sometimes so-called bone pain is actually pain associated with significant osteoarthritis at joints adjacent to pagetic bone; such arthritis may be due to the presence of pagetic bone deformity in one or both parts of the joint. An example of this is the situation in which there is Paget's disease of the pelvis causing a deformity of the acetabulum; a normal femur may comprise the other component of the arthritic hip joint, with a joint deformity from the pelvis causing classic pain symptoms in the thigh or the knee. In this case the thigh pain is from a pagetic hip, not a pagetic femur. An analysis of such symptoms of pain becomes more complex in the individual who has a narrowed hip joint due to deforming Paget's disease of the femur, who has a painful thigh in association with the bowed femur, with evidence of small fissure fractures on the convex surface of the bow, and some non-pagetic degenerative disease of the lumbar spine. In this patient the thigh pain may originate in several possible places, including a non-pagetic site (i.e. radicular pain from the lumbar spine). A decision to treat such a patient with bisphosphonates must take into account the likely cause of the pain and whether treatment of the pagetic bone remodelling abnormality is likely to alleviate the symptom.

Warmth or heat in the skin overlying a site of Paget's disease, as shown in Table 2, is best appreciated in a long bone or the skull. This symptom, which may be an annoying one for many patients, appears to be a result of the increased vascularity associated with active increased pagetic bone turnover. It is readily reduced with successful treatment that reduces bone turnover.

A variety of neurological complications may occur in association with Paget's disease affecting the skull or the vertebrae. Skull involvement, particularly when there is substantial thickening of bone noted on radiographs, is frequently associated with hearing loss of a mixed conduction and sensorineural type in most cases. There is little evidence that suppression of pagetic activity with any agent can reverse this problem, but it seems possible that successful treatment of the remodelling abnormality might slow or prevent further progression. Headache, also most commonly associated with skull thickening or deformity and often described as a 'band-like' tightening or simply sharp pain, may be substantially improved if there is successful suppression of elevated bone turnover. However, it has been our experience that some pagetic headache symptoms do not respond well to bisphosphonate therapy, even when there is a dramatic lowering of very high initial levels of serum alkaline phosphatase and urinary hydroxyproline or pyridinium cross-links, because the condition had previously caused such severe deformity of the skull bones that mechanical factors were producing the pain.

A very serious, but fortunately rare, complication of skull involvement is the development of hydrocephalus due to an obstruction of cerebrospinal fluid flow as a consequence of the thickened pagetic bone. This problem, usually associated with basilar invagination that can be seen on plain radiographs, may present with one or more parts of the triad of slowly progressive dementia, ataxia and urinary incontinence. It is crucial to consider the diagnosis of hydrocephalus in patients with one or more of these symptoms, as much of the clinical problem may be reversible with prompt intervention. Use of intravenous bisphosphonate therapy (which in the

USA at this time would include either pamidronate or etidronate) in association with dexamethasone (up to 16 mg per day in divided doses) and expeditious performance of a shunt procedure by a neurosurgeon is, in our experience, a generally successful approach to management.

Pagetic vertebrae may also be the source of neurological complications, for which bisphosphonate therapy may be extremely helpful. Back pain ascribable to an area of pagetic bone often is ameliorated in response to bisphosphonate treatment in association with a decline in biochemical indices. Many investigators also relate case histories of patients with moderate to markedly elevated indices and signs of spinal cord or nerve root compression whose symptoms resolve without surgical decompression after a course of oral or intravenous bisphosphonate. Those of us who have witnessed this invariably dramatic type of response assume that a rapid suppression of bone resorption is accompanied by a shrinkage of the vascular engorgement of the bone and adjacent soft tissue. This decompression of the neural tissue (or, possibly, the elimination of a vascular steal phenomenon [2]) allows recovery of neural function.

Radiculopathy or localized back pain in the setting of increased biochemical indices frequently responds to bisphosphonate therapy with any of the currently available agents. Unfortunately, in some cases of bone enlargement and thickening causing spinal stenosis, bisphosphonate therapy may be less helpful because established mechanical factors rather than ongoing increases of bone turnover and associated hypervascularity are a cause of the symptom. Particularly when the initial increase in biochemical indices is minimal despite a large area of skeletal involvement in the spine and perhaps elsewhere, bisphosphonates may not alleviate symptoms, even while producing some decrease in the indices. None the less, an attempt to treat should be made whenever there are symptoms likely to have arisen in the setting of pagetic bone in the hope that some benefit can be achieved. Moreover, if the symptoms do not respond to medication and surgery is required, the reduction of pagetic hypervascularity after medical therapy (indicated by a reduction in indices of bone turnover) may lead to substantially less blood loss at operation.

A beneficial role for bisphosphonate therapy in the prevention of fracture of pagetic bone remains unproven. However, examples of filling in of areas of lytic predominance in association with the use of second or third generation bisphosphonates may imply that the risk of fracture through such bone is reduced. In the setting of impending fracture, careful assessment by an orthopaedic surgeon is necessary to determine if some type of internal or external fixation device is required; addition of a bisphosphonate other than etidronate (the single member of the class that is contraindicated in this setting due to the potential for a worsening of lytic alterations in structure or impairment of mineralization) may be of benefit in speeding bone healing. Finally, after a pathologic or traumatic fracture through pagetic bone, there is some controversy about the use of agents that alter bone turnover. It is not entirely clear whether addition of a non-etidronate bisphosphonate would enhance healing through suppression of abnormal remodelling or hinder resolution through a general slowing of the repair process. While many experts would add such an agent (and there is evidence anecdotally that the addition of calcitonin does not impair healing), it is our view that bisphosphonate-treated patients should be monitored closely with radiographic assessment.

III. Indications for treatment

Based upon the preceding discussion, one can consider the indications for use of bisphosphonate therapy. First, treatment is appropriate when symptoms are present that are likely to be ameliorated by the suppression of increased bone turnover. Many types of pagetic pain (i.e. from bone, from secondary arthritis, from neurologic compression, from excessive warmth) will respond to treatment. If the cause of pain is related to severe deformity — as in the case of vertebral compression, spinal stenosis from bone overgrowth, or major joint deformity and joint space obliteration — the mechanical aspects of the problem may be so great that medical therapy alone is incapable of alleviating the problem.

A second indication for treatment is the presence of active Paget's disease (i.e. associated with an increase in biochemical indices) at skeletal sites where progression over time is likely to lead to future complications. For example, asymptomatic monostotic involvement of the proximal tibia with even a mild increase above normal in the serum alkaline phosphatase is likely to progress over time, eventually producing a bowed lower leg that is shorter that the contralateral leg and is susceptible to pain, arthritic change at the ankle or knee and a risk of fracture. Thus, we would recommend treatment when there is pagetic involvement of (a) long bones, with the potential for bowing deformity; (b) the skull, with the risk of future hearing loss, cranial nerve abnormalities and rare compressive syndromes; (c) the vertebrae, with the risk of compression fractures, spinal stenosis, radiculopathy, and rare thoracic level cord compression; and (d) other skeletal sites adjacent to major joints, in an attempt to avoid the development of progressive joint deformity (although in this instance it is not clear whether suppression of activity is preventive).

Three other indications for therapy include the need for reduction of abnormal bone turnover and subsequent decrease in hypervascularity prior to elective surgery on pagetic bone (generally not etidronate if a long bone is involved), the prevention of hypercalcaemia in an immobilized patient with severe polyostotic disease and very high pagetic indices, and the presence of angina or congestive heart failure in a patient with severe Paget's disease and underlying heart disease for whom a high output state due to the Paget's disease may be contributing to the cardiac problem.

IV. Specific bisphosphonate therapy

1. General considerations

The literature is replete with numerous reports of the effects of etidronate and pamidronate in the management of Paget's disease. A smaller number of studies discuss more limited clinical experiences with clodronate, alendronate, tiludronate, risedronate, dimethyl-APD and aminohexane bisphosphonate. The primary issues involved in assessing the use of a bisphosphonate are those of efficacy and safety. Efficacy considerations include the ability of the agent to decrease symptoms, requiring placebo-controlled trials in general to establish this point, and the ability of the agent to lower the indices of increased bone turnover, providing evidence of a reduction in the ongoing bone remodelling abnormality that produces the architectural changes in bone. The duration of the period of lowered indices, the dosage of drug required to be effective (reflecting the intrinsic pharmacology of the drug, as considered elsewhere in this volume), and the extent to which indices are suppressed are all parts of the effectiveness component.

Safety considerations take into account the adverse effects that may be associated with the use of these drugs and are best evaluated when the study design is placebo-controlled. In terms of these agents the major side-effects are related to possible deleterious effects on bone mineralization as well as gastrointestinal symptoms and certain changes in laboratory tests (leucocyte counts and liver enzyme levels) without obvious clinical or physiological significance in this setting.

2. Etidronate

A number of well-controlled early studies of etidronate clearly established that this agent was effective in lowering pagetic indices (the serum alkaline phosphatase and urinary excretion of total hydroxyproline) in the majority of patients with pagetic bone [3–6]. Initially, these studies employed orally administered drug at dosages ranging from 5 to 20 mg/kg per day for 6 months. It became apparent quite quickly that although the higher dosages were associated with up to 80% suppression of the indices, new pain and histological evidence of a defect in the mineralization of newly forming bone occurred in some of these patients. It was soon determined that the optimal approach to therapy with etidronate was a 6-month course of 5 mg/kg (generally 400 mg in most patients) per day for 6 months followed by 6 months of no therapy before any re-treatment was considered [3]. This approach led to an average 50% reduction in the indices of Paget's disease in perhaps two-thirds of patients and a treatment-related relief of a variety of symptoms in a similar number. As with other bisphosphonates etidronate required administration on an empty stomach, due to the poor gastrointestinal absorption of these compounds. Although the 400 mg dose given for 6 months may cause some impairment of mineralization, this is not of clinical significance in most patients. Presumably, the defect is repaired during the off-treatment period. Moreover, a careful study of fracture rates in etidronate-treated patients has found that the use of this agent is not associated with increased fractures in patients who receive the 5 mg/kg per day dose for no more than 6 months [7].

Clinical experience indicates that a minority of patients may experience new or worsened bone pain while receiving etidronate, particularly in the setting of osteolytic predominance in a weight-bearing bone; osteolytic progression may occur in this setting. In our experience this has been most likely in patients with relatively limited extent of disease localized to a weight-bearing bone with some lytic change.

It seems likely that much of the absorbed dose may be directed to the site, perhaps increasing the amount of drug to which the bone is exposed in comparison to what might go to a single site in a patient with more extensive, polyostotic disease.

The relatively long experience with etidronate has revealed a rather benign adverse effects profile for most patients who received repeated cycles of 6 months on/6 months off for 5 to 8 years [6, 8]. It is commonly appreciated, however, that a substantial number of subjects experience decreasing efficacy (i.e. serum alkaline phosphatase levels rise and/or are no longer suppressed to the same degree with repeated courses [5]). Moreover, the most severely affected patients may have a minimal biochemical response to the preferred 5 mg/kg/day regimen. This has led to experimentation with regimens involving 20 mg/kg/day for 1 month followed by 3 months of no treatment [6], but ongoing concerns about mineralization problems despite the shorter course of the higher dose and the recent availability of newer bisphosphonates has eliminated the need for this approach, in our view. Intravenous regimens are effective short-term, but very limited data on this approach exist [9].

Other effects associated with oral etidronate use include diarrhoea, typically when higher dosages than 400 mg per day are used, and a dose-dependent rise in the serum phosphate due to an enhanced renal tubular reabsorption of phosphate [10].

3. Clodronate

Dichloromethylene bisphosphonate, or clodronate, offers several advantages over etidronate. It is a more potent inhibitor of bone resorption than etidronate and causes relatively little suppression of mineralisation of bone at dosages that are effective in suppressing pagetic activity. Effective regimens, studied and reported primarily by European investigators, indicate that oral dosing regimens of 800 to 1600 mg daily for 3 to 6 months are associated with 50–80% decreases in pagetic biochemical indices that may be maintained for many months in most and up to several years in a few cases [11–13]. Intravenous clodronate, 300 mg per day for 5 days, may also effectively suppress the indices for many months [14].

Like other potent bisphosphonates (and unlike etidronate), clodronate may cause transient hypocalcaemia due to marked reductions in bone resorption, with a delay before new bone formation is also reduced. This leads to a secondary increase in parathyroid hormone levels and has led investigators to suggest that oral calcium and vitamin D supplements be given to patients receiving this and other potent bisphosphonates during treatment. The increases in parathyroid hormone may explain in part the lack of a rise in serum phosphate with clodronate and other, newer bisphosphonates. Like etidronate, clodronate at the 1600 mg per day dose may cause diarrhoea.

4. Pamidronate

More potent than either clodronate or etidronate, APD or pamidronate has been the subject of extensive study in Paget's disease, particularly in Europe and South America [15–19]. It is possible to summarize this broad experience by noting that pamidronate is extremely effective in rapidly suppressing the increased bone turnover of the disorder. With the introduction of pamidronate, the term 'remission' of Paget's disease — meaning a period of normalization of biochemical indices — has entered the language of specialists in this field.

The most confusing aspect of the successful pamidronate story, however, has been the amazing extent of the dosing regimens, both oral and intravenous, that have been applied with this agent [20, 21]. Oral regimens ranging from 1.2 g daily for 5 days to 600 mg daily for 6 months and intravenous regimens including single 60-mg infusions or multiple single infusions of 5 to 60 mg have all been utilised. The optimal regimen is not yet defined, and it may be that dosing will need to be individualized to the patient [21a]. It would appear that the severity of the process may be a rough indicator of the total dose needed, as cases with lower elevations of indices may attain marked reductions even into the normal range with less medication.

When indices fall, bone biopsies clearly show an improvement in bone histology, strongly supporting the concept expressed earlier that this agent may not only relieve symptoms but may truly improve long-term prognosis with a reduction in at least some complications through effective suppression of abnormal bone turnover. Even when indices do not fall into the normal range (as is still the experience with most moderately active cases, given the lack of clear guidelines for treatment), a sustained reduction in the indices for a number of months is to be expected. Although the response to re-treatment has been described as no different from the initial one [22], we and others have noted less striking results with repeated intravenous courses after escape from a period of initial suppression.

Many investigators are wary of oral regimens due to the problem of upper gastrointestinal irritation, including frank oesophageal ulceration, with daily doses in the range of 600 mg. Intravenous pamidronate, like most of the later aminobisphosphonates, is associated with a low-grade fever in many patients after the first dose, as is the early treatment period with the oral formulation. Transient lymphopenia (or leukopenia) and mild hypocalcaemia and secondary hyperparathyroidism may also occur following treatment.

Although the risk of a mineralisation problem should be remote with pamidronate, there has been a report of transient and asymptomatic early mineralisation defects with cumulative dosages of 180–360 mg of pamidronate given intravenously [23].

5. Other bisphosphonates

Tiludronate and aminohexane bisphosphonate (neridronate) appear to offer results similar to those with etidronate but do not cause mineralisation problems at therapeutic dosages. Limited clinical trials with dosages of 200, 400 and 800 mg of tiludronate per day orally for 3 to 6 months resulted in a 40–60% decrease in indices [24–26a]. Intravenous (50 mg for 5 days) or oral (400 mg per day for 1 month) aminohexane bisphosphonate showed similar short-term results [20, 27]. Published studies with alendronate (aminobutane bisphosphonate), a more potent inhibitor of bone resorption, are also limited, primarily describing short-term intravenous dosing regimens [28–30] that produce rapid suppression of urinary hydroxyproline and the characteristic delayed suppression of alkaline phosphatase, both in the range of at least 50% in these early trials. Limited oral treatment studies using 20 or 40 mg daily for up to 6 months indicate suppression of indices of bone turnover by 50–70% [30a, b] and normalization of alkaline phosphatase in 62% of subjects receiving 40 mg for 6 months [30b].

Dimethyl-APD has been investigated in the Netherlands [31] over a range of oral and intravenous dosing regimens. Published results suggest that suppression of indices by 80% on average and into the normal range in a subset of patients is possible with this potent agent. Finally, among the most potent of the newer agents now in clinical trials is risedronate, another compound capable of suppressing indices by 70–80% and into the normal range in some patients after oral dosing with 20–30 mg for periods of 2 to 6 months [32].

Two other newer bisphosphonates with a potency equal to or greater than risedronate and now in the early stages of clinical testing are BM 21.0955 (ibandronate) [33] and CGP 42446 (zoledronate) [34].

V. Summary

The role of bisphosphonates in the treatment of active and symptomatic disease and in the prevention of at least some long-term complications is rapidly becoming established. The early placebo-controlled trials with etidronate demonstrated the potential for symptomatic benefit at appropriate doses. The bisphosphonates that followed etidronate largely eliminated the problem with mineralisation defects and osteomalacia through their greater potency as inhibitors of bone resorption with no significant impairment of mineralisation at clinically effective doses. Suppression of biochemical indices by up to 80% even in patients with very high initial values is being observed with several of the newer agents, and periods of maintenance of these lowered levels may last many months. We still need to learn whether these agents will continue to be effective with re-treatment. Evidence of healing of lytic disease and the alteration of bone histology toward normal suggest that healthier bone is being formed after successful treatment. Although we do not yet speak of cure, the capacity to sustain the indices in the normal range — suggesting that normal remodelling is occurring — has brought the word remission into the vocabulary of Paget's disease specialists.

Adverse effects of the newer agents, particularly some of the amino derivatives, seem limited to mild temperature elevations early in treatment, an acute-phase reaction (lymphopenia or leukopenia) that is transient, and gastrointestinal irritation with the oral compounds. Mild elevations of liver transaminases may occasionally be seen, but these are transient and not clinically significant in the great majority of cases. Hypocalcaemia is typically temporary and asymptomatic, and it can be ameliorated by use of oral calcium supplements. Rarely, iritis may occur.

During the next few years, optimal dosing regimens will need to be developed that will permit individualised treatment, hopefully to bring the indices in most patients to within the normal range for prolonged periods. While patients with established deforming bone disease may not see a dramatic benefit in many cases, there is currently great hope that early and effective treatment may prevent the severe problems that some patients with this disorder must now endure.

References

1. Siris, E., Indications for medical treatment of Paget's disease of bone. In: Singer, F.R. and Wallach, S., eds., Paget's disease of bone. Clinical assessment, present and future therapy. New York: Elsevier, 1991; 44–56.
2. Herzberg, L. and Bayliss, E., Spinal cord syndrome due to non-compressive Paget's disease of bone: a spinal artery steal phenomenon reversible with calcitonin. Lancet 1980; 2: 13–15.
3. Canfield, R.E., Rosner, W., Skinner, J. et al., Diphosphonate therapy of Paget's disease of bone. J. Clin. Endocrinol. Metab. 1977; 44: 96–106.
4. Khairi, M.R.A., Altman, R.D., DeRosa, G.P. et al., Sodium etidronate in the treatment of Paget's disease of bone. Ann. Intern. Med. 1977; 87: 656–663.
5. Altman, R.D., Long-term follow-up of therapy with intermittent etidronate disodium in Paget's disease of bone. Am. J. Med. 1985; 79: 583–590.
6. Siris, E.S., Canfield, R.E., Jacobs, T.P. et al., Clinical and biochemical effects of EHDP in Paget's disease of bone: patterns of response to initial treatment and to long-term therapy. Metab. Bone Dis. Rel. Res. 1981; 4 and 5: 301–308.
7. Johnston, C.C., Altman, R.D., Canfield, R.E. et al., Review of fracture experience during treatment of Paget's disease of bone with etidronate disodium (EHDP). Clin. Orthop. 1983; 172: 186–194.
8. Meunier, P.J. and Ravault, A., Treatment of Paget's disease with etidronate disodium. In: Singer, F.R. and Wallach, S., eds., Paget's disease of bone. Clinical assessment, present and future therapy. New York: Elsevier, 1991; 86–99.
9. Meunier, P.J., Chapuy, M.-C., Delmas, P. et al., Intravenous disodium etidronate therapy in Paget's disease of bone and hypercalcemia of malignancy. Am. J. Med. 1987; 82 (suppl 2A): 71–78.
10. Recker, R.R., Hassing, G.S., Lau, J.B. et al., The hyperphosphatemic effect of disodium ethane-1-hydroxyl-1,1-diphosphonate (EHDP); renal handling of phosphorus and the renal response to parathyroid hormone. J. Lab. Clin. Med. 1973; 81: 258–266.
11. Meunier, P.J., Chapuy, M.C., Alexandre, C. et al., Effects of disodium dichloromethylene diphosphonate on Paget's disease of bone. Lancet 1979; 2: 489–492.
12. Douglas, D.L., Duckworth, T., Kanis, J. et al., Biochemical and clinical responses to dichloromethylene diphosphonate in Paget's disease of bone. Arthritis Rheum. 1980; 23: 1185–1192.
13. Delmas, P., Chapuy, M.C., Vignon, E. et al., Long term effects of dichloromethylene diphosphonate in Paget's disease of bone. J. Clin. Endocrinol. Metab. 1982; 54: 837–844.
14. Yates, A.J.P., Percival, R.C., Gray, R.E.S. et al., Intravenous clodronate in the treatment and retreatment of Paget's disease of bone. Lancet 1985; 1: 1474–1477.
15. Frijlink, W.B., te Velde, J., Bijvoet, O.L.M. et al., Treatment of Paget's disease with 3-amino-1-hydroxypropylidene-1,1-bisphosphonate (APD). Lancet 1979; 1: 799–803.
16. Harinck, H.I.J., Bijvoet, O.L.M., Blanksma, H.J. et al., Efficacious management with aminobisphosphonate (APD) in Paget's disease of bone. Clin. Orthop. 1987; 217: 79–98.
17. Thiebaud, D., Jaeger, P., Gobelet, C. et al., A single infusion of the bisphosphonate AHPrBP (APD) as treatment of Paget's disease of bone. Am. J. Med. 1988; 85: 207–212.
18. Mautalen, C., Gonzalez, D. and Ghiringhelli, G., Efficacy of the bisphosphonate APD in the control of Paget's bone disease. Bone 1985; 6: 429–432.
19. Cantrill, J.A., Buckler, H.M. and Anderson, D.C., Low dose intravenous 3-amino-1-hydroxypropylidene-1,1-bisphosphonate (APD) for the treatment of Paget's disease of bone. Ann. Rheum. Dis. 1986; 45: 1012–1018.
20. Kanis, J.A., Pathophysiology and treatment of Paget's disease of bone. Durham: Carolina Academic Press/Martin Dunitz, 1991; 159–216.
21. Bijvoet, O.L.M., Disodium pamidronate therapy of Paget's disease. In: Singer, F.R. and Wallach, S., eds., Paget's disease of bone. Clinical assessment, present and future therapy. New York: Elsevier, 1991; 100–111.

21a. Siris, E.S., Perspectives: a practical guide to the use of pamidronate in the treatment of Paget's disease. J. Bone Miner. Res. 1994; 9: 303–304.

22. Harinck, H.I.J., Pappoulos, S.E., Blanksma, H.J. et al., Paget's disease of bone: early and late responses to three different modes of treatment with amino-hydroxypropylidene bisphosphonate (APD). Br. Med. J. 1987; 295: 1301–1305.

23. Adamson, B.B., Gallacher, S.J., Byars, J. et al., Mineralisation defects with pamidronate therapy for Paget's disease. Lancet 1993; 342: 1459–1460.

24. Reginster, J.Y., Jeugmans-Huynen, A.M., Albert, A. et al., Biological and clinical assessment of a new bisphosphonate, (chloro-4 phenyl) thiomethylene bisphosphonate, in the treatment of Paget's disease of bone. Bone 1988; 9: 349–354.

25. Audran, M., Clochon, P., Etghen, D. et al., Treatment of Paget's disease of bone with (4-chloro-phenyl) thiomethylene bisphosphonate. Clin. Rheum. 1989; 8: 71–79.

26. Reginster, J.Y., Colson, F., Morlock, G. et al., Evaluation of the safety and efficacy of oral tiludronate in Paget's disease of bone. Arthritis Rheum. 1992; 35: 967–974.

26a. Reginster, J.Y., Treves, R., Renier, J.C. et al., Efficacy and tolerability of a new formulation of oral tiludronate (tablet) in the treatment of Paget's disease of bone. J. Bone Miner. Res. 1994; 9: 615–619.

27. Atkins, R.M., Yates, A.J.P., Gray, R.E.S. et al., Aminohexane diphosphonate in the treatment of Paget's disease of bone. J. Bone Miner. Res. 1987; 2: 273–279.

28. Adami, S., Salvagno, G., Guarrera, G. et al., Treatment of Paget's disease of bone with intravenous 4-amino-1-hydroxybutylidene-1,1-bisphosphonate. Calcif. Tissue Int. 1986; 39: 226–229.

29. O'Doherty, D.P., Bickerstaff, D.R., McCloskey, E.V. et al., Treatment of Paget's disease of bone with aminohydroxybutylidene bisphosphonate. J. Bone Miner. Res. 1990; 5: 483–491.

30. O'Doherty, D.P., Gertz, B.J., Tindale, W., et al., Effects of five daily 1 h infusions of alendronate in Paget's disease of bone. J. Bone Miner. Res. 1992; 7: 81–87.

30a. Adami, S., Mian, M., Gatti, P., et al., Effects of two oral doses of alendronate in the treatment of Paget's disease of bone. Bone 1994; 15: 415–417.

30b. Tucci, J., Lyles, K., Rude, R., et al., Comparison of alendronate and etidronate in the treatment of Paget's disease. J. Bone Miner. Res. 1994; 9 (Suppl. 1): S294.

31. Pappoulos, S.E., Hoekman, K., Clemens, W.G.M. et al., Application of an in vitro model and a clinical protocol in the assessment of the potency of a new bisphosphonate. J. Bone Miner. Res. 1989; 4: 775–781.

32. Brown, J.P., Kylstra, J., Bekker, P.J. et al., Risedronate in Paget's disease: preliminary results of a multicenter study. Semin. Arthritis Rheum. 1994; 23: 272.

33. Grauer, A., Knaus, J., Seibel, M., et al., Treatment of Paget's disease of bone with the new bisphosphonate BM 21.0955 by intravenous bolus injection. J. Bone Miner. Res. 1994; 9 (Suppl. 1): S430.

34. Arden-Cordone, M., Lyles, K.W., Knieriem, A., Anti-resorptive effect of COP 42,446 in Paget's disease of bone. J. Bone Miner. Res. 1994; 9 (Suppl. 1); S295.

Bisphosphonate on bones
O. Bijvoet, H.A. Fleisch, R.E. Canfield and G. Russell (eds.)
© 1995 Elsevier Science B.V. All rights reserved.

CHAPTER 20

Mechanisms of hypercalcaemia in malignancy and its clinical evaluation

D.J. Hosking

City Hospital, Hucknall Road, Nottingham NG5 1PB, UK

I. Introduction

The management of mild-moderate hypercalcaemia (<3.0 mmol/l) can often follow an orderly sequence from diagnosis to treatment. Above this level the condition tends to be intrinsically unstable (disequilibrium hypercalcaemia) so that treatment may need to be started before diagnosis is complete [1]. Under these circumstances it is important to be able to identify, and quantitate, the mechanisms which have contributed to the development of the hypercalcaemia. Fortunately, in most cases of severe hypercalcaemia, where the need for treatment is pressing, the diagnosis can usually be established fairly rapidly by routine techniques.

II. Differential diagnosis of hypercalcaemia

1. Common causes and prevalence

The common causes of hypercalcaemia are summarized in Table 1. In both the general population and in hospital, malignancy and hyperparathyroidism account for over 90% of hypercalcaemia. In the general population, malignancy and hyperparathyroidism have a relative prevalence of about 1:2, whereas in hospital the position is reversed [2–4]. Since hypercalcaemia is often a late feature of malignancy, by which time it is usually clinically apparent, most patients referred to hospital for the diagnosis of hypercalcaemia prove to have hyperparathyroidism [3, 5]. In hospitals with a renal dialysis and transplantation service, the prevalence of hypercalcaemia among these patients may be particularly high probably due to hyperparathyroidism unmasked by the switch from aluminium-containing phosphate binders to calcium carbonate [6].

The mainstay of diagnosis is a careful history including physical examination,

Table 1.

Differential Diagnosis of Hypercalcaemia

Primary hyperparathyroidism Malignant disease	} Table 2
Sarcoidosis	Clinical features. Hepatosplenomegaly Glucocorticoid-responsive hypercalcaemia
TB Leprosy Fungal	Clinical features diagnostic
Vitamin D Vit. A Toxicity Aluminium Lithium Thiazides Milk alkali syndrome	Glucocorticoid-sensitive hypercalcaemia Hepatosplenomegaly Complicates TPN, dialysis, biliary tract disease ↑ PTH in 20% of cases Responds to rehydration, drug withdrawal Renal impairment + metabolic alkalosis
Immobilisation Paget's disease Hyper-, hypothyroidism Addison's disease VIPoma, phaeochromocytoma Chronic renal failure Post renal transplantation Diuretic phase of acute renal failure	Clinical features diagnostic
Familiar hypocalciuric Hyperparathyroidism	Onset early in childhood. Family history Stable mild hypercalcaemia ↑ PTH in 20% Urinary calcium < 5 mmmol/day Cca/Ccreat < 0.01

which will often identify many of the characteristics of the conditions listed in Table 1. This should be supplemented by standard laboratory investigations including full blood count, sedimentation rate, serum calcium, phosphate, alkaline phosphatase, liver function tests, creatinine, urea, electrolytes and myeloma screen. Thyroid function tests should probably be included since the clinical features of thyrotoxicosis may not be apparent in the elderly and may also be obscured by hypercalcaemia [7]. Additional specific investigations should be added depending on the findings from the history and physical examination.

A chest radiograph should be included in the initial evaluation, and although isotope bone scans have a high sensitivity, they have low specificity and a low yield in the absence of skeletal symptoms or biochemical markers of abnormal turnover. Skeletal radiology should be reserved for symptomatic sites or foci of abnormality detected on scintigraphy.

2. Role of PTH and PTHrP assays in diagnosis

Measurements of intact PTH, PTHrP, osteocalcin, $25OHD_3$, $1,25(OH)_2D$ and nephrogenous cyclic AMP have added greatly to the understanding of the mechanisms of hypercalcaemia, they are, however, rarely available as a routine service,

Table 2.

Distinction between Hyperparathyroidism and Malignancy

Hyperparathyroidism	Malignancy
Commonly postmenopausal women Mild hypercalcaemia Stable. Long history	Both sexes Severe hypercalcaemia Unstable. Short history
Good general health Renal stones. Peptic ulcer Hypertension	Clinical features of malignancy -breast, bronchus, head and neck urogenital tract, myeloma
Normal albumin. Hb. ESR	↓ albumin ↓ Hb ↑ ESR
Family history of hyperparathyroidism Childhood head/neck irradiation	↓ Intact PTH

and this often precludes their use in the early diagnosis and management of severe hypercalcaemia. A particular problem may be the differentiation between granulomatous disease and lymphoma. Both conditions may present with lymphadenopathy, hepatosplenomegaly, hypercalcaemia and elevated serum levels of $1,25(OH)_2D$ [8–10]. Although many of these features are glucocorticoid-responsive, clinical distinction often depends upon a tissue diagnosis.

It is in the differentiation between hyperparathyroidism and malignancy (Table 2) that the recent development of assays for PTH and PTHrP have considerable potential [11, 12]. Current assays for PTH (1–84) are reliable and show consistent suppression in the hypercalcaemia of malignancy except where there is the simultaneous occurrence of both malignancy and hyperparathyroidism [12–15]. PTHrP is present in the circulation as both N-terminal and C-terminal fragments [11]. Two site assays for PTHrP show detectable levels in 80–90% of patients with cancer and hypercalcaemia but undetectable (or occasionally very low) levels in hyperparathyroidism [11, 12]. This helps greatly in the differential diagnosis of these two conditions. These studies also show that PTHrP secretion is extremely prevalent in the hypercalcaemia of cancer and may co-exist with the presence of osteolytic metastases [11, 12, 16].

III. Pathogenesis of the hypercalcaemia of malignancy

1. Bone

The normal physiology of bone has been discussed in detail elsewhere and will not be considered further. The pathophysiology of increased bone resorption has been described earlier; what has to be considered here are the quantitative implications of this change. In malignancy the normally tightly coupled components of bone turnover are so disrupted that there is a net efflux of calcium out of bone. Moreover, this is of such a magnitude that the homeostatic defences are overwhelmed, and hypercalcaemia develops. This can best be approached by considering each of the cell systems which preserve skeletal-calcium homeostasis.

(a) Increased bone resorption

Once osteoclastic bone resorption has been completed (after about 1 month), there is a phase of reversal where the resorption cavity is invaded by mononuclear cells, probably macrophages. Their role is uncertain, but they may complete resorption by removing collagenous and non-collagenous material prior to the initiation of formation. At this moment in time there will be a focal deficit of bone (the resorption space) which will progressively diminish over the subsequent 3–4 months due to osteoblastic bone formation [17, 18]. The magnitude of the resorption space at a tissue level will depend on the activation frequency and life-span of the BMUs as well as the depth of resorption [19–21]. Since total bone turnover is made up of a number of BMUs which are temporally asynchronous, then calcium removed by resorption at one site will be utilised by formation at another so that at the tissue level, calcium balance will be in equilibrium.

However, where osteolysis is increasing rapidly, as may occur with some tumours, there will inevitably be a temporal imbalance between resorption and formation (which takes longer to adapt to changes in turnover). This will release calcium in excess of that needed for the prevailing level of bone formation so that there will be a net efflux of calcium out of bone.

(b) Decreased bone formation

The above scenario will be much worse if bone formation is unable to increase to match the change in resorption. There are a number of reasons why this adaptive response may be impaired in malignancy.

In addition to increasing bone resorption, some factors inhibit bone formation. This is best seen in multiple myeloma [22, 23] but is also seen in other tumours [24, 24]. In myeloma the resorption is mediated by osteoclast activating factors (OAFs) which include tumour necrosis factor α (cachectin) and β (lymphotoxin) and interleukins 1 and 6 [26–29]. The reduced osteoblastic activity may be related to the ability of osteoclast-activating factors to inhibit osteoblastic activity. A similar situation may arise with primary tumours which secrete PTHrP [21].

Another mechanism which may inhibit bone formation is the destruction of trabecular architecture by metastatic deposits or increased bone resorption. As the trabecular plates become destroyed or perforated, part of the surface upon which osteoblastic bone formation would occur is lost [30]. Bone formation can only occur at sites of previous resorption and only rarely occurs on otherwise quiescent surfaces [18].

Increased bone resorption per se will also have a similar effect. Under normal circumstances the average resorption depth in trabecular bone is approximately 65 μm, and since the average trabecular thickness is about 150 μm, there should be little risk of perforation [19, 20]. However, where resorption depth is increased (direct or indirect effect of malignancy) or trabeculae are thinned (age or osteoporosis), there will be an increased risk of perforation. The risk of physical disruption of bone formation is also a function of increased activation frequency, which in addition will increase the risk of perforation by increasing the chance of simultaneous resorption cavities occurring on opposing trabecular surfaces.

Finally, bone formation may also be inhibited by immobilisation. Skeletal metastases frequently lead to pathological fractures causing bone pain and immobility. Gravitational stress is an important stimulus to bone formation, and when it is removed there will be a relative excess of resorption with a consequent calcium load to be excreted [31, 32]. Since pathological fractures often occur in these patients with aggressive metastases, any inhibition of formation (which acts as a 'sump' for resorbed calcium) is particularly unfortunate.

(c) Lining cell-osteocyte function

Bone ECF (ionized calcium 0.4 mmol/l) is separated from bulk ECF (ionized calcium 1.25 mmol/l) by an intact layer of lining cells which show many characteristics of osteocytes and are in contact with osteocytes within the lacunar system of bone. Calcium diffuses down its concentration gradient into bone and is returned to the bulk ECF by a PTH- and CT-responsive transport system. The capacity of this system has been estimated to be 25–150 mmol/day, substantially greater than that due to bone turnover [18, 34, 35].

It has been suggested that this process, coupled to a similar system in the renal tubule, is primarily responsible for the maintenance of ECF calcium homeostasis [35]. If this is true, then the way is open for this system to be influenced by hormonal factors such as PTHrP and thereby contribute to the hypercalcaemia of malignancy. In this hypothesis there would be an increased efflux of calcium across the lining cells of bone into bulk ECF. Hypercalcaemia would be maintained by renal tubular reabsorption responding to the same hormonal stimulus. The hypercalcaemia would lead to increased back diffusion into bone because of the increased gradient, but an equilibrium would be established at a new (raised) set point serum calcium. The contribution that these three components make to the calcium load which must be excreted will vary between individuals: the absolute fluxes of calcium are, however, difficult to quantitate.

2. Intestine

(a) Normal physiology

Calcium is absorbed by an active transport process in the upper small intestine. This is energy-dependent and regulated by $1,25(OH)_2D$, probably at multiple sites including luminal permeability, intracellular calcium transport and active extrusion at the basolateral membrane. In the distal intestine calcium is absorbed by facilitated diffusion, which also may be carrier-mediated and $1,25(OH)_2D$-modulated, and by passive diffusion down an electrochemical gradient. The proximal mechanism is saturable, while that in the distal bowel is partly dependent on the luminal calcium concentration. Although the former segments are more active in terms of calcium transport, substantial amounts of calcium are absorbed in the distal bowel because of the slower transit time of the luminal contents. PTH has no direct effect on intestinal absorption but regulates its efficiency through the influence on the renal 1α hydroxylase, thereby linking calcium absorption to the needs of homeostasis.

(b) Calcium absorption in malignancy
   Calcium intake. Most patients have a reduced intake of calcium in the hypercalcaemic phase of malignancy, largely due to the effects of the tumour and because of nausea and vomiting.
   Vitamin D metabolism. Serum $1,25(OH)_2D$ is usually low or undetectable in hypercalcaemia complicating solid tumours but is normal in normocalcaemic malignancy [36, 37]. This is what would be expected from the homeostatic response where PTH is suppressed and, together with any hypercalcaemic renal damage, in turn leads to decreased renal 1α hydroxylase activity. However, two factors might be expected to exert a stimulatory effect, namely tumour production of PTHrP and hypophosphataemia.
   Although PTHrP stimulates the production of $1,25(OH)_2D$ in animal models [38], it does not seem to do so in human hypercalcaemia [39]. The reason for this is uncertain, but it fits into a pattern of differences between the effects of PTH and PTHrP in various cell types and test systems [40]. Hypophosphataemia is a variable occurrence in the hypercalcaemia of malignancy [39] but was a constant finding in one study where $1,25(OH)_2D$ levels were preserved in hypercalcaemic patients with renal cell carcinoma [37]. However, in general there is no correlation between the presence of hypophosphataemia and serum $1,25(OH)_2D$ concentrations.
   The other group of hypercalcaemic patients in whom $1,25(OH)_2D$ levels are preserved or elevated are those with lymphomo/leukaemia. Tumours which appear capable of producing $1,25(OH)_2D$ include T-cell lymphomas [8, 10, 37, 38], non-Hodgkin's lymphoma [8–10], and Hodgkin's disease [9, 10, 41]. This is not an invariable occurrence but is independent of PTH suppression and renal impairment and responds to treatment of the primary tumour [8, 9, 41].
   $1,25(OH)_2D$ may not be the only vitamin D sterol implicated in the hypercalcaemia of malignancy since there is an isolated report of a product resembling $1,25(OH)_2D$ being isolated from a small cell carcinoma of lung [42]. This metabolite has equal potency to $1,25(OH)_2D$ in terms of the stimulation of intestinal transport and skeletal mobilisation of calcium [43]. Dietary calcium restriction in the patient did not reduce the degree of hypercalcaemia, which was therefore assumed to be due to increased bone resorption. This may be a general phenomenon of $1,25(OH)_2D$ production in malignancy where its relevance may be much greater as a factor stimulating bone resorption rather than as a mediator of increased dietary calcium absorption.

3. Kidney

(a) Normal physiology [44–46]
   (i) Glomerular filtration. Approximately 60% of the calcium in serum is ultrafilterable, and with a glomerular filtration rate (GFR) of 100 ml/minute this results in

a filtered load of about 190 mmol/day, of which all but 6–8 mmol are reabsorbed. The filtered load of phosphate is equivalent to the product of the serum phosphate and GRF and allows for the Donnan equilibrium and the ultrafilterable (87%) phosphate concentration.

(ii) Proximal nephron. In the proximal convoluted tubule (PCT) and the medullary loop of Henle, 80% of the filtered load of calcium is reabsorbed through tight junctions. The driving force is the gradient established by active sodium and water transport. Calcium reabsorption in this part of the nephron is therefore critically dependent on ECF volume homeostasis. About 60–70% of the filtered load of phosphate is reabsorbed in the PCT linked to a specific sodium-phosphate co-transporter in the luminal membrane. The co-transporter is inhibited by PTH, increased plasma phosphate concentration and perhaps also by metabolic acidosis. In the presence of PTH the tubular concentration of phosphate stabilises at about 70% of the plasma concentration, while in the absence of PTH it falls to approximately 30%. These effects may be more prominent in deep as compared with superficial nephrons.

(iii) Distal nephron. Calcium is reabsorbed in the cortical thick ascending limb, the cortical diluting segment and the early cortical collecting tubule. It is here that PTH exerts its major homeostatic function, acting on receptors in the basolateral membrane of a relatively small number of cells in discreet cortical segments of the nephron. Calcium enters passively at the luminal membrane and is actively extruded at the basolateral membrane, probably by a Ca-ATPase pump. The permeability of the luminal membrane for calcium is increased by a PTH-mediated increase in intracellular cAMP, which acts through specific receptors at this site. It is currently uncertain whether other intracellular messengers such as phosphoinositides are also involved in this process. $1,25(OH)_2D$ may also play a role in this transport process through the induction of calcium binding protein, which may facilitate entry of calcium across the luminal membrane [47, 48]. Although the effect of PTH on the PCT is to increase the delivery of calcium and sodium to the distal nephron, there is preferential calcium reabsorption at this latter site.

In the presence of PTH there is no phosphate reabsorption between the late PCT and the early distal convoluted tubule, although in the absence of PTH there may be some reabsorption in the pars recta. There is current uncertainty as to whether, and to what extent, phosphate is reabsorbed in more distal segments. Excretion of phosphate largely seems to depend on proximal reabsorption and the consequent delivery to the distal nephron.

(b) Calcium and phosphate reabsorption in malignancy

(i) Glomerular filtration. Reduction in GFR usually follows the development of hypercalcaemia but may occur simultaneously. Once established, renal damage may take months to regress completely but usually begins once the hypercalcaemia is corrected. A number of factors which commonly operate in malignancy may singularly or collectively act to impair GFR, and these are summarized in Table 3.

Table 3.

Factors Reducing GFR in Malignancy

ECF volume contraction:	Nausea, vomiting, diarrhoea
	Nephrogenic diabetes insipidus
	Impaired sodium chloride reabsorption
Hypercalcaemia:	Vasoconstriction? direct toxicity
Drugs used in malignancy:	Cytotoxics
	Non-steroidal anti-inflammatory drugs
	Antibiotics, antiviral agents
	Bisphosphonate toxicity
Hyperuricaemia	Direct toxicity, tubular damage
	Obstruction

Hypercalcaemia has a vasoconstrictor effect on blood vessels, and this might lead to a reduction in GFR [49]. However, the specific role of hypercalcaemia may be difficult to separate from accompanying factors such as volume depletion (Table 3). For example, in steady-state primary hyperparathyroidism or familial hypocalciuric hyperparathyroidism where volume depletion is unusual, a given level of hypercalcaemia is associated with less renal impairment than the equivalent level in malignancy, sarcoidosis or vitamin D intoxication, where other factors are operative [50, 51].

(ii) Proximal nephron. Two different mechanisms act on this segment of the nephron to disturb calcium and phosphate reabsorption, namely ECF volume contraction and PTHrP production.

ECF volume contraction. Volume depletion [49, 52] due to reduced fluid intake or increased losses through vomiting and diarrhoea is counteracted by enhanced proximal tubular reabsorption of sodium. Since calcium, phosphate and sodium share a common co-transport system in this portion of the nephron [53, 55], the increased sodium reabsorption will also decrease the delivery of calcium and phosphate to more distal nephron sites.

Hypercalcaemia may also have a direct inhibitory effect on the Na^+/K^+-ATPase in the thick ascending limb of the loop of Henle, and more distal nephron segments [56, 57] which will impair sodium chloride reabsorption, contribute to ECF volume contraction and thereby further enhance proximal calcium and phosphate reabsorption.

Parathyroid Hormone related Peptide (PTHrP). PTHrP is a 141 amino acid peptide encoded on chromosome 12 in a position homologous to that of PTH on chromosome 11 [58]. There is considerable homology with PTH in that 8 of the first 13 residues at the amino-terminal are identical. Thereafter, the peptides diverge, and this provides the potential for producing effects which are distinct from those of PTH [40].

In the kidney the 1–34 amino-terminal peptide of PTH and PTHrP have similar actions in terms of the generation of cAMP, promotion of calcium reabsorption and phosphaturia, presumably due to their action through the PTH receptor. However, in contrast to primary hyperparathyroidism where there is often hyperchloraemic acidosis, in the humoral hypercalcaemia of malignancy the plasma chloride levels are often low and bicarbonate elevated [40].

PTHrP may be produced by squamous cell carcinoma of the lung, skin, head and neck, renal cortical carcinoma, some breast tumours and adult cell leukaemia/ lymphoma [59–62]. The clinical importance of PTHrP secretion in malignancy is two-fold. Firstly, by acting like PTH it can maintain the serum calcium above normal by enhanced calcium reabsorption irrespective of whether the filtered load of calcium is increased. However, where there is also increased bone destruction, the need to excrete the increased calcium load will be impaired by PTHrP-mediated tubular reabsorption.

Although exceedingly rare, there have been isolated reports of ectopic secretion of PTH by small cell lung carcinoma [64, 65] and by ovarian carcinoma [66]. This was supported by evidence of mRNA encoding of PTH in the tumour and by a precipitous fall in serum PTH when the primary tumour was removed [64, 66].

(iii) Distal nephron. The major effect of hypercalcaemia on the distal nephron is to impair the concentrating capacity of the kidney [42], and this nephrogenic diabetes insipidus contributes to the ECF volume contraction which stimulates proximal tubular calcium reabsorption. Hypercalcaemia impairs the action of ADH on the collecting duct by inhibiting the production of cAMP in response to ADH, impairing the incorporation of tubulin into cytoplasmic microtubules and by reducing the generation of ATP by glycolytic enzymes. These effects are made worse by the high urinary flow 'washing out' urea from the renal medulla which is needed to provide the gradient for distal water reabsorption [62].

IV. Clinical assessment of the hypercalcaemia of malignancy

Although an understanding of the likely pathogenetic mechanisms is helpful in predicting the components of an individual patients hypercalcaemia, it is not essential. What must be established are the separate contributions of intestine, bone and kidney.

1. Two compartment model of hypercalcaemia

In theory the intestine may contribute to the calcium load to be excreted, but in practice it rarely does so for a variety of reasons. In most solid tumours PTH secretion and $1,25(OH)_2D$ production are suppressed by the hypercalcaemia so that the driving force to active calcium absorption is lost. Even though some haematological tumours produce $1,25(OH)_2D$, this may have little consequence if dietary calcium intake is reduced. This often occurs because anorexia, nausea and vomiting are common early features of moderate-severe hypercalcaemia and in some cases may also be due to local effects of the primary tumour. Even where calcium intake is rela-

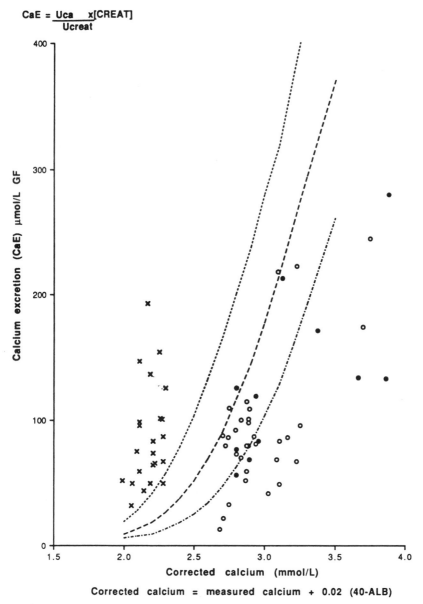

Fig. 1. Relationship between serum calcium and calcium excretion (CaE in treated hypoparathyroidism (X) and untreated primary hyperparathyroidism (○ serum creatinine <120 μmol/L, ● serum creatinine > 120μmol/L). Mean and range for normal subjects during calcium infusion shown by dotted lines.

tively preserved, the role of the intestine can be effectively eliminated by basing all measurements on fasting serum and urine samples. Thus, for practical purposes, the hypercalcaemia of cancer resolves into a two-compartment model depending on the balance between net calcium efflux from bone and elimination by the kidney. This has enormous practical advantages since these two components can be relatively easily separated using routine laboratory techniques.

2. Quantitation of the renal and skeletal components of hypercalcaemia

In the severely hypercalcaemic patient there is usually a pressing need to start treatment, and it is rarely possible to perform detailed studies of calcium homeostasis. Provided that less sophisticated tests give information about the type of treatment needed and its effectiveness, then their use can be fully justified.

When normal subjects are infused with calcium, there is a predictable relationship between the serum concentration and the urinary excretion rate (expressed in μmol/l glomerular filtrate) [67, 68]. These studies showed that for a given serum calcium level, patients with hyperparathyroidism have a relatively low calcium excretion rate compared with normal subjects, while in hyperparathyroidism there is an inappropriate hypercalciuria (Fig. 1). These changes reflect the respective excess or deficiency of PTH action on calcium resorption. As the calcium load to be excreted increases, then so does the absolute value of CaE. This relationship between serum calcium and CaE can therefore be resolved into two components. A shift in the horizontal direction reflects changes in the setting of renal tubular reabsorption: movement to the right indicates increased reabsorption, while movement to the left reflects the converse. Movement along or parallel to the mean value for normal subjects is due to changes in the calcium load per unit of renal function at a constant setting of tubular reabsorption. Although this relationship has shown considerable utility in practice, it has a number of limitations.

3. Steady states and transients

The disadvantage of data derived from acute calcium infusions is that as hypercalcaemia develops, there will be a progressive suppression of PTH secretion as well as a natriuresis. The setting of renal tubular calcium reabsorption will therefore also change but is unlikely to be detected in hourly urine collections with the same time trends that operate at the level of the parathyroid gland. That this transient state of hyperparathyroidism differs from the established condition is shown by the relative hypercalciuria of patients with hyperparathyroidism as compared with normal controls [67]. The inability of urinary measurements to accurately reflect short-term changes in parathyroid secretion may also account for the overlap between normal subjects and those with mild primary hyperparathyroidism [52], although the separation becomes better at more elevated levels of serum calcium (Fig. 1).

4. Renal impairment

The degree of renal impairment may also exert a significant influence on the ability to assess the renal components of hypercalcaemia. Serum creatinine and creatinine clearance may not always reflect the true GFR, and this problem may

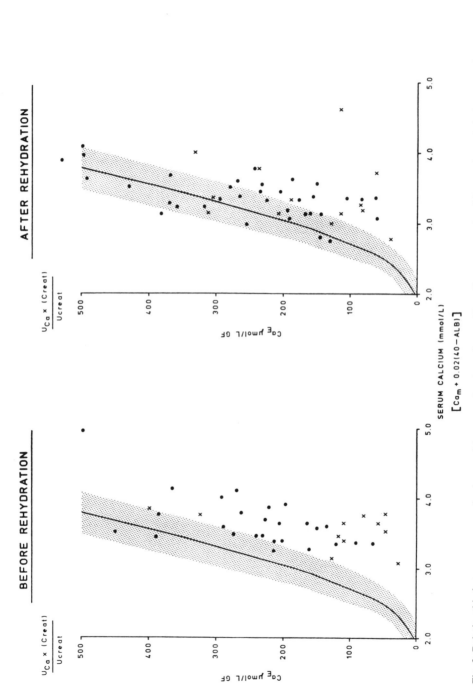

Fig. 2. Relationship between serum and urinary calcium excretion in patients with malignancy associated hypercalcaemia before and after rehydration (O bone metastases, X no bone metastases). Reproduced with permission from Hosking D.J. (71)

be made worse where there is substantial weight loss as in malignancy [69]. When calcium excretion rates are expressed per unit of glomerular filtrate (GFR being measured by [124]I-iothalamate clearance), they are raised in patients with moderate renal failure by comparison with normal subjects [70]. The use of reference ranges based on normal subjects rather than controls with renal impairment, comparable to that seen in hypercalcaemia, will tend to underestimate the renal component in malignancy-associated hypercalcaemia. Even so, separation is difficult at modest levels of hypercalcaemia but improves with increasing serum calcium. This is probably largely due to suppression of PTH in the normal controls but persistence of the effect of PTHrP or other factors in malignancy. In a practical sense this is less of a problem because it is at the higher levels of calcium that these measurements will be used. Extreme caution is needed, however, when using this method of analysis to detect small changes in calcium physiology.

5. Inter-relationship between calcium and sodium reabsorption

The ability to excrete a calcium load is strongly influenced by constraints due to the need to maintain sodium and ECF homeostasis. ECF volume depletion and the need to conserve sodium will result in an increase in the setting of renal tubular calcium reabsorption, which will be reflected by a horizontal displacement to the right in the relationship between serum calcium and CaE [71] (Fig. 2). Identical shifts are produced by PTH and PTHrP, and it may be difficult to separate these two mechanisms in clinical practice. Separation can best be achieved by careful measurements during the initial phase of treatment with saline rehydration. Reduction in the stimulus to proximal sodium and calcium reabsorption leads to a leftward shift in the relationship between serum calcium and CaE (Fig. 2) and a clearer impression of the relative contributions of bone and kidney to the hypercalcaemia. The practical use of this approach is illustrated in Fig. 3. The pretreatment position is represented by point A. Adequate rehydration restores ECF volume, improves GFR, diminishes the drive to proximal sodium (and calcium) reabsorption, and the serum calcium falls from 3.5 mmol/l to 3.0 mmol/l (point C). This can be resolved into two components: A-B (drawn parallel to the normal regression line) reflects the consequences of an improved GFR (reduction in serum creatinine from 135 μmol/l to 100 μmol/l); B-C, drawn horizontally, reflects the change in serum calcium at a constant calcium excretion rate and indicates the consequence of a sodium-mediated reduction in calcium reabsorption. The remaining hypercalcaemia is due to an increased calcium load from bone resorption, and the likely benefit from anti-resorptive therapy is indicated by the line C-D (assuming no further change in GFR or the setting of calcium reabsorption). The extent to which point C lies to the right of the normal relationship after adequate rehydration is an indication of the likely effect of tumoural factors (PTHrP) on tubular reabsorption [52, 70, 71, 73].

Unless hypercalcaemia is immediately life-threatening, there is much to be gained by separating an initial phase of rehydration from the introduction of

	Calcium (mmol/L)	Creatinine μmol/L	CaE μmol/LGF
Pretreatment	3.5	135	150
Post rehydration	3.0	100	110

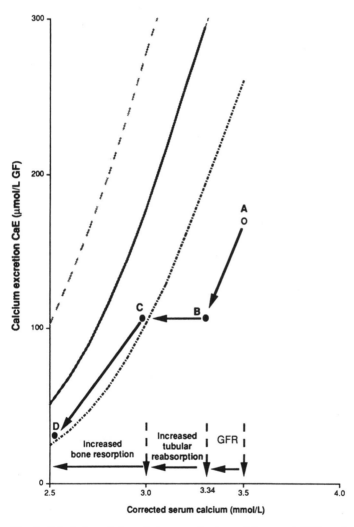

Fig. 3. Calculation of the relative contributions of improved GFR, reduced renal tubular calcium reabsorption and bone resorption to the fall in serum calcium. See text for details.

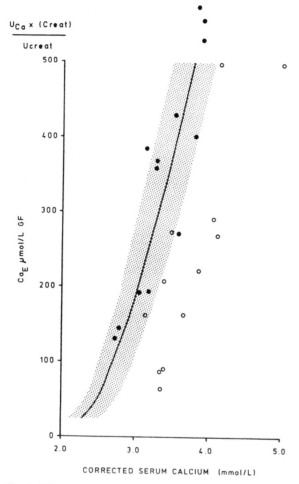

Fig. 4. Effects of sodium excretion on the relationship between serum calcium and CaE in patients with solid tumours which have metastasized to bone (● sodium excretion >3 mmol/L GF, ○ sodium excretion <1 mmol/L GF). Reproduced with permission from Hosking D.J. (71)

anti-osteolytic therapy. The clinical condition often improves, the forces leading to disequilibrium hypercalcaemia diminish, and both GFR and hypercalcaemia improve [52, 72].

The effect of sodium excretion on that of calcium is illustrated by data from patients with a variety of solid tumours which have metastasized to bone (Fig. 4). Those patients with the higher sodium excretion rates lie to the left of those who are conserving sodium because of dehydration. This has implications both for the choice of intravenous replacement therapy as well as conceptually in terms of the factors regulating calcium reabsorption.

More detailed analysis of the extent to which renal tubular reabsorption is af-

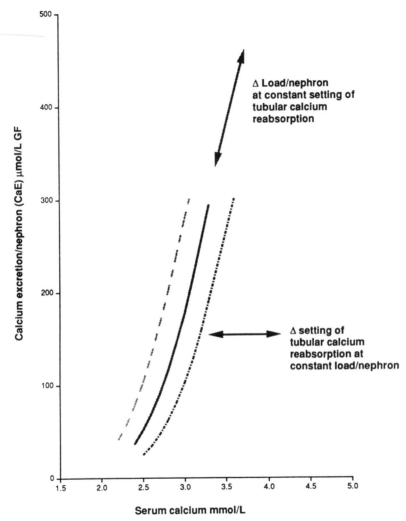

Fig. 5. Resolution of hypercalcaemia into a two compartment model

fected by sodium handling or humeral factors has been attempted but probably makes assumptions which become increasingly tenuous. Factorisation of urinary calcium excretion for that of sodium suggests that the ability of patients to excrete a calcium load depends more on the degree of hypercalcaemia than the tumour type [52]. This might operate through an increase in renal vascular tone, decreased peritubular hydrostatic pressure with enhanced fluid and electrolyte reabsorption [70]. Calculation of a calcium reabsorption index (TRCaI) and the notional setting of calcium reabsorption (TmCa/GFR) have shown variable correlations with the post rehydration sodium excretion rate [68, 74–76]. While shifts in the relationship between serum calcium and CaE due to clinically important changes in

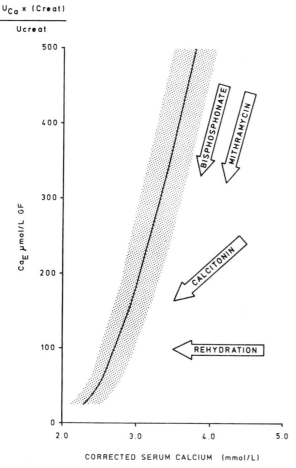

Fig. 6. Summary of therapeutic options to resolve hypercalcaemia and their influence on the relationship between serum calcium and CaE.

sodium excretion can easily be demonstrated, caution is needed when pushing the interpretation of this relationship beyond their physiological limits [52, 71].

VI. Summary

Simple biochemical measurements combined with an understanding of the likely mechanisms by which hypercalcaemia develop provides the basis for planning therapy. Separation of hypercalcaemia into its renal and skeletal components (Fig. 5) has important implications for the choice of therapy. Rehydration restores GFR by reducing the proximal tubular drive to sodium reabsorption, increasing the renal elimination of calcium. Bisphosphonates have a pure effect on bone resorption [52, 74], while calcitonin may reduce both renal and skeletal components of hypercalcaemia [77, 78] (Fig. 6). Although these measurements may be simplistic, they work well in clinical terms but may not be sufficiently robust for more detailed physiological investigations.

References

1. Parfitt, A.M., Equilibrium and disequilibrium hypercalcaemia: New light on an old concept. Metab. Bone Dis. Rel. Res. 1979; 1: 279–293.
2. Christensson, T., Hellstrom, K., Wengle, B., Alveryd, A. and Wikland, B., Prevalence of hypercalcaemia in a health screening in Stockholm. Acta. Med. Scand. 1976; 200: 131–137.
3. Fisken, R.A., Heath, D.A. and Bold, A.M., Hypercalcaemia in a hospital survey. Q. J. Med. 1980; 196: 405–418.
4. Fisken, R.A., Heath, D.A., Somers, S. and Bold, A.M., Hypercalcaemia in hospital patients. Lancet 1981; i: 202–206.
5. Heath, D.A. and Heath, E.M., Conservative management of primary hyperparathyroidism. J. Bone Min. Res. 1991; 6 (Suppl. 2): S117–S120.
6. Greaves, I., Grant, A.J., Heath, D.A., Michael, J. and Adu, D., Hypercalcaemia: changing causes over the past 10 years. Br. Med. J. 1992; 304: 1284.
7. Lafferty, F.W., Differential diagnosis of hypercalcaemia. J. Bone Min. Res. 1991; 6 (Suppl. 2): S51–S59.
8. Breslau, N.A., McGuire, J.L., Zerwekh, J.E., Frenkel, E.P. and Pak, C.Y.C., Hypercalcaemia associated with increased serum calcitriol levels in three patients with lymphoma. Ann. Intern. Med. 1984; 100: 1–6.
9. Rosenthal, N., Insogna, K.L., Godsall, J.W. et al., Elevations in circulating 1,25 dyhydroxy vitamin D in three patients with lymphoma associated hypercalcaemia. J. Clin. Endocrinol. Metab. 1985; 60: 29–33.
10. Adams, J.S., Fernandez, M., Gacad, M.A. et al., Vitamin D metabolite-mediated hypercalcaemia and hypercalciuria in patients with AIDS and non AIDS associated lymphoma. Blood 1989; 73: 235–239.
11. Burtis, W.J., Brady, T.G., Orloff, J.J. et al., Immunochemical characterisation of circulation parathyroid hormone-related protein in patients with humoral hypercalcaemia of cancer. N. Engl. J. Med. 1990; 322: 1106–1112.
12. Ratcliffe, W.A., Hutchesson, A.C.J., Bundren, N.J. and Ratcliffe, J.G., Role of assays for parathyroid-hormone related protein in investigation of hypercalcaemia. Lancet 1992; 339: 164–167.
13. Drezner, M.K. and Lebovitz, H.E., Primary hyperparathyroidism in paraneoplastic hypercalcaemia. Lancet 1978; i: 1004–1006.
14. Farr, H.W., Fahey, T.J., Nash, A.G. and Farr, C.M., Primary hyperparathyroidism and cancer. Am. J. Surg. 1973; 126: 539–543.
15. Stone, M.J., Lieberman, Z.H., Chakmakjian, Z.H. and Mathews, L., Co-existent multiple myeloma and primary hyperparathyroidism. J.A.M.A. 1982; 247: 823–824.
16. Budayr, A.A., Nissenson, R.A., Klein, R.F. et al., Increased serum levels of a parathyroid hormone-like protein in malignancy-associated hypercalcaemia. Ann. Intern. Med. 1989; 111: 807–812.
17. Parfitt, A.M., The actions of parathyroid hormone on bone; relation to bone remodeling and turnover, calcium homeostasis, and metabolic bone disease. Part III: PTH and osteoblasts, the relationship between bone turnover, and bone loss and the state of the bones in primary hyperparathyroidism. Metabolism 1976; 25: 1033–1069.
18. Parfitt, A.M., Quantum concept of bone remodeling and turnover: implications for the pathogenesis of osteoporosis. Calcif. Tissue Int. 1979; 28: 1–5.
19. Eriksen, E.F., Melsen, F. and Mosekilde, L., Reconstruction of the resorptive site in iliac and trabecular bone: A kinetic model for bone resorption in 20 normal individuals. Metab. Bone Dis. Rel. Res. 1984; 5: 35–242.
20. Eriksen, E.F., Mosekilde, L. and Melsen, F., Trabecular bone remodeling and balance in primary hyperparathyroidism. Bone 1986; 7: 213–221.
21. Mosekilde, L., Eriksen, E.F. and Charles, P., Hypercalcaemia of malignancy: pathophysiology, diagnosis and treatment. Crit. Rev. Oncol. Hematol. 1991; 11: 1–27.

22. Bataille, R., Chappard, D., Marcelli, C. et al., Abnormal bone remodeling in multiple myeloma: I. The importance of an unbalanced process in determining the severity of lytic bone disease. J. Clin. Oncol. 1989; 7: 1909–1914.

23. Bataille, R., Delmas, P.D., Chappard, D. and Sany, J., Abnormal serum bone Gla protein levels in multiple myeloma. Cancer 1990; 66: 167–172.

24. Delmas, P.D., Demiaux, B., Malaval, L. et al., Serum bone gamma carboxy glutamic acid-containing protein in primary hyperparathyroidism and in malignant hypercalcaemia. Comparison with bone histomorphometry. J. Clin. Invest. 1986; 77: 985–991.

25. Insogna, K.L. and Broadus, A.E., Hypercalcaemia of malignancy. Ann. Rev. Med. 1987; 38: 241–256.

26. Mundy, G.R., Raisz, L.G., Cooper, R.A., Schechter, G.P. and Salmon, S.E., Evidence for secretion of an osteoclast stimulating factor in myeloma. N. Engl. J. Med. 1974; 291: 1041–1046.

27. Garrett, I.R., Durie, B.G.M., Nedwin, G.E. et al., Production of the bone resorbing cytokine lymphotoxin by cultured human myeloma cells. N. Engl. J. Med. 1987; 317: 526–532.

28. Gowen, M., Wood, D.W., Ihrie, E.J., McGuire, M.B. and Russell, R.G.G., An interleukin 1-like factor stimulates bone resorption in vitro. Nature 1983; 306: 378–380.

29. Black, K., Mundy, G.R. and Garrett, I.R., Interleukin-6 causes hypercalcaemia in vivo, and enhances the bone resorbing potency of Interleukin-1 and tumour necrosis factor by two orders of magnitude in vitro. J. Bone Miner. Res. 1990; 5 (Suppl. 2): S271 (abstract 787).

30. Parfitt, A.M., Mathews, C.H.E., Villaneuva, A.R. et al., Relationships between surface, volume and thickness of iliac trabecular bone in aging and in osteoporosis. J. Clin. Invest. 1983; 72: 1396–1409.

31. Lanyon, L.E., The success and failure of the adaptive response to functional load bearing in averting bone fracture. Bone 1992; 13 (Suppl. 2): S17–21.

32. Evans, R.A., Lawrence, P.J., Thanakrishnan, G. et al., Immobilization hypercalcaemia due to low bone formation and responding to intravenous sodium sulphate. Postgrad. Med. J. 1986; 62: 395–398.

33. Parfitt, A.M., The action of parathyroid hormone on bone: relation to bone remodeling and turnover, calcium homeostasis and metabolic bone disease II PTH and bone cells: bone turnover and calcium regulation. Metabolism 1976; 25: 909–955.

34. Talmage, R.V., Cooper, C.W. and Toverud, S.U., The physiological significance of calcitonin. In: Peck, W.A. (Editor), Bone and mineral research 1. Excerpta Medica, Amsterdam, 1983; 74–143.

35. Parfitt, A.M., Plasma calcium control at quiescent bone surfaces: a new approach to the homeostatic function of bone lining cells. Bone 1989; 10: 87–88.

36. Stewart, A.F., Horst, R., Deftos, L.J. et al., Biochemical evaluation of patients with cancer-associated hypercalcaemia. N. Engl. J. Med. 1980; 303: 1377–1383.

37. Yamamoto, I., Kitamaru. N. Aoki, J. et al., Circulating 125-dihydroxy vitamin D concentrations in patients with renal cell carcinoma-associated hypercalcaemia are rarely suppressed. J. Clin. Endocrinol. Metab. 1987; 64: 175–179.

38. Fetchick, D.A., Bertolini, D.R., Sarin, D.S. et al., Production of 125-dihydroxy vitamin D3 by human T cell lymphotrophic virus-I-transformed lymphocytes. J. Clin. Invest. 1986; 78: 592–596.

39. Godsall, J.W., Burtis, W.J., Insogna, K.L., Broadus, A.E. and Stewart, A.F., Nephrogenous cyclic AMP, adenylate cyclase-stimulating activity, and the humoral hypercalcaemia of malignancy. Recent Prog. Horm. Res. 1986; 42: 705–750.

40. Martin, T.J. and Ebeling, P.R., A novel parathyroid hormone-related protein: role in pathology and physiology. Prog. Clin. Biol. Res. 1990; 332: 1–37.

41. Mercier, R.J., Thompson, J.M., Harman, G.S. and Messerschmidt, G.L., Recurrent hypercalcaemia and elevated 125-dihydroxy vitamin D levels in Hodgkins disease. Am. J. Med. 1988; 84: 165–168.

42. Shigeno, C., Yamamoto, I., Dokoh, S. et al., Identification of 125 (R)-dihydroxy vitamin D3-like boneresorbing lipid in a patient with cancer associated hypercalcaemia. J. Clin. Endocrinol. Metab. 1985; 61: 761–768.

43. Ishizuka, S., Bannai, K., Naruchi, T et al., Studies on the mechanism of action of 125-dihydroxy vitamin D3. I. Synthesis of 125 (R)- and 124 (S)- dihydroxy- (24-3H) vitamin D3 and their metabolism in the rat. J. Biochem. 1980; 88: 87–95.

44. Rose, D.B., Clinical physiology of acid-base and electrolyte disorders. McGraw-Hill, New York, 1989; 103–106, 143.

45. Habener, J.F. and Potts, J.T. Jr., Fundamental considerations in the physiology, biology and biochemistry of parathyroid hormone. In: Alvioli, L.V. and Krane, S.M. (Editors), Metabolic bone disease and clinically related disorders. W.B. Saunders, Philadelphia, 1990; 69–130.

46. Hruska, K.A. and Kurnik, B.R., Regulation of renal phosphate transport. In: Alvioli, L.V. and Krane, S.M. (Editors), Metabolic bone disease and clinically related disorders. W.B. Saunders, Philadelphia, 1990; 222–243.

47. Borke, J.L., Minami, J., Verma, A. et al., Co-localisation of erythrocyte Ca^{++}/Mg^{++}-ATPase and Vitamin D dependent 28-KDa calcium binding protein. Kidney Int. 1988; 34: 262–267.

48. Bronner, F. and Stein, W.D., CaBP facilitates intracellular diffusion for Ca pumping in distal convoluted tubules. Am. J. Physiol. 1988; 255: F558–562.

49. Benabe, J.E. and Martinez-Maldonado, M., Hypercalcaemic nephropathy. Arch. Intern. Med. 1978; 138: 777–779.

50. Lins, L.E., Renal function in hypercalcaemia. Acta. Med. Scand. 1979; 632 (Suppl.): 1–46.

51. Menko, F.H., Bijvoet, O.L.M., Fronen J.L.H.H. et al., Familial Benign hypercalcaemia study of a large family. Q. J. Med. 1983; S2 L11: 120–140.

52. Harink, H.I.J., Bijvoet, O.L.M., Plantinqh, A.S.T. et al., Role of bone and kidney in tumour-induced hypercalcaemia and its treatment with bisphosphonate and sodium chloride. Am. J. Med. 1987; 82: 1133–1142.

53. Walser, M., Calcium clearance as a function of sodium clearance in the dog. Am. J. Physiol. 1961; 200: 1099–1104.

54. Agus, S., Renal tubular transport of calcium: update. Adv. Exp. Med. Biol. 1987; 103: 37–49.

55. Suki, W.N., Calcium transport in the nephron. Am. J. Physiol. 1979; 237: F1-6.

56. Epstein, F.H. and Whittam, R., The mode of action of inhibition of calcium of cell-membrane adenosine-triphosphatase activity. Biochem. J. 1966; 99: 232–238.

57. Gutman, Y. and Katzper-Shamir, Y., The effect of urea, sodium and calcium on microsomal ATPase activity in different parts of the kidney. Biochem. Biophys. Acta 1971; 233: 133–136.

58. Mangin, M., Webb, A.C., Dreyer, B.E. et al., Identification of a cDNA encoding a parathyroid hormone-like peptide from a human tumour associated with humoral hypercalcaemia of malignancy. Proc. Natl. Acad. Sci. USA 1988; 85: 597–601.

59. Stewart, A.F., End, K.L., Burtis, W.J. et al., Frequency and partial characterization of adenylate cyclase stimulating activity and the humoral hypercalcaemia of malignancy. J. Bone Miner. Res. 1986; 1: 267–276.

60. Stewart, A.F., Wu, T., Goumas, D., Burtis, W.J., and Broadus, A.E., N-terminal amino acid sequence of two novel tumour-derived adenylate cyclase-stimulating proteins: identification of parathyroid hormone-like and parathyroid hormone-unlike domains. Biochem. Biophys. Res. Commun. 1987; 146: 672–678.

61. Strewler, G.J., Stern, P.H., Jacobs, J.W. et al., Parathyroid hormone like protein from human renal carcinoma cells. Structural and functional homology with parathyroid hormone. J. Clin. Invest. 1987; 80: 1803–1807.

62. Motokura, T., Fukumoto, S., Matsumoto, T. et al., Parathyroid hormone-relation protein in adult T cell leukaemia-lymphoma. Ann. Intern. Med. 1989; III: 484–488.

63. Stephenson, J.L., Countercurrent transport in the kidney. Ann. Rev. Biophys. Bioeng. 1978; 7: 315–339.

64. Schmelzer, H.J., Hesch, R.D. and Mayer, H., Parathyroid hormone and PTH mRNA in a human small cell lung cancer. Cancer Res. 1985; 99: 88–93.

65. Yoshimoto, K., Yamasaki, R., Sakai, H. et al., Ectopic production of parathyroid hormone by small cell lung cancer in a patient with hypercalcaemia. J. Clin. Endocrinol. Metab. 1989; 68: 976–981.

66. Nussbaum, S.R., Gaz, R.D. and Arnold, A., Hypercalcaemia and ectopic secretion of parathyroid hormone by an ovarian carcinoma with re-arrangement of the gene for parathyroid hormone. N. Engl. J. Med. 1990; 323: 324–1328.

67. Peacock, M., Robertson, W.G. and Nordin, B.E.C., Relation between serum and urinary calcium with particular reference to parathyroid activity. Lancet 1969; i: 384–386.

68. Nordin, B.E.C., Plasma calcium and magnesium homeostasis. In: Nordin, B.E.C. (Editor), Calcium, phosphate and magnesium metabolism. Churchill Livingstone, Edinburgh, 1976; 182–216.

69. Doolan, P.O., Alpen, E.L. and Thiel, G.B., A clinical appraisal of the plasma concentration and endogenous clearance of creatinine. Am. J. Med. 1962; 32: 65–79.

70. Tuttle, K.R., Kunau, R.T., Loveridge, N. and Mundy, G.R., Altered renal calcium handling in hypercalcaemia of malignancy. J. Am. Soc. Nephrol. 1991; 2: 191–199.

71. Hosking, D.J., Assessment of renal and skeletal components of hypercalcaemia. Calcif. Tissue Int. 1990; 46: S11–S19.

72. Hosking, D.J., Cowley, A.J. and Bucknall, C.A., Rehydration in the treatment of severe hypercalcaemia. Q. J. Med. 1981; 50: 473–481.

73. Bonjour, J.P. and Rizzoli, R., Pathophysiological aspects and therapeutic approaches of tumoral osteolysis and hypercalcaemia. Recent Results Cancer Res. 1989: 116: 29–39.
74. Bonjour, J.P., Philippe, J., Guelpa, G. et al., Bone and renal components in hypercalcaemia of malignancy and response to a single infusion of clodronate. Bone 1988; 9: 123–130.
75. Buchs, B., Rizzoli, R. and Bonjour, J.P., Evaluation of bone resorption and renal tubular reabsorption of calcium and phosphate in malignant and non malignant hypercalcaemia. Bone 1991; 12: 47–56.
76. Heller, S.R. and Hosking, D.J., Renal handling of calcium and sodium in metastatic and non metastatic malignancy. Br. Med. J. 1986; 292: 583–586.
77. Hosking, D.J. and Gilson, D., Comparison of the renal and skeletal action of calcitonin in the treatment of severe hypercalcaemia of malignancy. Q. J. Med. 1984; 53: 359–368.
78. Hosking, D.J., Stone M.D. and Foote, J.W., Potentiation of calcitonin by corticosteroids during treatment of the hypercalcaemia of malignancy. Eur. J. Clin. Pharmacol. 1990; 38: 37–41.

Bisphosphonate on bones
O. Bijvoet, H.A. Fleisch, R.E. Canfield and G. Russell (eds.)
© 1995 Elsevier Science B.V. All rights reserved.

CHAPTER 21

The suppression of hypercalcaemia of malignancy

D. Thiébaud and P. Burckhardt

Department of Internal Medicine, University Hospital, CHUV, CH-1011 Lausanne, Switzerland

I. Introduction

Hypercalcaemia is the cause of severe clinical symptoms, such as nausea and vomiting, dehydration, renal failure, disorientation and coma, and it can be lethal. Because of its clinical relevance, treatment is usually indicated. Its magnitude is a key consideration in determining the need for immediate and aggressive therapy. When the serum calcium concentration is greater than 3.5 mmol/l, immediate treatment is indicated, regardless of symptoms since they vary between patients for a similar degree of hypercalcaemia. This variability is due to the age of the patient, the presence of concurrent medical conditions, the duration of hypercalcaemia and the rate of increase in serum calcium concentration. When the serum calcium is only moderately elevated, the clinical manifestations rather than the calcium level should serve as a guide for therapy. The underlying condition must also be considered. When the patient has an incurable, widely disseminated cancer for which no specific therapy exists (as in the case of carcinoma of the lung where hypercalcaemia is commonly an agonal event), less aggressive or even no antihypercalcaemic treatment may be appropriate. In contrast, a substantial proportion of breast cancer or myeloma patients survive for long periods with adequate treatment [1, 2]. A recent analysis concluded that antihypercalcaemic therapy has an important palliative role, because symptoms are usually markedly improved and allow many patients to be discharged during the terminal phase of their illness [3]. Immediate effective treatment might also allow early administration of chemotherapy due to the improvement in renal function.

The treatment of hypercalcaemia would be obviously best achieved by specific treatment of the underlying disorder, but unfortunately is often not possible or there is not time enough in malignant conditions to alleviate symptoms of the disorder. Malignant hypercalcaemia is mostly due to increased bone resorption and in some tumours to a lesser degree to a PTHrP-induced increase in renal tubular reabsorption of calcium. This renal component of hypercalcaemia may be potentiated by dehydration and by a decrease in glomerular filtration rate, both consequences of hypercalcaemia itself [4, 5]. Therefore, a non-specific management of the hypercalcaemia has to be instituted to correct the dehydration and to restore the intravascular volume. The ideal treatment has to enhance the renal excretion of calcium, mostly through saline infusion promoting sodium diuresis, and to inhibit accelerated bone resorption. The reasons to restore the intravascular volume with saline administration have been extensively reviewed in the previous chapter and are the basis of the management of any hypercalcaemic condition [4]. Therefore, the present chapter focus on treatments aimed at decreasing bone resorption, such as mithramycin, calcitonin, gallium nitrate and bisphosphonates.

Although glucocorticoids have been widely used in the treatment of hypercalcaemic patients, it has become evident that they are generally ineffective in patients with carcinomas, and that their main use resides in the treatment of lymphoproliferative malignancies, particularly myeloma where they act through specific anti-tumoural effects [6]. Intravenous phosphate can rapidly lower the serum calcium concentration. However, this treatment is dangerous, because it acts through precipitation of calcium-phosphate complexes that will be deposited in blood vessels, lungs and kidneys, leading to severe organ damage [7, 8]. Oral phosphate is of limited value due to diarrhoea at the dose required to be effective to lower plasma calcium.

II. Mithramycin

Mithramycin (plicamycin), an inhibitor of RNA synthesis, is an effective treatment for hypercalcaemia by decreasing bone resorption [9]. It is given intravenously in a dose of 25 μg/kg body weight. The serum calcium concentration usually decreases 12 hours after the administration, and the maximal reduction occurs after 48–72 h [10]. Hypercalcaemia generally recurs within one week, however, and the use of repeated or multiple infusions (more than three) is limited by the risk of bone marrow, renal and hepatic toxicity, as well as immediate side-effects (mostly nausea). In a comparative randomized cross-over study, the bisphosphonate pamidronate was shown to be more effective and better tolerated than mithramycin [11]. Because of the concern over side-effects, the use of mithramycin has decreased as bisphosphonates have become available.

III. Calcitonin

Calcitonin produces a rapid inhibition of bone resorption which results in a moderate lowering of plasma calcium. In addition, it has a calciuretic effect, which potentiates the hypocalcaemic response, especially in patients with an increased tubular resorption of calcium [12]. The effect of calcitonin is only transient (24–72 h), a phenomenon also observed in vitro [13]. Its optimal use might be for severe hypercalcaemia in association with a bisphosphonate, because the latter is more potent and its effect lasts longer but starts later than calcitonin [14–15].

IV. Gallium nitrate

Gallium nitrate was shown to be effective in lowering plasma calcium when administered as a continuous intravenous infusion for 5 days. Its action is more delayed but more effective than calcitonin, or similar to etidronate in another study [16, 17]. It has not been compared to more potent bisphosphonates (clodronate or pamidronate). It is associated with nephrotoxicity. As the clinical experience with gallium nitrate is still limited and restricted mostly to one centre, it seems preferable to recommend the bisphosphonates which enjoy more than 10 years' clinical experience.

V. Bisphosphonates

Since the introduction of the use of bisphosphonates in the treatment of hyper-calcaemia in the late 1970s [18, 19], it became evident that these new compounds were extremely effective and well tolerated. Bisphosphonates have no direct effect on the renal handling of calcium; they act on hypercalcaemia exclusively by inhibit-ing bone resorption. Thus, they are especially effective in tumours in which the increase in blood calcium is due principally to bone destruction, such as myeloma, and their effect is less pronounced in tumours with an additional increase in tubu-lar reabsorption of calcium, such as seen in most squamous cell carcinomas, and due to the action of the paraneoplastic hormone PTHrP producing the humoral hypercalcaemia of malignancy [2, 20].

Most studies have been performed with etidronate, clodronate and pamidronate, and one or more of these three are now registered for therapeutic use in many countries. The present review focusses on the treatment of malignant hypercal-caemia. For more details on bisphosphonates in general, the reader is referred to other chapters, or recent reviews [21–23].

Etidronate decreased calcaemia in patients both with metastatic bone disease and with haematological malignancies such as myeloma [21]. Daily intravenous doses of 7.5 mg/kg for 3 days led to normalisation of calcaemia in 24% of patients [24], longer treatments being effective in more patients [25]. The effect on calcaemia and other biochemical parameters started after 48 hours, reaching a maximal effect after a week [24–26]. Etidronate was less effective than clodronate or pamidronate, a total dose of approximately 1500 mg (7.5 mg/kg for 3 days) being somewhat less active than 600 mg clodronate and much less active than 30 mg pamidronate [27]. The effect disappeared within days of discontinuation of the drug. Two studies have shown that the effect can be maintained in certain patients if the intravenous course is followed by oral treatment of 20 mg/kg/day [28, 29].

Etidronate is well tolerated, the side-effects being limited to some nausea and vomiting, mostly after oral administration. Patients may experience a metallic taste sensation [24, 29]. From what is known of the experience with etidronate in Paget's disease, with the dose required for treatment of hypercalcaemia, an inhibition of normal mineralisation will occur [22]. This could represent a problem if the compound is given for long periods. A rapid intravenous injection has led to renal failure, probably because of the formation of a solid phase of bisphosphonate in the bloodstream. Therefore, early bisphosphonates have to be administered in an infusion over a period of at least a few hours [21, 22].

Clodronate has been used since the late 1970s and was shown to be effective in the treatment of tumour-induced hypercalcaemia [19, 30]. When administered daily intravenously, its effect on calcaemia started after 2 days, normocalcaemia being usually obtained after 5 days [2, 22, 26, 31–35]. Hypocalcaemia occurred in some rare cases, but was usually asymptomatic. The treatment of patients with hypercalcaemia was most effective when 300 mg clodronate were given daily for about 5 days. It has been reported that the effect of a single intravenous infusion of 300 to 600 mg was almost similar to that of 3600 mg given over 12 days [31], and that 1 infusion of 500 mg was as active as multiple infusions of 500 mg [2]. One study showed that it is the total dose which is relevant, 1 infusion of 1500 mg being as efficient as 5 infusions of 300 mg, lower amounts being less effective [22]. As a compromise, one might use 300 mg/day for 2 to 3 days, or 600 mg for 1 day. An effect can also obtained by administering clodronate orally at a dose of generally 3200 mg/day until the calcaemia normalises [4, 19, 34, 35].

The effect usually lasted for the duration of the treatment, and relapses occurred a few days after stopping treatment. It is not known whether an increase in the total administered dose prolongs the effect. Therefore, the most practical procedure is to monitor the calcaemia and resume treatment when the blood calcium level increases again. Alternatively, an infusion of 300 mg may be administered weekly [31]. Another possibility is to give clodronate orally (1600–3200 mg/day) as maintenance therapy. However, this treatment is not effective in all patients, even when the dose is increased to 6400 mg/daily [31, 33, 35].

Clodronate is usually well tolerated. Some nausea and diarrhoea which can occur with oral therapy can be avoided by dividing the doses. Transient proteinuria has been observed in some cases [22, 27]. However, patients with impaired renal function showed no evidence of further deterioration of renal function [2].

Pamidronate (APD) is the most extensively tested compound in clinical trials among the bisphosphonates and is very effective to correct malignant hypercalcaemia (for extensive review, see [23]). The effect of pamidronate started after 24 hours, and normalisation of calcaemia occurred in the majority of patients on the third to fourth day [1, 4, 36–44]. The percentage of patients in whom calcaemia will normalise is difficult to assess, but appears to be close to 100% if a high enough dose is administered. Hypocalcaemia can develop [36, 42, 43] and is usually asymptomatic with rare exceptions [45].

Most studies have been performed using intravenous infusions. Initially between 15 to 30 mg were infused daily until calcaemia was normalised or reached a nadir [1, 2, 37, 38]. Later, it appeared that there is little difference in efficacy (as assessed by biochemical indices) between single dose (30 to 90 mg) and multiple doses (15 to 30 mg/day for $\leq$ 9 days) of intravenous pamidronate [39, 40, 41, 46, 47], and 1-day infusions became the treatment of choice.

Using a single intravenous pamidronate infusion, it was suggested that the reduction in serum calcium levels was unrelated to the pamidronate dose over ranges of 30 to 60 mg [46]. But this contrasted with the apparent dose-related effect of intravenous pamidronate 30 to 90 mg on the decrease in serum calcium levels, the incidence and duration of normocalcaemia and the frequency of hypercalcaemia relapse [43, 48]. Therefore, the optimal dose is still a matter of debate. There was a difference in the delay before relapse between 30 mg and 90 mg [43]. It has therefore been suggested that the dose should be adapted to the initial hypercalcaemia. A dose of 30 mg is proposed for an initial calcaemia below 3 mmol/l, 45 mg for 3–3.5 mmol/l, 60 mg for 3.5–4.0 mmol/l and 90 mg for a calcaemia above 4 mmol/l [43]. This controversy about the dose-response effect might be explained by the selection of patients in different studies: the demonstration of a dose dependency depends on the severity of malignant bone diseases and the respective role of the renal versus tumoral osteolysis components inducing hypercalcaemia. In a patient with a moderate hypercalcaemia (below 3.5 mmol/l) with an increased tubular reabsorption of calcium, the bone component is relatively minor, and varying the dose of pamidronate from 30 to 90 mg will not change the overall response in plasma calcium, because the 30 mg dose is sufficient. In contrast, a patient with severe hypercalcaemia with a normal tubular reabsorption of calcium might require at least 60 mg or more total dose to reach and maintain normocalcaemia. Increasing the dose to a total of 120 to 180 mg might be necessary to control hypercalcaemia in rare patients [49].

In the small number of patients in whom the duration of pamidronate-induced normocalcaemia could be assessed in the absence of concomitant anticancer therapy, hypercalcaemia recurred 1 to 10 (median 2 to 3) weeks after initiation of single [20, 41, 43, 46, 47] or multiple doses [1]. Therefore, the time after which patients relapse varies greatly and appears to depend both upon the severity of the disease and the dose of pamidronate given [43]. It is usual to administer one infusion of pamidronate, usually between 45 mg and 60 mg, and then to monitor calcaemia. A new infusion with a slight increase in the dose [20, 40] can be given if normocalcaemia is not attained or when calcium rises again.

Pamidronate is given by infusion, the rate usually not exceeding 7.5 to 15 mg/h, although recent data have shown that a single infusion of 60 mg over 1 hour is safe and had a similar biodisposability as that of a 24-h infusion [50].

Although it has been known for a long time that pamidronate is also active when given orally [18, 36], intravenous application has been preferred by most investigators, mostly because of gastrointestinal disturbances after oral administration and the urgency of the indication in malignant hypercalcaemia. A regimen of multiple infusions of pamidronate 30 mg/day for 6 days was of comparable efficacy to a multiple oral dose regimen of 1200 mg/day for 6 days, with normocalcaemia being achieved within 6 to 9 days in 100% of patients [51], which would indicate an absorption of 1–3%.

In the treatment of hypercalcaemia the side-effects of pamidronate are rare and of limited importance. Pamidronate induces an elevation of temperature and haematological changes (slight decrease in lymphocytes counts) during the first 24 to 48 hours in about 20–30% of patients [1, 4, 36, 42, 43]. These changes are transient and do not recur with a new treatment. Otherwise, parenteral administration is well tolerated if the drug is diluted to avoid phlebitis. Oral administration is often accompanied by gastrointestinal disturbances, such as nausea, vomiting and abdominal pain, especially at doses higher than 300 mg/day [36, 51]. The antihypercalcaemic response to bisphosphonates has been reported to be effective in all primary tumour types (lung, breast, head and neck, lymphoma, genitourinary, unknown). However, hypercalcaemia relapsed more frequently in cases of squamous cell cancer (a tumour typically associated with enhanced renal reabsorption of calcium) than in breast cancer [20, 47]. More recently, the concentration of parathyroid hormone-related protein (PTHrP) was shown to predict the response of humoral malignant hypercalcaemia to pamidronate [52]. Hence, as a determinant of renal calcium handling, for instance through PTHrP, the tumour type appears to influence the responsiveness. On the other hand, haematological malignancies, particularly myeloma with conserved renal function, seem to respond more rapidly to pamidronate than solid tumours [20, 47].

When other biochemical parameters than plasma calcium were measured, an early dramatic drop in urinary calcium was reported after all bisphosphonates. The effect on urinary hydroxyproline was less pronounced than on calcaemia and calciuria, probably due to production from soft-tissue metastases [1, 22, 36, 41, 43]. Plasma phosphate, as well as tubular reabsorption of phosphate assessed by the maximum reabsorption per unit of glomerular filtration rate (TmP/GFR), usually decreased transiently [39, 43]. This is probably the consequence of the observed increase in previously suppressed PTH [37, 39, 53] or a decrease of release of phosphate from the skeleton. Finally, renal function improved in most patients, probably secondary to the reduction of plasma calcium [4, 37, 39, 43].

VI. Comparative studies in the treatment of hypercalcaemia of malignancy

The therapeutic efficacy of pamidronate has been compared with that of plicamycine, prednisolone+calcitonin, and the bisphosphonates clodronate and etidronate in short-term studies [11, 27, 54, 55]. A single intravenous infusion of pamidronate (30 mg) was more effective in controlling hypercalcaemia of malignancy than a single infusion of clodronate (600 mg) or 3 consecutive daily intravenous infusions of etidronate (7.5 mg/kg/day) [17]. Pamidronate displayed a slightly more rapid onset of antihypercalcaemic action (day 1 vs day 2), a significantly greater reduction in serum calcium levels by day 6, and a more prolonged normocalcaemic remission. Consequently, normocalcaemia was achieved in a higher proportion of patients (88%) than with clodronate (38%) or etidronate (31%) within 6 days. In a recent study, a single intravenous infusion of pamidronate

60 mg was significantly superior to 3 consecutive daily infusions of etidronate 7.5 mg/kg/day with respect to the reduction in serum calcium levels, and the incidence and duration of normocalcaemia [55]. A similar advantage was recently shown in a comparison between pamidronate and clodronate given as a single dose [56].

In comparison with plicamycin (25 μk/kg as a single or repeated intravenous infusions) and with the combination of prednisolone (40 mg/day orally for 9 days) plus calcitonin (1200 U/day subcutaneously for 9 days), pamidronate exhibited a significantly more pronounced reduction in serum calcium levels after 6 to 9 days [54]. The effective and sustained control of hypercalcaemia obtained with pamidronate contrasted with the partial response to prednisolone+calcitonin and the transient response to plicamycine (indicated by a ca. 50% relapse rate by day 9). In another recent study involving 48 patents, a 24-h intravenous infusion of pamidronate 60 mg was more effective than a 30-minute infusion of plicamycine 20 μg/kg in restoring normocalcaemia and maintaining it for a longer period [11]. Moreover, the incidence of side-effects was lower in the pamidronate group.

The synergistic early antihypercalcaemic action of pamidronate and calcitonin has been confirmed in a comparative study involving matched groups of patients with hypercalcaemia of malignancy: combined therapy with a single intravenous infusion of pamidronate 45 to 60 mg and calcitonin suppositories (900 U/day for 3 days) resulted in a more rapid reduction in serum calcium levels and earlier achievement of normocalcaemia (day 3 vs day 6) than pamidronate monotherapy [15].

VII. Conclusion

Restoration of normocalcaemia is clinically relevant since it is associated with a general improvement in symptoms attributable to hypercalcaemia [5, 36, 39, 43, 44]. This comprises a marked improvement in polyuria/polydipsia, a variable improvement in neurological symptoms and gastrointestinal symptoms of nausea, vomiting, anorexia and constipation. This clinical benefit is less evident when serum calcium is lowered but not normalized [5]. Sustained normalisation of calcium can be achieved without side-effects with intravenous bisphosphonates. Therefore, bisphosphonates, especially of the new generation, are in many ways ideal antihypercalcaemic agents. They are effective in virtually all patients with increased bone resorption. Although it is difficult to draw clear conclusions about which bisphosphonates to use in which patient, and the optimal dose to administer, clodronate and pamidronate seems superior to etidronate [55], and new bisphosphonates with higher potency are undergoing clinical investigation (alendronate [57, 58] and ibandronate [59, 60]). The treatment can be given as a single dose over a few hours (and probably even shorter with new more potent bisphosphonates) and therefore may as well be given to outpatients if the hypercalcaemia is moderate and does not require intravenous rehydration. New bisphosphonates appear superior to plicamycine or gallium nitrate because they cause a more marked and prolonged decrease in calcaemia and have fewer side-effects. They have an excellent safety profile and appear to be the agents of choice for initial and long-term management of cancer-related hypercalcaemia.

References

1. Coleman, K.E. and Rubens, R.D., 3(amino-1,1-hydroxypropylidene) bisphosphonate (APD) for hypercalcaemia of breast cancer. Br. J. Cancer 1987; 56: 465–469.
2. Paterson, A.D., Kanis, J.A., Cameron, E.C., Douglas, D.L., Beard, D.L. et al., The use of dichloromethylene diphosphonate for the management of hypercalcaemia in multiple myeloma. Br. J. Haematol. 1983; 54: 121–132.
3. Ralston, S.H., Gallacher, S.J., Patel, U., Campbell, J. and Boyle, I.T., Cancer-associated hypercalcaemia: morbidity and mortality. Ann. Intern Med. 1990; 112: 499–504.
4. Harinck, H.I.J., Bijvoet, O.L.M., Plantingh, A.S.T., Body, J.J., Elte, J.W.F. et al., Role of bone and kidney in tumour-induced hypercalcaemia and its treatment with bisphosphonate and sodium chloride. Am. J. Med. 1987; 82: 1133–1142.
5. Bonjour, J.P., Philippe, J., Guelpa, G., Bisetti, A., Rizzoli, R. et al., Bone and renal components in hypercalcaemia of malignancy and responses to a single infusion of clodronate. Bone 1988; 9: 123–130.
6. Mundy, G.R., Wilkinson, R. and Heath, D.A., Comparative study of available medical therapy for hypercalcaemia of malignancy. Am. J. Med. 1983; 74: 421–432.
7. Breuer, R.I. and LeBauer, J., Caution in the use of phosphates in the treatment of severe hypercalcaemia. J. Clin. Endocrinol. 1967; 27: 695–698.
8. Shackney, S. and Hasson, J., Precipitous fall in serum calcium, hypotension, and acute renal failure after intravenous phosphate therapy for hypercalcaemia. Ann. Intern Med. 1967; 66: 906–916.
9. Minkin, C., Inhibition of parathyroid hormone-stimulated bone resorption in vitro by the antibiotic mithramycin. Calcif. Tissue Res. 1973; 13: 249–257.
10. Perlia, C.P., Gubish, N.J. and Walter, J., Mithramycin treatment of hypercalcaemia. Cancer 1970; 25: 389–394.
11. Thürlimann, B., Waldburger, R., Senn, H.J. and Thiébaud, D., Mithramycine and APD in symptomatic tumour related hypercalcaemia. A prospective randomised cross-over trial. Ann. Oncol. 1992; 3: 619–623.
12. Hosking, D.J. and Gilson, D., Comparison of the renal and skeletal actions of calcitonin in the treatment of severe hypercalcaemia of malignancy. Q. J. Med. 1984; 111: 359–368.
13. Wener, J.A., Gorton, S.J. and Raisz, L.G., Escape from inhibition of resorption in culture of fetal bone treated with calcitonin and parathyroid hormone. Endocrinology 1972; 90: 752–759.
14. Ralston, S.H., Alzaid, A.A., Gardner, M.D. and Boyle, I.T., Treatment of cancer associated hypercalcaemia with combined aminohydroxypropylidene diphosphonate and calcitonin. Br. Med. J. 1986; 292: 1549–1550.
15. Thiébaud, D., Jacquet, A.F. and Burckhardt, P., Fast and effective treatment of malignant hypercalcaemia. Arch. Intern Med. 1990; 150: 2125–2128.
16. Warrell, R.P. Jr., Israel, R., Gaynor, J.J. and Bockman, R.S., Gallium nitrate for acute treatment of cancer-related hypercalcaemia. J. Clin. Oncol. 1991; 9: 1467–1475.
17. Warrell, R.P. Jr., Murphy, W.K., Schulman, P., O'Dwyer, P.J. and Heller, G., A randomized double-blind study of gallium nitrate compared with etidronate for acute control of cancer-related hypercalcemia. J. Clin. Oncol. 1991; 9: 1467–1475.
18. Van Breukelen, F.J.M., Bijvoet, O.L.M. and Van Oosterom, A.T., Inhibition of osteolytic bone lesions by (3-amino-1-hydroxypropylidene)-1,1-bisphosphonate (APD). Lancet 1979; 1: 803–805.
19. Chapuy, M.C., Meunier, P.J., Alexandre, C.M. and Vignon, E.P., Effects of disodium dichloromethylene diphosphonate on hypercalcaemia produced by bone metastases. J. Clin. Invest. 1980; 65: 1243–1247.
20. Thiébaud, D., Jaeger, P. and Burckhard, P., Response to retreatment of malignant hypercalcaemia with the bisphosphonate AHPrBP (APD): respective role of kidney and bone. J. Bone Miner. Res. 1990; 5: 221–226.
21. Fleisch, H., Bisphosphonates. Pharmacology and use in the treatment of tumour-induced hypercalcaemic and metastatic bone disease. Drugs 1991; 42: 919–944.
22. Kanis, J.A. and McCloskey, E.V., The use of clodronate in disorders of calcium and skeletal metabolism. In: Kanis, J.A. (Editor), Calcium metabolism. Krager A.G., Basel, 1990; pp. 89–136
23. Fitton, A. and McTavish, D., Pamidronate: a review of its pharmacological properties and therapeutic efficacy in resorptive bone disease. Drugs 1991; 41: 289–318.
24. Singer, F.R., Ritch, P.S., Lad, T.E., Ringenberg, Q.S., Schiller, J.H. et al., Treatment of hypercalcaemia of malignancy with intravenous etidronate. Arch. Intern Med. 1991; 151: 471–476.

25. Ryzen, E., Martodam, R.R., Troxell, M., Benson, A., Paterson, A. et al., Intravenous etidronate in the management of malignant hypercalcaemia. Arch. Intern Med. 1985; 145: 449–452.
26. Jung, A., Comparison of two parenteral diphosphonates in hypercalcaemia of malignancy. Am. J. Med. 1982; 72: 221–226.
27. Ralston, S.H., Gallacher, S.J., Patel, U., Dryburgh, F.J., Fraser, W.D. et al., Comparison of three intravenous bisphosphonates in cancer-associated hypercalcaemia. Lancet 1989; 2: 1180–1182.
28. Schiller, J.H., Rasmussen, P., Benson, A.B., Witte, R.S., Bockman, R.S. et al., Maintenance etidronate in the prevention of malignancy-associated hypercalcaemia. Arch. Intern Med. 1987; 147: 963–966.
29. Ringenerg, Q.S. and Ritch, P.S., Efficacy of oral administration of etidronate disodium in maintaining normal serum calcium levels in previously hypercalcaemic cancer patients. Clin. Therapeut. 1987; 9: 318–325.
30. Jacobs, T.P., Siris, E.S., Bilezikian, J.P., Baquiran, D.C., Shane, E. et al., Hypercalcaemia of malignancy: treatment with intravenous dichloromethylene diphosphonate. Ann. Intern Med. 1981; 94: 312–316.
31. Adami, S., Bolzicco, G.P., Rizzo, A., Salvagno, G., Bertoldo, F. et al., The use of dichloromethylene bisphosphonate and aminobutane bisphosphonate in hypercalcaemia of malignancy. Bone Miner. 1978; 2: 395–404.
32. Percival, R.C., Paterson, A.D., Yates, A.J.P., Beard, D.J., Douglas, D.L. et al., Treatment of malignant hypercalcaemia with clodronate. Br. J. Cancer 1985; 51: 665–669.
33. Scharla, S.H., Minne, H.W., Sattar, P., Mende, U., Blind, E. et al., Therapie der Tumorhypercalciämie mit Clodronat. Dtsch. Med. Wochenschr. 1987; 112: 1121–1125.
34. Siris, E.S., Sherman, W.H., Baquiran, D.C., Schlatterer, J.P., Osserman, E.F. et al., Effects of dichloromethylene diphosphonate on skeletal mobilization of calcium in multiple myeloma. N. Engl. J. Med. 1980; 302: 310–315.
35. Rastad, J., Benson, L., Johannson, H., Knuutila, M., Pettersson, B. et al., Clodronate treatment in patients with malignancy-associated hypercalcaemia. Acta Med. Scand. 1987; 221: 489–494.
36. Van Breukelen, F.J.M., Bijvoet, O.L.M., Frijlink, W.B., Sleeboom, H.P., Mulder, H. et al., Efficacy of amino-hydroxypropylidene bisphosphonate in hypercalcaemia: observations on regulation of serum calcium. Calcif. Tissue Int. 1982; 34: 321–327.
37. Sleeboom, H.P., Bijvoet, O.L.M., Van Oosterom, A.T., Gleed, J.H. and O'Riordan, J.L.H., Comparison of intravenous (3-amino-1-hydroxypropylidene)-1,1-bisphosphonate and volume repletion in tumour-induced hypercalcaemia. Lancet 1983; 239–243.
38. Portmann, L., Häfliger, J.M., Bill, G. and Burckhardt, P., Un traitement simple de l'hypercalcémie tumorale: l'amino-hydroxypropylidène bisphosphate (APD) i.v. Schweiz. Med. Wochenschr. 1983; 113: 1960–1963.
39. Thiébaud, D., Jaeger, P., Jacquet, A.F. and Burckhard, P., A single-day treatment of tumour-induced hypercalcaemia by intravenous amino-hydroxypropylidene bisphosphonate. J. Bone Miner. Res. 1986; 1: 555–562.
40. Yates, A.J.P., Murray, R.M.L., Jerums, G.L. and Martin, T.J., A comparison of single and multiple intravenous infusions of 3-amino-1-hydroxypropylidene)-1,1-bisphosphonate (APD) in the treatment of hypercalcaemia of malignancy. Aust. NZ. J. Med. 1987; 17: 386–391.
41. Body, J.J., Magritte, A., Seraj, F., Sculier, J.P. and Borkowski, A., Aminohydroxypropylidene bisphosphonate (APD) treatment for tumour-associated hypercalcaemia: a randomized comparison between a 3-day treatment and single 24-hour infusions. J. Bone Miner. Res. 1989; 4: 923–928.
42. Body, J.J., Pot, M., Borkowski, A., Scoulier, J.P. and Klastersky, J., Dose/response study of amino-hydroxypropylidene bisphosphonate in tumour-associated hypercalcaemia. Am. J. Med. 1987; 82: 957–963.
43. Thiébaud, D., Jaeger, P., Jaquet, A.F. and Burckhardt, P., Dose-response in the treatment of hypercalcaemia of malignancy by a single infusion of the bisphosphonate AHPrBP. J. Clin. Oncol. 1988; 762–768.qtavol. no.?
44. Sawyer, N., Newstead, C., Drummond, A. and Cunningham, J., Fast (4-h) or slow (24-h) infusions of pamidronate disodium (aminohydroxypropylidene diphosphonate) (APD) as single shot treatment of hypercalcaemia. Bone Miner. 1990; 9: 122–128.
45. Jodrell, D.I., Iveson, T.J. and Smith, I.E., Symptomatic hypocalcaemia after treatment with high-dose aminohydroxypropylidene diphosphonate. Lancet 1987; 4: 622.
46. Davis, J.R.E. and Heath, D.A., Comparison of different dose regimes of aminohydroxypropylidene-1,1-bisphosphonate (APD) in hypercalcaemia of malignancy. Br. J. Clin. Pharmacol. 1989; 28: 269–274.

47. Morton, A.R., Cantrill, J.A., Craig, A.E., Howell, A., Davies, M. et al., Single-dose versus daily intravenous aminohydroxypropylidene bisphosphonate (APD) for the hypercalcaemia of malignancy. Br. Med. J. 1988; 296: 811–814.
48. Nussbaum, S.R., Younger, J., Gagel, R.F., Zubler, M.A., Chapman, R. and Malette, L.E., Single-dose intravenous therapy of hypercalcaemia of malignancy with pamidronate (APD). Comparison of 30-, 60-, and 90-mg dosages. Am. J. Med. 1993; 95: 297–304.
49. Pecherstorfer, M. and Thiébaud, D., Treatment of resistant tumour-induced hypercalcaemia with escalating doses of pamidronate (APD). Ann. Oncol. 1992; 3: 661–663.
50. Leyvraz, S., Hess, U., Flesch, G., Bauer, J., Hauffe, S., Ford, J.M. and Burckhardt, P., Pharmacokinetics of pamidronate in patients with bone metastases. J. Natl. Cancer Inst. 1992; 84: 788–792.
51. Thiébaud, D., Portmann, L., Jaeger, P.H, Jaquet, A.F. and Burckhardt, P., Oral versus intravenous AHPrBP (APD) in the treatment of hypercalcaemia of malignancy. Bone 1986; 7: 247–253.
52. Gurney, H., Grill, V. and Martin, T.J., Parathyroid hormone-related protein and response to pamidronate in tumour-induced hypercalcaemia. Lancet 1993; 341: 1611–1613.
53. Fraser, W.D., Fraser, C., Logue, Gallacher, S.J. et al., Direct and indirect assessment of the parathyroid hormone response to pamidronate therapy in Paget's disease of bone and hypercalcaemia of malignancy. Bone Miner. 1991; 12: 113–121.
54. Ralston, S.H., Gardner, M.D., Dryburgh, F.J., Jenkins, A.S., Cowan, R.A. et al., Comparison of aminohydroxypropylidene diphosphonate, mithramycin and corticosteroid/calcitonin in treatment of cancer-associated hypercalcaemia. Lancet 1985; 2: 907–910.
55. Gucalp, R., Ritch, P., Wiernik, P.H., Ravi Sarma, P., Keller, A. et al., Comparative study of pamidronate disodium and etidronate disodium in the treatment of cancer-related hypercalcaemia. J. Clin. Oncol. 1992; 10: 134–142.
56. Purohit, O.P., Anthony, C., Owen, J. and Coleman, R., A randomised double-blind comparison of single infusions of pamidronate or clodronate for hypercalcaemia of malignancy. Bone Miner. 1994; 25 (Suppl. 1): S81.
57. Bickerstaff, D.R., O'Doherty, D.P., McCloskey, E.V. et al., Effects of amino-butylidene diphosphonate in hypercalcaemia due to malignancy. Bone 1991; 12: 17–20.
58. Nussbaum S.R., Warrell, R.P., Rude, R., Stewart, A.F., Sacco, J.F., et al., Dose-response study of alendronate sodium for the treatment of cancer-associated hypercalcemia. J. Clin. Oncol. 1993; 11: 1618–1623.
59. Wurster, C., Schöter, K.H., Thiébaud, D., Scharla, S.H. et al., Methylpentylaminopropylidenebisphosphonate (BM 21.0955): a new potent and safe bisphoshonate for the treatment of cancer-associated hypercalcaemia. Bone Miner. 1993; 22: 77–85.
60. Pecherstorfer, M., Herrmann, Z., Body, J.J., Manegold, C., Thiébaud, D., A randomized phase II trial comparing different doses of the bisphosphonate Ibandronate (BM 21.0955) in the treatment of hypercalcemia of malignancy (submitted for publication).

Bisphosphonate on bones
O. Bijvoet, H.A. Fleisch, R.E. Canfield and G. Russell (eds.)
© 1995 Elsevier Science B.V. All rights reserved.

CHAPTER 22

Bone involvement in solid tumours

R.D. Rubens

Guy's Hospital, London SE1 9RT, UK

I. Patterns of metastasic bone disease

Primary bone cancer occurring predominantly in children and adolescents is rare, but secondary bone cancer, particularly from carcinomas of the breast, lung, prostate, kidney and thyroid, is common; the prevalent cancers of the colon and rectum do not usually lead to metastatic bone disease. The incidence of bone metastases from different primary sites recorded in postmortem studies is summarised in Table 1. While the variability in these metastatic patterns is probably related to molecular and cellular biological characteristics of both the tumour cells and the tissues to which they metastasise, other factors such as vascular pathways and blood flow are also important.

Given the high prevalence of carcinomas of the breast, bronchus and prostate, these cancers probably account for more than 80% of cases of metastatic bone disease. The distribution of bone metastases is predominantly to the axial skeleton, particularly the spine, pelvis and ribs, rather than the appendicular skeleton, although lesions in the humeri and femora are quite common [1].

Breast cancer, the most common malignancy in women of Western Europe and North America (which, in the areas of its highest incidence, accounts for some 10%

Table 1.

Incidence of Skeletal Metastases in Autopsy Studies [1]

Primary tumour size	Number of studies	Incidence (%) of bone metastases	
		Median	Range
Breast	5	73	47–85
Prostate	6	68	33–85
Thyroid	4	42	28–60
Kidney	3	35	33–40
Bronchus	4	36	30–55
Oesophagus	3	6	5– 7
Gastrointestinal tract	4	5	3–11
Rectum	3	11	8–13

of all cancers), is the tumour most often associated with metastatic bone disease. Because of the long clinical course this disease can follow, even after metastases have developed, the morbidity from bone deposits presents a major problem for health care systems. There are no powerful predictors of which patients are at high risk of developing skeletal disease, but the incidence of bone metastases has been found to be significantly raised in association with steroid receptor-positive and well-differentiated tumours [2]. A study of 587 patients dying from breast cancer showed that 69% had radiological evidence of skeletal metastases before death compared to 27% each for lung and liver metastases [2]. In this study, in which 2240 patients presented with breast cancer over a 10-year period, 681 (30%) had relapsed after a median follow-up of 5 years, of whom 395 (50%) had distant metastases. In all, 184 had a first relapse in bone, accounting for 47% of all those with first distant relapse, 24% of the total with any relapse (both local and distant) and 8% of the whole study population.

Although patients with first relapse in the skeleton did not differ from those with first relapse in the liver, in terms of age, menstrual status or median postoperative disease-free interval, the survival experience was markedly different in these two metastatic categories. Median survival after first relapse in bone was 20 months, compared with only 3 months after first relapse in liver (Fig. 1). In patients with metastatic bone disease apparently remaining confined to the skeleton, the median duration of survival was 24 months. These results show how protracted a problem bone metastases can be for many patients with breast cancer.

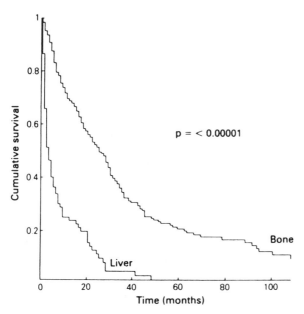

Fig. 1. Survival of patients with breast cancer after first relapse in bone compared to survival after first relapse in liver. (Reproduced with permission from [2]).

The skeleton is by far the most common site of metastatic disease in prostatic cancer. Unlike breast cancer, in which radiologically the lesions frequently show a mix of osteoblastic and osteolytic appearances, osteosclerotic disease predominates in prostatic cancer. Nevertheless, computed tomography often identifies lytic areas within these ostensibly sclerotic lesions. Histological studies have also demonstrated increased bone reabsorption in metastatic prostatic cancer [37]. Like breast cancer, metastatic bone disease in prostatic cancer can follow a relatively long course, with patients having a median survival prospect of about 17 months after the diagnosis of bone metastases [4].

In lung cancer, the incidence of bone metastases identifiable at the time of primary diagnosis is highest in the small cell variety and lowest with squamous cell tumours, but at autopsy the incidence of bone metastases is similar for all four main histological types of lung cancer (squamous cell, small cell, large cell anaplastic and adenocarcinoma) at about 30% [5]. Survival from the primary diagnosis of lung cancer is poor, and fewer than 10% of patients are alive at 5 years. Once metastatic disease is evident, most patients die within a few months. Bone metastases from lung cancer are usually of the osteolytic type, but, because of the poor survival prospects, morbidity from them is much less of a long-term health care problem than for either breast or prostatic cancers.

II. Complications of bone metastases

Several complications give rise to the substantial morbidity from bone metastases. They include pain, impaired mobility, pathological fracture, spinal cord compression, cranial nerve palsies, nerve root lesions, hypercalcaemia and suppression of bone marrow function. Pain is usually the presenting symptom and is caused by a variety of factors including periosteal stretching, compression of infiltration of nerve roots, reflex muscle spasm and the local effects of cytokines. In a study of 498 patients with first relapse in bone from breast cancer, 145 (29%) developed one or more of these complications of metastatic bone destruction [2]. A pathological fracture occurred in 78 patients (16%), spinal cord compression in 13 (3%) and hypercalcaemia in 86 (17%).

The precise incidence of pathological fracture in patients with metastatic bone disease is uncertain. In one series, 150 (8%) of 1800 patients with metastatic bone disease had fractures of either the femur (90%) or humerus (10%) [6]. The inclusion of rib and vertebral fractures in addition to those of long bones would show that pathological fractures affect a considerably higher proportion of patients with bone metastases. In this series, cancer of the breast was responsible for 53% of pathological fractures, kidney for 11%, lung 8%, thyroid and lymphoma each for 5% and prostatic cancer for 3%; a variety of other cancers accounted for the remainder. Radiological assessment of long bones suggests that when metastatic destruction involves over 50% of cortical thickness, the risk of fracture is so high that prophylactic surgery is indicated [7].

Compression of the spinal cord or cauda equina in patients with metastatic disease of the spine is a medical emergency necessitating prompt diagnosis and treatment. Its causes include pressure from an enlarging extradural mass, spinal angulation following vertebral collapse, vertebral dislocation following pathological fracture or, rarely, pressure from intradural metastases. The standard diagnostic test has been myelography, which often reveals multiple levels of compression. Similar information can also be obtained from magnetic resonance imaging, which in recent years has become the preferred investigation for diagnosing this complication of metastatic bone disease. Back pain is the most common initial symptom of spinal cord compression and affected 125 of 130 (96%) patients in one series [8]. Two types of pain may occur, local spinal or radicular. Radicular pain varies with the location of the tumour, being common in the cervical (79%) and lumbosacral (90%) regions and less so with thoracic lesions (55%). Both local spinal and radicular pain are experienced close to the site of the lesion identified at myelography. Motor weakness, sensory loss and autonomic dysfunction are all common at presentation of spinal cord or cauda equina compression, each affecting more than half of patients. The most common primary tumours producing this complication in decreasing order of frequency are carcinoma of the breast, lung cancer, prostatic cancer, lymphoma and renal carcinoma.

Hypercalcaemia is another emergency associated with metastatic bone disease. Its clinical features include nausea, vomiting, dehydration and confusion. While malignant hypercalcaemia is usually associated with demonstrable bone metastases, this is not always the case. In a review of 147 patients with advanced breast cancer having hypercalcaemia, 125 (85%) had definite radiographic evidence of bone metastases, but in 22 (15%) there was no such evidence of skeletal involvement. In the latter group, there was a significantly raised incidence of liver metastases and inappropriately high renal tubular reabsorption of calcium, which suggested that liver involvement could be facilitating a humoral component in the pathogenesis of hypercalcaemia in these patients [9].

Extensive infiltration of the bone marrow by metastatic disease causes leucoerythroblastic anaemia and pancytopenia, predisposing to infection and haemorrhage. Radiotherapy, often needed for the treatment of bone metastases, can exacerbate this problem, which in turn may comprise the ability effectively to give chemotherapy.

Animal experiments have shown that cytotoxic drugs can interfere with osteoblastic function and new bone formation [10], but the clinical significance of these findings is unknown. Other iatrogenic factors may also aggravate the morbidity from bone metastases. For example, ovarian ablation and corticosteroids used in the treatment of breast cancer may predispose to osteoporosis. This condition can present diagnostic problems in elderly patients in whom it may be difficult to distinguish between osteoporotic or metastatic disease as the cause of vertebral collapse.

III. Mechanisms of metastatic bone disease

The key characteristic of malignant cells is an ability to invade into surrounding tissues and to separate to form growths elsewhere. The mechanisms involved in the evolution of cancer are far from fully understood, but in recent years substantial progress has been made towards elucidating the complex underlying molecular and cellular processes. Although the development and behaviour of cancer are ultimately determined by the genetic control of cell regulation, permissive factors in the environment are undoubtedly important in determining the full expression of many cancers as clinical disease. Genes have been identified which are associated with malignant growth. Many encode either physiological growth factors or growth factor receptors, but their abnormal or amplified expression can result in cancerous proliferation. Homologues of these oncogenes are found in the genomes of carcinogenic viruses. Products of other genes function to regulate or inhibit cell division. Loss or mutation of these genes can also lead to uncontrolled growth, so they are referred to as tumour suppressor genes or anti-oncogenes.

Once the malignant process has been initiated in a cell, a complex series of mechanisms is necessary for a cancer to become established and manifested as clinical disease. Although a primary tumour itself can give rise to serious problems, it is usually distant metastases that are responsible for the lethal potential and which present the most difficulties for treatment. Secondary spread can occur in a variety of ways, including through lymphatic vessels, across serous cavities or along nerves, but blood-borne spread is of the greatest importance.

After a cell has acquired a malignant phenotype, it proliferates at its primary site. Initially, the nutrients needed for cellular growth are provided by simple diffusion from the bloodstream, but this soon becomes inadequate, and a new tumour vasculature is required. This develops by extension from the normal blood supply of the surrounding tissues. Experiments with tritiated thymidine-labelling and autoradiography have shown that tumour endothelial cells multiply with a doubling time of a few days, while endothelial cells of normal tissues rarely divide. Much evidence points to the malignant cells as the source of the stimulus for endothelial cell growth known as tumour angiogenesis factor. The continual presence of this factor is needed for the growth and maintenance of new tumour blood vessels [11].

The next step in the malignant process is the invasion of cancer cells into local structures, including their blood vessels. This process is facilitated by proteolytic enzymes. Once access to the blood circulation has been gained, tumour emboli can travel throughout the body. It seems likely that tumour cells are susceptible to a variety of host defence mechanisms in the blood stream including lysis by lymphocytes, monocytes and natural killer cells [12], in addition to mechanical damage from turbulence and trapping in capillaries. Studies with injected radiolabelled tumour cells suggest that fewer than one in a thousand entering the circulation actually survive and develop into metastases [13].

When disseminated cancer cells have arrived at sites of secondary growth, they adhere either to capillary endothelial cells or to exposed basement membrane [14]. The molecular mechanisms of cell to cell adhesion in both the detachment of malignant cells from primary tumours and their establishment at metastatic sites are still poorly understood, but it is of interest to note that a gene found to be deleted on chromosome 18 in some human colon cancers shows significant homology to those encoding for cell adhesion molecules and other cell surface glycoproteins [15]. For a metastasis to become established, the malignant cells adhering at the metastatic location have to extravasate into the tissues, perhaps by a process similar to invasion at the primary site. The ultimate establishment of metastases requires neo-vascularisation for proliferative growth to proceed.

The predominant distribution of bone metastases in the axial skeleton in which most of the red bone marrow is situated suggests that the slow blood flow at these sites could assist in the attachment of metastatic cells. This is in contrast to the circulation in the kidneys which accounts for a high proportion of the cardiac output and in which metastatic disease is extremely rare. This explanation alone does not, however, account adequately for metastatic patterns. It seems likely that molecular properties of both the malignant cells and those of the tissue in which metastases develop must also be important. Furthermore, the high incidence of bone metastases, without corresponding lesions in the lungs, has raised questions about the precise route cancer cells take from primary tumours to the skeleton. The absence of lung deposits makes it unlikely that malignant cells pass through the pulmonary circulation. Even if lung tissue is not receptive as a site for the establishment of metastatic disease, tumour cells are unlikely to pass through its narrow capillaries, particularly when aggregated as tumour emboli.

The experiments of Batson in animals and human cadavers which demonstrated the vertebral-venous plexus provide a good explanation for the predilection of metastatic spread from certain cancers to the skeleton [16]. He demonstrated how venous blood in both the pelvis and from the breast flowed not only into the venae cavae, but also directly into the vertebral-venous plexus. Moreover, the flow into the vertebral veins predominated when intrathoracic or intra-abdominal pressure was elevated, as for example during Valsalva's manoeuvre, and so presumably its clinical counterparts such as coughing.

These experiments helped to explain the tendency of prostatic and breast cancer to produce metastases in the axial skeleton and limb girdles. Further studies demonstrated the extent of this network of valve-less vessels which involve the epidural veins, perivertebral veins, veins of the thoraco-abdominal wall and veins of the head and neck, all carrying blood under low pressure [16]. In this system, blood is continually subjected to arrest and reversal of the direction of flow. This vertebral-venous system parallels, connects with and provides bypasses for the portal, pulmonary and caval system of veins and so provides a pathway for the spread of disease between distant organs. Primary lung tumours invade directly into the pulmonary venous system to gain access to the arterial circulation for dissemination.

IV. Pathophysiology

The damage to the skeleton caused by metastatic disease is often much more extensive than can be expected simply from the volume of tumour cells. Much evidence has accumulated leading to the conclusion that most of the skeletal destruction is mediated by osteoclastic cells. Although tumour masses may damage the skeleton in other ways, possibly by compression of vasculature and consequent ischaemia in the late stages of cancer, this is of lesser importance.

It has been demonstrated that malignant cells secrete many factors which stimulate, both directly and indirectly, osteoclastic activity [17]. They include prostaglandin E (PGE) and a variety of cytokines and growth factors such as transforming growth factor (TGF) α and β, epidermal growth factor (EGF), tumour necrosis factors (TNF) and interleukin-1 (IL-1). For example, IL-1, the most powerful stimulator of bone resorption *in vitro*, is produced by squamous carcinoma cells [18]. Several human breast cancer lines have also been shown to produce osteoclast-stimulating factors including TGF-α, TGF-β, EGF, parathyroid hormone-related peptide (PTHrP) and prostaglandins [19]. Procathepsin D, another osteoclast-stimulating factor, has also been shown to be a breast cancer cell product [20]; this enzyme is under the regulatory control of oestrogens in the MCF-7 cell line [21]. The active form of this enzyme stimulates bone resorption *in vitro* and is associated with proteolysis of collagen chains and the activation of TGF-β. Normal bone trabeculae are lined by a thin layer of uncalcified matrix which protects the calcified bone from osteoclastic activity, and the action of these proteolytic enzymes may be a prerequisite for osteoclastic bone resorption [22].

Malignant cells may also stimulate bone resorption by stimulating tumour-associated immune cells to release osteoclast-activating factors [23]. It has been shown that human melanoma cells produce a factor which stimulates macrophages to release TNF and IL-1 *in vitro* [24]. Furthermore, purification of a cytokine-releasing factor from medium conditioned by melanoma cells have identified it to be granulocyte-macrophage colony stimulating factor (GM-CSF) [25], which activates osteoclastic bone resorption.

In addition to the local paracrine factors described above, osteoclastic activity can also be stimulated in malignant disease by systemic factors, particularly PTHrP. This peptide is immunologically distinct from parathormone, but the two hormones have significant homology at the amino-terminus of the molecule which is necessary for osteoclast stimulation [26]. Ectopic production of this hormone, particularly in lung cancer, is a cause of osteoclastic bone resorption and hypercalcaemia even in the absence of bone metastases.

It appears that these factors act only indirectly on osteoclasts as these cells lack the required surface receptors. The receptors are, however, expressed on osteoblasts, and these appear to control bone resorption by their influence on osteoclasts. *In vitro* studies of isolated osteoclasts show that they are not stimulated when exposed to any of the stimulating factors alone [27]. However, when exposed to these factors in the presence of osteoblasts, osteoclastic activity is increased; this does not depend upon direct cell-cell contact and is due to a diffusible factor. A further function of osteoblasts in controlling bone resorption is probably the production of collagenase which can degrade the bone matrix [28].

Although osteolytic disease often predominates at the sites of bone metastases, osteosclerosis may predominate, particularly in prostatic cancer. In some instances, the new bone formation is not necessarily preceded by bone resorption [29].

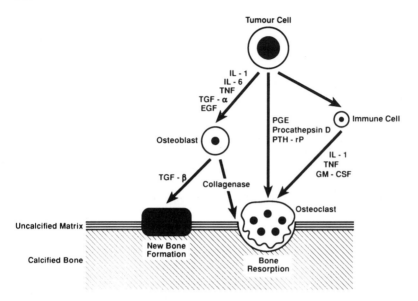

Fig. 2. Diagrammatic summary of the cellular and molecular interactions involved in bone resorption and new bone formation in metastatic disease of the skeleton.

Osteoblast growth factors such as TGF-β and platelet-derived growth factor have been purified from prostatic tumour cells [30].

The complex interaction between tumour cells, osteoblasts, osteoclasts and associated immune cells is summarised in Fig. 2.

V. Assessment of response of bone metastases to treatment

A variety of treatments, including radiotherapy, endocrine treatment, chemotherapy and bisphosphonates are used for the treatment of metastatic bone disease. Assessing the response to treatment of these sites is relatively difficult in comparison with disease in soft tissues. Response is usually judged by re-calcification of previously lytic disease on plain radiographs according to the UICC criteria [31]. However, this method does not observe tumour regression directly, but rather a delayed consequential healing. This results in reported response frequencies being lower in the skeleton compared with soft-tissue disease [2], but this is a reflection of the insensitivity of the assessment method rather than a true differences in response rate.

Imaging methods to be considered for the assessment of disease in the skeleton include isotopic bone scanning, plain radiography, computerised tomography and magnetic resonance imaging. The isotope bone scan is the most sensitive method for screening bone metastases, lesions being detectable from 3–12 months before becoming apparent radiographically [32]. The isotopic bone scan, which images function rather than structure, reflects osteoblastic activity. For this reason, it is not of value for the early assessment of response to treatment, because increased osteoblastic activity associated with either progression of bone disease or healing is indistinguishable [33]. The UICC criteria of response depend largely on plain radiography, but this method is insensitive, identifying the response according to re-calcification of previous lytic disease. Computerised tomography improves detection and can also be used to identify areas of lytic disease in predominantly osteoblastic lesions. Magnetic resonance imaging also enhances observation of structural detail and is particularly effective for defining the anatomy of the spinal cord or nerve root compression. Nevertheless, neither computerised tomography nor magnetic resonance imaging, which are complicated, expensive and time-consuming techniques, can identify a response within the first months of starting a new treatment.

Because of these limitations of imaging techniques, efforts have been made to identify other parameters of response in bone. Recently, particular attention has been paid to biochemical parameters. Biochemical factors studied have included serum calcium, the bone isoenzyme of alkaline phosphatase (ALP-BI), osteocalcin and acid phosphatase as well as urinary excretion of hydroxyproline and calcium. It has been found that the increased osteoblastic activity associated with an ultimate response according to UICC criteria is characterised by an elevation of the serum osteocalcin and ALP-BI one month after starting treatment, while at this time there is also a drop in the urinary calcium excretion [34]. These changes were seen in 14/16 patients with subsequent radiological evidence of bone healing, whilst similar biochemical changes at one month were seen in only 4/20 patients with progressive disease ($P < 0.001$). The combination of a more than 10% rise in ALP-BI and osteocalcin and a greater than 10% fall in urinary calcium excretion gave a diagnostic efficiency of 89% for discriminating between response and progression. Serum calcium and tartrate-resistant acid phosphatase and urinary hydroxyproline excretion were unhelpful in discriminating between response groups. Recently, preliminary observations on the urinary excretion of the cross-linking amino acids of collagen, pyridinoline and deoxypyridinoline, have shown a significant decrease in patients with bone metastases 4 weeks after starting treatment with the osteoclast-inhibiting agent pamidronate [35].

The importance of these results lies in the context of the treatment of bone metastases being palliative rather than curative. Early information at one month indicative of either response or progressive disease would be particularly helpful in determining whether or not treatment should be continued. This cannot be achieved if reliance is placed solely upon imaging tests. The desirability of identifying a probable ultimate response is emphasised when it is acknowledged that the aim of treatment in metastatic bone disease is to keep patients as symptom-free and as active for as along as possible with the fewest adverse effects from treatment.

References

1. Galasko, C.S.B., The anatomy and pathways of skeletal metastases. In: Weiss, L. and Gilbert, A.H. (Editors), Bone metastasis. G.K. Hall, Boston, 1981; pp. 49–63.

2. Coleman, R.E. and Rubens, R.D., The clinical course of bone metastases in breast cancer. Br. J. Cancer 1987; 55: 61–66.
3. Urwin, G.H., Percival, R.C., Harris, S., Beneton, M.N.C., Williams, J.L. and Kanis, J.A., Generalised increase in bone resorption in carcinoma of the prostate. Br. J. Urol. 1985; 57: 721–723.
4. Clain, A., Secondary malignant disease of bone. Br. J. Cancer 1965; 19: 15–29.
5. Muggia, F.M. and Chervu, L.R., Lung cancer: diagnosis in metastatic sites. Semin. Oncol. 1974; 1: 217–228.
6. Higinbotham, N.L. and Marcove R.C., The management of pathological fractures. J. Trauma 1965; 5: 792–798.
7. Fidler, M., Prophylactic internal fixation of secondary neoplastic deposits in long bones. Br. Med. J. 1973; 1: 341–343.
8. Gilbert, R.W., Kim, J.-H. and Posner, J.B., Epidural spinal cord compression from metastatic tumour diagnosis and treatment. Ann. Neurol. 1978; 3: 40–51.
9. Coleman, R.E., Fogelman I. and Rubens, R.D., Hypercalcaemia and breast cancer-an increased humoral component in patients with liver metastases. Eur. J. Surg. Oncol. 1988; 14: 423–428.
10. Friedlaender, G.E., Tross, R.B., Doganis A.C., Kirkwood, J.M. and Baron, R., Effects of chemotherapeutic agents on bone. 1. Short-term methotrexate and doxorubicin (Adriamycin) treatment in a rat model. J. Bone Joint Surg. (Am) 1984; 66: 602–607.
11. D'Amore, P.A., Growth factors, angiogenesis and metastasis. In: Welch, D.R., Bhuyahn, B.K. and Liotta, L.A. (Editors), Cancer metastasis: experimental and clinical strategies. Alan R. Liss Inc., New York, 1986; pp. 269–283 (Progress in clinical and biological research, vol. 212).
12. Hanna, N. and Fidler, I.J., Role of natural killer cells in destruction of circulating tumour emboli. J. Natl. Cancer Inst. 1980; 65: 801–809.
13. Fidler, I.J., Metastasis: quantitative analysis of distribution and fate of tumour emboli labelled with 12sI-5-iodo-2-deoxyridine. J. Natl. Cancer Inst. 1970; 45: 773–782.
14. Kramer, R.H., Gonzalez, R. and Nicolson, G.L., Metastatic tumour cells adhere preferentially to the extracellular matrix underlying vascular endothelial cells. Int. J. Cancer 1980; 26: 639–645.
15. Fearon, E.R., Cho, K.R., Nigro, J.M., Kern, S.E., Simons, J.W., Ruppert, J.M., Hamilton, S.R., Preisinger, A.C., Thomas, G., Kinzler, K.W. and Vogelstein, B., Identification of a chromosome 18q gene that is altered in colorectal cancers. Science 1990; 247: 49–56.
16. Batson, O.V., The role of the vertebral veins in metastatic process. Ann. Intern. Med. 1942; 16: 38–45.
17. Mundy, G.R., Hypercalcaemia of malignancy revisited. J. Clin. Invest. 1988; 82: 1–6.
18. Sato, K., Fujii, Y., Kasano, K., Tsushima, T. and Shizume, K., Production of Interleukin-1 alpha and a parathyroid hormone-like factor by a squamous cell carcinoma of oesophagus (EC-G1) derived from a patient with hypercalcaemia. J. Clin. Endocrinol. Metab. 1988; 67: 592–621.
19. Travers, M.T., Barrett-Lee, P.J., Berger, U. et al., Growth factor expression in normal, benign and malignant breast tissue. Br. Med. J. 1988; 296: 1621–1624.
20. Wo, Z., Bonewald, L.F., Oreffo, R.O.C. et al., The potential role of procathepsin D secreted by breast cancer cells in bone resorption. In: Cohn, D.V., Glorieux, F.H. and Martin, T.J. (Editors), Calcium regulation and bone metabolism. Elsevier, North-Holland, Amsterdam, 1990; pp. 304–310.
21. Cavailles, V., Garcia, M. and Rochefort, H., Regulation of cathepsin D and P52 gene expression by growth factors in MCF-7 human breast cancer cells. Mol. Endocrinol. 1989; 3: 552–558.
22. Chambers, T.J. and Fuller, K., Bone cells predispose endosteal surface to resorption by exposure of bone mineral to osteoclastic contact. J. Cell. Sci. 1985; 76: 155–163.
23. McBride, W.H., Phenotype and functions of intratumoral macrophages. Biochem. Biophys. Acta 1986; 865: 27–41.
24. Sabatini, M., Bonewald, L., Chavez, J. and Mundy, G.R., Production of GM-CSF by a human tumour associated with leukocytosis and hypercalcaemia induces cytokine production by host cells. J. Bone Miner. Res. 1989; 4 (Suppl. 1): S155 (Abstract).
25. Sabatini, M., Chavez, J., Mundy, G.R. and Bonewald, L.F., Stimulation of tumour necrosis factor release from monocyte cells by the A375 human melanoma via granulocyte-macrophage colony stimulating factor. Cancer Res. 1990; 50: 2673–2678.
26. Suva, L.J., Winslow, G.A., Moseley, J.M. et al., A parathyroid hormone-related protein implicated in malignant hypercalcaemia: cloning and expression. Science 1987; 237: 893–896.
27. Chambers, T.J., McSheehy, P.M.J., Thomson, B.M. and Fuller, K., The effect of calcium-regulating hormones and prostaglandine on bone resorption by osteoclasts disaggregated from neonatal rabbit bones. Endocrinology 1985; 116: 234–239.

28. Sakamoto, S. and Sakamoto, M., Bone collagenase, osteoblasts and cell-mediated bone resorption. In: Peck, W.A. (Editor), Bone and mineral research vol. 4. Elsevier, Amsterdam, 1986; pp. 49–102.
29. Valentin Opran, A., Edouard, C., Charhon, S. and Meunier, P.J., Histomorphometic analysis of iliac bone metastases of prostatic origin. In: Donath, A. and Huber, H. (Editors), Bone and tumours. Medicine et hygiène, Geneve, 1980; pp. 24–28.
30. Koutsilieris, M., Rabbini, S.A., Bennett, H.P.J. and Goltzman, D., Characteristics of prostate-derived growth factors for cells of the osteoblast phenotype. J. Clin. Invest. 1987; 80: 941–946.
31. Hayward, J.L., Carbone, P.P., Heuson, J.C., Kumaoka, S., Segaloff, A. and Rubens, R.D., Assessment of response to therapy in advanced breast cancer. Eur. J. Cancer Clin. Oncol. 1977; 13: 89–94.
32. Chaudary, M.A., Maisey, M.N., Shaw, P.J., Rubens, R.D. and Hayward, J.L., Sequential bone scans and chest radiographs in the postoperative management of early breast cancer. Br. J. Surg. 1983; 70: 517–518.
33. Coleman, R.E., Rubens, R.D. and Fogelman, I., The bone scan flare following systemic therapy for bone metastases. J. Nucl. Med. 1988; 28: 1354–1359.
34. Coleman, R.E., Whitaker, K.D., Moss, D.W., Mashiter, G., Fogelman, I. and Rubens, R.D., Biochemical monitoring predicts response in bone metastases to treatment. Br. J. Cancer 1988; 58: 205–210.
35. Coleman, R.E., Houston, S., James, I., Rodger, A., Rubens, R.D., Leonard, R.C.F. and Ford, J., Preliminary results of the use of urinary excretion of pyridinium crosslinks for monitoring metastatic bone disease. Br. J. Cancer 1992; 65: 766–768.

Bisphosphonate on bones
O. Bijvoet, H.A. Fleisch, R.E. Canfield and G. Russell (eds.)
© 1995 Elsevier Science B.V. All rights reserved.

CHAPTER 23

The treatment of metastatic bone disease

R.E. Coleman

Y.C.R.C. Department of Clinical Oncology, Weston Park Hospital, Sheffield S10 2SJ, UK

I. Introduction

Metastatic bone disease is a common clinical problem, and bone metastases account for 99% of all malignant tumours in bone. Typically, destructive metastatic involvement of the skeleton leads to pain and steadily increasing disability over several years, punctuated by episodes of hypercalcaemia, pathological fractures, and culminating in premature death. At any one time in the UK there are 15–20,000 women alive with bone metastases from breast cancer, and when one considers also that 85% of men with advanced prostate cancer and 65% of patients with lung cancer will develop skeletal metastases, the clinical importance of the condition becomes obvious.

In general, the treatment of bone metastases is aimed at palliating symptoms, with cure only rarely a realistic aim (e.g. lymphoma), and will vary depending on the underlying disease. External beam radiotherapy, endocrine treatments, chemotherapy and radioisotopes are all important modalities. In addition, orthopaedic intervention may be necessary for the structural complications of bone destruction, and some, although by no means all patients with bone metastases, will develop hypercalcaemia.

Underlying all the morbidity associated with skeletal metastases is the presence of an increased rate of bone resorption, mediated largely by the osteoclast [1]. Until recently, the management of osteolytic lesions and hypercalcaemia associated with malignancy has been far from ideal due to the toxicity or limited efficacy of the therapies available. In recent years, however, the bisphosphonates, agents with potent and sustained inhibitory effects on osteoclastic bone resorption, have emerged as an effective treatment for hypercalcaemia [2–4] and appear extremely promising in the management of osteolysis associated with malignancy [5–8].

II. Clinical and pathological features

Bone metastases are especially common from carcinomas arising in the breast, prostate and lung, and these three tumours alone account for 80% of patients with bone metastases [9]. These cancers, as well as multiple myeloma and carcinomas of the thyroid and kidney, demonstrate a phenomenon known as osteotropism, meaning they possess an extraordinary affinity for bone. In breast cancer this correlates with positive oestrogen binding receptors [10], and in prostate cancer with histological grade [11].

Irrespective of the tissue of origin of the cancer, the distribution of bone metastases is predominantly in the axial skeleton, particularly the spine, pelvis and ribs, rather than the appendicular skeleton, although lesions in the proximal femora and humeri are not uncommon. This distribution is similar to the red bone marrow in which slow blood flow possibly assists attachment of metastatic cells.

It is important to appreciate that metastatic bone disease can pursue a very indolent clinical course. For example, although the prognosis of patients with bone metastases from lung cancer is only a few months, the median survival of women with metastatic bone disease from breast cancer is 2 years [10], while up to 20% of men with advanced prostate cancer will survive 5 years [11]. In these two conditions particularly, effective palliative therapy is essential to maintain high quality and useful life.

Much progress has been achieved in understanding the mechanisms by which tumour cells cause invasion and destruction of bone. Histological examination of involved bone may show tumour cells in resorption bays on bone surfaces, and although cancer cells can erode bone directly through the production of proteolytic enzymes, the indirect action of cancer cells on osteoclast activity is much more important. It is now generally accepted that osteoclast activation is the key step in the establishment and growth of all bone metastases [12].

In some cancers, particularly multiple myeloma and most breast cancers, osteolysis predominates though areas of new bone formation are usually also identifiable on histological examination. In others, osteosclerosis is dominant, with either new bone being laid down away from the normal resorption bays and/or condensation of new bone within the infiltrated bone marrow stroma. It is this predominance of lysis or sclerosis which gives rise to the characteristic radiographic appearances of bone metastases. When bone resorption predominates, focal bone destruction occurs, and bone metastases gain a lytic appearance. Conversely, in bone metastases associated with increased osteoblast activity (e.g. prostate cancer), the lesions appear sclerotic on X-ray. Even when one element predominates, both processes are greatly accelerated in the surrounding bone [13]. This is radiographically typified by the appropriately termed 'mixed' lesions, seen most commonly in breast cancer, in which both lytic and sclerotic components are clearly visible.

Clinically, lytic bone metastases are much more frequent and cause the most morbidity. Pathological fractures and hypercalcaemia are seen less often in patients with sclerotic lesions, while pain, when present, is probably caused by a minor lytic component which is difficult to demonstrate on conventional radiographs.

III. Treatment of bone metastases

1. Radiation therapy for bone metastases

Localised external beam radiotherapy is the treatment of choice for the palliation of painful single sites. However, for the treatment of multiple involved sites, wide field irradiation such as hemibody treatment is a rational alternative to sequential treatments with standard fields. In addition, recently there has been great interest in the use of systemically administered radioisotopes which exhibit preferential uptake in bone metastases.

(a) External beam radiotherapy

Bones lying just below the skin surface such as the ribs, skull and clavicles can be efficiently treated with an orthovoltage beam of 250–300 KeV. The beam is directed by an applicator to suit the required area of treatment and will give sufficient penetration to adequately treat the affected area. For the long bones, pelvis and spine, which are more deeply seated, a megavoltage beam is required to achieve sufficient penetration.

Irradiation of bone can result in a number of pathological changes, including atrophy, osteitis, necrosis and sarcomatous change. Relatively small doses of irradiation will result in inhibition of bone growth, and in young children a single dose as low as 4 Gy may result in permanent shortening of a growing bone. Indeed, inhibition of bone growth has been used therapeutically to prevent heterotopic bone formation following total hip arthroplasty; postoperative radiotherapy with doses as low as 10 Gy in 10 daily fractions have been reported to be effective in suppressing reactive bone growth [14].

The structural effects of irradiation on bone containing metastases have only been studied post-mortem. Initially, there are degeneration and necrosis of tumour cells followed by a proliferation of collagen. Subsequently, a rich vascular fibrous stroma is produced within which intense osteoblast activity lays down newly woven bone. This is then gradually replaced by lamellar bone and the intratrabecular stroma repopulated by bone marrow tissue. Radiologically, it can be seen that recalcification of lytic areas begins 3–6 weeks after irradiation, with maximum recalcification occurring 2 months from the time of irradiation [15, 16].

There is no doubt that local irradiation is effective for bone pain. Overall response rates of around 85% are reported, with complete relief of pain achieved in one-half of patients [17]. Pain relief usually occurs rapidly, with more than 50% of responders showing benefit within 1 to 2 weeks. Improvement in pain 6 weeks or more after treatment is unusual.

Traditionally, treatment techniques and doses have varied considerably between different centres, with no particular approach appearing to be superior in terms of pain relief. In a large American study, the Radiation Therapy and Oncology Group (RTOG) reported the results of a prospective randomised study of more than 1000 treatments for metastatic bone pain. A variety of dose fractionation schedules were used, ranging from 15 Gy in 5 fractions to 40.5 Gy in 15. An overall response rate of 90% was observed, with approximately half of responders maintaining pain relief until death. Median duration of pain relief in the complete responders was 12–15 weeks. The complete response rate was 35% after 40.5 Gy in 15 fractions compared with only 28% after 25 Gy in 5 ($P = 0.0003$) [18, 19]. However, two other prospective randomised studies have shown no difference in response rates between single or short course radiotherapy and fractionated courses given over 2–3 weeks [20, 21].

When there are multiple scattered sites of painful bone metastases, wide field hemibody irradiation is often preferable to treating each site individually with local irradiation. Using single fractions of 6–7 Gy to the upper hemibody and 6–8 Gy to the lower hemibody, pain relief is reported in about 75% of patients, often occurring rapidly and sometimes within 24–48 hours of treatment [22].

(b) Targeted radioisotope therapy

The therapeutic use of radioactive label tracer molecules is currently an area of considerable interest and research. The principles of this technique are well established following decades of experience with iodine-131 for the treatment of follicular thyroid cancer which may metastasize to bone. Excellent results can be obtained, particularly in patients with a significant uptake of iodine-131 by the metastases. Long-term palliation is usually possible, with 25% and 10% of patients still alive at 10 and 15 years, respectively [23].

Neuroblastomas, and tumours of neuroectodermal origin in general, frequently metastasize to bone. Of these patients 90% will incorporate the radiopharmaceutical ^{131}I-meta-iodo-benzyl guanadine (MIBG), and this has now been used to treat many children with metastatic neuroblastoma. In all, 5% of patients have undergone complete remission, 40% have experienced partial remission and 10% progressed [24]. Bone marrow suppression is often severe, and ideally bone marrow harvesting should be performed in patients with extensive bone metastases as a precautionary measure.

Targeted radiotherapy has several theoretical advantages over external beam radiotherapy. Firstly, the intracellular uptake of therapeutic radiopharmaceuticals ensures that the radiation dose is delivered specifically to the tumour, and normal tissues are spared unnecessary irradiation, allowing repeated treatments if necessary. Secondly, given an adequate blood supply, the radiation dose should be evenly administered throughout the treatment volume. The α- or β-emitting radionuclides are the most suitable, but apart from iodine-131 they have been very expensive and technically difficult to produce, so that despite the theoretical attractions of radioisotope therapy, only relatively few have been evaluated clinically.

Strontium-89 imitates calcium and is preferentially taken up at sites of new bone formation. It has been shown to localise efficiently at the sites of prostatic bone metastases, with greater accumulation occurring in the metastatic lesions than is observed in normal bone [25]. The radiation dose to individual vertebral metastases from a single 150-MBq dose of strontium-89 has been shown to vary from 9–92 Gy, the variation depending on the extent of metastatic spread. Of great clinical importance is the low dose of radiation to the bone marrow, which is only about one-tenth of that to the bone metastases [26].

Strontium therapy provides pain relief in up to 80% of patients, with 10–20% becoming pain free [27, 28]. On average, the response lasts for 6 months with only mild haematological toxicity. A number of randomised clinical trials have been performed. These have included a double-blind trial comparing the effects of strontium-89 with strontium chloride (placebo) as palliative therapy. The radioactive strontium-89 was clearly superior in terms of pain relief ($P < .01$) [28]. In a more recent study, the addition of strontium-89 to conventional radiotherapy was shown to reduce the subsequent morbidity of bone metastases from prostatic cancer and improve the patients' quality of life [29].

Samarium-153 with its short half-life (46 hours) has recently been linked to ethylene diamine tetramethylene phosphonate (EDTMP) for use as a radiopharmaceutical [30]. Because of this linkage to EDTMP, samarium-153 also concentrates preferentially in skeletal metastases and, being both a β- and γ-ray emitter, is suitable for combined therapy and imaging. Early clinical reports indicate that ^{153}Sm-EDTMP can also provide excellent pain relief [31].

2. Systemic therapy for bone metastases

Systemic therapy for bone metastases may be directed against the tumour cell to reduce cell proliferation and, as a consequence, the production of cytokines and growth factors. Alternatively, systemic treatment is directed towards blocking the effect of these substances on host cells. Chemotherapy, endocrine treatments and bone-seeking isotopes have direct anti-tumour effects, whereas agents such as the bisphosphonates and calcitonin are effective by preventing host cells (primarily osteoclasts) from reacting to tumour products. Systemic therapy therefore has either direct or indirect actions.

(a) Direct anti-cancer therapy

In general, the systemic treatment for metastatic bone disease utilises the same treatments that are available for other metastatic manifestations of malignancy. Treatment therefore has to be discussed according to tumour type. Breast and prostate cancer are the most important, not only because they are common, but also because there are effective, albeit palliative, systemic treatments available.

(i) Breast cancer Endocrine therapy is the treatment of choice for the initial therapy of metastatic disease. Exceptions to this are when visceral disease is so extensive and/or aggressive that it is inadvisable to wait 6–8 weeks for a possible response, or in patients who are known to have hormone receptor-negative tumours and for whom response to endocrine therapy is unlikely [32]. In these two situations cytotoxic chemotherapy is the initial treatment of choice.

Significant (> 50%) tumour shrinkage (a complete or partial objective response) following endocrine treatment occurs in one-third of unselected patients but is more likely in those with either steroid-receptor-positive tumours, a long disease-free interval from diagnosis to relapse, and bone or soft-tissue metastases rather than visceral disease [33].

The median duration of response to endocrine therapy is around 15 months, but remissions of several years are occasionally seen. Eventual relapse to primary endocrine treatment is inevitable, but subsequent responses to second- or third-line endocrine therapy will occur in 20–25% of primary responders.

There are not major differences in efficacy between the available endocrine agents, but the toxicity profiles do differ. There have been reports in the literature claiming higher response rates in bone with aminoglutethimide [34] and medroxy-progesterone acetate [35], but these have not been confirmed and probably reflect the difficulty in accurately assessing response in bone.

Chemotherapy is not suitable for all patients but, when used appropriately, can produce very worthwhile palliation of symptoms without causing unacceptable toxicity. Furthermore, the recent improvements in supportive care have improved the quality of life of patients requiring chemotherapy for advanced disease. Toxicity of chemotherapy can be distressing but can be minimised by the use of modern anti-emetics, dosage modification and careful explanation of the intended treatment. Objectively responding patients will usually gain relief of symptoms and may be able to resume their previous activities. Response rates to single agents vary from 20–60%, and combination chemotherapy regimens achieve objective responses in about 40–60%. Most responses are partial, with a complete response rate of only 5–20%. The duration of response is probably also shorter than with endocrine therapy, with a median of 9–12 months. The precise choice of drugs and schedule of administration to obtain the best results are not yet certain and will vary from one patient or clinical problem to another. The anthracyclines, doxorubicin and epidoxorubicin, are particularly active but also are sometimes too toxic for elderly or frail patients.

Chemotherapy can be hazardous in patients with extensive bone disease due to poor bone marrow tolerance following replacement of functioning marrow by tumour and the effects of previous irradiation. In view of this, regimens with relatively little myelotoxicity are usually preferable, a combination of cyclophosphamide, methotrexate and fluorouracil (CMF) being the most widely used palliative regimen.

(ii) Prostate cancer Bone is the major site of metastatic disease in prostate cancer and in many patients the only symptomatic problem. At least 80% of prostate tumours exhibit some degree of hormone responsiveness [36], with surgical castration still the most commonly used form of endocrine manipulation. Many new forms of endocrine treatment have been introduced recently, including the LHRH agonists and the anti-androgens. These pharmacological alternatives are not necessarily any more effective than surgical orchidectomy [37, 38], but for many patients are aesthetically preferable.

Patients with advanced prostate cancer tend to be elderly and often of poor performance status. Because of this, their tolerance to toxic chemotherapy regimens is often poor, and this has significantly limited the use of this treatment modality.

(iii) Other tumours Skeletal morbidity is a major problem in multiple myeloma, and either widespread lytic metastases or diffuse osteopenia may occur. Around

50% of patients will respond to chemotherapy with a reduction in paraprotein levels and subjective improvement. Alkylating agents such as melphalan and the corticosteroids are the most frequently prescribed agents. Despite the subjective improvement that is seen, bone healing is rare, lytic lesions persisting despite control of the disease.

Bone involvement in curable malignancies is relatively uncommon. Bone metastases are occasionally seen in patients with germ cell tumours and may represent an adverse prognostic feature [39], but despite this, cure with chemotherapy is usual. Bone involvement at diagnosis in lymphoma is relatively uncommon. Localised bone involvement does not significantly affect the prognosis in Hodgkin's disease but does carry an adverse prognosis in non-Hodgkin's lymphoma. Curative therapy, however, is still possible, and there is no evidence that bone represents a 'sanctuary site'.

(b) Indirect anticancer therapy

The dominant role of the osteoclast in tumour-induced osteolysis (TIO) and the ability of bisphosphonates to block this osteoclast-mediated bone destruction provide the rationale for their use in patients with bone metastases. Over the past 5–10 years a number of studies have been conducted with three aims: firstly, the reduction of local osteolysis by the tumour, minimising structural damage, and reducing morbidity; secondly, the prevention of new metastatic lesions; and thirdly, the protection of bone from systemic mediators of resorption.

The early clinical studies with bisphosphonates for osteolysis were small and uncontrolled, but nevertheless, improvements in bone pain and biochemical responses were seen. Since these preliminary reports, five carefully evaluated phase-2 studies of intravenous pamidronate every 2 to 4 weeks as the sole treatment of osteolysis due to bone metastases from advanced breast cancer have been performed [5, 40–43]. They have all reported similar results, indicating strongly that, although these studies were also not placebo-controlled, real symptomatic, biochemical and radiological benefit was achieved. In summary, they showed that relief of pain occurs in one-half of patients, and bone healing, as evidenced by sclerosis of lytic lesions, is observed in about one-quarter. Selective inhibition of bone resorption occurred with a reduction in urinary calcium excretion but without inhibiting osteoblast activity.

Beneficial effects have not been confined to breast cancer. In a preliminary study of pamidronate for bone metastases from hormone-resistant prostate cancer, osteoclast inhibition resulted in pain relief, stabilisation of rising tumour markers and improvements in bone biochemistry [44]. Similarly, oral clodronate has been shown in an open phase-2 study to produce useful pain relief in patients with hormone-resistant bone metastases from prostate cancer [45].

Three large randomised studies have been published [6–8] (Table 1). In the first one from Leiden, pamidronate was given in combination with conventional anticancer therapy [6]. One hundred and seventy women with bone metastases from breast cancer were randomised to oral pamidronate or a control group, systemic therapy being left to the discretion of the physician. Impressive results in favour of the combined treatment were seen, with a statistically significant reduction in the incidence of hypercalcaemia, pathological fractures, pain and improved quality of

Table 1.

Results of randomised bisphosphonate trials in the treatment of bone metastases

	Bisphosphonate	Control	p
Pamidronate (breast cancer) [6]			
(event rate/100 patients years)			
Hypercalcaemia	7	16	<0.003
Fractures	7	9	0.27
Pain	26	37	<0.004
Radiotherapy	26	39	<0.002
Change in systemic treatment	41	63	<0.005
Clodronate (breast cancer) [7]			
(number of episodes)			
Hypercalcaemia	28	52	<0.01
Vertebral fractures	84	124	<0.03
All events	168	305	<0.001
Clodronate (myeloma) [8]			
(% of patients)			
Progression of lytic disease at 2 years	12%	24%	0.026
Progression of vertebral fractures at 2 years	30%	40%	N.S.
% Becoming pain free	30%	15%	<0.01

life [46]. The overall complication rate of bone involvement (per 100 patient years) was 61 for the treatment group and 81 for the control group ($P < 0.02$). However, the lack of a placebo treatment for the control group makes it impossible, albeit unlikely, to exclude the possibilities of observer bias and/or a placebo effect.

A second, more recent placebo-controlled study with clodronate in advanced breast cancer also reports an impressive reduction in skeletal morbidity. Both the frequency of hypercalcaemia (28 vs 52, $P < 0.01$) and the number of fractures and deformities of vertebral bodies were reduced (84 vs 124, $P < 0.03$) [7]. A reduction in the requirement for radiotherapy specifically to the spine was reported, but there was no significant difference between the two groups in the overall number of radiotherapy treatments prescribed.

Thirdly, a placebo-controlled study of oral clodronate as an adjunct to treatment with melphalan and prednisolone for the treatment of multiple myeloma has recently been published. Progression of osteolytic bone lesions was delayed, and bone pain and hypercalcaemia were significantly reduced [8].

Several small, randomised studies have also been reported. Elomaa et al. randomly assigned 34 patients with progressive bone metastases from breast cancer to receive either oral clodronate or placebo in addition to their most recent systemic therapy. Those who received oral clodronate required less analgesic, had fewer requirements for radiotherapy or episodes of hypercalcaemia, and developed fewer new bone lesions than patients receiving placebo [47]. A study in multiple myeloma, also with clodronate, showed a reduction in pain, fewer new lytic lesions and a non-significant improvement in survival in the bisphosphonate-treated group, but again, the study was not placebo-controlled [48]. Two negative randomised studies have been reported. A randomised, double-blind, placebo-controlled study of etidronate in 57 patients with hormone-resistant prostate cancer showed no advantage to oral etidronate in terms of symptom response or analgesic requirements [49]. Similarly, a preliminary report of aminoglutethimide as endocrine treatment with or without intravenous pamidronate for bone metastases from advanced breast cancer has failed to show any influence of pamidronate on the course of bone metastases over and above that achieved with endocrine therapy alone [50].

It is now clear from work in tumour-induced hypercalcaemia that there is a dose-response relationship, and higher doses of bisphosphonates may be necessary if intermittent intravenous treatment is to be used. Somewhat surprisingly, the bone healing observed with parenteral pamidronate has yet to be reported following continuous oral therapy with any of the three currently available compounds. New, more potent bisphosphonate analogues are in early clinical development and may be more effective. However, it may be that despite the obvious convenience of oral bisphosphonates, the high-dose intermittent intravenous treatment is superior.

There is great interest in the potential use of bisphosphonates for the prevention of bone metastases. Animal data and indirect clinical results suggest this is a rational hypothesis, and a number of placebo-controlled clinical trials of oral therapy as an adjunct to systemic therapy have recently started.

IV. Assessment of response

The objective assessment of response to treatment has been defined by the Union Internationale Contra la Cancer (UICC). In breast cancer, this is based on changes seen on serial plain radiographs, and therefore the precise effect of therapy is difficult to measure objectively [51]. It is generally accepted that sclerosis of lytic metastases with no radiological evidence of new lesions constitutes tumour regression (a partial response or PR). However, some patients will have a mixture of sclerotic and lytic lesions before starting therapy, making interpretation of serial radiographs difficult. In patients with sclerotic metastases, radiological assessment of response is almost impossible. Even when radiological evidence of response to successful therapy is obtained, it is often not evident for 6 months and may be delayed for more than a year. Complete response in non-osseous sites affected by breast cancer occurs in 10–20% of patients, but a complete response (CR) in bone with return of normal trabecular pattern or resolution of sclerotic metastases is rare. Radiographic assessment of response is clearly imprecise, as exemplified by the observation that patients with X-ray evidence of sclerosis and those with no change in radiographic appearances for at least 3 months have a similar outcome in terms of survival [52].

It is clear that alternative methods of response assessment are necessary. Without more precise criteria it is difficult both to compare different treatments or define the role of new treatment approaches such as bisphosphonate therapy. Complication rates, pain and quality of life measurements are important surrogates which enable treatment comparisons to be made but are less valuable in determining an individual patient's response to therapy.

Attention has turned recently to using biochemical markers of bone resorption and formation as alternative methods of response assessment [53]. Fasting urinary calcium excretion (UCCR) is a sensitive indicator of net calcium loss from the skeleton, cheap and easy to measure. Serial measurements have been shown to correlate with the response to endocrine and cytotoxic therapy for breast cancer [54, 55], and the UCCR is currently the most widely used biochemical parameter for comparing the efficacy and duration of action of different doses, schedules and formulations of the bisphosphonates.

Urinary hydroxyproline is a useful marker of osteolysis in benign bone disease but has proved unreliable in malignancy due to contributions from soft-tissue destruction, diet, collagen synthesis and complement activation. Recently, new markers of collagen breakdown, the amino acids pyridinoline and deoxypyridinoline which form the cross-links between collagen strands in hard connective tissues, have been proposed as more useful alternatives to hydroxyproline. Both pyridinoline and deoxypyridinoline are almost completely excreted during collagen degradation, are unaffected by diet and can be measured in the urine. Reduction in excretion of both of these markers has been demonstrated to occur within 4 weeks of commencing oral pamidronate for progressive bone metastases [56]. Further study is needed, but urinary excretion of the pyridinolines and/or the new radioimmunoassays for collagen metabolites [57] may prove to be useful indicators of bisphosphonate efficacy.

V. Complications of bone involvement

1. Hypercalcaemia of malignancy

Hypercalcaemia causes a number of unpleasant signs and symptoms, which vary considerably from patient to patient. These are often non-specific, affecting many systems in the body, and can be easily mistaken for symptoms of the underlying cancer or associated treatment if there is not acute awareness of the possibility of hypercalcaemia. If untreated, a progressive rise in serum calcium will occur, leading to a deterioration in renal function and conscious level. Death ultimately ensues as the result of cardiac arrhythmia and renal failure.

It is unusual for there to be doubt about the aetiology of hypercalcaemia in cancer patients, but non-malignant causes must be considered particularly in the absence of metastases. In the community, hyperparathyroidism is the most common cause of hypercalcaemia [58] and may be encountered also in cancer patients. Measurement of parathyroid hormone using a modern specific radioimmunoassay is therefore worthwhile if there is any doubt about the diagnosis, levels of PTH being low or undetectable in malignancy and inappropriately high in hyperparathyroidism.

All three bisphosphonates are effective for the treatment of hypercalcaemia and superior to other agents [2-4]. Etidronate and clodronate are usually given intravenously over 3-5 days whereas pamidronate is effective as a single intravenous infusion and is the current treatment of choice amongst oncologists. In the only randomised comparison of the three bisphosphonates for hypercalcaemia of malignancy, a single 30-mg infusion of pamidronate was most effective and had the longest duration of action when compared to etidronate 7.5 mg/kg body weight on three successive days and clodronate 600 mg as a single intravenous infusion [59]. Normocalcaemia following pamidronate is usually maintained for 10–28 days, the duration depending somewhat on the severity of hypercalcaemia and dose administered. Repeated administration every 2 to 3 weeks will usually prevent recurrence of the hypercalcaemia.

2. Pathological fractures

Metastatic destruction of bone reduces its load-bearing capabilities. Microfractures cause pain, and rib fractures are common. Vertebral collapse also frequently occurs, resulting in loss of height, kyphoscoliosis and a degree of restrictive lung disease. However, it is fracture of a long bone or fracture-dislocation and epidural extension of tumour in the spine which causes the most disability. Because the development of a fracture is so devastating to a cancer patient, increasing emphasis is being placed on attempts to predict metastases at risk of fracture and the use of pre-emptive surgery.

Fractures are common through lytic metastases and weight-bearing bones, the proximal femora being the most commonly affected sites. Damage to both trabecular and cortical bone is structurally important, but it is the relevance of cortical destruction which is most clearly appreciated. Over the years several radiological features have been identified which may predict imminent fracture. Fracture is likely if lesions are large, predominantly lytic and erode the cortex [60]. Prophylactic internal fixation is the treatment of choice for such lesions followed by radiotherapy [61]. It is easier to stabilise a bone while it is still intact, and rehabilitation and convalescence are much shorter and easier. If the patient is not fit for surgery, then radiotherapy and non-weight-bearing is indicated.

Untreated pathological fractures rarely heal, and although radiotherapy may achieve local tumour control, bony union remains unlikely. Radiotherapy inhibits chondrogenesis, a prerequisite for fracture healing, and with large areas of bone destruction there may be insufficient matrix remaining for adequate repair.

3. Spinal instability

Back pain is a frequent symptom in patients with disseminated carcinoma but in some patients is due to spinal instability. This can cause excruciating pain which is mechanical in nature. The patient is only comfortable when lying absolutely still and any movement produces severe pain. Consequently, the patient may not be able to sit, stand or walk even with the use of a spinal support.

Because the pain is due to the instability and not the metastasis, radiotherapy or systemic treatment will not alleviate it. As with pathological fractures of long bones, stabilisation is required for pain relief. This involves major surgery, but with careful selection of patients, excellent results can be obtained.

4. Spinal cord compression

Compression of the spinal cord or cauda equina may occur in association with spinal instability (see above) or in isolation. When there is more than a 50% vertebral collapse, compression of the spinal cord becomes more likely. Invasion of the epidural space with compression of the spinal cord and nerve roots necessitates urgent corticosteroids and radiotherapy or surgical intervention to reduce permanent neurological damage [62].

The choice between surgical decompression and radiotherapy depends on a variety of clinical features. Surgical decompression is indicated in patients with recent onset of symptoms with progressive paraplegia and urinary retention of < 30 hours duration. The site of compression should be localised to no more than 2 or 3 segments, and the patient should have a life expectancy of at least several weeks. In those patients where the paraplegia has been established for several days or urinary retention has been present for more than 30 hours, surgical decompression rarely results in the recovery of bladder or motor function. Radiotherapy is indicated for those who are either unfit for surgery or do not fulfill the criteria of surgical decompression and will at least usually relieve pain even if it is not able to improve neurological function.

VI. Summary

Bone metastases cause considerable morbidity, and the palliative and supportive treatment that sufferers require for many months, and sometimes years, constitutes a major health care problem. Optimum management requires a multidisciplinary team including not only medical and radiation oncologists, orthopaedic surgeons, general physicians, radiologists and nuclear medicine physicians but also symptom control and terminal care specialists. In recent years there have been many exciting developments in both our understanding of the pathophysiological processes involved and treatment options. Further research and refinement of treatment is needed to improve further the prospects for the many patients with skeletal metastases.

References

1. Scher, H.I. and Yagoda, A., Bone metastases: pathogenesis, treatment and rationale for use of resorption inhibitors. Am. J. Med. 1987; 82 (Suppl. 2A): 6–28.
2. Body, J.-J., Borkowski, A., Cleeren, A. et al., Treatment of malignancy-associated hypercalcaemia with intravenous aminohydroxypropylidene diphosphonate. J. Clin. Oncol. 1986; 8: 1177–1183.
3. Hasling, C., Charles, P. and Mosekilde, L., Etidronate disodium for treating hypercalcaemia of malignancy: A double blind, placebo-controlled study. Eur. J. Clin. Invest. 1988; 16: 433–437.
4. Bonjour, J.-P., Philippe, J., Guelpa, G. et al., Bone and renal components in hypercalcaemia of malignancy and responses to a single infusion of clodronate. Bone 1988; 9: 123–130.
5. Coleman, R.E., Woll, P.J., Miles, M. et al., 3-amino-1,1 hydroxypropylidene bisphosphonate (APD) for the treatment of bone metastases from breast cancer. Br. J. Cancer 1988; 58: 621–625.

6. van Holten-Verzantvoort, A.T., Kroon, H.M., Bijvoet, O.L.M., Cleton, F.J. et al., Palliative pamidronate treatment in patients with bone metastases from breast cancer. J. Clin. Oncol. 1993; 11: 491–498.
7. Paterson, A.H.G., Powles, T.J., Kanis, J.A. et al., Double-blind controlled trial of oral clodronate in patients with bone metastases from breast cancer. J. Clin. Oncol. 1993; 11: 59–65.
8. Lahtinen, R., Laakso, M., Palva, I., Virkkunen, P., Elomaa, I. for the Finnish Leukaemia Group, Randomised, placebo-controlled multicentre trial of clodronate in multiple myeloma. Lancet 1992; 340: 1049–1052.
9. Abrams, H.L., Spiro, R. and Goldstein, N., Metastases in Carcinomas: Analysis of 1000 autopsied cases. Cancer 1950; 23: 74–85.
10. Coleman, R.E. and Rubens, R.D., The clinical course of bone metastases from breast cancer. Br. J. Cancer 1987; 55: 61–66.
11. Nesbit, R.M. and Baum, W.C., Endocrine control of prostatic carcinoma: clinical and statistical survey of 1818 cases. J.N.C.I. 1984; 68: 507–517.
12. Boyce, B.F., Normal bone remodelling and its disruption in metastatic bone disease In: Rubens, R.D. and Fogelman, I. (Editors), Bone metastases — diagnosis and treatment. Springer-Verlag, London, 1991; pp. 11–30.
13. Galasko, C.S.B., Mechanisms of bone destruction in the development of skeletal metastases. Nature 1976; 263: 507–508.
14. Anthony, P., Keys, H., McCollister, C.E., Rubin, P. and Lush, C., Prevention of heterotopic bone formation with early postoperative irradiation in high risk patients undergoing total hip arthroplasty: comparison of 10.00 Gy vs 20.00 Gy schedules. Int. J. Radiat. Oncol. Biol. Phys. 1987; 13: 365–369.
15. Matsubayashi, T., Koga, H., Nishiyama, Y., Tominaga, S. and Sourada, T., The reparative process of metastatic bone lesions after radiotherapy. Jpn. J. Clin. Oncol. 1981; 11: 253–249.
16. Hoskin, P.J., Radiotherapy in the management of bone metastases. In: Rubens, R.D. and Fogelman, I. (Editors), Bone metastases — diagnosis and treatment. Springer-Verlag, London, 1991; pp. 207–222.
17. Hoskin, P.J., Scientific and clinical aspects of radiotherapy in the relief of bone pain. Cancer Surv. 1988; 7: 69–86.
18. Blitzer, P.H., Reanalysis of the RTOG study of the palliation of symptomatic osseous metastasis. Cancer 1985; 55: 1468–1472.
19. Tong, D., Gillick, L. and Hendrickson, F., The palliation of symptomatic osseous metastases: final results of the study by the Radiation Therapy Oncology Group. Cancer 1982; 50: 893–899.
20. Price, P., Hoskin, P.J., Easton, D., Austin, D., Palmer, S.G. and Yarnold, J.R., Prospective randomised trial of single and multifraction radiotherapy schedules in the treatment of painful bony metastases. Radiother. Oncol. 1986; 6: 247–255.
21. Madsen, E.L., Painful bone metastasis: efficacy of radiotherapy assessed by the patients: a randomised trial comparing 4 Gy x 6 versus 10 Gy x 2. Int. J. Radiat. Oncol. Biol. Phys. 1983; 9: 1775–1779.
22. Hoskin, P.J., Ford, H.T. and Harmer, C.L., Hemibody irradiation for metastatic bone pain. Clin. Oncol. 1989; 1: 41–42.
23. Charbord, P., L'heritier, C., Cukerstein, W., Lumbroso, J. and Tubiana, M., Radio-iodine treatment in differentiated thyroid carcinomas. Treatment of first local recurrences and of bone and lung metastases. Ann. Radiol. 1977; 20: 783–786.
24. Clarke, S.E.M., Isotope therapy for bone metastases In: Rubens, R.D. and Fogelman, I. (Editors), Bone metastases — diagnosis and treatment. Springer-Verlag, London, 1991; pp. 187–206.
25. Blake, G., Strontium-89 therapy: strontium kinetics in disseminated carcinoma of the prostate. Eur. J. Nucl. Med. 1986; 12: 447–454.
26. Blake, G.M., Zivanovich, M.A., Blaquiere, R.M. et al., Strontium-89 therapy: Measurement of absorbed dose to skeletal metastases. J. Nucl. Med. 1988; 29: 549–557.
27. Robinson, R., Spicer, J.A., Preston, D.F., Wegst, A.V. and Martin, N.L., Treatment of metastatic bone pain with strontium-89. Nucl. Med. Biol. 1987; 14: 219–222.
28. Lewington, V.J., McEwan, A.J., Ackery, D.M. et al., A prospective, randomised double-blind crossover study to examine the efficacy of strontium-89 in pain palliation in patients with advanced prostate cancer metastatic to bone. Eur. J. Cancer 1991; 27: 954–958.
29. Porter, A.T., McEwan, A.J.B., Powe, J.E., Reid, R., McGowan, D.G. et al., Results of a randomised phase-III trial to evaluate the efficacy of strontium-89 adjuvant to local field external beam irradiation in the management of endocrine resistant metastatic prostate cancer. Int. J. Radiat. Oncol. Biol. Phys. 1993; 25: 805–813.

30. Ketring, A., Sm-153-EHDP and rhenium-186 HEDP as bone therapeutic radiopharmaceuticals. Int. J. Radiat. Appl. Instrum. [B]. 1987; 14: 223–232.
31. Turner, J.H., Claringbold, B.G., Heatherington, E.L., Sorby, P. and Martindal, A.A., A phase I study of samarium-153 ethylenediamenetetramethylene phosphonate therapy for disseminated skeletal metastases. J. Clin. Oncol. 1989; 7: 1926–1931.
32. O'Reilly, S.M., Richards, M.A. and Rubens, R.D., Liver metastases from breast cancer: the relationship between clinical, biochemical and pathological features and survival. Eur. J. Cancer 1990; 26: 574–577.
33. Clark, G.M., Sledge, G.W., Osborne, C.K. and McGuire, W.L., Survival from first recurrence: Relative importance of prognostic factors in 1,015 breast cancer patients. J. Clin. Oncol. 1987; 5: 55–61.
34. Smith, I.E., Harris, A.L., Morgan, M. et al., Tamoxifen versus aminoglutethimide in advanced breast carcinoma: a randomised cross-over trial. Br. Med. J. 1981; 283:1432–1434.
35. Van Veelen, H., Willemse, P.H.B., Tjabbes, T., Scweitzer, J.H. and Sleijfer, D.T., Oral high-dose medroxyprogesterone acetate versus tamoxifen. Cancer 1986; 58: 7–13.
36. Solowat, M.S., Newer methods of hormonal therapy for prostate cancer. Urology 1984; 24 (Suppl. 5): 30–38.
37. Mauriac, L., Coste, P., Richaud, P., Lamarche, P., Mage, P. and Bonichon, F., Clinical study of an LHRH agonist (ICI 118.630, Zoladex) in the treatment of prostatic cancer. Am. J. Clin. Oncol. 1988; 11: 8117–8119.
38. Sogani, P.C., Vagaiwala, M.R. and Whitmore, W.F. Jr., Experience with flutamide in patients with advanced prostatic cancer without prior endocrine therapy. Cancer 1984; 54: 744–750.
39. Williams, S.D., Birch, R., Einhorn, L.H. et al., Treatment of disseminated germ-cell tumours with cisplatin, bleomycin and either vinblastine or etoposide. N. Engl. J. Med. 1987; 316: 1435–1440.
40. Burckhardt, P., Thiebaud, D., Perey, L. et al., Treatment of tumour induced osteolysis by APD. Rec. Res. Cancer Res. 1989; 116: 54–66.
41. Grabelsky, S., Lipton, A., Harvey, H. et al., Pamidronate disodium (APD) — A dose-seeking study in patients with breast cancer. Proc. ASCO. 1991; 10: 42 (abstract 41).
42. Morton, A.R., Cantrill, A., Pillai, G.V. et al., Sclerosis of lytic bone metastases after disodium aminohydroxypropylidene bisphosphonate (APD) in patients with breast cancer. Br. Med. J. 1988; 297: 772–773.
43. Tyrell, C.J. on behalf of the Aredia Multinational Coopertise Group. Role of pamidronate in the management of bone metastases from breast cancer. Results of a non-comparative multicenter phase II trial. Am. Oncol. 1994; 5 (Suppl. 1): 37–40.
44. Clarke, N.W., Holbrook, I.B., McClure, J. et al., Osteoclast inhibition by pamidronate in metastatic prostate cancer: a preliminary study. Br. J. Cancer 1991; 63: 420–423.
45. Vorreuther, R., Biphosphonates as an adjunct to palliative therapy of bone metastases from prostatic carcinoma: a pilot study on clodronate. Br. J. Urol. 1993; 72: 792–795.
46. van Holten-Verzantvoort, A.T., Zwinderman, A.H., Aaronson, N.K. et al., The effect of supportive pamidronate treatment on aspects of quality of life with advanced breast cancer. Eur. J. Cancer 1991; 27: 544–549.
47. Elomaa, I., Blomqvist, C., Porrka, L. et al., Diphosphonates for osteolytic metastases. Lancet 1985; i: 1155–1156.
48. Merlini, G., Parrinello, G.A., Piccinini, L. et al., Long-term effects of parenteral dichloromethylene diphosphonate (Cl2MDP) on bone disease of myeloma patients treated with chemotherapy. Haematol. Oncol. 1990; 8: 23–30.
49. Smith, J.R., Palliation of painful bone metastases from prostate cancer using sodium etidronate: results of a randomized, prospective, double-blind, placebo-controlled study. J. Urol. 1989; 141; 85–87.
50. Millward, M.J., Cantwell, B.M.J., Carmichael, J. et al., A randomised trial of the addition of disodium pamidronate (APD) to endocrine therapy for advanced breast cancer with bone metastases. Proc. ASCO. 1991; 10: 42.
51. Hayward, J.L., Carbone, P.P., Heuson, J.C., Humaoka, S., Segaloff, A. and Rubens, R.D., Assessment of response to therapy in advanced breast cancer. Eur. J. Cancer 1977; 13: 89–95.
52. Howell, A., Mackintosh, J., Jones, M. et al., The definition of the "no change" category in patients treated with endocrine therapy and chemotherapy for advanced carcinoma of the breast. Eur. J. Cancer 1988; 24: 1567–1572.
53. Coleman, R.E., Assessment of response to treatment. In: Rubens, R.D. and Fogelman, I. (Editors), Bone metastases — diagnosis and treatment. Springer-Verlag, London, 1991; pp. 99–120.

54. Coleman, R.E., Whitaker, K.D., Moss, D.W., Mashiter, G., Fogelman, I. and Rubens, R.D., Biochemical monitoring predicts response in bone metastases to treatment. Br. J. Cancer 1988; 58: 205–210.
55. Campbell, F.C., Blamey, R.W., Woolfson, A.M.J. et al., Calcium excretion CaE in metastatic breast cancer. Br. J. Surg. 1983; 70: 202–204.
56. Coleman, R.E., Houston, S., James, I. et al., Preliminary results of the use of urinary excretion of pyridinium crosslinks for monitoring metastatic bone disease. Br. J. Cancer 1992; 65: 766–768.
57. Kymala, T., Tammela, L., Risteli, L., Risteli, J., Taube, T. and Elomaa, I., Evaluation of the effect of oral clodronate on skeletal metastases with type ! collagen metabolites. A controlled trial of the Finnish Prostate Group. Eur. J. Cancer 1993; 29A: 821–825.
58. Fisken, R.A., Heath, D.A. and Bold, A.M., Hypercalcaemia — a hospital survey. Q. J. Med. 1980; 196: 405–418.
59. Ralston, S.H., Gallacher, S.J., Patel, U. et al., Comparison of three intravenous bisphosphonates in cancer-associated hypercalcaemia. Lancet 1989; ii: 1180.
60. Fidler, M.W., Pathological fractures of the spine including those causing anterior spinal cord compression: surgical management. In: Noble, J. and Galasko, C.S.B. (Editors), Recent developments in orthopaedic surgery: Festschrift to Sir Harry Platt. Manchester University Press, Manchester, 1987; pp. 94–103.
61. Galasko, C.S.B., The role of the orthopaedic surgeon in the treatment of skeletal metastases. In: Rubens, R.D. and Fogelman, I. (Editors), Bone metastases — diagnosis and treatment. Springer-Verlag, London, 1991; pp. 207–222.
62. Siegal, T. and Siegal, T., Vertebral body resection for epidural compression by malignant tumours. Results of forty-seven consecutive operative procedures. J. Bone Joint Surg. [Am] 1981; 67: 375–382.

Bisphosphonate on bones
O. Bijvoet, H.A. Fleisch, R.E. Canfield and G. Russell (eds.)
© 1995 Elsevier Science B.V. All rights reserved.

CHAPTER 24

Bisphosphonate treatment of metastatic bone disease from breast cancer

A.T.M. van Holten-Verzantvoort

Department of Endocrinology and Metabolic Diseases, University Hospital, Leiden, The Netherlands

I. Bone metastases and breast cancer: a description

Breast cancer is the most frequent malignant tumour and the main cause of death due to malignancy in women in Western Europe, North America, Latin America and Australasia. In North America and Europe, women have a 1:12 chance of developing breast cancer before the age of 75 years [1, 2]. Metastatic breast cancer cannot be cured; even 20 years and more after treatment for primary breast cancer, there is still an excess risk of mortality [3, 4].

At the time of the first diagnosis of breast cancer, 1–2% of patients present with bone metastases [5, 6]. The prevalence increases sharply with more advanced stages of disease: in stage IV at least 70% of patients experience symptoms from bone metastases. Post-mortem bone metastases are found in about 85% of patients.

The skeleton is the most frequent first site of distant metastasis (25–47%), and the sole site in 15–27% of patients with a first manifestation of metastasis from breast cancer [7–9]. Bone metastases are more common in oestrogen receptor positive (ER-positive) tumours and in well-differentiated tumours [10–12].

Bone metastases are seldom the direct cause of death in advanced breast cancer [13]. Often, the disease runs a protracted clinical course, and palliative treatment is frequently required. Median survival after first recurrence in bone is 16–24 months, compared with 6–12 months after first recurrence in visceral sites and 25–47 months after first recurrence in soft tissue [7, 14, 15]. Survival may be longer in patients with osteoblastic metastases or with limited skeletal involvement [12, 16, 17], and may even extend to several years if the metastases remain confined to the skeleton [18, 19].

The main pathogenetic mechanism of metastasis to bone in breast cancer is osteoclastic resorption of the bone, which is then followed by tumour invasion. Several factors such as transforming growth factor α (TGF-α) [20, 21], prostaglandin [22, 23] and proteases [24] may be produced by breast cancer or associated cells and cause enhancement of osteoclastic bone resorption. Transforming growth factor β (TGFβ) [25] and insulin-like growth factor (IGF) [26], factors which stimulate bone formation (with or without inhibition of resorption) were also found associated with breast cancer. Parathyroid hormone-related protein (PTHrP) was considered to be of minor importance, but recent evidence strongly suggests that it may frequently be involved in the aetiology of hypercalcaemia [27–29] and bone metastases [30]. The net balance of simultaneously produced, tumour-derived bone-forming and bone-resorbing factors probably determines the predominant clinical features of osteolysis or sclerosis of untreated metastases.

Less frequently, other mechanisms may also be involved in metastasis to bone: in vitro experiments showed direct, osteoclast-independent, bone resorption by breast cancer cells [31].

The majority of the patients have osteolytic metastases; pure osteoblastic disease and mixed osteolytic/osteoblastic disease are found in about 10% and 30%, respectively, of cases. The metastases usually occur multifocally and localise preferentially in the axial skeleton, most often in the thoracolumbar spine, ribs and pelvis [12, 18, 32].

Morbidity is common. Pain, the dominant symptom, is experienced by 70% of patients. Pathological fractures of the long bones occur in 9–25% [7, 16, 19], vertebral collapse in the majority of patients [16]. Spinal cord compression is encountered in ±5% of patients. Breast cancer accounts for 50% of all cases of radiotherapy for bone pain, for 30–50% of the total incidence of pathological fractures and for about 20% of all episodes of spinal cord compression in cancer [19, 33–35].

Hypercalcaemia develops in 10–15% of patients with metastatic disease [7, 19, 32]. Usually a sign of rapidly progressive, extensive bone involvement, it most often occurs as a pre-terminal event [7, 16]. In about 15% of patients bone metastases are not evident and humoral factors, notably PTHrP, seem causally involved [28, 36, 37]. Hypercalcaemia may also occur as part of a flare reaction after initiation of endocrine therapy.

Patients with metastatic breast cancer cannot be cured, and the quality of their life is often adversely affected by the frequency and severity of related morbid events [38, 39]. Although a recent statistical overview suggested otherwise [40], survival does not seem to improve significantly in patients responding to treatment [41–43]. Therefore, treatment of bone metastases should aim primarily at optimal palliation of the symptoms and improvement of quality of life and functional status with minimal treatment-related toxicity and psychosocial discomfort.

Response rates for bone metastases to systemic treatment, by UICC/WHO criteria, are quite low compared with those for other metastatic sites. This may be explained by the insensitivity of the defined categories of response, which consider only objective radiological regression and sclerosis of metastatic lesions as signs of response [44–45]. Subjective response criteria are not included in the definition of response. Yet prompt relief of bone pain occurs about as often as objective regression at non-osseous sites [45–47].

It is beyond the scope of this chapter to discuss in detail the diverse therapeutic approaches of metastatic breast cancer; some comments will be made only.

Bone metastases usually occur multifocally and as part of widespread disease. Therefore, systemic cancer treatment is the most rational approach to controlling both morbidity and disease progression.

Endocrine treatment is preferred for patients with hormone-sensitive breast cancer. Pain relief is effectuated in about 50%. an objective response, i.e. radiological regression of bone metastases, occurs in 10–20%, but radiological stabilization is found in an additional 30% of patients [7, 48]. Only 10% of patients with hormone-insensitive breast cancer can be expected to respond to endocrine therapy [41, 49, 50]. Tamoxifen, a synthetic anti-oestrogen, is the treatment of choice, at least for post-menopausal women [51].

Several chemotherapeutic regimens may be employed. The efficacy of combination chemotherapy is superior to that of single-agent therapy. In comparative studies, adriamycin-type combinations tended to yield slightly better response rates than CMF-type (cyclophosphamide, methotrexate, fluorouracil) combinations, but the toxicity was higher for the former [42, 43, 51]. Most patients experience relief of bone pain; an objective response in bone is reported in 15–35% of patients, and in about 45% the metastatic bone disease stabilises [43, 52]. Patients with only bone metastases respond more often to first line chemotherapy and for longer periods of time [18, 53].

Surgery, radiotherapy and radioisotope therapy may effectively control bone pain, pathological fractures and spinal cord compression. However, the former two measures are best suited for the management of one or a limited number of bone metastases. Half-body irradiation, effective pain therapy in case of multiple sites of symptomatic bone metastases, is associated with serious toxicity [32, 33]. Radioisotope therapy is gaining attention. Currently, several new drugs with a more favourable therapeutic index are being investigated [32].

Clearly, palliative care for morbidity due to bone metastases from breast cancer is far from optimal with the therapies currently available. It is worthwhile to continue the search for therapies that effectively control symptoms and progression of bone metastases without increasing toxicity. Recent investigations indicate that bisphosphonates may be valuable tools here.

II. Palliative treatment of bone metastases from breast cancer with bisphosphonates

Inhibition of tumour-induced bone resorption has been documented in vitro [54, 55] and in in vivo animal models [56–60]. Bisphosphonates have no effect on tumour growth [57–60]. They do not interfere with the anti-tumour activity of chemotherapeutic agents or host immunity [57].

The potent in vivo inhibition of malignancy-induced osteoclastic bone resorption supports the application of bisphosphonates in malignant diseases. The first publication in 1979 on the treatment of tumour-induced hypercalcaemia was actually also the first to describe inhibition of tumour-induced osteolysis in normocalcaemic patients [61]. It raised considerable interest in the treatment and/or prevention of bone metastases.

Two therapeutic strategies may be considered.

Episodes of severe symptoms, for example, tumour-induced hypercalcaemia, require rapid and maximal *suppression* of bone destruction. This may be achieved with high-dose bisphosphonate therapy because the initial rate of suppression of osteoclastic bone resorption is clearly dose-dependent [62]. The efficacy of suppressive treatment can be assessed by the prompt reversal of deranged clinical symptoms, as has repeatedly been shown in hypercalcaemia studies [63, 64]. If the bisphosphonate therapy is then continued, the suppression of resorption reaches a plateau level. The level of this plateau, and consequently also of the suppression of normal bone turnover, is again dose-dependent [62]. In principle, therefore, high-dose therapy should be of short duration to avoid long-term disturbances of normal bone remodelling or mineralisation.

However, many breast cancer patients with bone metastases, although incurable, survive for a long period of time. During this period, tumour-induced osteolysis, unopposed by bone formation, will persist, and the patients will continue to develop new bone metastases and to suffer from related morbidity. In these patients treatment should aim at *prevention* of disease progression and skeletal morbidity. This implies long-term bisphosphonate treatment, during which a balance must be found between preservation of normal bone integrity and remodelling on the one hand and inhibition of the pathological bone resorption on the other. During preventive treatment, the efficacy will therefore depend on the choice of bisphosphonate and the dose and duration of treatment as well as on the continuous driving force of metastatic osteolysis. A complicating factor is the lack of objective, sensitive and reproducible response criteria for bone metastases to treatment.

Since 1979, several publications have appeared, and evidence is accumulating that bisphosphonates are potentially powerful instruments for the treatment of established metastatic bone disease.

1. Etidronate

Few data on etidronate treatment of bone metastases in humans have been published; most studies concerned the treatment of hypercalcaemia. The well-documented impaired mineralisation noted during etidronate treatment makes this drug unfit for continuous long-term use. Moreover, two double-blind studies of patients suffering from multiple myeloma and prostatic cancer revealed no improvement in morbidity due to bone metastases during treatment with etidronate [65, 66].

2. Clodronate

More studies have been performed with clodronate. A beneficial effect on bone pain was shown for patients with multiple myeloma in a placebo-controlled cross-over study [67]. Since then, several open and placebo-controlled studies in breast cancer patients have been carried out (often, patients with other malignancies were also enrolled in the studies).

The drug was usually given orally, in daily doses of 1200–3200 mg. In two studies parenteral (intravenous and intramuscular) treatment preceded oral treatment [68, 69]; once a single 600-mg infusion was given in a placebo-controlled, cross-over design [70]. Clodronate therapy was added as a supplement to cancer therapy; in one study clodronate was administered as monotherapy in the initial parenteral phase [68]. In two studies the patients were treated long-term (1–3 years) [71, 72]; in the others treatment was limited to ≤ 4 months.

During clodronate therapy bone resorption decreased [67, 68, 70–73] and the calcium balance improved [69].

Skeletal morbidity decreased during clodronate therapy. Overall, a significant bone-pain-reducing effect was found for 60–85% of breast cancer patients [68, 70, 71, 73].

The two placebo-controlled, long-term studies, containing 34 [71, 74] and 174 patients [72], revealed also significant effects on other parameters of skeletal morbidity. Episodes of hypercalcaemia were reduced by 45–75% [71, 72]. A decrease of 70% in radiotherapy episodes for bone pain and pathological fractures was found in one study [71]; in the other study, although the prevalence of vertebral fractures decreased significantly by 35%, fractures of long bones occurred as often as in the placebo-treated control group [72]. A deceleration of the rate of radiological progression of bone metastases was found in the former study [71]. The longer survival found for clodronate-treated patients in one study [74] seemed to be due mainly to the prevention of severe hypercalcaemic periods in these patients compared with controls. This positive effect was not confirmed by the other long-term study [72].

Long-term clodronate treatment proved to be free of serious side-effects [68, 71, 72]. Patients suffering from osteoblastic metastases seemed prone to a transient hypocalcaemia after the start of clodronate treatment [68].

3. Alendronate

Preliminary results of a short-term trial revealed inhibition of bone resorption and a reduction in bone pain in the majority of patients during intravenous alendronate therapy. Compared with clodronate, alendronate seemed more potent [75].

Table 1 summarizes the results of treatment of osteolytic metastases from breast cancer with clodronate and alendronate.

4. Pamidronate

The first study describing pamidronate-induced inhibition of bone resorption in osteolytic metastases in normocalcaemic patients [61] generated clinical studies to assess the palliative benefit of pamidronate treatment of metastatic bone disease. Most studies consisted of breast cancer patients, some included also other types of

Table 1.

Palliative bisphosphonate treatment of metastatic bone disease in patients with breast cancer

N	Study[a] type	Dose(mg)	Oral/i.v.	Duration	Response[b] clinical	radiological	Ref.
Clodronate							
10	p	3200/day	oral	8+8 weeks cross-over	+	n.r.	[73]
24[c]	p	600	i.v. cross-over	1 infusion	+	n.r.	[70]
59[c]	o	1200/day[d]	oral	3 months	+	n.r.	[68]
34	p	1600/day	oral	12 months	+	+	[71, 74]
173	p	1600/day	oral	3 years	+	n.r.	[72]
Alendronate							
12[c]	o	2.5/day	i.v.	5 days	+	n.r.	[75]

[a] p = double blind placebo controlled, o = open, controlled.
[b] n.r.: not reported. Clinical response: favourable effects on bone pain, hypercalcaemia, (symptomatic impending) pathological fractures and/or treatment for bone metastases. Radiological response: regression of lytic lesions.
[c] Other tumour types were also included.
[c] Parenteral loading preceded oral treatment.

malignancy. Two studies were performed in a non-placebo controlled, randomized fashion [76, 77]; the others were open non-controlled. The treatment schedules employed varied considerably in dose and duration. In all studies except three [76, 78, 79], pamidronate was given intravenously.

Pamidronate therapy (oral and intravenous) had a significant, favourable effect on biochemical parameters of increased bone resorption [78–83].

Various regimens of intravenous pamidronate therapy have been used: 90 mg single infusion [84], 30 mg/2 weeks [85], 60 mg/2 weeks [80], 60 mg/4 weeks for 4 cycles followed by 60 mg/3 months [86] or 30 mg/week for 4 cycles and thereafter 30 mg fortnightly [78]. Objective radiological regression or stabilization of bone metastases with a good response of bone pain and improved mobility was found for 25% [78] to 55% of patients [84–86], and quality of life improved [84] (preliminary results in [80]). However, there appeared to be no correlation between the analgesic efficacy of pamidronate and objective radiological improvement [78].

Dosage studies suggested a dose-dependent effect of intravenous treatment on bone pain [81, 82, 87], radiological response [81] and quality of life [82, 87]. The lowest effective dose seemed to be >15 mg/week [82, 87]. A dose-dependent efficacy on biochemical parameters of bone resorption remains to be established [82, 83].

Most of the above-mentioned studies were conducted with pamidronate as monotherapy, some in combination with tumour treatment. In two studies standard tumour treatment was administered together with pamidronate. Refractory bone metastases from breast cancer improved as far as bone pain (all patients) and radiological extent of disease (70% of patients) were concerned during a combined course of pamidronate 60 mg/2 weeks intravenously and chemotherapy (epirubicin) [88]. During standard endocrine therapy (aminogluthetimide with hydrocortisone) with or without intravenous pamidronate 30 mg/3 weeks, no additional effect on morbidity due to bone metastases, attributable to pamidronate, was found. However, the pamidronate dose was very low, and this study is continuing with higher doses of pamidronate [77].

Parenteral pamidronate was well tolerated; there was only an occasional occurrence of local phlebitis, transient pyrexia or asymptomatic hypocalcaemia.

Overall, the studies, except one [77], followed the suppressive approach in an attempt to treat severe symptoms and achieve objective healing of bone metastases which generally were resistant to tumour treatment. However, most of these studies were open and uncontrolled, no specific regimen has been studied systematically, and treatment schedules have not been compared sufficiently to allow accurate definition of an optimal therapeutic regimen.

As argued at the beginning of this section, the long-term prevention of morbidity and new bone metastases in patients suffering from a disease like metastatic breast cancer, which is incurable but characterised by prolonged survival, implies long-term treatment, possibly extending over several years. In the 'intravenous' suppression studies, pamidronate was well tolerated, but durations exceeded 9 months only in a few cases. It is, however, conceivable that the quality of life for these patients might be impaired by intermittent parenteral drug administration over long periods of time. The only study cited above, which was designed as a 'prevention' study, limited the number of infusions on an outpatient basis to 12 [77].

One study reported on long-term, preventive, oral treatment in breast cancer patients.

This prospective study, median follow-up 18 to 21 months, contained 161 patients. It was performed in a non-placebo controlled, randomized fashion. Eighty-one patients were treated with 300 mg pamidronate per day (but 600 mg/day in the early phase of the study), which was added to unrestricted cancer treatment [76, 89]. Skeletal morbidity was significantly less in pamidronate-treated patients in comparison with control patients. Hypercalcaemia periods decreased by 65%. Reductions in episodes of severe bone pain, impending pathological fractures and therapeutic interventions (systemic treatment or radiotherapy) for osteolytic metastases were also significant but less pronounced: 30–50%. The effects of pamidronate were gradual in onset but persistent over time. A significant favourable effect on some aspects of quality of life, bone pain and mobility impairment was found [90]. However, both the radiological course of skeletal disease, assessed by the freedom-from-progression period, and overall survival were comparable in both groups. The unintended, but (due to gastrointestinal intolerance) necessary dose reduction in the early phase of the study allowed an analysis of effects of different doses. As for the intravenous treatment, a dose/effect relationship was suggested for clinical effects and quality of life improvement. It also became evident that the tolerance for oral pamidronate, at least of some galenic forms, is limited to doses of about 300 mg/day in patients in whom many cancer-related factors contribute also to gastrointestinal toxicity. This was confirmed in other studies [79].

Table 2 summarizes the studies of pamidronate treatment of osteolytic metastases from breast cancer.

Table 2.

Palliative bisphosphonate treatment of metastatic bone disease in patients with breast cancer: continued

N	Study[a] type	Dose(mg)	Oral/ i.v.	Duration	Response[b] clinical	radiological	Ref.
Pamidronate: suppressive treatment							
28	n	30/2 weeks	i.v.	variable[c]	+	+	[85]
25	n	30/2 weeks to 90/4 weeks	i.v.	variable[c]	+[d]	+[d]	[81]
22	n	30/week +30/2 weeks	i.v. i.v.	4 weeks 6 months	+	+	[78]
20	n	90	i.v.	1 infusion	+	+	[84]
22	n	60/2 weeks	i.v.	6 months	+	n.r.	[80]
34	n	30/4 weeks to 90/2 weeks	i.v.	variable[c]	+[d]	n.r.	[87]
20	n	60/2 weeks +standard chemotherapy	i.v.	6 months	+	+	[88]
28[e]	n	60/month +60/3 months	i.v. i.v.	4 months variable[c]	+	+	[86]
23[e]	o	60/3 weeks vs. 90/3 weeks	i.v. i.v.	variable[c] variable[c]	+[d]	n.r.	[82]
Pamidronate: preventive treatment							
82	o	30/3 weeks +standard endocrine treatment	i.v.	9 months	−	−	[77]
161	o	600 → 300/day	oral	lifelong	+[d]	−	[90,76]

[a] o = open, controlled; n = open, not controlled.
[b] n.r.= not reported. Clinical response: favourable effects on bone pain, hypercalcaemia, (symptomatic impending) pathological fractures and/or treatment for bone metastases. Radiological response: regression of lytic lesions.
[c] Duration not predetermined; usually treatment continued until disease progression.
[d] A dose-dependent efficacy was suggested.
[e] Other tumour types were also included.

III. Conclusion

Overall, the various studies indicate that bisphosphonates are potentially powerful tools in the battle against metastatic bone disease from breast cancer. Although the patients often suffered from advanced stages of metastatic bone disease which were refractory to tumour treatment, a response to bisphosphonate treatment in terms of relief of bone pain (generally in ≥50% of patients), reduction in periods of hypercalcaemia, (impending) pathological fractures and morbidity-related therapeutic interventions, and even of radiological regression of bone metastases was found.

The toxicity was limited. Clodronate was generally well tolerated. Tolerance of oral pamidronate was limited to low doses; intravenous pamidronate proved to be safe and non-toxic at pharmacological doses, even in doses well above the maximum tolerated oral dose.

However, the therapeutic efficacy of bisphosphonate treatment in the various studies was far from complete. The patient populations were heterogeneous, and generally the metastatic bone disease was well advanced. No one treatment was studied systematically, schedules were not compared, and the duration of treatment was often short. A dose-dependency for the effects, in particular for pamidronate, was suggested. Clearly, further research is mandatory to define the optimal treatment strategy and to improve treatment benefit. To this end it is of importance to distinguish suppressive and preventive approaches in the treatment of metastatic bone disease because they may differ in the choice of bisphosphonate, dose, duration and mode of administration.

The development of new bisphosphonates is of major significance. Treatment of tumour-induced hypercalcaemia with dimethyl-APD (both oral and intravenous) [91, 92], methylpentylaminopropylidene bisphosphonate (BM 21.0955) [93] and alendronate [94, 95] was found to be very efficaceous and non-toxic. The better therapeutic index of the parenteral and oral forms of these third-generation bisphosphonates may improve treatment efficacy in a convenient way.

Finally, one could consider 'preventive' therapy started some steps earlier in the treatment of those breast cancer patients who are at high risk of developing bone metastases. Data from in vivo studies suggest that prophylactic treatment with clodronate in metastases-free animals protects the skeleton against tumour-induced osteolysis [96]. This seems to be supported by preliminary findings from a human study [97]. However, there is certainly until now no convincing evidence about the potential benefit of long-term bisphosphonate treatment for metastases-free patients in terms of a delay or complete prevention of the development of bone metastases. Data from a few studies addressing this issue are expected to come up soon.

References

1. Tomatis, L., Cancer: causes, occurrence and control. (Scientific Publications no. 100) IARC, 1990.
2. Miller, A.B., Breast cancer epidemiology, etiology and prevention. In: Harris J.R., Hellman S., Henderson, I.C. and Kinne, D.W. (Editors), Breast diseases. Lippincott, Philadelphia, 1987; pp. 87–102.
3. Harris, J.R. and Henderson, I.C. Natural history and staging of breast cancer. In: Harris, J.R., Hellman, S., Henderson, I.C. and Kinne, D.W. (Editors), Breast diseases. Lippincott, Philadelphia, 1987; pp. 87–102.
4. Haybittle J.L., Curability of breast cancer. Br. Med. Bull. 1990; 47: 319–323.
5. Perez, D.J., Powles, T.J., Milan, J., et al., Detection of breast carcinoma metastases in bone: relative merits of X-rays and skeletal scintigraphy. Lancet 1983; ii: 613–616.
6. Rossing, N., Munck, O., Pors Nielsen, S. and West Andersen, K., What do early bone scans tell about breast cancer patients. Eur. J. Cancer Clin. Oncol. 1982; 18: 629-36.
7. Coleman, R.E. and Rubens, R.D., The clinical course of bone metastases from breast cancer. Br. J. Cancer 1987; 55: 61–66.
8. Kamby, C., Vejborg, I., Daugaard, S., et al., Clinical and radiologic characteristics of bone metastases in breast cancer. Cancer 1987; 60: 2524–2531.
9. Lee, Y.-T.M., Patterns of metastasis and natural courses of breast carcinoma. Cancer Metastasis Rev. 1985; 4: 153–172.
10. Lee, Y.-T.M., Correlation of estrogen receptor with site of recurrence or metastasis and breast cancer prognosis. Breast 1984; 10: 27–31.
11. Campbell, F.C., Blamey, R.W., Elston, C.W., Nicholson, R.I., Griffiths, K. and Haybittle, J.L., Oestrogen-receptor status and sites of metastasis in breast cancer. Br J Cancer 1981; 44: 456-9.

12. Kamby, C., Bruun Rasmussen, B. and Kristensen, B., Oestrogen receptor status of primary breast carcinomas and their metastases. Relation to pattern of spread and survival after recurrence. Br. J. Cancer 1989; 60: 252–257.

13. Hagemeister, F.B., Buzdar, A.U., Luna, M.A. and Blumenschein, G.R., Causes of death in breast cancer: a clinicopathologic study. Cancer 1980; 46: 162–167.

14. Clark, G.M., Sledge, G.W., Osborne, C.K. and McGuire, W.L., Survival from first recurrence: Relative importance of prognostic factors in 1015 breast cancer patients. J. Clin. Oncol. 1987; 5: 55–61.

15. Kamby, C., Ejlertsen, B., Andersen, J., et al., The pattern of metastases in human breast cancer. Influence of systemic adjuvant therapy and impact on survival. Acta Oncol. 1988; 27: 715–719.

16. Paterson, A.H.G., Bone metastases in breast cancer, prostate cancer and myeloma. Bone 1987; 8 Suppl. 1: S17–S22.

17. Vincent, M.D., Powles, T.J., Ashley, S., et al. An analysis of possible prognostic features of long term and short term survivors of metastatic breast cancer. Eur. J. Cancer Clin. Oncol. 1986; 22: 1059–1065.

18. Scheid, V., Buzdar, A.U., Smith, T.L. and Hortobagyi, G.N., Clinical course of breast cancer patients with osseous metastases treated with combination chemotherapy. Cancer 1986; 58: 2589–2593.

19. Sherry, M.M., Greco, F.A., Johnson, D.H. and Hainsworth, J.D., Breast cancer with skeletal metastases at initial diagnosis: distinctive clinical characteristics and favorable prognosis. Cancer 1986; 58: 178–182.

20. Ciardiello, F., Kim, N., McGeady, M.L., et al., Expression of transforming growth factor alpha (TGFα) in breast cancer. Ann. Oncol. 1991; 2: 169–182.

21. Derynck, R., Transforming growth factor α. Cell 1988; 54: 593–595.

22. Bringhurst, F.R., Bierer, B.E., Godeau, F., Neyhard, N., Varner, V. and Segre, G.V., Humoral hypercalcemia of malignancy. J. Clin. Invest. 1986; 77: 456–464.

23. Valentin-Opran, A., Eilon, G., Saez, S. and Mundy, G.R., Estrogens and antiestrogens stimulate release of bone resorbing activity by cultured human breast cancer cells. J. Clin. Invest. 1985; 75: 726–731.

24. Danø, K., Andreasen, P.A., Grøndahl-Hansen, J., Kristensen, P., Nielsen, L.S. and Skriver, L., Plasminogen activators, tissue degradation, and cancer. Adv. Cancer Res. 1985; 44: 139–266.

25. Knabbe, C., Lippman, M.E., Wakefield, L.M., et al., Evidence that transforming growth factor-β is a hormonally regulated negative growth factor in human breast cancer cells. Cell 1987; 48: 417–428.

26. Huff, K.K., Kaufman, D., Gabbay, K.H., Spencer, E.M., Lippman, M.E. and Dickson, R.B., Secretion of an insulin-like growth factor-1-related protein by human breast cancer cells. Cancer Res. 1986; 46: 4613–4619.

27 Burtis, W.J., Wu, T., Bunch, C., Wysolmerski, J.J., Insogna, K.L., Weir, E.C., et al., Identification of a novel 17,000-dalton parathyroid hormone-like adenylate cyclase-stimulating protein from a tumour associated with humoral hypercalcemia of malignancy. J. Biol. Chem. 1987; 262: 7151–7156.

28. Grill, V., Ho, P., Body, J.J., et al., Parathyroid hormone-related protein: elevated levels in both humoral hypercalcemia of malignancy and hypercalcemia complicating metastatic breast cancer. J. Clin. Endocrinol. Metab. 1991; 73: 1309–1315.

29. Southby, J., Kissin, M.W., Danks, J.A., et al., Immunohistochemical localization of parathyroid hormone-like protein in human breast cancer. Cancer Res. 1990; 50: 7710–7716.

30. Powell, G.J., Southby, J., Danks, J.A., et al., Localization of parathyroid hormone related protein in breast cancer metastases: increased incidence in bone compared with other sites. Cancer Res. 1991; 51: 3059–3061.

31. Eilon, G. and Mundy, G.R., Direct resorption of bone by human breast cancer cells in vitro. Nature 1978; 276: 726–728.

32. Nielsen, O.S., Munro, A.J. and Tannock, I.A., Bone metastases: Pathofysiology and management policy. J. Clin. Oncol. 1991; 9: 509–524.

33. Hoskin, P.J. and Hanks, G.W., Bone pain. Baillières Clin. Oncol. 1987; 1: 399–416.

34. Ford, H.T. and Yarnold, J.R., Radiation therapy — pain relief, and recalcification. In: Stoll, B.A. and Parbhoo, S. (Editors), Bone metastases: monitoring and treatment, Raven, New York, 1983: 343–354.

35. Sørensen, P.S., Børgesen, S.E., Rohde, K., et al., Metastatic epidural spinal cord compression. Results of treatment and survival. Cancer 1990; 65: 1502–1508.

36. Coleman, R.E., Fogelman, I. and Rubens, R.D., Hypercalcaemia and breast cancer — an increased humoral component in patients with liver metastases. Eur. J. Surg. Oncol. 1988; 14: 423–428.

37. Henderson, J.E., Shustik, C., Kremer, R., Rabbani, S.A., Hendy, G.N. and Goltzman, D., Circulating

concentrations of parathyroid hormone-like peptide in malignancy and in hyperparathyroidism. J. Bone Miner. Res. 1990; 5: 105–113.

38. Rubens, R.D., Towlson, K.E., Ramirez, A.J., et al., Appropriate chemotherapy for palliating advanced cancer. Br. Med. J. 1992; 304: 35–40.

39. de Koning, H.J., van Ineveld, B.M., de Haes, J.C.J.M., van Ootmarsum, G.J., Klijn, J.G.M. and van der Maas, P.J., Advanced breast cancer and its prevention by screening. Br. J. Cancer 1992; 65: 950–955.

40. A'Hern, R.P., Ebbs, S.R. and Baum, M.B., Does chemotherapy improve survival in advanced breast cancer? A statistical overview. Br. J. Cancer 1988; 57: 615–618.

41. Henderson, I.C., Hayes, D.F., Come, S., Harris, J.R. and Canellos, G., New agents and new medical treatments for advanced breast cancer. Semin. Oncol. 1987; 14: 34–64.

42. Coates, A., Gebski ,V., Bishop, J.F., et al., Improving the quality of life during chemotherapy for advanced breast cancer. N. Engl. J. Med. 1987; 317: 1490–1495.

43. Marsoni, S., Hurson, S. and Eisenberger, M., Chemotherapy of bone metastases. In: Garattini S, editor. Bone resorption, metastasis and diphosphonates. Raven, New York, 1985: 181–194.

44. Whitehouse, J.M.A., Site-dependent response to chemotherapy for carcinoma of the breast. J. R. Soc. Med. 1985; 78 Suppl. 9: 18–22.

45. Coombes, R.C., Dady, P., Parsons, C., et al., Assessment of response of bone metastases to systemic treatment in patients with breast cancer. Cancer 1983; 52: 610–614.

46. Coleman, R.E. and Rubens, R.D., Bone metastases and breast cancer. Cancer Treat. Rev. 1985; 12: 251–270.

47. Russell, J.R., Cytotoxic therapy — pain relief and recalcification. In: Stoll, B.A. and Parbhoo, S. (Editors), Bone metastases: monitoring and treatment. Raven, New York, 1983: 355–368.

48. Cocconi, G., Bisagni, G., Ceci, G., et al., Low-dose aminogluthetimide with and without hydrocortisone replacement as a first-line endocrine treatment in advanced breast cancer: a prospective randomized trial of the Italian Oncology Group for Clinical Research. J. Clin. Oncol. 1992; 10: 984–989.

49. Rose, C. and Mouridsen, H.T., Preferred sequence of endocrine therapies in advanced breast cancer. In: Santen, R.J. and Juhos, E. (Editors), Endocrine-dependent breast cancer: critical assessment of recent advances. Huber, Bern, 1988: 81–91.

50. Smith, I.E., Macaulay, V., Comparison of different endocrine therapies in the management of bone metastases from breast cancer. J. R. Soc. Med. 1985; 78 Suppl. 9: 15–17.

51. Monfardini, S., Brunner, K., Crowther, D., et al. (Editors), UICC manual of adult and paedriatic medical oncology. Springer, Heidelberg, 1987.

52. Tranum, B.L., McDonald, B., Thigpen, T., et al., Adriamycin combinations in advanced breast cancer. Cancer 1982; 49: 835–839.

53. Smalley, R., Mayer-Scogna, D. and Malmud, L., Prolonged response to chemotherapy (CAF) in patients with metastases to bone only in stage 4 breast cancer. Proc. Am. Assoc. Cancer Res. 1979; 20: 347–348.

54. Jung, A., Mermillod, B., Barras, C., Baud, M. and Courvoisier, B., Inhibition by two diphosphonates of bone lysis in tumor conditioned media. Cancer Res. 1981; 41: 3233–3237.

55. Galasko, C.S.B., Samuel, A.W., Rushton, S. and Lacey, E., The effect of prostaglandin synthesis inhibitors and diphosphonates on tumour-mediated osteolysis. Br. J. Surg. 1980; 67: 493–496.

56. Jung, W., Bornand, J., Mermillod, B., Edouard, C. and Meunier, P.J., Inhibition by diphosphonates of bone resorption induced by the Walker tumor of the rat. Cancer Res. 1984; 44: 3007–3011.

57. Guaitani, A., Polentarutti, N., Fillipeschi, S., et al., Effects of disodium etidronate in murine tumor models. Eur. J. Cancer Clin. Oncol. 1984; 20: 685–693.

58. Guaitani, A., Sabatini, M., Coccioli, G., Cristina, S., Garattini, S. and Bartošek, I., An experimental rat model of local bone cancer invasion and its responsiveness to ethane-1-hydroxy-1, 1-bisphosphonate. Cancer Res. 1985; 45: 2206–2209.

59. Radl, J., Croese, J.W., Zurcher, C., et al., Influence of treatment with APD-bisphosphonate on the bone lesions in the mouse 5T2 multiple myeloma. Cancer 1985; 55: 1030–1040.

60. Krempien, B., Wingen, F., Eichmann, T., Müller, M. and Schmähl, D., Protective effects of a prophylactic treatment with the bisphosphonate 3-amino-1-hydroxypropane-1,1-bisphosphonic acid on the development of tumor osteopathies in the rat: experimental studies with the Walker carcinosarcoma. Oncol. 1988; 45: 41–46.

61. van Breukelen, F.J.M., Bijvoet, O.L.M., van Oosterom, A.T., Inhibition of osteolytic bone lesions by (3-amino-1-hydroxypropylidene)-1,1-bisphosphonate (APD). Lancet 1979; i: 803–805.

62. Reitsma, P.H., Bijvoet, O.L.M., Verlinden-Ooms, H. and van der Wee-Pals, L.J.A., Kinetic studies

of bone and mineral metabolism during treatment with (3-amino-1-hydroxypropylidene)-1,1-bis-phosphonate (APD) in rats. Calcif. Tissue Int. 1980; 32: 145–157.

63. Harinck, H.I.J., Bijvoet, O.L.M., Planting, A.S.T., et al., Role of bone and kidney in tumor-induced hypercalcaemia and treatment with bisphosphonate and sodium chloride. Am. J. Med. 1987; 82: 1133–1142.
64. Kanis, J.A., McCloskey, E.V., O'Rourke, N., et al., Bisphosphonates in the management of hyper-calcaemia of malignancy. In: Russel, R.G.G. and Kanis, J.A. (Editors), Tumour-induced hypercal-caemia and its management. Royal Society of Medicine Services, London, 1991; pp. 59–70.
65. Belch, A.R., Bergsagel, D.E., Wilson, K., O'Reilly, S., Wilson, J., Sutton, D., et al., Effect of daily etidronate on the osteolysis of multiple myeloma. J. Clin. Oncol. 1991; 9: 1397–1402.
66. Smith, J.A., Palliation of painful bone metastases from prostate cancer using sodium etidronate: results of a randomized, prospective double-blind placebo controlled study. J. Urol. 1989; 141: 85–87.
67. Siris, E.S., Sherman, W.H., Baquiran, D.C., Schlattern, J.P., Osserman, E.F. and Canfield, R.E., Ef-fects of dichloromethylene disphosphonate on skeletal mobilization of calcium in multiple myeloma. N. Engl. J. Med. 1980; 302: 310–315.
68. Francini, G., Gonnelli, S., Petrioli, R., Conti, F., Paffetti, P. and Gennari, C., Treatment of bone metastases with dichloromethylene bisphosphonate. J. Clin. Oncol. 1992; 10: 591–598.
69. Jung, A., Chantraine, A., Donath, A., et al., Use of dichloromethylene diphosphonate in metastatic bone disease. N. Engl. J. Med. 1983; 308: 1499–1501.
70. Paterson, A.H.G., Ernst, D.S., Powles, T.J., Ashley, S., McCloskey, E.V. and Kanis, J.A., Treatment of skeletal disease in breast cancer with clodronate. Bone 1991; 12 Suppl. 1: S25–S30.
71. Elomaa, I., Blomqvist, C., Gröhn, P., et al., Long-term controlled trial with diphosphonate in patients with osteolytic bone metastases. Lancet 1983; i: 146–149.
72. Paterson, A.H.G., Powles, T.J., Kanis, J.A., McCloskey, E., Hanson, J. and Ashley, S., Double-blind controlled trial of oral clodronate in patients with bone metastases from breast cancer. J. Clin. Oncol. 1993; 11: 59–65.
73. Siris, E.S., Hyman, G.A. and Canfield, R.E., Effects of dichloromethylene diphosphonate in women with breast carcinoma metastatic to the skeleton. Am. J. Med. 1983; 74: 401–406.
74. Elomaa, I., Blomqvist, C., Porkka, L., et al., Diphosphonates for osteolytic metastases. Lancet 1985; i: 1155–1156.
75. Attardo-Parrinello, G., Merlini, G., Pavesi, F., Crema, F., Fiorentini, M.L. and Ascari, E., Effects of a new aminodiphosphonate (aminohydroxybutylidene diphosphonate) in patients with osteolytic lesions from metastases and myelomatosis. Arch. Intern. Med. 1987; 147: 1629–1633.
76. van Holten-Verzantvoort, A.T.M., Kroon, H.M., Bijvoet, O.L.M., et al., Palliative pamidronate (APD) treatment in patients with bone metastases from breast cancer. J. Clin. Oncol. 1993; 11: 491–498.
77. Millward, M.J., Cantwell, B.M.J., Carmichael, J. and Harris, A.L., A randomised trial of the addition of disodium pamidronate (APD) to endocrine therapy for advanced breast cancer with bone metastases. Proc. Asco. 1991; 10: 421.
78. Dodwell, D.J., Howell, A., Morton, A., Daley-Yates, P.T. and Hoggarth, C.R., Pamidronate (APD) treatment of skeletal metastases from breast cancer. In: Rubens, R.D. (Editor), The management of bone metastases and hypercalcaemia by osteoclast inhibition. Huber, Toronto, 1990: pp. 62–75.
79. Coleman, R.E., Dirix, L.Y., Dodwell, D., et al., Phase I/II evaluation of effervescent and enteric coated oral pamidronate for bone metastases. Eur. J. Cancer 1991; 27: 945–946.
80. Bachouchi, M., Bruning, P.F., Soukop, M., et al., Intravenous pamidronate (APD) in the treatment of osteolytic metastases of breast cancer — preliminary results of a multicentre study. In: Bijvoet, O.L.M. and Lipton, A. (Editors), Osteoclast inhibition in the management of malignancy-related bone disorders. Hogrefe and Huber, Lewiston, 1991: pp. 38–44.
81. Lipton, A., Glover, D., Harvey, H., et al., Disodium pamidronate (APD) — a dose seeking study in patients with breast and prostate cancer: preliminary report. In: Bijvoet, O.L.M. and Lipton, A. (Editors). Osteoclast inhibition in the management of malignancy-related bone disorders. Hogrefe and Huber, Lewiston, 1991: 33–37.
82. Radziwill, A.J. and Thürlimann, B., Significant improvement of quality of life in patients with malignancy-related bone disease and bone pain after high dose pamidronate: a randomized dose finding study. Ann. Oncol. 1992; 3 Suppl. 5: A725.
83. Body, J.J., Dumon, J.C., Magritte, A., et al., Pamidronate for bone metastases: a biochemical dose-response study. Eur. J. Cancer. 1991; 27 Suppl. 2: S292.
84. Hacking, A., Gudgeon, C.A., McNaughton, D. and Dent, D.M., Pamidronate (APD) as single

infusion monotherapy in the treatment of bone metastases from breast cancer. In: Bijvoet, O.L.M. and Lipton, A. (Editors), Osteoclast inhibition in the management of malignancy-related bone disorders. Hogrefe and Huber, Lewiston, 1991: 45–53.

85. Coleman, R.E., Woll, P.J., Miles, H., Scrivener, W. and Rubens, R.D., Treatment of bone metastases from breast cancer with (3-amino-1-hydroxypropylidene)-1,1-bisphosphonate (APD). Br. J. Cancer 1988; 58: 621–625.

86. Thiebaud, D., Leyvraz, S., von Fliedner, V., et al., Treatment of bone metastases from breast cancer and myeloma with pamidronate. Eur. J. Cancer 1991; 27: 37–41.

87. Thürlimann, B. and Morant, R., Pamidronate for osteolytic bone metastases: is there a dose effect? Eur. J. Cancer 1991; 27 Suppl. 2: S284.

88. Panagos, G., Boukis, H., Papadakou, M., et al., Treatment of extensive bone metastasis due to refractory breast cancer with combination of disodium palmidronate and epirubicin. Ann. Oncol. 992; 3 Suppl. 5: A352.

89. van Holten-Verzantvoort, A.T., Bijvoet, O.L.M., Cleton, F.J., et al., Reduced morbidity from skeletal metastases in breast cancer patients during long-term bisphosphonate (APD) treatment. Lancet 1987; ii: 983–985.

90. van Holten-Verzantvoort, A.T.M., Zwinderman, A.H. and Aaronson, N.K., et al., The effect of supportive pamidronate treatment on aspects of quality of life of patients with advanced breast cancer. Eur. J. Cancer 1991; 27: 544–549.

91. Papapoulos, S.E. and van Holten-Verzantvoort, A.T.M., Modulation of tumour-induced bone resorption by bisphosphonates. J. Steroid. Biochem. Mol. Biol. 1992; 43: 131–136.

92. Schweitzer, D.H., Hamdy, N.A.T. and Papapoulos, S.E., Single infusion of dimethyl-APD in malignancy-associated hypercalcaemia: factors affecting the calcium-lowering response. Bone Miner. 1994; 25 Suppl. 1: S82.

93. Wüster, Chr., Schöter, K.H., Thiébaud, D., et al., Methylpentylaminopropylidenebisphosphonate (BM 21.0955): a new potent and safe bisphosphonate for the treatment of cancer-associated hypercalcaemia. Bone Miner. 1993; 22: 77–85.

94. Rizzoli, R., Buchs, B. and Bonjour, J.-P., Effect of a single infusion of alendronate in malignant hypercalcemia: dose dependency and comparison with clodronate. Int. J. Cancer 1992; 50: 706–712.

95. Adami, S., Bolzicco, G.P., Rizzo, A., et al., The use of trichloromethylene bisphosphonate and aminobutane bisphosphonate in hypercalcemia of malignancy. Bone Miner. 1987; 2: 395–404.

96. Krempien, B. and Manegold, Chr., Prophylactic treatment of skeletal metastases, tumour-induced osteolysis, and hypercalcaemia in rats with the bisphosphonate Cl2MBP. Cancer 1993; 72: 91–98.

97. Krempien, B. and Diel, I., Histomorphological changes in trabecular bone in patients with primary breast cancer after continuous long term oral treatment with Cl2MBP. Bone Miner. 1994; 25 Suppl. 1: S80.

Bisphosphonate on bones
O. Bijvoet, H.A. Fleisch, R.E. Canfield and G. Russell (eds.)
© 1995 Elsevier Science B.V. All rights reserved.

CHAPTER 25

Bisphosphonates and prostatic carcinoma with bone metastases

Silvano Adami

University of Verona, Policlinico, 37134 Verona, Italy

I. Introduction

Prostatic cancer is one of the most common causes of bone metastases [1]. Androgen withdrawal by surgical or medical castration can induce substantial objective responses for some time, but the final outcome is almost invariably progressive skeletal disease [2]. In these patients the pain related to metastatic bone disease is very disabling and represents a major problem in the conservative treatment of most patients with prostatic carcinoma.

Several bisphosphonates have been shown to reduce bone resorption due to malignancy, and this is associated with clinical benefit: improvement in bone pain, decreased morbidity from skeletal complications, and possibly a survival advantage.

In the last seven years several reports have been published on the symptomatic benefit of bisphosphonate therapy in patients with bone metastases owing to prostatic carcinoma [3–13]. This is somewhat surprising since these metastases are almost exclusively osteoblastic in nature, and the only recognized effect of bisphosphonates on bone is the inhibition of osteoclastic bone resorption.

II. Rationale for using bisphosphonates

The osteosclerotic metastases of prostatic carcinoma are characterized by an increase of bone density adjacent to tumour tissue, and over time, uninvolved bones rarify as the involved bone become denser [14]. This may be due to the prostatic synthesis of a humoral factor stimulating both growth and differentiation of osteoblastic-like cells [15, 16]. This factor has been recently identified as an amino-terminal fragment of urokinase-type plasminogen activator [17], and it is produced by humoral prostatic cancer cell lines and by postpubertal but not prepubertal normal prostate [16].

However, more recently it has become apparent that in osteoblastic metastases there is a synchronous increase in bone resorption. This could be recognized from the frequently raised urinary hydroxyproline excretion which acutely decreases as a consequence of administration of inhibitors of bone resorption [18]. A direct demonstration of increased bone resorption came also from extensive histological studies. Bone biopsies taken for diagnostic purposes might include either tumour-free or tumour-infiltrated areas. In a study of 13 patients with carcinoma of the prostate and skeletal metastases, it was observed that bone-forming surfaces and active osteoblast numbers were increased in skeletal sites adjacent to tumour tissue, and indices of bone resorption were significantly increased at sites adjacent to tumour. Contrary to expectation, indices of bone resorption were also increased in bone distant from skeletal metastases [19]. In a larger series of patients, the fraction of trabecular surfaces with sign of erosions was consistently well above the normal range and directly proportional to the severity of tumour infiltration (from completely free to total infiltration). The severity of tumour infiltration was also inversely related to lamellar bone volume. Thus, in the totally infiltrated areas, lamellar bone was almost absent, and the normal bone was replaced by a large excess of woven bone, which explains the osteosclerotic appearance of these skeletal lesions [20].

It remains to be established whether increased bone resorption is secondary to osteoblastic overactivity or is due to a direct stimulatory activity of tumoural origin. The latter hypothesis appears to be more attractive for two reasons. In patients with prostatic carcinoma osteolytic lesions can also be detected; the osteosclerotic lesions are made up of woven bone [20], and this indicates the preceding resorption of normal lamellar bone. Thus, inhibition of bone resorption at the level of tumour infiltration might inhibit the progression of the secondary osteosclerotic skeletal lesion.

III. Clinical studies

In 1985 we showed in an uncontrolled study that clodronate may represent an important form of supporting treatment in patients with bone metastases owing to prostatic carcinoma, providing sustained relief of pain: four patients who had been bedridden became ambulatory, and reversal of paralysis was also noted in one of the patients [3]. Percival et al. [10] reported reversal of paraplegia in a patient with prostatic cancer treated with clodronate and mithramycin. The efficacy of clodronate was also tested in controlled, dose-finding studies [4]. Fifty-six patients with bone metastasis owing to prostatic carcinoma were randomly allocated to 4 single-blind, controlled therapeutical trials, assessing bone pain by daily consumption of analgesic drugs and by visual analogue scale. In the first protocol the effects of 2 weeks' treatment with i.v. infusion of either 300 mg clodronate dissolved in 500 ml of saline (7 patients) or 500 ml saline (6 patients) were compared. The differences in both pain score and analgesic consumption were so striking that the trial was not extended for ethical reasons, and all patients on placebo were given clodronate i.v. The oral administration of 1200 mg clodronate for 2 weeks was completely ineffective in 11 patients. In the 13 patients given clodronate i.v. for 2 weeks, bone pain relapsed fairly quickly in most of them. However, in 18 patients a maintenance therapy with 1200 mg clodronate/day for at least 6 weeks after a 2-week i.v. treatment course did prevent the relapse of bone pain.

Experience with etidronate is more extensive. Symptomatic improvement has been reported in both prostate cancer patients given 5–7 mg/kg/day [13] and in 3 of 4 administered 5–20 mg/kg/day [11]. Carey and Lippert [6] studied 12 patients treated with etidronate at an oral daily dose of 15 mg/kg for 2 weeks followed by an oral maintenance dose of 5 mg/kg a day. Substantial pain relief was observed in 10 patients after 7 to 10 days of therapy. However, these results have been disputed by Smith [21] in a randomized, prospective, double-blind, placebo-controlled study involving 57 patients, treated with etidronate at doses of 7.5 mg/kg intravenously for 3 days, followed by 400 mg orally (possibly not under strictly fasting conditions) per day. The author concluded that at these doses etidronate was ineffective for palliation of bone pain from prostate cancer.

Favourable results on bone pain have been also reported in patients treated with pamidronate [5, 7, 8, 22]. Clarke et al. [5] conducted a controlled, non-blind trial on 42 patients, 27 of whom were given i.v. pamidronate 30 mg weekly for 4 weeks, then 30 mg every 2 weeks for 5 months. Forty-four per cent of treated patients showed an improvement in pain score during the study, a finding not observed in controls. Similar trends were recorded for performance status, while skeletal scintigraphy showed stabilization or regression in 6 of 18 pamidronate-treated patients whose scans were deteriorating at the start of the trial. In a proportion of both treated and control patients, the histomorphometric changes were also evaluated. Both the indices of bone resorption and osteoblastic activity, which were abnormally raised before therapy, significantly fell in response to i.v. pamidronate.

In an ongoing pilot study we have treated 10 patients with metastatic prostate cancer with i.v. alendronate (Istituto Gentili, Italy) 5 mg daily for 7 days, then 5 mg weekly for 2–5 months. Seven patients experienced significant relief of pain sustained for as long as the treatment was continued (Figure 1).

In most of the above-mentioned studies, the biochemical effects of bisphosphonate therapy have been reported. There is a general agreement that bisphosphonate administration lowers the indices of bone resorption (usually urinary excretion of hydroxyproline and calcium) [3, 18, 22], which are above the normal range in 50–80% of the patients [3, 23]. However, raised urinary hydroxyproline rarely decreases to the normal range [3] since much of the amino acid produced in these patients is by destruction of soft tissue rather than bone.

Serum alkaline phosphatase does not change or even rises within the first 2–4 weeks of therapy [3], and its changes are not consistent thereafter [7]. This might suggest the occurrence of an 'uncoupling' between the overall rate of bone resorption and formation, leading to transient mild hypocalcaemia [22], which is rarely symptomatic. A similar pattern of changes in the indices of bone turnover as a result of clodronate therapy have been recently detected by measuring serum

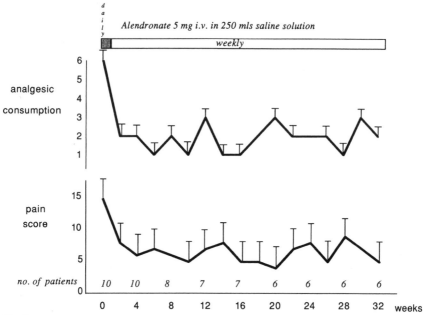

Fig. 1.

Table 1.

Mean daily bioavailable dose of bisphosphonate (clodronate equivalents) given over 2 weeks to patients with metastatic prostate cancer. In the patients to whom the bisphsophonate was not given daily, the total dose administered over 2 weeks was divided by 14, in order to extrapolate the daily dose

Reference	Actual bisphosfonate	Bioavailable daily dose (mg clodr. Eq)	Reported efficacy
Adami et al. 1987	Clodronate/i.v.	300	+ + +
Adami and Mian [4]	Clodronate/os	36	− − −
Clarke et al. [7]	Pamidronate/i.v.	60	+ + −
Smith, 1988	Etidronate/os	60	− − +
Lippert et al. 1988	Etidronate/i.v and os	30	+ + −
Adami (this chapter)	Alendronate/i.v.	430	+ + +

type I collagen metabolites: the propeptide and the cross-linked telopeptide which reflect the synthesis and degradation of bone collagen, respectively [12].

IV. Conclusions

With only one exception [21] all studies agree that bisphosphonate administration has a favourable effect on bone pain in patients with metastatic prostate cancer; this is probably due to inhibition of abnormally raised bone resorption, which precedes the apposition of excess woven bone and the appearance of osteosclerotic skeletal lesions. It has been suggested that the patients who show the best symptomatic responses to bisphosphonate treatment are those with coexistent lytic bone metastases [9] or increased indices of bone resorption [12], but this is definitely not our experience. The variability in the magnitude, duration and time of appearance might depend on the large variability of the doses adopted in the different studies. In Table 1 are listed the mean bioavailable, clodronate-equivalent, daily dose given in 6 different trials, over 2 weeks, which is the time usually required in order to observe symptomatic improvement. The intestinal absorption of bisphosphonates has been assumed to be 3% and the potency ratio as follows: 1 alendronate = 10, pamidronate = 150, clodronate = 200 etidronate.

In our experience the dose of bisphosphonate required in order to obtain a substantial and consistent therapeutical effect is relatively high, and this can be easily obtained only by intravenous administration.

References

1. Abrams, H.L., Spiro, R. and Goldstein, N., Metastases in carcinomas: analysis of 1000 autopsied cases. Cancer 1950; 3: 74–85.
2. Geller, J., Overview of enzyme inhibitors and anti-androgens in prostatic cancer. J. Androl. 1991; 12: 364–371.
3. Adami, S., Salvagno, G., Guarrera, G., Bianchi, G., Dorizzi, R., Rosini, S., Mobilio, G. and Lo Cascio, V., Dichloromethylene-diphosphonate in patients with prostatic carcinoma metastatic to the skeleton. J. Urol. 1985; 134: 1152–1154.
4. Adami, S. and Mian, M., Clodronate therapy of metastatic bone disease in patients with prostatic carcinoma. Recent results in cancer Research 1989; 116: 67–72.
5. Clarke, N.W., McClure, J. and George, N.J.R., Clinical and metabolic effects of disodium pamidronate in metastatic prostate cancer. In: Bijvoet, O.L.M. and Lipton, A. (Editors), Osteoclastic inhibition in the management of malignancy-related bone disorders. Hogrefe and Huber Publishers, Toronto, 1991; pp. 54–63.
6. Carey, P.O. and Lippert, M.C., The treatment of painful prostatic bone metastases with oral etidronate sodium. Urology 1988; 32: 403–407.
7. Clarke, N.W., McClure, J. and George, N.J.R., Subjective and metabolic effects of aminohydroxy-prpylidene bisphosphonate (APD) in patients with advanced cancer of the prostate-preliminary report. In: Rubens, R.D. (Editor), The management of bone metastases and hypercalcemia by osteoclast inhibition. Hogrefe and Huber Publishers, Toronto, 1990; pp. 81–89.
8. Masud, T. and Slevin, M.L., Pamidronate to reduce pain in normocalcemic patients with disseminated prostatic carcinoma. Lancet 1989; 1: 1021–1022.
9. Lipton, A., Grabelsky, S., Glover, D., Harvey, H., Simeone, J. and Seaman, S., Pamidronate disodium (APD): The American experience in breast and prostate cancer. Bone Miner. 1992; 17 (suppl.1): S27.
10. Percival, R.C., Watson, M.E., Williams, J.L. and Kanis, J.A., Carcinoma of the prostate: remission of paraparesis with inhibitors of bone resorption. Postgrad. Med. J. 1985; 61: 551–553.
11. Scher, H.I. and Yagoda, A., Bone metastases: Pathogenesis, treatment and rationale for use of resorption inhibitors. Am. J. Med. 1987; 82 (suppl 2A): 6–28.
12. Kilmälä, T., Tammela, T., Risteli, L., Risteli, J. and Elomaa, I., A controlled study with clodronate in patients with prostate cancer with emphasis to monitore bone metastases using type 1 collagen metabolites. Bone Miner. 1992; 17 (suppl.1): S27.
13. Schnur, W., Etidronate for the relief of metastatic bone pain. J. Urol. 1984; 131: 404–407.
14. Hosking, D.J., Chamberlain, M.J. and Shortland-Webb, W.R., Osteomalacia and carcinoma of the prostate with major re-distribution of skeletal calcium. Br. J. Radiol. 1975; 48: 451–456.
15. Simpson, E., Harrod, J., Eilon, G., Jacobs, J.W. and Mundy, G.R., Identification of a messenger ribonucleic acid fraction in human prostatic cancer cells coding for a novel osteoblast-stimulating factor. Endocrinology 1985; 117: 1615–1620.

16. Koutsilieris, M., Rabbani, S.A., Bennett, H.P. and Goltzman, D., Characteristics of prostate-derived growth factors for cells of the osteoblast phenotype. J. Clin. Invest. 1987; 80: 941–946.
17. Rabbani, S.A., Desjardins, J., Bell, A.W., Banville, D., Mazar, A. and Goldzman, D., An amino-terminal fragment of urokinase isolated from a prostate cancer cell line (PC-3) is mitogenic for osteoblast-like cells. Biochem. Biophys. Res. Commun. 1990; 173: 1058–1064.
18. Percival, R.C., Urwin, G.H., Watson, M.E. et al., Biochemical and histological evidence that carcinoma of the prostate is associated with increased bone resorption. Eur. J. Surg. Oncol. 1987; 13: 41–49.
19. Urwin, G.H., Percival, R.C., Harris, S., Beneton, M.N.C., Williams, J.L. and Kanis, S.A., Generalized increase in bone resorption in carcinoma of the prostate. J. Urol. 1985; 57: 721–723.
20. Clarke, N.W., McClure, J. and George, N.J.R., Morphometric evidence for bone resorption and replacement in prostate cancer. Br. J. Urol. 1991; 68: 74–80.
21. Smith, J.A., Palliation of painful bone metastases from prostate cancer using sodium etidronate: results of a randomized, prospective, double blind, placebo-controlled study. J. Urol. 1989; 141: 85–87.
22. Pelger, R.C.M., Lycklama, A., Nijeholt, A.A.B. and Papapoulos, S.E., Short-term metabolic effects of pamidronate in patients with prostatic carcinoma and bone metastases. Lancet 1989; 2: 865.
23. Bishop, M. and Fellows, G., Urinary hydroxyproline excretion — a marker of bone metastases in prostae carcinoma. Br. J. Urol. 1977; 49: 711–718.

Bisphosphonate on bones
O. Bijvoet, H.A. Fleisch, R.E. Canfield and G. Russell (eds.)
© 1995 Elsevier Science B.V. All rights reserved.

CHAPTER 26

Bone pathology in myeloma

Régis Bataille *

Laboratoire d'Hématologie, Institut de Biologie, 9, quai Moncousu, 44035 Nantes cédex 01, France

I. Introduction

Lytic bone lesions and hypercalcemia are common features in patients with multiple myeloma. Few patients with multiple myeloma do not develop lytic bone lesions. Exceptionally, some patients present with osteosclerotic lesions. In contrast, other B-cell malignancies (except for hairy cell leukaemia) are not associated with bone involvement despite bone marrow invasion. It is thus critical to clarify the mechanisms of bone lesions in multiple myeloma (and those of bone protection observed in a minority of multiple myeloma patients) and to understand why bone involvement is restricted to multiple myeloma.

II. Multiple myeloma induces an excessive osteoclastic resorption in the close vicinity of malignant cells

An increased osteoclastic resorption on quantitative bone biopsy is a char-acteristic feature of patients with active multiple myeloma [2, 17, 23, 33]. This excessive bone resorption is observed in the close vicinity of myeloma cells in all patients with active disease regardless of the presence (or absence) of lytic bone lesions on radiography. This excessive bone resorption is related to an increase of both trabecular osteoclast number, which is easily quantified in 75% of the patients [5], and single osteoclast activity. This excessive osteoclastic resorption is not observed on non-invaded biopsy and/or on biopsy from patients in remis-sion. Multiple myeloma-activated osteoclasts have normal length, in contrast to the large multinucleated osteoclasts encountered in primary hyperparathyroidism and Paget's disease of bone [11]. The increased osteoclastic resorption explains the high sensitivity of myeloma patients to the acute effects of calcitonin, a potent

---

* Supported by grants from la Ligue Nationale Contre le Cancer (Paris, France).

anti-osteoclastic agent [9, 10], and supports the potentially beneficial effects of bisphosphonates in the treatment of myeloma-induced bone changes, as illustrated by published results [1, 12, 25, 31] and in agreement with previous mouse studies [27]. When quantitative bone biopsies were performed in individuals with early (i.e. infraclinical) multiple myeloma, an excessive bone resorption was also observed, as marked as that in patients with overt multiple myeloma [5]. On the other hand, this abnormal remodelling was not found in individuals with either benign monoclonal gammopathy or smoldering multiple myeloma [5]. These critical data have shown that the excessive osteoclastic resorption was an early phenomenon in multiple myeloma which could be observed several years before the first clinical symptoms of the disease and thus is a useful parameter to discriminate between benign monoclonal gammopathy or smoldering multiple myeloma and early active multiple myeloma [5].

III. An uncoupling bone remodelling explains lytic bone lesions in multiple myeloma

That an increased osteoclastic resorption was observed in almost all patients with multiple myeloma demonstrated that lytic bone lesions could not simply be explained by an increased bone resorption [3]. At diagnosis, when we compared the histomorphometric features of patients with lytic bone lesions to those of patients lacking such lesions, it was evident that both subsets of patients had an opposing bone profile. An uncoupling bone process (i.e. increased bone resorption with decreased bone formation) was a characteristic feature of patients with lytic bone lesions. Such an uncoupling was not observed in patients lacking lytic bone lesions [3]. Thus, these data have shown that the inhibition of bone formation was as critical in the occurrence of lytic bone lesions as the excessive bone resorption [3]. This concept was further supported by studies we performed in 10 patients who had never developed lytic bone lesions or who presented with sclerotic multiple myeloma [4]. Eight of these patients had increased parameters of both bone resorption and bone formation, whereas 2 had a selective increase of parameters of bone formation. Serial biopsies (performed in a same patient) have confirmed the occurrence of an uncoupling process during bone destruction and conversely the maintenance of a coupling process in patients lacking lytic bone lesions despite active disease. The critical role of bone formation in the occurrence of lytic bone lesions in patients with multiple myeloma was further supported by our studies with the bone gla protein (BGP) [6, 7]. A good correlation was found between BGP serum levels and bone formation rates (evaluated on bone biopsies) in patients with either early or overt multiple myeloma [4, 5, 7]. Extensive studies of serum BGP in multiple myeloma have shown an inverse correlation between BGP serum levels and the lytic potential of the tumour [6, 7]. Patients lacking lytic bone lesions had significantly higher BGP serum levels than those with lytic bone lesions.

IV. What is the mechanism of myeloma-induced bone changes?

The generation of new osteoclasts with increased osteoclastic resorption (at the single-cell level) in the close vicinity of myeloma cells is an early and characteristic feature of myeloma bone marrow [5]. With advanced disease, bone formation is suppressed, whereas in early disease osteoblastic activity is maintained or rather stimulated [5]. Another critical observation is the strong natural killer (NK) cell activity which has been found in the bone marrow of patients with multiple myeloma and not in that of patients with B-cell malignancies other than multiple myeloma [32]. Thus, accelerated maturation of both osteoclasts and NK cells are the most specific features of multiple myeloma when compared to other B-cell malignancies and could be related abnormalities.

Since Mundy et al.'s first study [23], several works have confirmed the presence of a strong bone-resorbing activity in the bone marrow of patients with multiple myeloma [13–16, 18, 20, 29, 30, 35]. In 3 of these studies, IL-1β rather than TNFα or β was shown to be the cytokine supporting the bone-resorbing activity present in the bone marrow of patients with multiple myeloma [16, 20, 35]. We and others have shown that interleukin-6 was an essential paracrine rather than autocrine myeloma cell growth factor [8, 19, 21, 22, 26, 36]. The recent demonstrations of (i) the bone resorbing activity of IL-6 in vitro and in vivo (in mouse), (ii) the induction of IL-6 by IL-1β, (iii) the synergy between IL-1β and IL-6 in vitro in terms of bone-resorbing activity and (iv) the IL-6 mediation of IL-1β bone-resorbing activity show that IL-6 and IL-1β, which are overproduced in the microenvironment of multiple myeloma, are the most critical and final products involved in myeloma-induced bone changes [28]. Intensive research has to be devoted to the nature of known and unknown factors produced by the myeloma cells themselves and able to both stimulate the production of IL-6 by the tumoural microenvironment and synergize with IL-6 and IL-1β to increase bone resorption and myeloma cell growth. M-CSF could be a critical factor in this process. Indeed, myeloma cell lines do produce M-CSF in vitro [24], and M-CSF is overproduced in vivo in multiple myeloma, in relation to disease severity [34]. Taken together, these data suggest that M-CSF, which is overproduced in vivo, perhaps by the myeloma cells themselves, could be important in the pathogenesis of myeloma-induced bone changes.

V. Conclusions

Bone involvement, mainly bone destruction, is a characteristic and usual feature of multiple myeloma. On the other hand, it is exceptional in B-cell malignancies other than multiple myeloma. Bone destruction is the consequence of an uncoupling process associating an increased osteoclastic resorption with an inhibition of bone formation. Conversely, patients lacking lytic bone lesions or those with sclerotic multiple myeloma have an increased bone resorption but maintain a normal or have an increased bone formation (coupling process). This excessive osteoclastic resorption is an early phenomenon, as opposed to the inhibition of bone formation. It is observed several months or years before the occurrence of the first clinical symptoms of the disease. Thus, it is an early criterion of malignancy, useful for discriminating between benign monoclonal gammopathy or smoldering multiple myeloma and early active multiple myeloma. Several osteoclast-activating factors, produced either by the myeloma cells themselves or the haematopoietic microenvironment, are probably involved in the pathogenesis of such bone lesions. At the present time, IL-6 and IL-1β appear to be the most critical factors. Indirect arguments suggest that other haematopoietic growth factors (mainly M-CSF) could play a role. Taken together, these data demonstrate a close relationship between myeloma cell growth factors and osteoclast-activating factors.

References

1. Ascari, E., Attardo-Parrinello, G. and Merlini, G., Treatment of painful bone lesions and hypercalcemia. Eur. J. Haematol. 1989; 43: 135–138.
2. Bataille, R., Chappard, D., Alexandre, C. and Sany, J., Importance of quantitative histology of bone changes in monoclonal gammopathy. Br. J. Cancer 1986; 53: 805–810.
3. Bataille, R., Chappard, D., Marcelli, C. et al., Mechanism of bone destruction in multiple myeloma. The importance of an unbalanced process in determining the severity of lytic bone disease. J. Clin. Oncol. 1989; 7: 1909–1914.
4. Bataille, R., Chappard, D., Marcelli, C. et al., Osteoblast stimulation in multiple myeloma lacking lytic bone lesions. Br. J. Haematol. 1990; 76: 484–487.
5. Bataille, R., Chappard, D., Marcelli, C. et al., The recruitment of new osteoblasts and osteoclasts is the earliest critical event in the pathogenesis of human multiple myeloma. J. Clin. Invest. 1991; 88: 62–66.
6. Bataille, R., Delmas, P. and Sany, J., Serum bone gla-protein (osteocalcin) in multiple myeloma. Cancer 1987; 59: 329–334.
7. Bataille, R., Delmas, P.D., Chappard, D. and Sany, J., Abnormal serum bone gla-protein levels in multiple myeloma: crucial role of bone formation and prognostic implications. Cancer 1990; 66: 167–172.
8. Bataille, R., Jourdan, M., Zhang, X.G. and Klein, B., Serum levels of interleukin-6, a potent myeloma cell growth factor, as a reflect of disease severity in plasma cell dyscrasias. J. Clin. Invest. 1989; 84: 2008–2011.
9. Bataille, R. and Sany, J., Clinical evaluation of myeloma osteoclastic bone lesions: II. Induced hypocalcemia test using salmon calcitonin. Metab. Bone Dis. Rel. Res. 1982; 4: 39–42.
10. Bataille, R., Legendre, C. and Sany, J. Acute effects of salmon calcitonin in multiple myeloma: a valuable method for serial evaluation of osteoclastic lesions and disease activity. A prospective study of 125 patients. J. Clin. Oncol. 1985; 3: 229–236.
11. Chappard, D., Rossi, J.F., Bataille, R. and Alexandre, C., Cytomorphometry of osteoclasts demonstrates an abnormal population in B-cell malignancies but not in multiple myeloma. Calcif. Tissue Int. 1991; 48: 13–17.
12. Delmas, P.D., Charrhon, S., Chapuy, M.C. et al., Long-term effects of dichloromethylene diphosphonate (Cl2MDP) on skeletal lesions in multiple myeloma. Metab. Bone Dis. Rel. Res. 1982; 4: 163–167.
13. Durie, B.G.M., Salmon, S.E. and Mundy, G.R., Relation of osteoclast activating factor production to extent of bone disease in multiple myeloma. Br. J. Haematol. 1981; 47: 21–30.
14. Gailani, S., McLimans, W.F., Mundy, G.R., Nussbaum, A., Roholt, O. and Zeigel, R., Controlled environment culture of bone marrow explants from human myeloma. Cancer Res. 1976; 36: 1299–1304.
15. Garrett, J.R., Durie, B.G.M., Nedwin, G.E. et al., Production of lymphotoxin, a bone resorbing cytokine, by cultured human myeloma cells. N. Engl. J. Med. 1987; 317: 526–532.
16. Gozzolino, F., Torcia, M., Aldinucci, D.L. et al., Production of interleukin-1 by bone marrow myeloma cells. Blood 1989; 74: 380–387.

17. Grauer, J.L., Blanc, D., Zagala, A. et al., L'histomorphométrie osseuse dans les dysglobulinémies monoclonales. Rev. Rhum. 1986; 53: 517–523.
18. Josse, R.G., Murray, T.M., Mundy, G.R., Jez, D. and Heershche, J.N.M., Observations on the mechanism of bone resorption induced by multiple myeloma marrow culture fluids and partially purified osteoclast-activating factor. J. Clin. Invest. 1981; 67: 1472–1481.
19. Kawano, M., Hirano, T., Matsuda, T. et al., Autocrine generation and essential requirement of BSF/2 IL-6 for human multiple myeloma. Nature 1988; 322: 83–85.
20. Kawano, M., Yamamoto, I., Iwato, K. et al., Interleukin-I beta rather than lymphotoxin as the major bone resorbing activity in human multiple myeloma. Blood 1989; 73: 1646–1649.
21. Klein, B., Widjenes, J., Zhang, X.G. et al., Murine, anti-Interleukin-6 monoclonal antibody therapy for a patient with plasma cell leukemia. Blood 1991; 78: 1198–1904.
22. Klein, B., Zhang, X.G., Jourdan, M. et al., Paracrine rather than autocrine regulation of myeloma cell growth and diffentiation by interleukin-6. Blood 1989; 73: 517–526.
23. Mundy, G.R., Raisz, L.G., Cooper, R.A., Schechter, G.P. and Salmon, S.E., Evidence for the secretion of an osteoclast stimulating factor in myeloma. N. Engl. J. Med. 1974; 291: 1041–1046.
24. Nakamura, M., Merchav, S., Carter, A. et al., Expression of a novel 3-5-kb macrophage colony-stimulating factor transcript in human myeloma cells. J. Immunol. 1989; 143: 3543–3547.
25. Paterson, A.D., Kanis, J.A., Cameron, E.C. et al., The use of dichloromethylene diphosphonate for the management of hypercalcemia in multiple myeloma. Br. J.. Haematol. 1983; 54: 121–132.
26. Portier, M., Rajzbaum, G., Zhang, X.G. et al., In vivo paracrine but not autocrine interleukin-6 gene expression in multiple myeloma. Eur. J. Immunol. 1991; 21: 1759–1762.
27. Radl, J., Croese, J.W., Zurcher, C. et al., Influence of treatment with APD-bisphosphonates on the bone lesions in the mouse 5T2 multiple myeloma. Cancer 1985; 55: 1030–1040.
28. Roodman, G.D., Interleukin-6: an osteotropic factor? J. Bone Miner. Res. 1992; 7: 475–477.
29. Rossi, J.F. and Bataille, R., In vitro osteolytic activity of human myeloma plasma cells and the clinical evaluation of myeloma osteoclastic bone lesions. Br. J. Cancer 1984; 50: 119–121.
30. Schecter, G.P., Wahl, L.M. and Horton, J.E., In vitro bone resorption by human myeloma cells. In: Potter, M. (Editor), Progress in myeloma. Biology of myeloma. North-Holland. 1980; pp. 67–80.
31. Siris, E.S., Sherman, W.H., Baquiran, D.C., Schlatterer, J.P., Osserman, E.F. and Canfield, R.E., Effects of dichloromethylene diphosphonate on skeletal mobilization of calcium in multiple myeloma. N. Engl. J. Med. 1980; 302: 310–315.
32. Uchida, A., Yagita, M., Sugiyama, H., Hoshino, T. and Moore, M., Strong natural killer (NK) cell activity in bone marrow of myeloma patients: accelerated maturation of bone marrow NK cells and their interaction with other bone marrow cells. Int. J. Cancer 1984; 34; 375–382.
33. Valentin-Opran, A., Charhnon, S.A., Meunier, P.J., Edouard, C.M. and Arlot, M.E., Quantitative histology of myeloma-induced bone changes. Br. J. Haematol. 1982; 52: 601–610.
34. Wieczorek, A.J., Belch, A.R., Jacobs, A. et al., Increased circulating colony-stimulating factor-1 in patients with pre leukemia, leukemia and lymphoid malignancies. Blood 1991; 77: 1796.
35. Yamamoto, I., Kawano, M., Sone, T. et al., Production of interleukin-1β, a potent bone resorbing cytokine, by cultured myeloma cells. Cancer Res. 1989; 49: 4242–4246.
36. Zhang, X.G., Klein, B. and Bataille, R., Interleukin-6 is a potent myeloma-cell growth factor in patients with aggressive Multiple Myeloma. Blood 1989; 74: 11–13.

Bisphosphonate on bones
O. Bijvoet, H.A. Fleisch, R.E. Canfield and G. Russell (eds.)
© 1995 Elsevier Science B.V. All rights reserved.

CHAPTER 27

Bisphosphonates in multiple myeloma

E. McCloskey

WHO Collaborating Centre for Metabolic Bone Diseases, Department of Human Metabolism and Clinical Biochemistry, University of Sheffield Medical School, Beech Hill Road, Sheffield S10 2RX, UK

I. Introduction

Multiple myeloma accounts for approximately 1% of all malignancies and about 10% of haematological malignancies. The incidence is highest in the seventh decade of life, and the disease usually has a rapidly progressive course with a median survival of 2–3 years. Chemotherapy is the preferred initial treatment for overt symptomatic myelomatosis. Though chemotherapy can have a significant effect on the morbidity associated with skeletal complications, and advances in chemotherapy have led to some improvement in the median survival of patients with myelomatosis, skeletal disease frequently continues to progress throughout the course of the disease. Palliative radiotherapy is useful but has a limited role in the management of bone pain in myeloma, usually in patients with disabling pain from a well-defined focal process that has failed to respond to chemotherapy. The knowledge that progressive osteolysis is mediated by normal osteoclasts and the development of specific inhibitors of osteoclast activity such as the bisphosphonates have led to the use of these agents in the short and long-term management of myelomatous skeletal complications. This chapter summarises the available evidence for the efficacy of the bisphosphonates in myeloma.

II. Clinical and radiological features of multiple myeloma

Symptoms related to osteolytic bone destruction are the most prominent feature at the time of diagnosis of multiple myeloma, and skeletal complications arise in up to 80% of patients during the course of their disease [1]. The three cardinal features of osteolysis in myelomatosis are bone pain, pathological fractures and hypercalcaemia. Bone pain is present in approximately 70% of patients at the time of diagnosis, with back pain, the most frequent site, occurring in almost half

Prevalence (%)

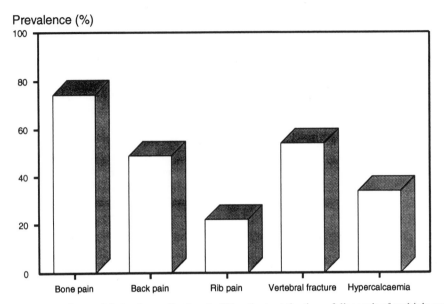

Fig. 1. Prevalence of skeletal complications in 254 patients at the time of diagnosis of multiple myeloma. Bone pain, particularly in the spine, is the predominant feature. The prevalences of bone pain in the upper and lower limbs were 7% and 11%, respectively.

(Fig. 1) [1–3]. Other frequently painful sites include the rib cage, shoulder girdle and hips. The pain is characteristically exacerbated by movement and is less at night. The mechanism(s) of bone pain in myelomatosis, as in other malignancies, remains obscure. There is a strong relationship between the presence of vertebral fracture and the severity and prevalence of back pain [4], but radiological evidence of disease is not always present at sites of bone pain [5]. It is well recognised that the sensitivity of skeletal scintigraphy for bone lesions in myelomatosis is inferior to that of radiography, detecting only about 50% of lesions demonstrated on x-rays [6, 7]. However, increased uptake of isotope has been demonstrated at sites of bone pain [8], and the sensitivity of scintigraphy is similar to radiography in the spine and ribs [6]. It has been suggested that the increased uptake may reflect bone infarction and/or increased osteoblastic activity at sites of pathological fracture.

Radiological evidence of osteolysis is present in approximately 80% of patients at presentation. Bone loss may be focal, diffuse or mixed. The characteristic osteolytic lesions show well-defined margins, are of a fairly uniform size and occur most frequently in the axial skeleton. Focal or diffuse osteosclerosis, rather than osteolysis, may occur but is rare. Pathological fractures were observed in 60% of patients in the series from the Mayo Clinic [1]. In a recent series of 250 patients, pathological fractures at appendicular and axial sites were reported in approximately 50% of patients at diagnosis [3]. In the same series, the prevalence of vertebral fracture was 56% when assessed by a specific and sensitive method for defining vertebral fracture on lateral spine radiographs [9]. The extent of skeletal disease on radiographs at presentation appears to relate to the total myeloma cell burden. There is also a good correlation between skeletal involvement and prognosis and the extent of skeletal destruction or its effects on performance status are used in systems for clinical staging of the disease and estimation of prognosis [10, 11].

Hypercalcaemia is an important cause of morbidity at the time of presentation of myelomatosis, occurring in up to one-third of patients [1, 3]. Osteolysis is the predominant underlying mechanism, but marked osteolytic bone destruction is not invariably associated with hypercalcaemia. Other mechanisms, particularly the frequent impairment of renal glomerular function in myelomatosis, are also important in the development and maintenance of hypercalcaemia in myelomatosis [12].

III. Mechanisms of osteolysis in myelomatosis

Increased osteoclast activity is frequently observed in close proximity to myeloma cells in histological specimens obtained from patients with myelomatosis (Fig. 2) [13–15]. The increase in osteoclastic activity appears to be correlated with the tumour cell burden [15] and results from the local generation of one or more osteoclast-activating factors (OAF) by the myeloma cells and/or by normal marrow cells in response to the presence of myeloma cells [16]. Though the exact nature of OAF remains unknown, it is likely that it represents the activity of a number of local factors rather than being a single substance, and recent evidence suggests that at least three cytokines may be implicated in the increased osteoclastic activity of myelomatosis. Tumour necrosis factor β (TNF-β) or lymphotoxin, produced by myeloma cells, is a potent stimulator of osteoclastic bone resorption which can induce hypercalcaemia in vivo [17]. Neutralising antibodies to lymphotoxin have been shown to inhibit much, but not all, of the bone-resorbing activity of myeloma cells [17]. Increased bone-resorbing activity in mixed cultures of myeloma and normal marrow cells has also been suppressed by neutralising antibodies to interleukin-1 (IL-1), suggesting that the local collaboration of this cytokine is important in the pathogenesis of osteolysis [18]. Finally, the concentration of the paracrine growth factor, IL-6, is also increased in the serum of patients with myelomatosis [19]. In vivo, it is known to be a powerful stimulator of bone resorption and can also induce hypercalcaemia [20]. There is increasing evidence that the effects of many factors known to increase osteoclastic activity, such as TNF-β and IL-1, are mediated by changes in IL-6 production and can be blocked using neutralising antibodies to IL-6 [21].

In contrast to osteoclast activity, the activity of osteoblasts in myeloma is characteristically reduced despite a similar increase in osteoblast and osteoclast number [13, 15]. The mechanism for the relative suppression of bone formation is poorly understood. Possible mediators may include the decreased circulating levels of parathyroid hormone and calcitriol which have been documented in myeloma and which are known to have trophic effects on osteoblasts. The reduction in calcitriol is probably multifactorial, reflecting in part the suppression of PTH secretion by increased efflux of calcium from bone, the frequent use of glucocorticoids in the

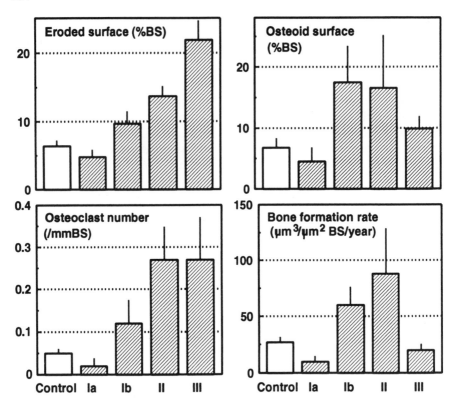

Fig. 2. Histological indices of bone resorption and formation in iliac crest biopsies from patients with multiple myeloma according to the degree of marrow involvement by plasma cells. Advanced disease is associated with a more marked imbalance between the eroded surface and the osteoid surface, suggesting possible uncoupling of bone resorption and formation. Open bars = controls, hatched bars = myeloma, Stage Ia-III (from [15]).

management of myeloma, and possibly the effects of renal impairment and hyperphosphataemia on 1α-hydroxylase activity. Inhibitors of bone resorption have been shown to increase circulating levels of calcitriol in hypercalcaemia patients with myeloma, probably by restoration of circulating levels of PTH. Successful chemotherapy is also often associated with an increase in serum alkaline phosphatase activity, suggesting a decrease in the inhibition of osteoblast activity. Though it is possible that this is mediated indirectly by changes in the calcium-regulating hormones, the production of a factor by myeloma cells which directly suppresses osteoblastic activity has been demonstrated [22, 23].

IV. Biochemical markers of bone turnover in myelomatosis

The uncoupling of bone resorption and formation which occurs in myeloma is reflected biochemically in the disproportionate increase in markers of resorption and the normal or suppressed markers of formation. Thus, the fasting urinary excretion of calcium and hydroxyproline are characteristically increased in patients with myelomatosis [24, 25]. There is also increasing evidence that excessive bone resorption continues in normocalcaemic patients in plateau phase after chemotherapy, and that this is not always detectable using traditional biochemical indices of resorption [15, 24, 26]. A similar pattern is observed in other tumours, e.g. metastatic breast cancer, where the prevalence of fasting hypercalciuria (40%) is significantly higher than the prevalence of hypercalcaemia (10%) [27]. In contrast to resorptive indices, serum activity of alkaline phosphatase is normal or only slightly increased in up to 80% of patients. More recently, serum levels of osteocalcin, a more specific marker of osteoblast function, have also been reported to be reduced, with the lowest values being associated with a poor prognosis [28]. A significant correlation has been observed between fasting urinary hydroxyproline excretion and the degree of radiological disease [24]. Successful treatment with chemotherapy is associated with a large and significant reduction in bone resorption as judged by fasting hydroxyproline excretion. The level of hydroxyproline excretion, however, frequently remains elevated above normal limits [24]. Whether this represents continuing bone resorption and/or tumour-derived hydroxyproline is not clear. The effect of chemotherapy on the fasting urinary Ca/Cr ratio is similar. Further reductions in fasting calcium and hydroxyproline excretion can be induced by specific inhibitors of bone resorption, suggesting that resorption continues despite adequate chemotherapy [26, 29]. Increased bone formation may also occur as a response to successful chemotherapy, and the normalisation of the Ca/Cr ratio may reflect a correction of the imbalance between bone resorption and formation.

V. Clinical use of bisphosphonates in myelomatosis

The imbalance between bone resorption and formation underlies the progressive bone loss in myelomatosis [30]. Although decreased bone formation may contribute to increased skeletal fragility, for example, by impairing the ability to repair microfractures leading to structural disruption of bone, it is probably of little qualitative importance in the presence of the massive increases in bone resorption. The increased osteolysis gives rise to the common clinical complications of myeloma, namely hypercalcaemia, bone pain and pathological fracture. The bisphosphonates, potent inhibitors of osteoclast activity, have been used very successfully in the treatment of hypercalcaemia in myeloma. There is, however, very few data on their efficacy in the acute management of bone pain and, until recently, their ability to decrease the incidence of pathological fracture and other skeletal complications in the long-term.

1. Bisphosphonates in the acute management of hypercalcaemia in myeloma

Increased bone resorption is the predominant mechanism underlying the induction of hypercalcaemia in malignancy. The induction and progression of hypercalcaemia are enhanced by impairment of renal function, predominantly a decrease in GFR and an impaired ability to concentrate urine in the distal nephron [12]. Renal impairment may be induced by hypercalcaemia itself or by factors related to the myelomatosis, including amyloidosis and paraprotein-induced tubular damage. The effects of intravascular volume depletion and hyponatraemia are largely reversed by adequate volume expansion with saline, and this remains the first line of therapy in the vast majority of patients [31]. The use of loop diuretics should be limited to patients in whom congestive cardiac failure might be induced during rehydration. If hypercalcaemia persists despite adequate hydration, the bisphosphonates are the next choice for therapy. Three bisphosphonates, etidronate, clodronate and pamidronate are currently licensed in many countries for the treatment of hypercalcaemia. Both clodronate and etidronate are available in oral and intravenous formulations. Though there are few studies which have exclusively examined the efficacy of bisphosphonates in myeloma, most studies of malignant hypercalcaemia have included one or more patients with myeloma. In these patients, the response to bisphosphonate therapy is usually more complete than that in patients with solid tumours, and serum calcium values are restored to well within normal limits in the vast majority of patients [32–34] (Fig. 3). In many solid tumours, with or without skeletal metastases, the increase in extracellular calcium is partially induced by increased renal tubular reabsorption of calcium [35, 36]. The latter is mediated by factors elaborated by tumour cells, such as PTHrP, which act directly on the

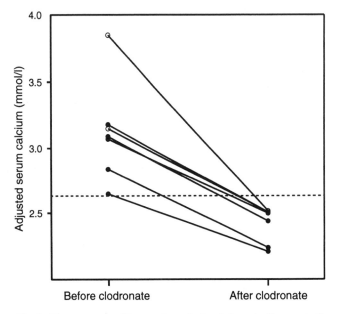

Fig. 3. The response of hypercalcaemia to clodronate therapy in 7 patients with myelomatosis. Clodronate was administered either intravenously (300 mg daily for 5 days, solid circles) or by mouth (800–1600 mg daily for 11 days, open circles). Serum calcium values were restored to normal in all patients.

renal tubule and is not amenable to therapy with bisphosphonates [37]. In contrast, haematological malignancies, including myeloma, are not associated with the production of such factors.

The efficacy of bisphosphonates in myeloma is such that any failure of the hypercalcaemia to respond should raise suspicion of another underlying cause. A possible explanation is the finding of elevated values of total serum calcium in the presence of normal values of ionised calcium. The increase in total calcium reflects increased abnormal binding of calcium by paraproteins. This 'pseudohypercalcaemia' is a relatively rare cause of hypercalcaemia but occurs most commonly in multiple myeloma, particularly those associated with excessive production of IgG.

In contrast to hypercalcaemia associated with solid tumours, hypercalcaemia in patients with haematological malignancy is usually responsive to therapy with corticosteroids [38]. This is probably mediated by an anti-tumour effect and/or inhibition of the activity of some bone-resorbing factors [39]. The time-course of response to corticosteroids, and of other systemic chemotherapy, is much longer than that occurring after bisphosphonate therapy, and normalisation of serum calcium can take several weeks to occur [12].

2. Bisphosphonates in the acute management of bone pain in myeloma

A number of studies have shown that the administration of bisphosphonates, either intravenously, intramuscularly or orally, can reduce bone pain in malignancy [40–44]. Most experience has been gained with clodronate, but it is likely that other bisphosphonates would have similar effects. The mechanism(s) of the reduction in bone pain remain unclear. A reduction in local blood flow, similar to that observed following bisphosphonate therapy in Paget's disease of bone, may play a role. In hypercalcaemic patients, the increased ionised calcium concentration is thought to increase sensitivity to pain, so that reducing serum calcium may have an analgesic effect. The latter mechanism is unlikely to be implicated in prostatic malignancy, in which a marked effect of clodronate to reduce bone pain has been demonstrated in controlled studies [43]. The onset of analgesic response is similar to that of inhibition of bone resorption, suggesting that local factors involved in bone resorption by some tumours may be important in the pathophysiology of bone pain.

To date, there are relatively few data on the acute effects of bisphosphonates on bone pain in myeloma. A regime of intravenous clodronate (300 mg daily for 7 days) followed by intramuscular clodronate (100 mg daily for 10 days) significantly reduced bone pain in 30 patients with myeloma compared with 30 patients treated with standard chemotherapy. This effect occurred within 7 days of commencing therapy and persisted for an average of 3 months (range 15 days to 5 months). Similar results were obtained by the same workers using intravenous aminohydroxybutylidene diphosphonate [45] (Fig. 4). The major drawback of these studies is their open design and the lack of placebo, which may introduce bias and tend to overstate the analgesic effect. The results are sufficiently encouraging, however, to suggest that the bisphosphonates might play a useful role in the acute

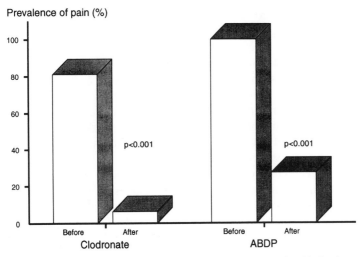

Fig. 4. The effect of intravenous clodronate (300 mg daily for 10 days) or aminohydroxybutylidene diphosphonate (2.5 mg daily for 5 days, ABDP) on bone pain in myeloma. The proportions of patients experiencing moderate or severe bone pain before and 7–15 days after the start of treatment are shown (adapted from [45]).

management of bone pain in myelomatosis, and there is clearly a need for further well-controlled clinical trials.

3. Bisphosphonates in the long-term management of skeletal disease in myeloma

There is good evidence that destructive bone disease progresses in myeloma despite apparently successful responses to systemic chemotherapy. New pathological fractures, persistent or de novo bone pain and recurrent hypercalcaemia give rise to a significant clinical burden during the course of the disease. The ability of the bisphosphonates to suppress bone resorption in the acute management of hypercalcaemia has prompted interest in their ability to modify the progression of skeletal disease in malignancy [14, 27, 29, 41, 46]. During the last decade a number of small studies have examined the effect of long-term treatments with bisphosphonates, particularly clodronate or etidronate, in myelomatosis. Delmas et al. carried out a double-blind, placebo-controlled trial of oral clodronate, 1600 mg daily, and monitored patients over a period of up to 18 months [14]. Histologically, clodronate therapy was associated with a marked reduction in osteoclast number (4.27 + 3.05 to 1.51 + 0.99 after 1 year) compared with patients receiving placebo (2.00 + 1.89 to 2.57 + 2.00). Clinically, the severity of bone pain and the incidence of vertebral and non-vertebral fractures were significantly reduced by clodronate, whereas the severity of bone pain increased in the placebo-treated patients. The assessment of the anti-fracture efficacy of clodronate in this study is limited by the study size (13 patients in total), which could not exclude the possibility of a statistical error. The controlled nature of the study, however, suggests that a moderate degree of clinical benefit could be derived. Ascari et al. examined the use of an intermittent regime of intravenous (300 mg daily for 7 days) and intramuscular (100 mg daily for 10 days) clodronate repeated at a mean interval of 4 months [42]. In 30 patients with myeloma, treatment with clodronate reduced the number of hypercalcaemic events (6 vs 18 per 100 patient years, $P < 0.06$), bone pain (8 vs 40 events per 100 patient years, $P < 0.001$), pathological fractures (6 vs 30 per 100 patients years, $P < 0.001$) and new osteolytic lesions (9 vs 42 per 100 patient years, $P < 0.001$) over a median follow-up of 24 months (range 8–36 months) compared with 30 patients treated with chemotherapy alone. Thus, skeletal morbidity appeared to be reduced by 60–80%. It is important to note, however, that this was an open study in which biases may have tended to overstate the clinical benefit.

A double-blind, placebo-controlled study of the effect of long-term oral etidronate on skeletal disease has been carried out by the National Cancer Institute of Canada [47]. In this study, 166 patients were randomised to receive either etidronate (5 mg/kg/day; $n=92$) or placebo ($n=74$) as well as standard chemotherapy at the time of diagnosis with treatment continuing until death. There was no significant benefit derived from the etidronate therapy in terms of height loss, progressive vertebral deformity, bone pain, pathological fracture or hypercalcaemia. It is possible that the lack of effect of etidronate related to the low dose and the poor bioavailability of the bisphosphonates. There was, however, a significant rise in serum phosphate in etidronate-treated patients, suggesting that some absorption had occurred. Etidronate can induce a mineralisation defect at the dose used in this study [48], and it is likely that this effect would be more marked during long-term therapy. This raises the possibility that osteomalacia-related fractures and bone pain may have masked any beneficial effect of decreased bone resorption. In the absence of biochemical markers of bone turnover or histological assessment of mineralisation, it is not possible to confirm or refute this hypothesis. The role of etidronate in disorders which require high dose or long-term continuous therapy has been superseded by the availability of bisphosphonates which do not impair mineralisation during long-term therapy [14, 26].

Long-term clodronate therapy was examined in a large Finnish double-blind, placebo-controlled trial which has recently been published [29]. In this study, patients with myeloma were randomised to receive either oral clodronate 2400 mg daily ($n = 168$) or an identical placebo ($n = 168$) in addition to standard chemotherapy with melphalan-prednisolone. The proportion of patients with progressive osteolytic bone lesions on repeat skeletal radiographs after 24 months of therapy was significantly reduced in the clodronate-treated group (24 vs 12%, $P = 0.026$) (Table 1). A 25% reduction in the number of patients with progressive vertebral fractures was also demonstrated (30% vs 40%), though this did not achieve statistical significance. There was no apparent effect on the incidence of appendicular fracture, similar to results obtained in a recent placebo-controlled trial in metastatic breast cancer [27]. The proportion of patients who were pain-free at 24 months of follow-up increased from 24% at entry to 54% during clodronate therapy ($P < 0.001$) compared with an increase from 29% to 44% in the placebo group ($P < 0.01$), but the difference between the groups was not statistically significant. There

Table 1.

The effect of long-term oral clodronate therapy on the progression of skeletal disease in 336 patients with myeloma treated for 2 years. Clodronate (2400 mg daily) reduced the progression of osteolytic lesions and appeared to decrease the rate of new vertebral fractures

	Placebo (%)	Clodronate (%)	P-value
Progressive osteolytic bone lesions	24	12	0.026
Progression of vertebral fractures	40	30	NS
Progression of non-vertebral fractures	23	24	NS

were no significant adverse effects attributable to clodronate treatment, and survival was similar in the two treatment groups.

VI. Summary

The rationale for the use of the bisphosphonates in myeloma-induced osteolysis is well established [49]. There is no doubt about their efficacy in the acute management of hypercalcaemia. It is probable that they could play a significant role in the acute management of bone pain, but further controlled trials are necessary. In the long-term, treatment with clodronate has been shown to modify the progression of skeletal disease. Results are awaited from a further double-blind, placebo-controlled trial with oral clodronate 1600 mg daily which is currently being carried out as part of the MRC VIth Myeloma Trial in the UK. The evidence to date supports the view that the bisphosphonates will prove a useful adjunct in the management of skeletal disease in myeloma.

References

1. Kyle, R.A., Multiple myeloma: Review of 869 cases. Mayo Clinic Proc. 1975; 50: 29.
2. Kyle, R.A., Multiple myeloma. An update on diagnosis and management. Acta Oncol. 1990; 29: 1–8.
3. McCloskey, E.V., O'Rourke, N., MacLennan, I., Chapman, C., Beneton, M., Greaves, M., Preston, F.E. and Kanis, J.A., Natural history of skeletal disease in multiple myelomatosis and treatment with clodronate. Bone Miner. 1992; 17 (Suppl. 1): S27.
4. Kanis, J.A. and McCloskey, E.V., The detection of vertebral fracture. RPR manuscript, 1993.
5. Whitelaw, D.M., Pain in multiple myeloma. Can. Med. Assoc. J. 1963; 88: 1242–1243.
6. Lindstrom, E. and Lindstrom, F.D., Skeletal scintigraphy with technetium diphosphonate in multiple myeloma — a comparison with skeletal x-ray. Acta Med. Scand. 1980; 208: 289–291.
7. Tamir, R., Glanz, I., Lubin, E., Vana, D. and Pick, A.I., Comparison of the sensitivity of 99mTc-methyl diphosphonate bone scan with the skeletal x-ray survey in multiple myeloma. Acta Haematol. 1983; 69: 236–242.
8. Charles, N.D., Durant, J. and Barry, W.E., Bone pain in multiple myeloma. Studies with radioactive 87Sr. Arch. Intern. Med. 1973; 130: 53–58.

9. McCloskey, E.V., Spector, T.D., Eyres, K.S., Fern, D.E., O'Rourke, N., Vasikaran, S. and Kanis, J.A., The assessment of vertebral deformity-a method for use in population studies and clinical trials. Osteoporosis Int. 1993; 3: 138–147.

10. Durie, B.G.M. and Salmon, S.E., A clinical staging system for multiple myeloma: Correlation of measured myeloma cell mass with presenting clinical features, response to treatment, and survival. Cancer 1975; 36: 842.

11. MRC Working Party on Leukaemia in Adults. Prognostic features in the third myelomatosis trial. Br. J. Cancer 1980; 42: 831–840.

12. Kanis, J.A., Yates, A.J.P. and Russell, R.G.G., Hypercalcaemia and skeletal complications of myeloma. In: Delamore, I.W. (Editor), Multiple myeloma and other paraproteinaemias. Churchill Livingstone, Edinburgh, 1986; 307–322.

13. Valentin-Opran, A., Charhon, S.A., Meunier, P.J., Edouard, M.C. and Arlot, M., Quantitative histology of myeloma-induced bone changes. Br. J. Haematol. 1982; 52: 601–610.

14. Delmas, P., Charhon, S., Chapuy, M.C., Vignon, E., Briancon, D., Edouard, C. and Meunier, P.J., Long-term effects of dichloromethylene diphosphonate (Cl2MDP) on skeletal lesions in multiple myeloma. Metab. Bone Dis. Rel. Res. 1982; 4: 163–168.

15. Taube, T., Beneton, M.N.C., McCloskey, E.V., Rogers, S., Greaves, M. and Kanis, J.A., Abnormal bone remodelling in patients with myelomatosis and normal biochemical indices of bone resorption. Eur. J. Haematol. 1992; 49: 192–198.

16. Mundy, G.R., Raisz, L.G., Cooper, R.A., Schecter, G.P. and Salmon, S.E., Evidence for secretion of an osteoclast stimulating factor in myeloma. N. Engl. J. Med. 1974; 291: 1041–1046.

17. Garrett, I.R., Durie, B.G.M., Nedwin, G.E., Gillespie, A., Bringman, T., Sabatini, M., Benolini, D.R. and Mundy, G.R., Production of lymphotoxin, a bone resorbing cytokine, by cultured human myeloma cells. N. Engl. J. Med. 1987; 317: 526–532.

18. Kawano, M., Yamamoto, I. and Iwato, K., Interleukin-1 beta rather than lymphotoxin as a major bone resorbing activity in human multiple myeloma. Blood 1989; 73: 1646–1649.

19. Bataille, R., Jourdan, M., Zhang, X.G. and Klein, B., Serum levels of interleukin-6, a potent myeloma cell growth factor, as a reflection of disease severity in plasma cell dyscrasias. J. Clin. Invest. 1989; 84: 2008–2011.

20. Black, K., Mundy, G.R. and Garrett, I.R., Interleukin-6 causes hypercalcaemia in-vivo, and enhances the bone resorbing potency of interleukin-1 and tumor necrosis factor by two orders of magnitude in vitro. J. Bone Miner. Res. 1990; 5: 787.

21. Garrett, I.R., Black, K.S. and Mundy, G.R., Interactions between interleukin-6 and interleukin-1 in osteoclastic bone resorption in neonatal mouse calvaria. Calcif. Tissue Int. 1990; 46 (Suppl. 2): S140–149.

22. Evans, C.E., Galasko, C.S.B. and Ward, C., Does myeloma secrete an osteoblast inhibiting factor? J. Bone Joint Surg. [Br] 1989; 71: 288–290.

23. Evans, C.E., Ward, C., Rathour, L. and Galasko, C.S.B., Myeloma affects both the growth and function of human osteoblast-like cells. Clin. Exp. Metastasis 1992; 10: 33–38.

24. Stepan, J.J., Neuwinova, R., Pacovsky, V., Forrnankova, J. and Silinkova-Malkova, E., Biochemical assessment of bone disease in multiple myeloma. Clin. Chem. Acta 1984; 142: 203–209.

25. Siris, E.S., Sherman, W.H., Baquiran, D.C., Schlatterer, J.P., Osserman, E.F. and Canfield, R.E., Effects of dichloromethylene diphosphonate on skeletal mobilisation of calcium in multiple myeloma. N. Engl. J. Med. 1980; 302: 305–310.

26. McCloskey, E.V., Beneton, M.N.C., Harris, S., Greaves, M., Preston, F.E. and Kanis, J.A., Diphosphonates in multiple myelomatosis. Calcif. Tissue Int. 1989; 44 (Suppl.): S106.

27. Paterson, A.H.G., Powles, T.J., Kanis, J.A., McCloskey, E.V., Hanson, J. and Ashley, S., Double-blind controlled trial of oral clodronate in patients with bone metastases from breast cancer. J. Clin. Oncol. 1993; 11: 59–65.

28. Bataille, R., Delmas, P., Chappard, D. and Sany, J., Prognostic implications of serum bone gla-protein levels in multiple myeloma: crucial role of bone formation. Cancer 1990; 66: 167–172.

29. Lahtinen, R., Laakso, M., Palva, I., Virkkunen, P. and Elomaa, I., Randomised placebocontrolled multicentre trial of clodronate in multiple myeloma. Lancet 1992; 340: 1049–1052.

30. Bataille, R., Chappard, D., Marcelli, C. et al., Mechanisms of bone destruction in multiple myeloma: the importance of an unbalanced process in determining the severity of lytic bone disease. J. Clin. Oncol. 1989; 7: 1909–1914.

31. Hosking, D.J., Cowley, A.J. and Bucknall, C.A., Rehydration in the treatment of severe hypercalcaemia. Q. J. Med. 1981; 50: 473–481.

32. Paterson, A.D., Kanis, J.A., Cameron, E.C. et al., The use of dichloromethylene diphosphonate for the management of hypercalcaemia in multiple myeloma. Br. J. Haematol. 1983; 54: 121–132.
33. Percival, R.C., Paterson, A.D., Yates, A.J.P., Douglas, D.L., Neal, F.E., Russell, R.G.G. and Kanis, J.A., Treatment of malignant hypercalcaemia with clodronate. Br. J. Cancer 1985; 51: 665–669.
34. Bonjour, J.P., Philippe, J., Guelpa, G., Bisetti, A., Rizzoli, R. and Jung, A., Bone and renal components in hypercalcaemia of malignancy and response to a single infusion of clodronate. Bone 1989; 9: 123–130.
35. Stewart, A.F., Horst, R., Deftos, L.J., Cadman, E.C., Lang, R. and Broadus, A.E., Biochemical evaluation of patients with cancer-associated hypercalcaemia: evidence for humoral and non-humoral groups. N. Engl. J. Med. 1980; 303: 1377–1383.
36. Percival, R.C., Yates, A.J.P., Gray, R.E.S. et al., Mechanism of malignant hypercalcaemia in carcinoma of the breast. Br. Med. J. 1985; 291: 776-779.
37. Mundy, G.R., Mechanisms of osteolytic bone destruction. Bone 1991; 12 (Suppl.): S1–6.
38. Percival, R.C., Yates, A.J.P., Gray, R.E.S., Neal, F.E., Forrest, A.R.W. and Kanis, J.A., The role of glucocorticoids in the management of malignant hypercalcaemia. Br. Med. J. 1984; 289: 287.
39. Trumpf, M., Kowalski, M.A. and Mundy, G.R., Effects of glucocorticoids on osteoclastactivating factor. J. Lab. Clin. Med. 1978; 92: 772–778.
40. Siris, E.S., Hyman, G. and Canfield, R.E., Effects of dichloromethylene diphosphonate in women with breast carcinoma metastatic to the skeleton. Am. J. Med. 1983; 74: 401–406.
41. Elooma, I., Blomquist, C., Porkka, L. et al., Long-term controlled trial with diphosphonate in patients with osteolytic bone metastases. Lancet 1983; 1: 146–148.
42. Ascari, E., Attardo-Parrinello, G. and Merlini, G., Treatment of painful bone lesions and hypercalcaemia. Eur. J. Haematol. 1989; 43 (Suppl. S1): 135–139.
43. Adami, S. and Mian, M., Clodronate therapy of metastatic bone disease in patients which prostatic carcinoma. In: Bisphosphonates and tumour osteolysis. Recent Results Cancer Res. 1989; 116: 67–72.
44. Ernst, D.S., MacDonald, R.N., Paterson, A.H.G., Jensen, J. and Bruera, E., A double-blind cross-over trial of IV clodronate in metastatic bone pain. J. Pain Sympt. Man. 1992; 7: 4–11.
45. Attardo-Parrinello, G., Merlini, G., Pavesi, F., Crema, F., Fiorentini, M.L. and Ascari, E., Effects of a new aminodiphosphonate (aminohydroxybutylidene diphosphonate) in patients with osteolytic lesions from metastases and myelomatosis. Comparison with dichloromethylene diphosphonate. Arch. Intern Med. 1987; 147: 1629-1633.
46. Van Holten-Verzantvoort, A.T., Bijvoet, O.L.M., Cleton, F.J. et al., Reduced morbidity from skeletal metastases in breast cancer patients during long-term bisphosphonate (APD) treatment. Lancet 1988; ii: 983–985.
47. Belch, A.R., Bergsagel, D.E., Wilson, K. et al., Effect of daily etidronate on the osteolysis of multiple myeloma. J. Clin. Oncol. 1991; 1397–1402.
48. Boyce, B.F., Fogelman, I., Ralston, S., Smith, L., Johnston, E. and Boyle, I.T., Focal osteomalacia due to low-dose diphosphonate therapy in Paget's disease. Lancet 1984; 1: 821–824.
49. Kanis, J.A., McCloskey, E.V., Taube, T. and O'Rourke, N., Rationale for the use of bisphosphonates in bone metastases. Bone 1991; 12 (Suppl. 1): S13–S18.

Bisphosphonate on bones
O. Bijvoet, H.A. Fleisch, R.E. Canfield and G. Russell (eds.)
© 1995 Elsevier Science B.V. All rights reserved.

CHAPTER 28

Treatment of established osteoporosis with bisphosphonates

Socrates E. Papapoulos

Department of Endocrinology and Metabolic Diseases, University Hospital, Leiden, The Netherlands

I. Introduction

Bisphosphonates were first given to patients with osteoporosis about 20 years ago, but it is only recently that this application has been systematically explored. Although the slow progress of the disease (requiring long-term observations) is partly responsible, issues related to bisphosphonate pharmacology and to the complexity of the osteoporotic syndrome had to be considered carefully and have contributed to this slow development. In this chapter the background of bisphosphonate treatment of established osteoporosis will be discussed and the results of controlled and open trials with various bisphosphonates reviewed.

II. Theoretical considerations

1. Contrary to other indications, the rationale for the use of bisphosphonates in the treatment of osteoporosis is not immediately obvious. It is generally believed that osteoporosis results from an imbalance between bone formation and bone resorption. When this is accompanied by an increase in the activation of new bone remodelling units — high bone turnover — bone loss increases further. Agents which suppress bone resorption and reduce bone turnover, such as the bisphosphonates, are, therefore, expected to help restore the balance and to be beneficial to patients with osteoporosis. This generalization fails, however, to take into account the complexity and the heterogeneity of the osteoporotic syndrome. Although there are forms of osteoporosis associated with high rates of bone loss which will respond favourably to the suppressive action of the bisphosphonates (Figure 1), in the majority of elderly patients with established osteoporosis, bone turnover is generally not increased, and there is no evidence for an accelerated bone loss.

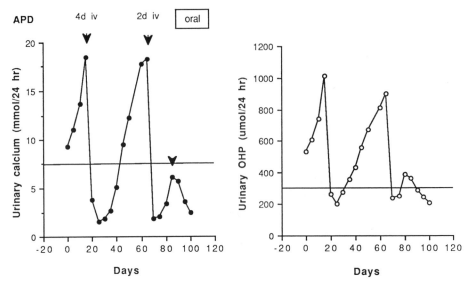

Fig. 1. Sequential changes of urinary calcium and hydroxyproline (OHP) excretions in a 65-year-old woman with postmenopausal osteoporosis before and after treatment with bisphosphonate. Two courses of intravenous bisphosphonate followed by oral bisphosphonate were given. Note the progressively increasing rates of bone resorption before therapy during admission to the metabolic ward while on a constant cacium intake and a gelatin-free diet. APD = pamidronate, iv = intravenous, d = days; horizontal lines represent the upper limit of the normal range. Five years later the patient is well, and no underlying cause for the excessive resorption was ever found.

2. According to current knowledge of bone cellular dynamics, suppression of bone resorption will be followed by suppression of bone formation to an equal extent, leading to a state of lower bone turnover. If this is excessive, it may reduce the ability of bone to remodel, thus increasing the risk of skeletal failure and damage, something which is obviously undesirable in patients with osteoporosis. Animal experiments have, indeed, shown that rigorous long-term suppression of bone turnover with bisphosphonate increases the number of pathological fractures [1].

3. As discussed earlier in this volume, bisphosphonates given at doses which suppress bone resorption effectively can have prolonged effects on bone metabolism which appear to depend on the dose of the compound as well as on the rate of bone resorption and turnover. In addition, 30–50% of the administered bisphosphonate is excreted in the urine, while nearly all the rest accumulates in the skeleton where it is retained for a long time, and there is uncertainty about its long-term effects on bone metabolism. Questions are raised about the dose, the duration of response, as well as the metabolic fate and the removal of bisphosphonate from the bone surface in relation to bone remodelling.

These issues together with the lack, until recently, of pharmacokinetic information in humans necessitated the design of extensive pilot studies, sometimes of long duration, to assess the feasibility and mode of treatment of patients with osteoporosis with bisphosphonates. A number of such studies have been performed and helped to formulate several concepts regarding the use of bisphosphonates in the prevention and therapy of established osteoporosis.

III. Protocol design

Initial long-term studies in animals treated with bisphosphonate at doses which strongly suppressed bone resorption revealed an increase in pathological fractures [1]. Heany and Saville [2] and Jowsey et al [3] studied the effect of high-dose etidronate (20 mg/kg/d) on calcium balance and bone histology in patients with osteoporosis. Although a slight but significant increase in calcium balance was found after one year, the dose used suppressed bone turnover by about 50% and led to the development of osteomalacia. It was, therefore, clear that this was not the right approach. Reitsma et al. [4] treated growing rats with daily subcutaneous injections of different doses of pamidronate and followed the changes in bone resorption and in calcium balance. Treatment suppressed bone resorption and significantly increased calcium retention. Both the rate and degree of suppression of bone resorption were dose-dependent (Figure 2). More important was the finding that with all doses used, suppression of resorption reached a plateau, also dose-dependent, which did not decrease further despite the continuous administration of the bisphosphonate.

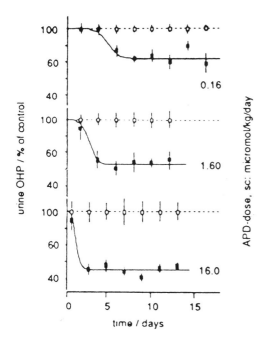

Fig. 2. Rate and degree of suppression of bone resorption in groups of 6 rats each during treatment with daily injections of pamidronate. (O) control animals; (●) treated animals; OHP = hydroxyproline. Reproduced from [4].

These results suggested for the first time that it may be possible to modulate bone remodelling mildly and induce significant increases in calcium balance with low-dose bisphosphonate and that uninterrupted administration is not necessarily accompanied by a progressive suppression of bone resorption. Frijlink et al. [5] examined the effects of uninterrupted bisphosphonate (pamidronate) administration on calcium balance in patients with Paget's disease in whom increased bone resorption is associated with increased bone formation. Pamidronate given orally (600 mg/day) to these patients induced a rapid suppression of bone resorption without any measurable effects on bone formation. During the initial phase of treatment there was a dissociation between bone resorption and bone formation in favour of the latter, resulting in an increase in calcium balance to about 8 mmol/day (Figure 3). This dissociation was, however, transient, and the suppression of resorption was subsequently followed by suppression of formation until a new equilibrium was reestablished. Yet after 6 to 9 months of treatment, the equilibrium calcium balance was about 1 mmol more positive than before treatment started. This suggested persistence of the effect of treatment on calcium retention. As these studies were performed in models characterized by increased bone turnover, the question was

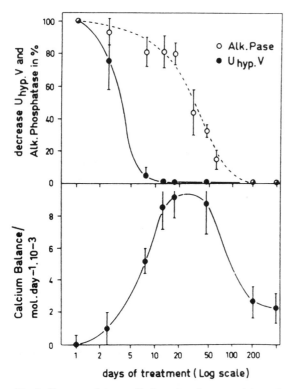

Fig. 3. Changes of serum alkaline phosphatase activity, urinary hydroxyproline excretion and external calcium balance in patients with Paget's disease treated with oral pamidronate 600 mg/day. Reproduced from [5].

whether the effects of bisphosphonate treatment could be reproduced in patients with osteoporosis and normal or low bone turnover.

In an initial study 7 patients with osteoporosis and normal bone turnover were treated with pamidronate orally 600 mg/day, a dose which, as expected, suppressed bone resorption effectively (decrease of urinary hydroxyproline excretion by 40%). During 15 days of treatment the calcium balance increased significantly from -0.49 ± 1.0 mmol/day to 4.99 ± 0.53 mmol/day [6]. Thus, the short-term effect of pamidronate treatment observed in patients with Paget's disease could be reproduced in patients with osteoporosis and normal bone turnover as a result of the forced transient uncoupling of bone resorption and bone formation. The dose used was, however, rather high for long-term administration to patients without increased bone turnover, and a lower dose (150 mg/d) was given to 14 patients with osteoporosis for a year. This mode of treatment induced a mild suppression of bone resorption which was not compensated by a proportional decrease in bone formation, leading to a positive calcium balance after one year (mean calcium balance was -0.72 ± 0.59 mmol/day before treatment and rose to 1.33 ± 0.87 mmol/day after one year, $P < 0.005$). This increase may seem small, but it corresponds to a yearly gain in bone mass of about 3% in a patient with osteoporosis.

The mechanism underlying these responses is not entirely clear. In the short-term and with the higher doses of bisphosphonate, the following sequence of events is possible: suppression of resorption induces a decrease in serum calcium, which in turn stimulates PTH secretion. This increases renal tubular reabsorption of calcium and the renal production of calcitriol, which acts on the intestine and increases intestinal absorption of calcium. The combined effects of PTH and calcitriol increase calcium retention. In the long-term, however, with the establishment of a new steady state, other explanations must be sought. In the original studies with low-dose pamidronate, a significant decrease in TmP/GFR was found after one year of treatment, indicating persistently increased PTH activity [7]. However, in more recent studies employing sensitive and specific assays for the measurement of PTH (IRMA), no changes in circulating concentrations of PTH, measured 6-monthly, were found during a 2-year follow-up of osteoporotic patients treated with 150 mg pamidronate daily [8]. It is, therefore, unlikely that chronic PTH hypersecretion is responsible for the changes observed. Furthermore, net calcium absorption had returned to pretreatment levels after one year of treatment [7], supporting the idea that calcitriol was also not increased in the long run. The answer should therefore be sought in the bone tissue itself. Bijvoet et al. [9] suggested that formation and resorption cycles should be considered as mutually dependent elements of a cybernetic equilibrium. Resetting of the equilibrium in a cyclical process is as a rule incomplete, and continuous low-grade suppression of resorption will result in a continuing positive bone balance. This can be achieved by long-term administration of low-dose bisphosphonate. Alternatively, it may also be hypothesized that low doses of certain bisphosphonates exert not only a mild anti-resorptive effect but may also have an additional anabolic action on the skeleton, as some in vitro studies have previously suggested.

Another approach to treatment, which has been much more intensively explored, takes into consideration the cyclic nature of bone biodynamics. Bone remodelling is thought to be achieved through cycles of non-synchronized bone resorption and bone formation sequences taking place at sundry sites of the bone surface. Frost proposed that an increase in trabecular bone volume can be achieved by temporally coherent activation of bone remodelling units with a pulse of a stimulatory drug followed by suppression of the resulting resorptive phase by a short course of an inhibitory drug, allowing bone formation to proceed normally after the resorptive phase has been curtailed [10]. The resulting positive transients in bone balance can be exploited time and again by repeating these treatment cycles at appropriate intervals. This is the so-called ADFR regimen (activation-depress-free-repeat). Anderson et al. [11] treated 5 osteoporotic patients in this way for 9–24 months and reported improvements in trabecular bone volume (histologically) and in bone remodelling dynamics. Oral phosphate was used as an activator of osteoclast activity, followed by etidronate for 2 weeks as depressor and then by a 70-day treatment-free period. The cycle was repeated. Subsequent studies, however, in a larger number of patients from the same institution failed to confirm these preliminary observations, and it was concluded that this regimen results in short-term improvement in trabecular bone mass with no evidence at a cellular level that long-term improvements in bone remodelling occurred [12]. This was also confirmed in a large, double-blind, placebo-controlled study with etidronate which failed to show any additional benefit when a stimulator of osteoclastic activity was added to a regimen of intermittent bisphosphonate administration [13]. Although it may be argued that these regimens did not apply the concepts in practice exactly as formulated by Frost, there is at present no evidence to suggest that use of bisphosphonates in ADFR regimens will confer any advantage over the use of the drug alone. The concept, however, of discontinuous administration supported by some principles of bisphosphonate pharmacology has led to the design of regimens with intermittent administration. Apart from the theoretical consideration that a short period of suppression of bone resorption will be followed by a period during which bone formation will proceed normally, leading to a positive bone balance, this approach was thought to have some practical advantages as it is expected to reduce the exposure of the skeleton to the drug and to decrease the chances of an adverse effect on the mineralization of newly formed bone (a problem relevant to the use of etidronate) or to diminish possible risks associated with the accumulation of bisphosphonates in the skeleton because of their long skeletal half-life.

These two protocols, namely the discontinuous and the uninterrupted administration of bisphosphonates, have been tested in long-term studies of patients with established osteoporosis, but results of controlled trials exceeding 2 years are presently available only with bisphosphonate given intermittently.

IV. Effects on bone mass

1. Intermittent administration of bisphosphonate

The first randomized trial with bisphosphonate (etidronate) in osteoporosis was reported by Pacifici et al. [14]. Postmenopausal women with osteoporosis were treated with a form of coherence therapy regimen consisting of phosphate for 3 days, followed by etidronate (400 mg/day) for 14 days, followed by 8 weeks of neither drug plus continuous calcium carbonate therapy (1 g/day). Results were compared to those obtained in two other groups of women receiving either hormonal replacement therapy (HRT) together with calcium supplements or calcium carbonate alone. At the end of the study the bone loss at the spine was significantly higher in the phosphate/etidronate-treated patients than in the hormone/calcium group, who did not lose any bone. The authors concluded that this regimen was not as effective as HRT in preventing trabecular bone loss in osteoporosis, nor was it any more effective than calcium supplementation alone. This study has been criticized in that no care was taken in the administration of calcium supplements, which should not be taken together with the bisphosphonate. Calcium may bind the bisphosphonate in the intestine and reduce further its already low intestinal absorption. A different picture emerged in two double-blind, placebo-controlled trials of the effect of intermittent etidronate in patients with postmenopausal osteoporosis [13, 15]. In both studies etidronate was given orally 400 mg/day for 2 weeks followed by a rest period of 11–13 weeks. In the first study vitamin D and calcium supplements were given continuously throughout the treatment period, while in the second only calcium supplements were given during the bisphosphonate-free period. In both studies a modest but significant increase in trabecular bone mineral density was found with no significant change in cortical bone mass. This increase was around 5% and occurred during the first 2 years of treatment, a finding consistent with the expected effect of an anti-resorptive agent on bone cellular dynamics. This level could be maintained for up to 5 years of treatment.

The effects of intermittent administration of other bisphosphonates are less well documented. Clodronate given intermittently (1200–1600 mg/day) in a placebo-controlled study induced an increase in total body calcium measured by neutron activation analysis by about 6% after 18 months [16]. In another small, uncontrolled, long-term study with oral clodronate, the same pattern of response was observed, but there was a tendency for values to revert to baseline after 4 years [17]. In a more recent study clodronate 400 mg/day for 1 month every 3 months induced an increase in lumbar mineral density by about 3 to 4% after one year of treatment, while there was a decrease of about 2% in a control group of patients who received no specific treatment for their osteoporosis [18]. Pamidronate was given orally, 250–300 mg/day for 2 months followed by a 2-month drug-free period, to 18 patients with osteoporosis for at least 3 and up to 5 years [19]. There was an increase in the BMD of the lumbar spine by 2.4% the first year and 2.5% the second year, but no further change in the following 3 years. These results are similar to those obtained with intermittent etidronate treatment though with a higher total dose of a more potent bisphosphonate. Passeri et al. [20] treated osteoporotic patients with intermittent infusions of alendronate (5 mg/day for 2 days every 3 months) and reported prolonged effects on bone metabolism and increases in spinal mineral density of about 9% after 1 year of treatment. The recently reported findings of Thiebaud et al. [21] who treated 16 osteoporotic patients with i.v. pamidronate 30 mg every 3 months for 2 years as part of a randomized study comparing the effects of this regimen to sodium fluoride, were similar. There was an increase in bone mineral density of the spine of about 10.5% after 2 years associated with a significant increase (4.5%) in the BMD of the neck of the femur (primarily cortical bone). The total dose of bisphosphonate given in the last two studies was low, but the effects were quite impressive despite the relatively short duration of the studies. This emphasises the importance of a different approach to the treatment of osteoporosis in the elderly compared with other indications of bisphosphonate therapy. It will also be interesting to follow these patients to observe the long-term effects of these regimens on bone metabolism as the suppression of resorption induced in some of these studies was nearly 50% of starting values.

2. Uninterrupted administration of bisphosphonate

The effectiveness of continuous administration of bisphosphonates was originally examined in open studies with pamidronate. In an initial study Valkema et al. [6] measured the BMC of the lumbar spine by DPA in 24 patients with osteoporosis treated with oral pamidronate 150 mg/day. Another group of 19 patients with osteoporosis and similar clinical and densitometric findings who received the same conventional care and treatment, but no pamidronate, served as control. In the pamidronate group BMC increased by $6.8 \pm 1.7\%$ over a mean period of measurements of 2.2 years ($P < 0.0005$), while no significant change occurred in the control group. The latter finding is consistent with results obtained in control groups in other studies of osteoporosis and shows that conventional care can stabilize trabecular bone mass in elderly patients with established osteoporosis. This study was extended and included more patients and showed a yearly increase in BMC of the lumbar spine of about 3% per year for at least 4 years of treatment [6, 22, 23]. Similar results have also been reported in other open studies of shorter duration with uninterrupted administration of pamidronate [24]. These results, if confirmed, raise the possibility of an additional, possibly anabolic effect of this regimen on skeletal tissue. This concept is currently being tested in controlled studies with pamidronate and alendronate. Recently published reports of 2 and 1 year placebo-controlled studies with oral pamidronate and alendronate, respectively, are in agreement with the results of the open studies [25, 26].

In summary, all bisphosphonates tested so far, independently of route and mode of administration, increase significantly the bone mineral density of the spine in patients with established osteoporosis. This increase is not due to a redistribution of calcium in the skeleton as mineral density at sites with predominantly cortical bone either does not change or increases with treatment. The fundamental question is whether these effects of bisphosphonate therapy on bone mass are associated with an increased resistance of the skeleton to new fractures.

V. Prevention of fractures

In contrast to the unequivocal effect of bisphosphonate therapy on mineral density in patients with established osteoporosis, its ability to protect skeletal integrity against new fractures has not yet been fully established. Long-term controlled data on fracture frequency have only been obtained in the two randomized, double-blind, placebo-controlled trials with intermittent etidronate. Because of the different patient populations included in these studies and because the trials continued either in double-blind or in open design, several conclusions about the effectiveness of this regimen in the prevention of new fractures in patients with vertebral osteoporosis can be drawn. In the study of Storm et al. [15] fewer patients with much severer osteoporosis were included. The latter was evident from the high fracture frequency during the trial, the bone loss in the placebo-treated patients, and the biochemical and histological evidence of higher bone turnover in the group as a whole. Furthermore, the high mortality rate (10 deaths, equally distributed between the two groups of 66 patients in total) suggests that this was a separate group of patients, possibly with an underlying cause for the osteoporosis in a number of them. Therefore, bisphosphonate treatment given as anti-resorptive therapy can be expected to be effective. In this study there was no significant difference in the rate of new vertebral fractures between placebo-treated and etidronate-treated patients after 3 years of treatment. When, however, the results of the first year were compared with those after the third year, there was a significant reduction in the frequency of new fractures. This lower fracture rate was sustained for another 2 years, during which all patients were treated with active drug [27]. Despite reservations about the sample size, way of analysing fracture rates and statistical treatment of data, it can be concluded that in this study there was a clear tendency for a decrease in the rate of new vertebral fractures. The bisphosphonate had, therefore, a therapeutic effect. The results of the large American, multicentre study [13] which included more patients with milder disease are much more difficult to interpret. Although in the initial publication a significant reduction in the frequency of new vertebral fractures was reported, both the number of fractures and the follow-up period were inadequate to support this conclusion. Comparison, for example, of the rate of new fractures in placebo-treated patients (68/1000 patient years, $n = 91$) against that of etidronate-treated patients (44.2/1000 patient years, $n = 98$) revealed no significant difference. A marginal level of significance was obtained only when the patients who received additional phosphate were included in the analysis. The authors analysed further the frequency of new vertebral fractures according to the bone mass at the start of treatment and found significant differences but only in the patients with low bone mass. Additional data obtained during extension of this trial in a double-blind design for a third year revealed a higher rate of new vertebral fractures in patients being actively treated than in those on placebo [28].

Overall, no statistical difference in the rate of new vertebral fractures over 3 years was documented. This trial was continued with an open design for an additional year, and it was reported that patients with 3 or more vertebral fractures and low bone mass at study entry were the most likely ones to show a favourable response to treatment [29]. These accounted for about one-fifth of the population studied. The combined results of these studies strongly suggest that this form of bisphosphonate treatment may offer protection against new vertebral fractures in patients with severe vertebral osteoporosis and possibly accelerated bone loss, as would be expected from the pharmacological properties of these drugs. No evidence has been presented yet about the anti-fracture efficacy of etidronate therapy in patients with mild osteoporosis [30].

Controlled studies of fracture frequency during treatment with other bisphosphonates are not yet available. In the open studies with uninterrupted pamidronate, a rate of new vertebral fractures of 50.5/1000 patient years was reported after a mean period of treatment of 53 months, and all new fractures occurred in patients who entered the study with 4 or more vertebral fractures [23]. However reassuring this low rate of new fractures, the lack of a parallel placebo-treated group does not allow any further conclusions to be drawn about the efficacy of this regimen in the prevention of new vertebral fractures.

In summary, there is sufficient evidence in support of the anti-fracture efficacy of bisphosphonate treatment in patients with severe osteoporosis and possibly unopposed bone loss. The preventive effect of these drugs in patients with milder disease and no underlying cause for their osteoporosis needs to be established. There is no information yet on the efficacy of bisphosphonate treatment in the prevention of hip fractures. The mechanism underlying the protective action of bisphosphonates on fracture development requires further consideration. Is the modest increase in bone mass responsible for that, or is the anti-resorptive effect per se preventing the perforation of new trabecular structures? For the design of optimal treatment regimens with bisphosphonates, these questions need to be addressed. At present, it is certainly reassuring that patients most likely to benefit from this treatment can be identified.

VI. Effects on bone quality

During long-term therapy with bisphosphonates two additional issues of clinical importance need to be considered. The first concerns the quality of the newly formed bone and the second, the possible adverse effects of the drug on bone metabolism due to its prolonged residence in the skeleton. The first is particularly relevant to etidronate, which is known to induce osteomalacia. Analysis of bone biopsies obtained in the two placebo-controlled trials with intermittent etidronate reported no evidence of a defect in the mineralization of newly formed osteoid [31, 32]. Similarly, in bone biopsies from the open studies with pamidronate, no evidence of mineralization defects were found after 5 or more years of continuous treatment (unpublished). Long-term exposure of the skeleton to bisphosphonate may theoretically lead to suppression of bone turnover to a degree which may reduce the ability of the bone to remodel, thus increasing the risk of fractures. Detailed evaluation of the bone biopsies obtained in the Danish trial with intermittent etidronate reported a significant decrease in the activation frequency of new bone remodelling units and of the depth of resorption cavities after 60 weeks of treatment. The interesting relevant finding of this study was the reversal of the activation frequency at sites of the iliac crest which had been previously biopsied to pretreatment levels after 150 weeks of treatment. This finding supports the idea that bone is still capable of responding to stimuli and that there is no risk for inducing 'frozen bone' with long-term treatment. On the other hand, it raises questions about treatment efficacy in the long term, as this may also be interpreted as treatment escape. Detailed reportage of the long-term results of the American study may shed light on this issue.

Follow-up of biochemical parameters of bone metabolism in studies with other bisphosphonates showed decreases in serum alkaline phosphatase activity and in urinary hydroxyproline excretion in the first year of treatment but no additional suppression in the following years [23]. An example during treatment of patients with osteoporosis for 5 years with uninterrupted pamidronate is shown in Figure 4.

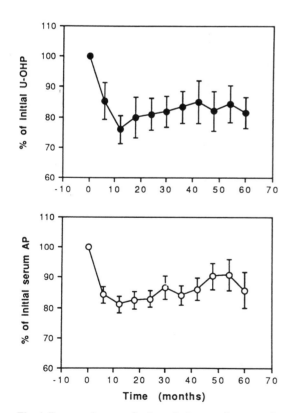

Fig. 4. Percent changes of urinary hydroxyproline excretion and serum alkaline phosphatase activity in patients with osteoporosis treated with oral pamidronate 150 mg/day for 5 years. Reproduced from [23].

These results strongly suggest that the accumulation of the bisphosphonate in the skeleton is not necessarily accompanied by a cumulative effect on bone metabolism and strengthen the view that surface-bound bisphosphonate is biologically active while the drug which is buried in bone is biologically inert. In support of these clinical observations, there is mounting evidence from animal experiments demonstrating either improvement or no change in the biomechanical competence of bone which appears to depend on the dose and class of bisphosphonate used. In planning treatment with uninterrupted bisphosphonate, care should be taken to avoid excessive suppression of bone turnover, as shown in Figure 4. If suppression of resorption is excessive, dose adjustment may be necessary. This recommendation is based on data obtained with the use of hydroxyproline as the biochemical parameter of bone resorption. Relative ranges of newer parameters for assessing bone resorption (e.g. collagen cross-links) need to be established. A subject which is usually not discussed in relevant publications is the possible additive effect of calcium supplements on bone resorption, and care should be taken to titrate the dose as in short-term studies even with relatively low-dose bisphosphonate, profound suppression of bone resorption has been reported. This subject has not yet been addressed in detail.

VII. Side-effects of therapy

Apart from possible adverse effects on bone metabolism, which as already discussed can be dose- and compound-related and can be avoided by careful planning and follow-up, side-effects of treatment are unremarkable. Gastrointestinal side-effects have been reported mainly with the use of aminobisphosphonates. With pamidronate given in enteric-coated pellets, some cases of severe oesophagitis have been observed. Although the incidence of this complication appears to be low, it was considered by the responsible pharmaceutical industry to be of sufficient severity to justify discontinuation of clinical trials in the prevention and treatment of osteoporosis with this formulation. Nitrogen-containing bisphosphonates, especially when given intravenously, may also induce a mild, transient acute-phase reaction on first exposure to the drug.

VIII. Bisphosphonates and the growing skeleton

Osteoporosis in children is usually secondary to endocrine, genetic or haematological disorders or is drug-induced (e.g. glucocorticoids). Primary osteoporosis, or idiopathic juvenile osteoporosis, is rare; it occurs usually in prepubertal children who present with vertebral and metaphyseal fractures, especially of the distal femur and tibia [33]. Metaphyseal fractures may be considered typical of juvenile osteoporosis and may help differentiate the disease from other forms of osteoporosis in children, though this is not always the case. There is very limited experience in treating osteoporosis in children, and efforts have been concentrated on identifying possible underlying causes and improving calcium intake and absorption. There are, however, cases in which the primary cause is unknown (juvenile osteoporosis), it cannot be treated (osteogenesis imperfecta), or it cannot be removed (stopping steroid therapy). In severe cases osteoporosis may progress rapidly, causing considerable invalidity and requiring urgent management. Nitrogen-containing bisphosphonates have been tried with success in some children presenting with progressive vertebral osteoporosis of varying aetiologies.

Encouraged by the clinical, biochemical and radiological responses to bisphosphonate (pamidronate) in a child with severe juvenile osteoporosis and multiple metaphyseal and vertebral fractures [34], we treated a number of children with progressive vertebral osteoporosis with nitrogen-containing bisphosphonates for long periods [35]. Diagnoses included juvenile osteoporosis, osteogenesis imperfecta, steroid-induced osteoporosis and juvenile arthritis. Clinically, all children improved impressively, with marked decreases in bone pains. Treatment given continuously for up to 6 years was associated with a normal pattern of linear growth. There was a dramatic increase in external calcium balance associated with increases in bone mineral density of the spine along a slope different from that of their healthy peers and a tendency for the bone mass to catch up with normal values. This was paralleled by increases in bone mineral density measured at cortical sites. Radiological changes were striking and consisted of band-like metaphyseal sclerosis and concentric epi- and apophyseal sclerosis [36, 37]. The extent of sclerosis depends on the duration of treatment and is related to growth activity. Most remarkable was the finding of complete reversal of spinal deformities with treatment in three patients. Improvement in the shape of vertebrae has been previously observed in children with juvenile arthritis on steroids after altering the treatment regimen [38] or with Cushing's disease after successful treatment. It appears that vertebrae in children have the potential to restore their structure as soon as the adverse stimulus is removed or the process is successfully treated. It is, therefore, important to initiate treatment early as there is no chance to reverse spinal deformities after closure of the epiphyses, as occurs in adults with spinal osteoporosis. The best results are obtained when treatment starts before puberty. When bisphosphonate is given later, the changes, though still of significant magnitude, are less impressive, and the chances of attaining a normal bone mass are minimal. These long-term, but clearly preliminary studies strongly suggest that bisphosphonates can be beneficial to children with osteoporosis for whom very limited therapeutic options are currently available. They further strengthen the notion that the accumulation of the bisphosphonate in the skeleton is not accompanied by long-term adverse effects on calcium metabolism. The growing skeleton is particularly sensitive to factors which adversely affect bone metabolism, and any potential deleterious effects of long-term bisphosphonate administration may thus be best identified in children. No such effects were seen during long-term bisphosphonate treatment. In addition, the quick relapse and reversal of treatment effects in some children after stopping treatment is in line with the notion that bisphosphonates affect a bone surface-related process, whereas the drug which is buried in bone is biologically inactive.

IX. Conclusions and unresolved issues

Bisphosphonates are clearly efficaceous in the management of patients with osteoporosis. A distinction should be made between therapeutic and preventive regimens, and the presentation of osteoporosis should not be considered pathophysiologically the same in all patients. In osteoporosis characterized by increased rates of bone loss, treatment schedules similar to those employed in other clinical indications of bisphosphonate therapy can be used. The optimal preventive regimen for the majority of patients with vertebral osteoporosis still needs to be established. All regimens used induced an increase or a stabilization of spinal mineral density for a number of years without any significant side-effects. Bisphosphonates appear further to protect the skeleton against new fractures, but more studies are needed to demonstrate this unequivocally. Issues remaining to be addressed in future studies include the efficacy of bisphosphonate therapy in the prevention of hip fractures, the mode of administration (intermittent versus continuous), and consequently the choice of the bisphosphonate class, duration of treatment and finally changes in bone metabolism following treatment arrest.

Acknowledgements. Our studies have been supported by a programme grant from the Dutch Organization for Scientific Research (NWO 900-541-191).

References

1. Flora, L., Hassing, G.S., Cloyd, G.G., Bevan, J.A., Parfitt, A.M. and Villanueva, A.R., The long-term skeletal effects of EHDP in dogs. Metab. Bone Dis. Rel. Res. 1981; 4: 289–300.
2. Heaney, R.P. and Saville, P.D., Etidronate disodium in postmenopausal osteoporosis. Clin. Pharmacol. Ther. 1976; 20: 593–604.
3. Jowsey, J., Riggs, B., Kelly, P.J., Hossman, D.L. and Bordier, P., The treatment of osteoporosis with disodium ethane-1-hydroxy-1, 1-diphosphonate. J. Lab. Clin. Med. 1971; 78: 574–584.
4. Reitsma, P.H., Bijvoet, O.L.M., Verlinden-Ooms, H. and Wee van der Plas, L.J.A., Kinetic studies of bone and mineral metabolism during treatment with (3-amino-1-hydroxypropylidene)-1, 1-bisphsphonate (APD) in rats. Calcif. Tissue Int. 1980; 32: 145–157.
5. Frijlink, W.B., te Velde, J., Bijvoet, O.L.M. and Heynen, G., Treatment of Paget's disease with (3-amino-1-hydroxypropylidene)-1,1-bisphosphonate (APD). Lancet 1979; i: 799–803.
6. Valkema, R., Vismans, F.J.F.E., Papapoulos, S.E., Pauwels, E.K.J. and Bijvoet, O.L.M., Maintained improvement in calcium balance and bone mineral content in patients with osteoporosis treated with the bisphosphonate APD. Bone Miner. 1989; 5: 183–192.
7. Vismans, F.-J.F.E., APD, parathyroid hormone and osteoporosis. PhD Thesis, University of Leiden, 1984.
8. Landman, J.O. and Papapoulos, S.E., Uninterrupted oral bisphosphonate (pamidronate) therapy of patients with osteoporosis is not associated with chronic stimulation of parathyroid hormone (PTH) secretion. Osteoporosis Int. 1995; 5: 93–96.
9. Bijvoet, O.L.M., Valkema, R., Löwik, C.W.G.M. and Papapoulos, S.E., The use of bisphosphonates in osteoporosis. In: DeLuca, H.F. and Mazess, R. (Editors), Osteoporosis: Physiological basis, assessment and treatment. Elsevier Science, New York, 1990; pp. 331–338.
10. Frost, H.M., Treatment of osteoporosis by manipulation of coherent bone cell populations. Clin. Orthop. 1979; 143: 227–244.
11. Anderson, C., Cape, R.D., Crilly, R.G., Hodsman, A.B. and Wolfe, B.M., Preliminary observations of a form of coherence therapy for osteoporosis. Calcif. Tissue Int. 1984; 36: 341–343.
12. Hodsman, A.B., Effects of cyclical therapy for osteoporosis using an oral regimen of inorganic phosphate and sodium etidronate: a clinical and bone histomorphometric study. Bone Miner. 1989;

5: 201–212.
13. Watts, N.B., Harris, S.T., Genant, H.G. et al., Intermittent cyclical etidronate treatment of post-menopausal osteoporosis. N. Engl. J. Med. 1990; 323: 73–79.
14. Pacifici, R., McMurtry, C., Vered, I., Rupich, R. and Avioli, L.V., Coherence therapy does not prevent axial bone loss in osteoporotic women: a preliminary comparative study. J. Clin. Endocrinol. Metab. 1988; 66: 855–866.
15. Storm, T., Thamsborg, G., Steiniche, T., Genant, H.K. and Sorensen, O.H., Effect of intermittent cyclical etidronate therapy on bone mass and fracture rate in women with postmenopausal osteoporosis. N. Engl. J. Med. 1990; 322: 1265–1271.
16. Chesnut, C.H., Synthetic salmon calcitonin, diphosphonates and anabolic steroids in the treatment of postmenopausal osteoporosis. In: Christiansen, C. et al. (Editors), Osteoporosis. Glostrup Hospital, Copenhagen, 1984; pp. 549–555.
17. Montagnani, M., Agnusdei, D., Cepollaro, C., Zacchei, F., Civitelli, R. and Gennari, C., Increase in bone mineral density and duration of antiresorptive treatment in established osteoporosis. Bone Miner. 1992; 17 (suppl 1): S23.
18. Giannini, S., D'Angelo, A., Malvasi, L. et al., Effects of one year cyclical treatment with clodronate on bone mass and mineral metabolism in postmenopausal osteoporosis. Bone 1993; 14: 137–141.
19. Devogelaar, J.P. and Nagant de Deuxchaisnes, C., Treatment of involutional osteoporosis with the bisphosphonate APD (disodium pamidronate); non-linear increase of lumbar bone mineral density. J. Bone Miner. Res. 1990; 5: S97.
20. Passeri, M., Baroni, M.C., Pedrazzoni, M. et al., Intermittent treatment with intravenous 4-amino-1-hydroxybutylidene-1,1-bisphosphonate (AHBuBP) in the therapy of postmenopausal osteoporosis. Bone Miner. 1991; 15: 237–248.
21. Thiebaud, D., Burckhardt, P., Melchior, J. et al., Two years' effectiveness of intravenous pamidronate (APD) versus oral fluoride for osteoporosis occurring in the menopause. Osteoporosis Int. 1994; 4: 76–83.
22. Papapoulos, S.E., Bijvoet, O.L.M., Valkema, R. et al., New bisphosphonates in the treatment of osteoporosis. In: Christiansen, C. and Overgaard, K. (Editors), Osteoporosis 1990. Osteopress ApS, Copenhagen, 1990; pp. 1294–1300.
23. Papapoulos, S.E., Landman, J.O., Bijvoet, O.L.M. et al., The use of bisphonates in the treatment of osteoporosis. Bone 1992; 13: S41–S49.
24. Fromm, G.A., Vega, E., Plantalech, L., Galich, A.M. and Mautalen, C.A., Differential action of pamidronate on trabecular and cortical bone in women with involutional osteoporosis. Osteoporosis Int. 1991; 1: 129–133.
25. Reid, I.R., Wattie, D.J., Evans, M.C., Gamble, G.D., Stapleton, J.P. and Cornish, J., Continuous therapy with pamidronate in postmenopausal osteoporosis. Bone Miner. 1994; 25: S75.
26. Adami, S., Baroni, M.C., Broggini, M. et al., Treatment of postmenopausal osteoporosis with continuous daily oral alendronate in comparison with either placebo or intranasal salmon calcitonin. Osteoporosis Int. 1993; 3 (suppl 3): 21–27.
27. Storm, T., Thamsborg, G., Sorensen, H.A., Kollerup, G., Genant, H.K. and Sorensen, O.H., Long-term treatment with intermittent, cyclical etidronate: effect on bone mass and fracture. J. Bone Miner. Res. 1992; 7: S117.
28. Jackson, R.D., Harris, S.T., Genant, H.K. et al., Cyclical etidronate treatment of postmenopausal osteoporosis: 4 years experience. Bone Miner. 1992; 17 (suppl 1): 154.
29. Harris, S.T., Watts, N.B., Jackson, R.D. et al., Four-year study of intermittent cyclic etidronate treatment of postmenopausal osteoporosis: Three years of blinded therapy followed by one year of open therapy. Am. J. Med. 1993; 95: 557–567.
30. Papapoulos, S.E., The role of bisphosphonates in the prevention and treatment of osteoporosis. Am. J. Med. 1993; 95 (5A): 48S–52S.
31. Storm, T., Steiniche, T., Thamsborg, G. and Melsen, F., Changes in bone histomorphometry after long-term treatment with intermittent, cyclic etidronate for postmenopausal osteoporosis. J. Bone Miner. Res. 1993; 8: 199–208.
32. Ott, S.M., Woodson, G.C. and Huffer, W., Bone histomorphometric changes in women with post-menopausal osteoporosis treated with etidronate. In: Christiansen, C. and Overgaard, K. (Editors), Osteoporosis 1990. Osteopress ApS, Copenhagen, 1990; pp. 1318–1322.
33. Papapoulos, S.E., Idiopathic juvenile osteoporosis. In: Nordin, B.E.C., Need, A.G. and Morris, H.A. (Editors), Metabolic bone and stone disease. Churchill Livingstone, London, 1993; pp. 81–82.
34. Hoekman, K., Papapoulos, S.E., Peters, A.C.B. and Bijvoet, O.L.M., Characteristics and bisphos-phonate treatment of a patient with juvenile osteoporosis. J. Clin. Endocrinol. Metab. 1985; 61:

952–956.
35. Papapoulos, S.E., Hamdy, N.A.T., Valkema, R., Pauwels, E., Kroon, H. and Papapoulou, V., The effects of long-term uninterrupted treatment with bisphosphonates on the growing skeleton. In: Christiansen, C. and Riis, B. (Editors), Osteoporosis 1993. Handelstrykkeriet ApS, Aalborg, 1993; pp. 210–211.
36. van Persijn-van Meerten, E.L., Kroon, H.M. and Papapoulos, S.E., Epi- and metaphyseal changes in children caused by administration of bisphosphonates. Radiology 1992; 184: 249–254.
37. Devogelaar, J.P., Malghem, J., Maldague, B. and Nagant de Deuxchaisnes, C., Radiological manifestations of bisphosphonate treatment with APD in a child suffering from osteogenesis imperfecta. Skeletal Radiol. 1987; 16: 360–363.
38. Varonos, S., Ansell, B.M. and Reeve, J., Vertebral collapse in chronic arthritis; its relationship with glucocorticoid therapy. Calcif. Tissue Int. 1989; 41: 75–78.

Bisphosphonate on bones
O. Bijvoet, H.A. Fleisch, R.E. Canfield and G. Russell (eds.)
© 1995 Elsevier Science B.V. All rights reserved.

CHAPTER 29

Bisphosphonates and osteoporosis

O. Helmer Sørensen

The Osteoporosis Research Centre, Copenhagen Municipal Hospital, 1399 Copenhagen K, Denmark

I. Introduction

During the last few years a number of clinical studies have shown that bisphosphonate treatment is able to increase bone mass in postmenopausal osteoporosis. The increases have mainly been registered in the lumbar spine, while minor or no changes have been observed in the peripheral skeleton [1–18].

Etidronate, pamidronate and clodronate are the three bisphosphonates that predominantly have been used in human studies. They are registered in many countries for the treatment of Paget's disease and malignant hypercalcaemia, conditions that are characterized by an excessive osteoclastic bone resorption. Etidronate has been approved in several countries for the treatment of established osteoporosis. New and more potent bisphosphonates are currently under clinical investigation, including risedronate, tiludronate and alendronate.

II. Treatment of established osteoporosis

Continuous treatment with etidronate implies a risk of a mineralization defect if large doses are used [19]. A similar risk has not been found with pamidronate [20].

ADFR (activate-depress-free-repeat) has been tried using oral phosphate [2–4, 7, 9, 12, 21], thyroid hormone [10] or PTH [22] as activators. None has proved superior to an intermittent, cyclical treatment without activator.

Cyclical treatments with pamidronate, clodronate or etidronate have been effective in increasing spinal bone mass in most studies [5, 7, 11, 13, 15, 17].

Table 1 illustrates the effect of bisphosphonates on spinal bone mass. The negative results reported by Pacifici et al. [2] were probably due to lack of spacing between the calcium and the etidronate intake. In a later study the same group found an increase in the spinal bone mass of 6.6% in postmenopausal women after 18 months of treatment [11].

Table 1.

Effects of bisphosphonates on spinal bone mass

		Years of treatment	% Change
Etidronate			
Genant et al.	1987 [1]	2	+7.2
Pacifici et al.	1988 [2]	2	−8.0
Hodsman	1989 [3]	1	+8.3
Mallette et al.	1989 [4]	1	+8.2
Storm et al.	1990 [5]	3	+5.3
Storm et al.	1992 [6]	5	+6.7
Watts et al.	1990 [7]	2	+4.2/+5.2
Jackson et al.	1992 [8]	3	+5.0
Miller et al.	1991 [9]	2	+15.7
Steiniche et al.	1991 [10]	1	NS
Stark et al.	1992 [11]	1 1/2	+6.6
Evans et al.	1993 [12]	2	+3.1
Clodronate			
Chesnut	1984 [13]	1 1/2	+6
Pamidronate			
Valkema et al.	1989 [14]	2	+6.8
Devogelaer et al.	1990 [15]	2	+4.9
Fromm et al.	1991 [16]	1	+5.3
Thiébaud et al.	1993 [17]	2	+10.5
Alendronate			
Passeri et al.	1991 [18]	1	+9.0

Table 2.

Effects of bisphosphonates on peripheral bone mass

		Years of treatment	Site	% Change
Etidronate				
Genant et al.	1987 [1]	2	Forearm	NS
Pacifici et al.	1988 [2]	2	Forearm	NS
Storm et al.	1990 [5]	3	Forearm	NS
Storm et al.	1992 [6]	5	Forearm	NS
Watts et al.	1990 [7]	2	Trochanter	+2.5
			Ward's Triangle	NS
			Femoral neck	NS
Jackson et al.	1992 [8]	3	Trochanter	+2.7
			Ward's Triangle	+2.2
			Femoral neck	NS
Pamidronate				
Devogelaer et al.	1990 [15]	2	Forearm	NS
Papapoulos et al.	1992 [20]	2	Forearm	NS
Fromm et al.	1991 [16]	1	Forearm	NS
			Femoral neck	NS
			Ward's Triangle	NS
Thiébaud et al.	1993 [17]	2	Forearm	+7
			Hip	+4.8
Alendronate				
Passeri et al.	1991 [18]	1	Forearm	NS

The effect on the peripheral skeleton is much less pronounced (Table 2). This might be due to the slower turnover in cortical than in trabecular bone or to a reduced responsiveness of cortical osteoclasts to bisphosphonates [23].

III. Etidronate

Etidronate has been evaluated in randomised, double-blind, prospective studies in postmenopausal osteoporosis. In a multicentre trial conducted by Watts and co-workers [7], half of the etidronate-treated patients received oral phosphate for 3 days prior to each etidronate cycle in order to stimulate the activation frequency. This did not seem to affect the outcome, so the two etidronate arms of the study were pooled and the results compared with those from the two placebo groups. After 2 years the patients receiving etidronate had significant increases in the spinal bone density. The most striking effect was observed in a subgroup of patients with the lowest bone density in whom the vertebral fracture rate was reduced by two-thirds. The positive effect of cyclical etidronate treatment was maintained in a 4-year follow-up study [24].

In the Danish study [5,6] cyclical etidronate treatment (400 mg/day for 2 weeks/ off for 13 weeks, cycle repeated) was compared to placebo in a group of elderly women with severe osteoporosis. The spinal bone mass increased significantly (+5.3%) in the treated group compared with a fall (− 2.7%) in the placebo group after 3 years of treatment. Some authors have expressed concern that these patients might be suffering from other diseases with severe ongoing bone loss [25], but we are not aware that a bone loss of less than 1% per year is unusual in postmenopausal women. On the contrary, we regard this as a very moderate bone loss, which was also supported by the normal baseline values of serum alkaline phosphatase and urinary hydroxyproline excretion in the two groups. The same authors [20, 25] have expressed criticism concerning the mortality among our patients. Several studies have shown that bone mineral content is a good predictor of survival [26, 27]. The bone mass was markedly reduced in our patients, so we consider a mortality of 59/1000 years in the present study very close to what could be expected considering the general mortality in Copenhagen for women aged 70–79 years was 34/1000 years in 1987. The rate of new vertebral fractures was not affected by the treatment during the first year. In the following 2 years a significant reduction in the rate of new vertebral fractures was seen in the treated group.

After a 3-year study all patients were asked to continue in an open-labelled cyclical etidronate regimen for another 2 years. Seventeen patients from the former etidronate group and 19 patients from the placebo group entered treatment, and 13 and 17 patients, respectively, completed the study. The spinal bone mass increased slightly in the etidronate group to a 5-year value of 6.9% above the baseline level. In the former placebo group the spinal bone mass increased from a 3-year value of−2.7% to +5.3% above baseline after 5 years.

The reduced vertebral fracture rate was maintained in the former etidronate group, indicating that the treatment seems to be effective for at least 5 years. The vertebral fracture rate was reduced significantly in the former placebo group after 2 years of active treatment.

A reduction in vertebral fracture rate was also reported by Hodsman [3] who studied ADFR therapy with etidronate as the depressor. The study was not placebo-controlled, and the vertebral fracture rate was estimated in the same patients in the middle and at the end of the study, which inevitably involves statistical problems.

Silberstein and Schnur [28] reported an increase in bone mass not only in the spine but also in the femoral neck, Ward's triangle and greater trochanter in postmenopausal women treated with etidronate in an ADFR regimen. The results are difficult to compare with other studies since the patients were divided into responders and non-responders. The vertebral fracture rate was compared with that seen in a retrospectively selected, small control population. Fractures were defined as more than a 20% decrease in vertebral height as evaluated by dual photon absorptiometry, which might create methodological problems, but by this method the investigators registered 83% fewer lumbar vertebral fractures in the treatment group than in the control population.

Histomorphometry. An early study using large doses of etidronate in a few patients indicated a risk of a mineralization defect resembling osteomalacia [19]. Consequently, etidronate was administered in smaller doses and in cyclical regimens in later studies. No mineralization defects have been observed with these regimens [29, 30]. Bone histomorphometry has shown a decrease in activation frequency and resorption depth, both of which will contribute to a reduced risk of new perforations of the trabecular network and thus to a maintenance of the remaining bone strength [28, 29]. In a recent study Steiniche et al. [31] examined the bone histomorphometric changes after 5–7 years of cyclical etidronate treatment. The depth of the resorption lacunae was still significantly reduced, indicating that the preventive effect on trabecular perforations can be maintained for at least 7 years. Furthermore, it was found that the activation frequency returned towards normal, pointing at reversibility rather than at a constant suppression of bone remodelling

Side-effects. No severe side-effects have been described.

In conclusion, cyclical etidronate therapy increases spinal bone mass, whereas minor or no changes occur in the peripheral skeleton. There is strong evidence that the vertebral fracture rate decreases during treatment, while there is no evidence of either negative or positive effects on other fracture types. Bone histomorphometry has not shown any signs of osteomalacia with the intermittent regimens.

IV. Pamidronate

This bisphosphonate has been successfully used in patients with Paget's disease and malignant hypercalcaemia. The experience with the compound in osteoporosis is more limited, and published studies have so far only been open and non-randomised in a limited number of patients.

Valkema et al. [14] showed a positive calcium balance during one year of continuous pamidronate treatment of patients with miscellaneous bone diseases.

They also found that the bone mass increased in 24 patients receiving pamidronate 150 mg/day. These patients constituted a rather mixed population of both sexes and on concomitant treatments including oestrogens and active vitamin D compounds. The study was further biased by the fact that 10 patients had been on pamidronate treatment for a mean of 1.6 years before the first bone density measurements were performed. A proper control group was lacking. The investigators concluded that the patients had an annual gain of 3% in lumbar density. Upon reanalysis of their data, the authors later came to the conclusion that the gain was 2.4% per year and that it continued for at least 4 years [20]. These results differed from those of Devogelaer et al. [15] who followed 18 patients treated for 3–5 years with pamidronate given intermittently (250–300 mg/day for 2 months/2 months off, cycle repeated). In accordance with similar studies with etidronate, they registered an increase of lumbar bone mass of 2.5% annually during the first 2 years followed by a stable plateau. Fromm et al. [16] studied the effect of pamidronate given continuously to 35 patients for 18 months. Bone mineral density could be evaluated throughout the course of treatment in only 14 patients who showed an increase in the lumbar spine and the greater trochanter.

In an open and partially randomised study Thiébaud et al. [17] compared the effect of intermittent, intravenous pamidronate with oral fluoride in 16 and 27 osteoporotic women, respectively. Pamidronate was administered at a dose of 30 mg every third month. Marked increases were seen in the bone density of the lumbar spine (10%), the forearm and the femoral neck (average 5%) after 2 years of treatment.

Data on fracture in osteoporotic patients on pamidronate treatment are very limited. Papapoulos et al. [20] evaluated the spine deformity index in a mixed group of patients on continuous pamidronate treatment for at least 2 years and came to the conclusion that no significant progression was seen. However, the authors pointed out that the significance of the results was difficult to assess due to lack of a control group.

Histomorphometry. To our knowledge there are no data on bone histology in osteoporotic patients treated with pamidronate.

Side-effects. A few patients developed oesophageal erosions and gastric ulcers during oral treatment, which makes use of the compound less attractive for chronic and relatively benign conditions such as postmenopausal osteoporosis. A Danish study in more than 150 patients has thus recently been interrupted after more than 3 years of therapy due to the above-mentioned risk.

However, the intermittent, intravenous pamidronate regimen is promising. Apart from transient fever and flu-like symptoms in 30% of the patients, this regimen was well tolerated [17]. Continuous pamidronate treatment does not, in contract to etidronate, involve any mineralization defect.

In conclusion, oral pamidronate increases lumbar bone mass. Controlled studies, fracture data and histomorphometry are lacking. Oral therapy involves a risk of oesophageal and gastric erosions, which makes the treatment unattractive. Intermittent, intravenous therapy might become a future alternative.

V. Other bisphosphonates

Only a few data are available on clodronate [13] and alendronate [18] in the treatment of postmenopausal osteoporosis. A very large US study on alendronate involving more than 6000 women has recently been initiated.

References

1. Genant, H.K., Harris, S.T., Steiger, P., Davey, P.F. and Block, J.E., The effect of etidronate therapy in postmenopausal osteoporotic women: Preliminary studies. In: Christiansen, C., Johanansen, J.S. and Riis, B.J. (Editors), Osteoporosis 1987. Nørhaven, Viborg, 1987; pp. 1177–118.
2. Pacifici, R., McMurtry, C., Vered, I., Rupich, R. and Avioli, L.V., Cohorence therapy does not prevent axial bone loss in osteoporotic women: a preliminary comparative study. J. Clin. Endocrinol. Metab. 1988; 66: 747–753.
3. Hodsman, A.B., Effects of cyclical therapy for osteoporosis using an oral regimen of inorganic phosphate and sodium etidronate: a clinical and bone histomorphometric study. Bone Miner. 1989; 5: 201–212.
4. Mallette, L.E., LeBlanch, A.D., Pool, J.L. and Mechanick, J.L., Cyclical therapy of osteoporosis with neutral phosphate and brief, high-dose pulses of etidronate. J. Bone Miner. Res. 1989; 4: 143–148.
5. Storm, T., Thamsborg, G., Steiniche, T., Genant, H.K. and Sørensen, O.H., Effect of intermittent cyclical etidronate therapy on bone mass and fracture rate in women with postmenopausal osteoporosis. N. Engl. J. Med. 1990; 322: 1265–1271.
6. Storm, T., Thamsborg, G., Kollerup, G. et al., Five years of intermittent cyclical etidronate therapy increases bone mass and reduces vertebral fracture rate in postmenopausal osteoporosis. Bone Miner. 1992; 17 (suppl. 1): S24.
7. Watts, N.B., Harris, S.T., Genant, H.K. et al., Intermittent cyclical etidronate treatment of postmenopausal osteoporosis. N. Engl. J. Med. 1990; 323: 73–79.
8. Jackson, R.D., Harris, S.T., Genant, H.K. et al., Cyclical etidronate treatment of postmenopausal osteoporosis: 4 year experience. Bone Miner. 1992; 17 (suppl. 1): 154.
9. Miller, P.D., Neal, B.J., McIntyre, D.O., Yanover, M.J., Anger, M.S. and Kowalski, L.J., Effect of cyclical therapy with phosphorus and etidronate on axial bone mineral density in postmenopausal osteoporotic women. Osteoporosis Int. 1991; 1: 171–176.
10. Steiniche, T., Hasling, C., Charles, P., Eriksen, E.F., Melsen, F. and Mosekilde, L., The effects of etidronate on trabecular bone remodeling in postmenopausal spinal osteoporosis: A randomised study comparing intermittent treatment and an ADFR regime. Bone 1991; 12: 155–163.
11. Stark, R., Civitelli, R., Avioli, L. and Pacifici, R., Comparison of etidronate therapy to calcium and estrogen therapy in postmenopausal women. Bone Miner. Res. 1992; 7 (suppl.1): S 329.
12. Evans, R.A., Somers, N.M., Dunstan, C.R., Royle, H. and Kos, S., The effect of low-dose etidronate and calcium on bone mass in early postmenopausal women. Osteoporosis Int. 1993; 3: 71–75.
13. Chesnut, C.H., Synthetic salmon calcitonin, diphosphonate and anabolic steroids in the treatment of postmenopausal osteoporosis. In: Christiansen, C., Arnaud, C.D., Nordin, B.E.C., Parfitt, A.M., Peck, W.A. and Riggs, B.L. (Editors), Osteoporosis 1984, Aalborg Stiftstrykkeri, 1984; pp. 549–555.
14. Valkema, R., Vismans, F.-J.F.E., Papapoulos, S.E., Pauwels, E.K.J. and Bijvoet, O.L.M., Maintained improvement in calcium balance and bone mineral content in patients with osteoporosis treated with bisphosphonate APD. Bone Miner. 1989; 5: 183–192.
15. Devogelaer, J.P. and Nagant de Deuxchaisnes, C., Treatment in involutional osteoporosis with the bisphosphonate APD (disodium pamidronate): Non-linear increase of lumbar bone mineral density. In: Christiansen, C. and Overgaard, K. (Editors), Osteoporosis 1990, Handelstrykkeriet Aalborg, 1990; pp, 1507–1509.
16. Fromm, G.A., Vega, E., Plantalech, L., Galich, A.M. and Mautalen, C.A., Differential action of pamidronate on trabecular and cortical bone in women with involutional osteoporosis. Osteoporosis Int. 1991; 1: 129–133.
17. Thiébaud, D., Burckhardt, P., Melchior, J., Lamy, O. and Gobelet, C., 2 years effectiveness of intravenous pamidronate (APD) versus oral fluoride in postmenopausal osteoporosis. In: Christiansen, C. and Riis, B. (Editors), Osteoporosis. Fourth international symposium on osteoporosis

and consensus development conference. Proceedings 1993. Handelstrykkeriet, Aalborg, 1993; pp. 125–127.

18. Passeri, M., Baroni, M.C., Pedrazzoni, M. et al., Intermittent treatment with intravenous 4-amino-1.hydroxybutylidene-1,1-bisphosphonate (AHBuBP) in the therapy of postmenopausal osteoporosis. Bone Miner. 1991; 15: 237–248.

19. Jowsey, J., Riggs, B.L., Kelly, P.J., Hoffmann, D.L. and Bordier, P., The treatment of osteoporosis with disodium ethane-1-hydroxy-1,1-diphosphonate. J. Lab. Clin. Med. 1971; 78: 574–584.

20. Papapoulos, S.E., Landman, J.O., Bijvoet, O.L.M. et al., The use of bisphosphonates in the treatment of osteoporosis. Bone 1992; 13: S 41–49.

21. Anderson, C., Cape, R.D.T., Crilly, R.G., Hodsman, A.B. and Wolfe, B.M.J., Preliminary observations of a form of coherence therapy for osteoporosis. Calcif. Tissue Int. 1984; 36: 341–343.

22. Hesch, R.D., Heck, J., Delling, G. et al., Results of a stimulatory therapy of low bone metabolism in osteoporosis with (1-38) h PTH and diphosphonate EHDP. Klin. Wschr, 1988; 66: 976–984.

23. Chappard, D., Petitjean, M., Alexandre, C., Vico, L., Minaire, P. and Riffat, G., Cortical osteoclasts are less sensitive to etidronate than trabecular osteoclasts. J. Bone Miner. Res. 1991; 6: 673–680.

24. Chesnut, C.H., Genant, H.K., Harris, S.T., Jackson, R.D., Licata, A.A., Miller, P.D. et al., Etidronate cyclical therapy for treatment of postmenopausal osteoporosis: 4 years experience. J. Bone Miner. Res. 1992; 7 (suppl 1): S 143.

25. Bijvoet, O.L.M., Valkema, R., Löwik, C.W.G.M. and Papapoulos, S.E., Bisphosphonates in osteoporosis? Osteoporosis Int. 1993; 3 (suppl 1): S 230–236.

26. Browner, W.S., Seeley, D.G., Vogt, T.M. and Cummings, S.R., Non-trauma mortality in elderly women with low bone mineral density. Lancet 1991; 338: 355–358.

27. Mellström, D., The older osteoporotic patient. In: Christiansen, C. and Riis, B. (Editors), Osteoporosis. Fourth international symposium on osteoporosis and consensus development conference. Proceedings 1993. Handelstrykkeriet, Aalborg, 1993; pp. 315–316.

28. Silberstein, E.B. and Schnur, W., Cyclic oral phosphate and etidronate increase femoral and lumbar bone mineral density and reduce lumbar spine fracture rate over three years. J. Nucl. Med. 1992; 33: 1–5.

29. Steiniche, T., Hasling, C., Charles, P., Eriksen, E.F., Melsen, F. and Mosekilde, L., The effects of etidronate on trabecular bone remodeling in postmenopausal osteoporosis: A randomized study comparing intermittent treatment and ADFR regime. Bone 1991; 12: 155–163.

30. Storm, T., Steiniche, T., Thamsborg, G. and Melsen, F., Changes in bone histomorphometry after long-term treatment with intermittent, cyclic etidronate for postmenopausal osteoporosis. J. Bone Miner. Res. 1993; 8: 199–207.

31. Steiniche, T., Storm, T., Thamsborg, G., Sørensen, O.H., Sørensen, H.A. and Melsen, F., Histomorphometric evaluation of bone biopsies after long-term cyclical etidronate treatment. In: Christiansen, C. and Riis, B. (Editors) Osteoporosis. Fourth international symposium on osteoporosis and consensus development conference. Proceedings 1993. Handelstrykkeriet, Aalborg, 1993; pp. 137–138.

Bisphosphonate on bones
O. Bijvoet, H.A. Fleisch, R.E. Canfield and G. Russell (eds.)
© 1995 Elsevier Science B.V. All rights reserved.

CHAPTER 30

Effects on destructive joint diseases

F. Eggelmeijer and F.C. Breedveld

Department of Rheumatology, University Hospital, Leiden, The Netherlands

I. Introduction

Several forms of chronic arthritis may cause joint destruction. The disease with the highest prevalence and most destructive course is rheumatoid arthritis (RA). The disease is characterised by a chronic inflammation located in the synovial tissue of joints and affects bone in various ways. In the earlier stages of the disease, periarticular osteopenia occurs around the inflamed joints. This is probably caused by soluble mediators produced in the arthritic process. In the more advanced stages of the disease, the articular cartilage and subchondral bone are eroded by an invasion of proliferating synovium (pannus). In a considerable percentage of patients with RA, the erosive changes progress slowly over years until gross joint deformity and/or ankylosis is reached. Finally, RA is complicated by generalised osteopenia, which is often symptomatic. Whether generalised osteopenia in RA is just related to age, sex, menopausal status, reduced mobility and steroid treatment, or to the inflammatory process itself is still unresolved.

Patients with RA are treated with so-called slow-acting or disease-modifying drugs. These include e.g. anti-malarials, gold compounds and cytotoxic drugs (azathioprine, methotrexate and cyclophosphamide). Their mechanism of action is uncertain but probably related to an influence on immune mechanisms involved in chronic arthritis. Although all these drugs are effective in controlling disease activity and some retard the progression of joint destruction, the evidence that these drugs improve the long-term outcome of joint destruction is limited. Bisphosphonates, via their powerful capacity to inhibit bone resorption, have the potential to influence joint destruction and thereby the severest consequence of RA, i.e. loss of joint function. The effects of drugs that may be useful in the treatment of RA have been frequently studied in animal models. Animal models of chronic arthritis share many clinical and histologic features with RA. The main difference concerns the fact that experimentally induced arthritis is a fulminating disease, which produces severe bone and joint destruction within weeks. The effect of bisphosphonates on the course of RA and experimentally induced chronic arthritis in animals has been the subject of a number of studies.

II. Bisphosphonates in experimentally induced arthritis

1. Adjuvant arthritis

Adjuvant arthritis can be provoked in rats by an injection of oil containing a preparation that possesses adjuvant activity [1]. In this system, heat-killed and desiccated *Mycobacterium tuberculosis*, several other non-viable bacteria, bacterial cell walls, and isolated peptidoglycans, as well as several synthetic compounds are known to be arthritogenic. Adjuvant arthritis resembles RA both clinically and histologically in man. The clinical expression of the adjuvant arthritis varies among different strains of rats. In general, arthritis develops 10 to 16 days after a subcutaneous adjuvant injection. Flagrant articular inflammation resulting in prominent swelling of the hindpaws especially persists for 4 to 8 weeks, culminating in ankylosis of the involved joints. Histologically, the initial alterations, occurring around day 5 after immunisation, consist of activation changes in the synovial lining cells, perivascular accumulation of mononuclear cells, and fibrin deposition within and upon the surface of the synovium and articular cartilage. These changes are followed by a sequence of synovial cell hyperplasia, intra- and subsynovial neovascularisation, and pannus extrusion over the surface of the cartilage. Pannus formation continues for several days, and by the time the lysozymes of synoviocytes have filled with debris, polymorphonuclear leucocytes and macrophages are present in the granulation tissue. The synovial pannus next appears to erode the cartilage and subchondral bone. A protracted inflammatory stage follows, characterised by a persistent, hyperplastic synovium packed with dense aggregates of mononuclear cells and granulomatous areas. In the late stage of adjuvant arthritis, periosteal bone formation occurs, resembling the bone changes observed in ankylosing spondylitis in man.

Disodium etidronate (EHDP) administered at 4 mg/kg/day subcutaneously from the time of adjuvant injection in female Wistar rats markedly inhibited the inflammatory response [2]. Histologically, pannus formation, erosion of the cartilage and osteoclastic resorption of the subchondral bone were almost completely prevented. In some of the animals, unmineralised periarticular substances with a structure similar to bone were observed, presumably osteoid. EHDP administered at 1 mg/kg/day greatly inhibited, but did not totally prevent, the bone changes induced. The histological changes in the joints of animals treated with EHDP at 0.2 mg/kg/day were indistinguishable from control animals with adjuvant arthritis. Radiologically, bone resorption and pathologic calcification in the soft tissue surrounding the joints was completely prevented by the administration of EHDP at 4 mg/kg/day. Discontinuation of EHDP administration (4 mg/kg/day) after 3 weeks resulted in rapid calcification of the joint areas, similar to the calcifications found in the control animals. In contrast to this, EHDP treatment started 3 weeks after the initial adjuvant injection hardly altered the course of the radiological changes.

A comparative study of EHDP and dichloromethane diphosphonate (Cl_2MDP) administered subcutaneously from the time of adjuvant injection in male Sprague-Dawley rats demonstrated that both bisphosphonates were able to inhibit the arthritic response [3]. EHGP and Cl_2MDP both effectively inhibited pedal swelling, bone resorption and pathological mineralisation. At dose levels of 0.5 and 1 mg/kg/day Cl_2MDP appeared to be more effective than EHDP. However, the effect of EHDP was clearly dose-dependent, while the effectiveness of Cl_2MDP did not show much improvement with the higher dose levels (i.e. 2, 4 and 8 mg/kg/day). High dosages of EHGP (4 mg/kg/day) totally blocked pathologic mineralisation, whereas Cl_2MDP only partially blocked these changes.

Disodium-3-amino-1-hydroxypropylidene-1,1-diphosphonate (APD) was administered subcutaneously in adjuvant arthritis, either throughout the whole experiment, or on days 5 to 9, or on days 17 to 20 following adjuvant injection [4, 5]. In both studies APD was shown to reduce hindpaw swelling efficiently. ADP appeared to be more effective than EHDP and Cl_2MDP.

4-Chlorophenyl thiomethylene diphosphonate administered at 0.16 mmol/kg/day orally on days 14 to 35 following adjuvant injection markedly reduced the severity and progression of adjuvant arthritis as measured by clinical, biochemical and histological parameters [6].

The use of monosodium [2-(3-pyridinyl) ethylidene] hydroxy diphosphonate in adjuvant arthritis has been studied in two strains of rats [7]. Treatment with either 14.8 mg/kg/day orally or 0.148 mg/kg/day subcutaneously starting on the day of adjuvant injection in Lewis rats reduced, both clinically and histologically, the arthritic response. Treatment with 0.148 mg/kg/day subcutaneously starting on day 14 after adjuvant injection in Sprague-Dawley rats resulted in a reduction in paw swelling and preservation of the architecture of the tibio-tarsal joints.

2. Collagen arthritis

Collagen arthritis can be provoked in rats, mice or monkeys by an intradermal injection of native heterologous or homologous type II collagen, derived from cartilage or the vitreous humour of the eye, emulsified in oil [1]. The resulting joint disease is similar to adjuvant arthritis.

APD and dimethyl-APD administered subcutaneously from the time of collagen injection in female Sprague-Dawley rats did not have any effect on the incidence and severity of collagen arthritis [8]. Hindlimb radiographs of all arthritis rats at 42 days showed equivalent destruction in those treated with APD, dimethyl-APD and saline. The cellular and humoral immune responses were also similar in the treated and untreated animals.

III. Bisphosphonates in rheumatoid arthritis

The clinical, biochemical and radiological effects of bisphosphonates in RA have been investigated in several clinical studies [9–13]. The first investigation consisted of an open study on five patients with severe erosive disease [9]. APD was administered as adjuvant therapy in a dose of 60 μmol/kg/day for 14 days and continued at 30 μmol/kg/day (approximately 750 mg per day). All patients had active disease and were treated with non-steroidal anti-inflammatory drugs (NSAIDs). Two patients received disease-modifying anti-rheumatic drugs (DMARDs). In the first week of treatment a marked inhibitory effect on bone resorption was seen, as reflected by a decrease in fasting urinary calcium/creatinine (Ca/Cr) and hydroxyproline/creatinine (Hp/Cr) ratios. During the second week of treatment the patients reported a decrease in morning stiffness and pain. There was an increase in the range of movement of the joints and a rapid decrease of the Ritchie articular index. The amelioration continued with prolonged treatment (7 to 17 weeks). Joint swelling decreased less rapidly, as did erythrocyte sedimentation rate (ESR), but both displayed a steady regression toward the normal range.

The aforementioned study was extended to 2 years of follow-up [10]. The beneficial clinical effects remained throughout the follow-up period, and no exacerbations of the joint disease were seen. Radiographic examination of hands and feet after 2 years showed progression of the established erosions in those joints that retained some inflammatory activity. However, no new erosions had developed. Healing of erosions, although scarce, was observed in joints in which the inflammatory activity had abated.

APD administered at a dose of 250 mg b.i.d. in an open study on 9 patients with active RA treated with NSAIDs and DMARDs resulted in an inhibition of bone resorption similar to that in patients treated with higher dosages of APD [10]. However, no amelioration in parameters of disease activity was noted during the 3 months of treatment.

EHDP was evaluated in 15 patients with active RA at a dose of 5 mg/kg/day rounded up or down to the nearest 200 mg [11]. Herewith most patients were treated with 400 mg EHDP/day for a period of 24 weeks. Apart from a slight improvement in the Ritchie articular index that just reached significance at weeks 4 and 20, no beneficial clinical effects were seen. Serial laboratory measurements, including ESR and C-reactive protein (CRP), demonstrated no significant changes, except for an increase in serum phosphate throughout the whole study period.

The effect of intravenous APD on disease activity and bone metabolism was investigated in a phase-1 study with 7 RA patients [12]. All patients had active disease and were taking NSAIDs, but had discontinued DMARDs for at least 3 months. APD was administered in courses of 5 days (0.25 mg/kg/day) at 6-week intervals. A total of three or four courses were given. There was no consistent trend in the indices of disease activity. Three of 7 patients improved with a reduction in the number of tender joints and a fall in ESR, but no change in other indices (pain score, CRP, blood cell counts, serum immunoglobulins and Rose-Waaler titres). In the other four patients the disease remained active. Bone resorption, as measured by fasting urinary Ca/Cr and Hp/Cr ratios, was reduced after the first course of APD. With successive courses the reduction of the Ca/Cr and Hp/Cr ratios was maintained only in the patients with clinical improvement.

The two placebo-controlled, double-blind trials on the effects of bisphosphonates in patients with RA was performed with APD [13, 14]. In the first study 40 RA patients were investigated, all of whom were already stabilised by treatment with one DMARD (i.e. penicillamine) and/or NSAIDs. They were randomly allocated on a double-blind basis to receive an intravenous infusion of either APD 30 mg in 500 ml 0.9% saline or a matching placebo, administered over a 2-h period. The infusion was repeated every 4 weeks over a follow-up period of 48 weeks. There was no significant difference in disease activity between the APD and placebo group as judged by clinical (grip strength, morning stiffness, pane score) and laboratory (ESR, CRP, blood cell counts) criteria. Progression of radiological joint damage of hands and feet, as judged by the Sharp index, was also similar in both groups. As in the previous studies bone resorption was markedly suppressed in the patients treated with the bisphosphonate. In a more recent study 30 patients with active RA were randomly allocated to receive a single intravenous infusion of placebo, 20 or 40 mg pamidronate. Pamidronate treatment resulted in a rapid and sustained reduction in urinary calcium and hydroxyproline excretions. A sustained reduction in serum corrected calcium was only noted in the 40 mg pamidronate group. In both pamidronate-treated groups a temporary increase in serum parathyroid hormone was noted. Compared with the placebo group clinical parameters of disease activity improved significantly in both APD-treated groups. The erythrocyte sedimentation rate and serum C-reactive protein levels improved significantly in patients treated with 40 mg pamidronate. No serious side-effects were documented.

IV. Comments

The aforementioned studies have shown that in the adjuvant arthritis model, bisphosphonates are able to inhibit the overall inflammatory response, bone re-sorption and pathologic calcification. Whilst the effects of bisphosphonates on bone resorption and pathologic calcification have been extensively studied and (partially) elucidated, the mechanism of the anti-inflammatory effect is unknown. Several mechanisms have been proposed. In chronic arthritis the massive proliferation of synovial tissue causes destruction of the subchondral bone. The resulting release of calcium, phosphate and matrix components originates a diffusional flux toward the synovial cavity. Increased concentrations of calcium and phosphate may result in precipitation of crystals which are able to generate an inflammatory response in an-imal models. Furthermore, elevated levels of calcium as such are able to stimulate cell proliferation, and several matrix components may generate an inflammatory response. Bisphosphonates with their powerful capacity to inhibit bone resorption are able to prevent a diffusional flux of calcium, phosphate and matrix components toward the synovial cavity. As a consequence, powerful stimuli for the initiation and enhancement of the inflammatory response are eliminated.

In contrast with the striking effects of bisphoshonates on the course of adjuvant arthritis, APD and dimethyl-APD were unable to alter the cellular and humoral immune responses in the collagen arthritis model. Whether the different effects of bisphosphonate administration in these arthritis models are due to differences in type and/or dosages used or to pathogenetic differences in the adjuvant and collagen arthritis model remains to be determined.

Studies on the effects of bisphosphonates in the treatment of RA are unequivocal. Most studies were able to demonstrate biochemical evidence of an inhibitory effect on bone resorption. Anti-inflammatory effects were observed only in studies using relatively high dosages of APD in patients with active disease [9, 10, 12, 14]. One study (with the longest follow-up, i.e. 2 years) suggests that APD administered as adjuvant therapy in RA patients with active disease is able to retard the progression of joint erosions [10]. Another study in which APD was administered intravenously in RA patients with stabilised disease (follow-up of 48 weeks) could not detect any effect on the radiological joint destruction [13]. None of the studies discussed has investigated the effects of bisphosphonates on periarticular or generalised osteopenia in RA.

In conclusion, bisphosphonates have proven to be effective in the treatment of adjuvant arthritis. At present there are insufficient data to judge the effects in RA. However, the data available are encouraging enough to justify further controlled studies on the potential beneficial effects of bisphosphonates on disease activity, joint erosions, periarticular and generalized osteopenia in patients with RA.

References

1. Breedveld, F.C. and Trentham, D.E., Progress in the understanding of inducible models of chronic arthritis. Rheum. Dis. Clin. North Am. 1987; 13: 531–544.
2. Francis, M.D., Flora, L. and King, W.R., The effects of disodium ethane-1-hydroxy-1,1-diphosphonate on adjuvant induced arthritis in rats. Calcif. Tissue Res. 1972; 9: 109–121.
3. Flora, L., Comparative anti-inflammatory and bone protective effects of two diphosphonates in adjuvant arthritis. Arthritis Rheum. 1979; 22: 340–346.
4. Kong, A.S., Shao, J., Rappo, R. and Leibowitz, M., Effects of diphosphonates on rat adjuvant arthritis. Int. J. Immunopharmacol. 1982; 4: 311 (abstract).
5. Glatt, M., Blätter, A., Bisping, M. and Bray, M.A., Effects of diphosphates (APD, EHDP) on inflammation and bone turnover in adjuvant arthritis rats. Experientia 1983; 39: 681 (abstract).
6. Barbier, A., Brelière, J.C., Remandet, B. and Roncucci, R., Studies on the chronic phase of adjuvant arthritis: effect of SR-41319, a new diphosphonate. Ann. Rheum. Dis. 1986; 45: 67–74.
7. Francis, M.D., Hovancik, K. and Boyce, R.W., NE-58095: a diphosphonate which prevents bone erosion and preserves joint architecture in experimental arthritis. Int. J. Tissue React. 1989; 11: 239–252.
8. Markusse, H.M., Lafeber, G.J.M. and Breedveld, F.C., Bisphosphonate in collagen arthritis. Rheumatol. Int. 1990; 9: 281–283.
9. Bijvoet, O.L.M., Frijlink, W.B., Jie, K. et al., APD in Paget's disease of bone. Role of the mononuclear phagocyte system? Arthritis Rheum. 1980; 23: 1 93–1204.
10. De Vries, E., Bijvoet, O.L.M. and Van Paassen, H.C., The use of bisphosphonates in inflammation. VIIe Séminaire d'Immunopathologie Rhumatismale. Nouveaux traitements de la polyarthrite rhumatoïde. Clermond-Ferrand, October 2nd, 1987.
11. Bird, H.A., Hill, J., Sitton, N.G., Dixon, J.S. and Wright, V., A clinical and biochemical assessment of etidronate disodium in patients with active rheumatoid arthritis. Clin. Rheumatol. 1988; 7: 91–94.
12. Tan, P.L.J., Ames, R., Yeoman, S., Ibbertson, H.K. and Caughey, D.E., Effects of aminobisphosphonate infusion on biochemical indices of bone metabolism in rheumatoid arthritis. Preliminary report. Br. J. Rheumatol. 1989; 28: 325–328.
13. Ralston, S.H., Hacking, L., Willocks, L., Bruce, F. and Pitkeathly, D.A., Clinical, biochemical and radiographic effects of amminohydroxypropylidene bisphosphonate treatment in rheumatoid arthritis. Ann. Rheum. Dis. 1989; 48: 396–399.
14. Eggelmeijer, F., Papapoulos, S.E., Van Paassen, H.C., Dijkmans, B.A.C. and Breedveld, F.C., Clinical and biochemical response to single infusion of pamidronate in patients with active rheumatoid arthritis. J. Rheumatol. 1994; 21: 2016–2020.

Bisphosphonate on bones
O. Bijvoet, H.A. Fleisch, R.E. Canfield and G. Russell (eds.)
© 1995 Elsevier Science B.V. All rights reserved.

CHAPTER 31

Ectopic calcification and ossification

Roger Smith

Nuffield Orthopaedic Centre and John Radcliffe Hospital, Headington, Oxford, UK

I. Introduction

Deposition of calcium in the soft tissues (ectopic calcification; Table 1) and on ectopic bone matrix (ossification; Table 2) has many causes [1]. Experimental work showed that etidronate could inhibit ectopic mineralisation in animal systems [2], but this has not been confirmed in man, and the current emphasis on bisphosphonates with a selective effect on bone resorption has diverted attention away from etidronate-like compounds. This chapter will concentrate on ectopic ossification.

II. Ectopic calcification

Calcification can result from previous damage in soft tissues (dystrophic calcification) or from an increase in circulating concentration of calcium or phosphate — or both (metastatic calcification). Rarely, it has no recognisable cause (idiopathic calcification) [1, 3].

1. Dystrophic calcification

This occurs in inherited and acquired disorders involving connective tissue, such as alkaptonuria (intervertebral discs), pseudoxanthoma elasticum (blood vessels), systemic sclerosis and dermatomyositis and also after infection, tumours and trauma. In systemic sclerosis, subcutaneous calcification, often around the phalanges, may be part of the syndrome, with Raynaud's phenomena and telangiectases. The calcific deposits can be sufficiently extensive to break through the skin as toothpaste-like material. In dermatomyositis, sheets of subcutaneous calcification can be deposited some time after the initial inflammatory episode (with a systemic illness and painful weak muscles); the calcification can be very extensive (calcinosis universalis), but can also disappear rapidly — sometimes in adolescence. Rarely, this is associated with hypercalcaemia [4].

Table 1.

The main causes of ectopic calcification

In damaged tissue (dystrophic, biochemistry normal)	After inflammation haemorrhage, etc.	Localised to site of injury
	Systemic sclerosis	Particularly around the fingers
	Dermatomyositis	Widespread subcutaneous
In undamaged tissues (metastatic, biochemistry abnormal)	Low calcium	Hypoparathyroidism Pseudohypoparathyroidism
	High calcium	Hyperparathyroidism Vitamin D overdose
	High phosphate	Tumoral calcinosis
	Low phosphate	Inherited hypophosphataemia
Idiopathic	Calcinosis circumscripta	

Table 2.

Causes of ectopic ossification

Acquired	After local injury. For example hip replacement After neurological injury, especially paraplegia In tumours Other disorders
Inherited	Myositis (fibrodysplasia) ossificans progressiva Familial osteoma cutis

2. Metastatic calcification

The distribution varies inexplicably with its cause; for example, subcutaneous and basal ganglia calcification in hypoparathyroidism and vascular calcification in hyperparathyroidism, suggesting that metastatic calcification is not simply related to the Ca:P product.

(a) Calcification and hypocalcaemia

This occurs in idiopathic, post-surgical, pseudo-hypoparathyroidism (PHP) and pseudopseudo-hypoparathyroidism (PPHP), in which the skeletal abnormalities of PHP co-exist with normal biochemistry. There is extensive subcutaneous calcification, calcification within the basal ganglia (and outside it [5]) and cataract formation. PHP is inherited as an autosomal dominant disorder with variable expression; in addition to ectopic calcification, its features include mental simplicity, round face, short stature and short 3rd and 4th metacarpals [6].

End-organ resistance to parathyroid hormone may be due to mutations in the gene responsible for one component (Gsα) of the G-protein signalling system [7]. Ossification occurs as well as calcification (below).

(b) Calcification and hypercalcaemia

This occurs in hyperparathyroidism, especially where there is renal glomerular failure. Their combination produces a high Ca × P product, and calcification occurs in the soft tissues, around the phalanges and larger joints, and also in the small and medium-sized arteries. There is calcification of the cornea, initially at the lateral and medial borders of the limbus. Acute hypercalcaemia due to vitamin D poisoning can produce conjunctival calcification.

(c) Calcification in hyperphosphataemia

Idiopathic hyperphosphataemia is a rare autosomal recessive disorder condition with an increase in the maximal tubular reabsorption of phosphate and sometimes with an inappropriate increase in plasma $1,25(OH)_2D$. Large masses of ectopic mineral which form around the joints from childhood onwards may discharge through the skin. Treatment with large oral doses of aluminium hydroxide can reduce the plasma phosphate and the size of the deposits [8].

(d) Calcification in hypophosphataemia

A particular feature of inherited hypophosphataemia, an X-linked dominant disorder, is widespread calcification of ligaments and tendons at their insertion into the periosteum (forming the so-called Sharpey fibres). This is termed an enthesiopathy. Calcification and new bone formation in the ligamenta flava may produce spinal cord compression [9, 10] (also see under ossification).

3. Idiopathic soft-tissue calcification

This includes calcific tendinitis and so-called calcinosis circumscripta.

III. Ectopic ossification

Acquired ossification occurs at the site of injury, such as after hip replacement or at a distance (following neurological injury such as paraplegia), in tumours and in a variety of other disorders [11]. The very rare condition of fibrodysplasia (myositis) ossificans progressiva is inherited as an autosomal dominant.

1. Acquired ectopic ossification

(a) Post-traumatic ossification

Aside from ectopic ossification at the site of accidental injury, total hip replacement is an important cause. The quoted incidence of periarticular ossification after total hip replacement varies greatly depending on the method used to detect it. It is said to occur more often in men than women and in certain individuals; for instance, where ossification follows hip replacement on one side, it is likely to occur if the contralateral hip is replaced. The reason for this is unknown. There is no confirmed association with HLA B27. The bone mainly forms in the hip abductors.

Disodium etidronate may delay mineralisation but only whilst it is being given [12]. More recently, it has been shown that non-steroidal anti-inflammatory drugs can reduce this form of ossification, being more effective when it is central (i.e. around the stem of the prostheses) than lateral in position [13, 14].

(b) Ossification after neurological injury

Extensive myositis ossificans can occur 1–4 months after injuries to the head and spinal cord, often in muscles distant from it such as the major ones of the thigh. Affected muscles become swollen, red and warm, and unless the cord lesion is complete, pain and tenderness also occur. At this time the differential diagnosis may include cellulitis, arthritis and thrombophlebitis. Radiologic calcification is initially absent, but an isotope bone scan will show increased uptake. Later there is progressive mineralisation with the eventual appearance of organised bone. Because this affects the major periarticular muscles, it leads to joint fixation, particularly of the hips. The plasma alkaline phosphatase may be increased in the early stages.

Attempted removal of ectopic bone is often difficult and produces little increase in movement. The ectopic bone recurs especially if it is removed too early. Oral etidronate in full dose (20 mg/kg body weight daily) may delay the onset of mineralisation, but only whilst it is being given. Although myositis ossificans is most commonly described after traumatic paraplegia, it can occur in other neurological disorders such as poliomyelitis and meningitis, and also after prolonged coma. The reason why ectopic ossification forms after head injury is unknown [15]. Similar effects of head injury are an increased rate of fracture healing and excessive callus formation. In such patients the serum contains an increased mitogenic activity for osteoblast-like cells [16]; the source of this activity is unknown, but there could be an increase in bone morphogenetic proteins [17].

(c) Ossification in tumours

Apart from primary bone tumours, ossification can occur in those of soft tissue such as parosteal sarcoma, soft-tissue sarcoma, lipoma and haemangioma. Of relevance is pseudomalignant myositis ossificans (also known as myositis ossificans circumscripta and non traumatic myositis ossificans). This condition affects people under the age of 30 and produces a painful, expanding lesion within muscle, particularly in the lower limbs, which enlarges for about 2–3 weeks. At this time radiographs show widespread, flocculent opacities which later become even and dense. There is a zoning pattern with peripheral maturation. Angiography distinguishes this lesion from bone tumours. The cause is unknown; it is self-limiting, benign and does not recur [1].

(d) Soft-tissue ossification in other disorders

In some of these, such as hypoparathyroidism, ectopic calcification also occurs. This often involves the ligaments of the spine, as in the spondyloarthropathies, particularly in ankylosing spondylitis, but also in psoriatic arthropathy, Reiter's syndrome and various forms of enteropathic arthritis.

In diffuse idiopathic skeletal hyperostosis (DISH) there is excessive ossification along the front of the vertebrae, especially in the upper thoracic spine, with bony protuberances at the junctions of the vertebral bodies and intervertebral discs; ossification also occurs around the ligaments of the pelvis and at the site of their attachments elsewhere.

Extensive ossification of the spinal ligaments of hypoparathyroidism leads to progressive stiffness. The enthesiopathy in inherited hypophosphataemia (vitamin-D-resistant rickets) is a form of ectopic ossification. Ossification of the posterior longitudinal ligament and sternoclavicular hyperostosis are particularly described from Japan [18]. Ligamentous ossification has been noted in patients treated with vitamin A analogues such as etetrinate for dermatological disorders [19]. The term osteoma cutis covers a number of rare conditions of uncertain cause.

Finally, ectopic bone may complicate varicose veins, chronic venous insufficiency and surgical incisions.

2. Inherited ectopic ossification

(a) Fibrodysplasia ossificans progressiva (myositis ossificans progressiva)

The main inherited cause of ectopic ossification is myositis ossificans progressiva (MOP) [20–22]. Histology suggests (to some) that the connective tissue within muscles is primarily involved, and the alternative term fibrodysplasia ossificans progressiva (FOP) is, therefore, widely used [23].

FOP is rare, with an incidence of about 1 per million, which increases with paternal age. Since patients rarely reproduce, most represent new mutations. The few family histories and affected monozygotic twins demonstrate that the mutant gene is inherited as a dominant with full penetrance but variable expression. Diagnosis depends on the combination of progressive myositis, leading to ossification in the major muscles, and characteristic skeletal abnormalities.

(i) Pathology Initially, there is oedema and round cell infiltration throughout the muscle with myofibrillar breakdown. Later, endochondral ossification leads to mature bone within which haemopoietic marrow is found. Information on the earliest histological appearances is scanty because biopsies are often taken after the acute phase of myositis; for this reason, there is still doubt about the primary lesion.

(ii) Clinical features Myositis. Episodes of myositis are the non-skeletal hallmark of this disease. Typically, the affected muscle becomes swollen and hard, sometimes after trauma; after a week or two these features subside, but the apparent improvement is followed in a month or so by ossification within the muscle and progressive joint fixation. Myositis usually begins in the upper paraspinal muscles. By late childhood or adolescence ossification will have occurred within the muscles around the shoulders, hips and knees to fix these joints and to complete the disability (Fig. 1). It is the large striated muscles which are affected; ossification does not involve the small muscles of the hands and feet, the diaphragm, the cardiac and smooth muscles. Ossification in the muscles around the jaw fixes it almost completely.

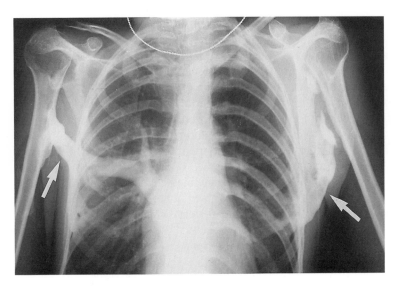

Fig. 1. Myositis (fibrodysplasia) ossificans progressiva. To show ossification in the thoracic muscles (arrows) fixing the movement of the shoulders.

Although the overall sequence of ossification is characteristic from large upper paraspinal to lower limb muscles, it varies considerably in its rate. For instance, neonates may have sufficient ossification to produce torticollis, whilst in contrast late and slow ossification producing stiffness may delay the correct diagnosis until adolescence.

Skeletal abnormalities. These affect the big toes (and to a lesser extent the thumbs) (Fig. 2), the cervical spine (Fig 3) and the metaphyses. The big toes are always abnormal; in the infant hallux valgus is associated with various bony abnormalities; in the adult they fuse to produce a short, fixed, monophalangic big toe. In the cervical spine the vertebral bodies are small and the laminae large. Both are variably fused, and this fusion is independent of nearby ossification of the cervical muscles [24]. Finally, the femoral necks are short and wide, and there are exostoses from the metaphyses.

Inconstant clinical features include early onset baldness, difficulty in hearing and mental retardation [20].

(iii) Differential diagnosis In the neonate bilateral hallux valgus should suggest the possibility of MOP. In childhood myositis may be mistaken for soft-tissue sarcoma; and the biopsy showing oedema and small round cell infiltration can be misinterpreted. Painful swelling of the masticatory muscles simulates mumps, and progressive stiffness with a fixed abnormal neck suggests the Klippel-Feil syndrome or childhood rheumatoid arthritis.

(iv) Management Once the diagnosis is made, and this is often delayed, there are four main questions: can the myositis be prevented; if myositis does occur

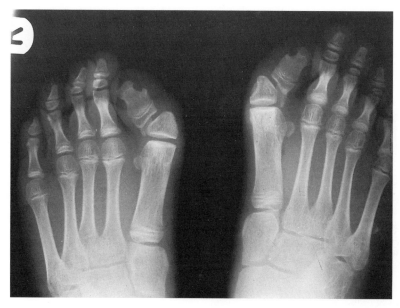

Fig. 2. FOP. Characteristic abnormal appearance of the big toes. They are short and deviated. Fusion to form a monophalangic hallux will occur later.

can subsequent ossification be prevented; what will be the eventual disability; and should ectopic bone be removed?

Since the onset of myositis is quite unpredictable, it is almost impossible to assess the effect of any form of therapy. Corticosteroids have been used, sometimes associated with symptom-free periods. Sometimes myositis follows injury, which should be avoided where possible. It seems likely, but difficult to prove, that myositis is inevitably followed by ossification. It is to prevent or slow down this ossification that the bisphosphonate EHDP (disodium etidronate) can be given in full doses (20 mg/kg bodyweight daily by mouth), but there is little evidence that this is effective [21]. Continued high-dose etidronate interferes with mineralisation, disorganises the growth plates, and delays fracture healing so it is not an acceptable long-term treatment. The disability produced by FOP is severe. The body moves as in one piece with the legs particularly fixed in partial extension, so that the help of a specialised rehabilitation centre is essential.

Removal of ectopic bone is technically difficult and rarely produces the expected increase in mobility; recurrence cannot be prevented.

(b) Familial osteoma cutis

This has been reported as a dominantly inherited disorder in a New Zealand family. The proposita had extensive subcutaneous ossification in one leg; relatives had insignificant multifocal subcutaneous ossification in childhood [25].

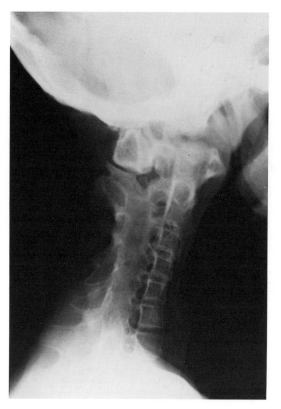

Fig 3. FOP. The cervical spine. The pedicles are large and fused and the vertebral bodies are abnormally small.

IV. Bisphosphonates in ectopic ossification and calcification

Ironically, bisphosphonates were first developed in the hope that they would be useful in preventing or retarding ectopic ossification. The first time a bisphosphonate was given to man was for fibrodysplasia ossificans progressiva. It is to prevent or slow down ossification after injury that the bisphosphonate EHDP (disodium etidronate), but not other bisphosphonates, was given in full doses (20 mg/kg bodyweight daily by mouth), but there is little evidence that this is effective [21]. The reason for the administration of EHDP (disodium etidronate) is that this drug at the given dose inhibits mineralisation of new bone. Since EHDP (disodium etidronate) also inhibits mineralisation of normal bone and since lower doses are not effective, the drug should not be given for longer than 3 months, preferably for shorter periods of a few weeks and only when a new exacerbation occurs.

Results may be somewhat more encouraging with other types of heterotopic ossification. Etidronate has been found to diminish the appearance of ossifications in patients with spinal cord injury, after cranial trauma, and after total hip replacement. EHDP (disodium etidronate) should be given in full doses (20 mg/kg bodyweight daily by mouth starting from before surgery and until 3 months after. Although ectopic bone formation reappears, at least partially, after discontinuation of the drug, the mobility of the hip seems nevertheless to be improved in the etidronate-treated patients. However, these results have been questioned by other authors [12, 29–33]. More recently, it has been shown that non-steroidal anti-inflammatory drugs can reduce this form of ossification, being more effective when it is central (i.e. around the stem of the prostheses) than lateral in position [13, 14].

Etidronate has been given in some cases of scleroderma, dermatomyositis, idiopathic infantile arterial calcification and calcinosis universalis. In none of these instances of ectopic calcification was any benefit observed.

V. Discussion

Ectopic ossification occurs when mesenchymal or stromal cells take on the behaviour of osteoblasts. This form of cell differentiation could result from an increase in bone-inducing substances or (for unknown reasons) a change in stromal cell expression [26].

The formation of ectopic bone after neurological damage could result from the first change, but so far this has not been clearly demonstrated [16].

In FOP the situation is potentially more informative since it is apparently due to a new mutation which affects both the formation of the skeleton and the behaviour of extraskeletal stromal cells. Although the timing of myositis differs widely from one affected patient to another, there is an order in which the muscles are affected from the upper paraspinal muscles to the lower and from the centre to the periphery. In looking for models which might give clues to FOP, the search has been wide; thus, it has been pointed out that the *Drosophila* decapentaplegic model could repay study [27]. Similarly, the effects of mutations in the homeobox genes which produce a striking change in the segmentation of the cervical spine could be relevant [28].

At present, it seems likely that ectopic ossification is a problem of cell biology rather than of mineralisation. In this sense the use of phosphonates, such as EHDP, which slow mineralisation represents only a superficial approach to the problem.

VI. Summary

Our understanding of the causes and treatment of ectopic calcification is still very primitive. It is not known why calcification occurs in damaged tissues, and metastatic calcification is often regarded merely as a form of mineral precipitation due to an increased Ca:P product, but its distribution in the tissues is not explained. In contrast, study of the inherited and acquired causes of ectopic ossification could illuminate the problem of the origin and differentiation of osteogenic cells.

References

1. Connor, J.M., Soft tissue ossification, 1st edn. Springer Verlag, Berlin, 1983.
2. Francis, M.D., Russell, R.G.G. and Fleisch, H., Diphosphonates inhibit formation of calcium phosphate crystals in vitro and pathological calcification in vivo. Science 1969; 165: 1264–1266.
3. Smith, R., Biochemical disorders of the skeleton. Butterworths, London, 1979.
4. Ostrov, B.E., Goldsmith, D.P., Eichenfield, E.H. and Athreya, B.H., Hypercalcaemia during the resolution of calcinosis universalis in juvenile dermatomyositis. J. Rheumatol. 1991; 18: 1730–1734.
5. McLoed, D.R., Hanley, D.A. and McArthur, R.G., Autosomal dominant hypoparathyroidism with intracranial ossification outside the basal ganglia. Am. J. Med. Gen. 1989; 32: 32–35.
6. Speigel, A.M., Pseudohypoparathyroidism. In: Scriver, C.R., Beaudet, A.L., Sly, W.S. and Valle, D. (Editors), The metabolic basis of inherited disease, 6th edn. McGraw Hill, New York, 1989; pp. 2013–2027.
7. Levine, L.A., Ahn, T.G., Klupt, S.F., Kaufman, K.D., Smallwood, P.M., Bourne, H.R., Sullivan, K.A. and Van Dop, C., Genetic deficiency of the alpha subunit of the guanine nucleotide-binding protein Gs as the molecular basis for Albright hereditary osteodystrophy. Proc. Natl. Acad. Sci. USA 1988; 85: 619–621.
8. Davies, M., Clements, M.R., Mawer, E.B. and Freemont, A.J., Tumoral calcinosis, clinical and metabolic response to phosphorous deprivation. Q. J. Med. 1987; 63: 493–503.
9. Adams, J.E. and Davies, M., Intraspinal new bone formation and spinal cord compression in familial hypophosphataemic vitamin D resistant osteomalacia. Q. J. Med. 1986; 61: 1117–1129.
10. Polisson, R.P., Martinez, S., Khoury, M., Harrell, R.M., Lyles, K., Friedman, N., Harrelson, J.M., Reisner, E. and Drezner, M.K., Calcification of entheses associated with x-linked hypophosphataemic osteomalacia. N. Engl. J. Med. 1985; 313: 1–6.
11. Nuovo, M.A., Norman, A., Chumas, J. and Ackerman, L.V., Myositis ossificans with atypical clinical, radiographic or pathologic findings, A review of 23 cases. Skeletal Radiol. 1992; 21: 87–101.
12. Thomas, B.J. and Amstutz, H.C., Results of the administration of diphosphonate for the prevention of heterotopic ossification after total hip arthroplasty. J. Bone Joint Surg. 1985; 67A: 400–403.
13. Schmidt, S.A., Kjaersgaard-Andersen, P., Pedersen, N.W., Kristensen, S.S., Pedersen, P. and Nielsen, J.B., The use of indomethacin to prevent the formation of heterotopic bone after total hip replacement. A randomised double-blind clinical trial. J. Bone Joint Surg. 1988; 70A: 834–838.
14. Kjaersgaard-Andersen, P., Sletgard, J., Gjerloff, C. and Lund, F., Heterotopic bone formation after non-cemented total hip arthroplasty. Clin. Orthop. Rel. Res. 1990; 252: 156–162.
15. Smith, R., Head injury, fracture healing and callus. J. Bone Joint Surg. 1987; 69B: 518–520.
16. Bidner, S.M., Rubins, I.M., Desjardins, J., Zukor, D.J. and Goltzman, D., Evidence for a humoral mechanism for enhanced osteogenesis after head injury. J. Bone Joint Surg. 1990; 72A: 1144–1149.
17. Tabas, J.A., Zasloff, M., Wasmuth, J.J., Emanuel, B.S., Altherr, M.R., McPherson, J.D., Wozney, J.M. and Kaplan, F.S., Bone morphogenetic protein, chromosomal localisation of human genes for BMPI, BMP 2A and BMP 3. Genomics 1991; 9: 283–289.
18. Seichi, A., Hoshino, Y. and Ohnishi, I., The role of calcium metabolism abnormalities in the development of ossification of the posterior longitudinal ligament of the cervical spine. Spine 1992; 17: 530–532.
19. Burge, S. and Ryan, T., Diffuse hyperostosis associated with etetrinate. Lancet 1985; ii: 397–398.
20. Connor, J.M. and Evans D.A.P., Fibrodyplasia ossificans progressiva. The clinical features and natural history of 34 patients. J. Bone Joint Surg. 1982; 64B: 76–83.
21. Smith, R., Russell, R.G.G. and Woods, C.G., Myositis ossificans progressiva. Clinical features of eight patients and their response to treatment. J. Bone Joint Surg. 1976; 58B: 48–57.
22. Cohen, R.B., Hahn, G.V., Tabas, J.A., Peeper, J., Levitz, C.L., Sando, A., Sando, N., Zasloff, M. and Kaplan, F.S., The natural history of heterotopic ossification in patients who have fibrodysplasia ossificans progressiva. A study of forty-four patients . J. Bone Joint Surg. Am. 1993; 75A: 215–219.
23. McKuslck, V.A., Heritable disorders of connective tissue, 4th Edn. C.V. Mosby, St. Louis, 1972.
24. Connor, J.M. and Smith, R., The cervical spine in fibrodysplasia ossificans progressiva. Br. J. Radiol. 1982; 55: 492–496.
25. Gardner, R.J.M., Yun, K. and Craw, S.M., Familial ectopic ossification. J. Med. Gen. 1988; 25: 113–117.
26. Smith, R. and Triffitt, J.T., Bones in muscles. Q. J. Med. 1986; 61: 985–990.
27. Kaplan, F.S., Tabas, J.A. and Zasloff, M.A., Fibrodysplasia ossificans progressiva, a clue from the fly? Calcif. Tissue Int. 1990; 47: 117–125.

28. Lufkin, T., Mark, M., Hart, C.P., Dolle, P., Lemeur, M. and Chambon, P., Homeotic transformation of the occipital bones of the skull by ectopic expression of a homeobox gene. Nature 1992; 359: 835–841.
29. Slooff, T.J.J.H., Feith, R., Bijvoet, O.L.M. and Nollen, A.J.G., The use of a diphosphonate in para-articular ossifications after total hip replacement. A clinical study. Acta Orthop. Belg. 1974; 40: 820–828.
30. Finerman, G.A.M. and Stover, S.L., Heterotopic ossification following hip replacement or spinal cord injury. Two clinical studies with EHDP. Metab. Bone Dis. Rel. Res. 1981; 4: 337–342.
31. Geho, W.B. and Whiteside, J.A., Experience with disodium etidronate in diseases of ectopic calcification. In: Frame, B., Parfitt, A.M. and Duncan, H. (editors), Clinical aspects of metabolic bone disease. Excerpta Medica, Amsterdam, 1973; pp. 506–511.
32. Reiner, M., Sautter, V., Olah, A., Bossi, E., Largiader, U. and Fleisch, H., Diphosphonate treatment in myositis ossificans progressiva. In: Caniggia, A. (editor), Etidronate. Istituto Gentili, Pisa, 1980; pp. 237–241.
33. Thomas, B.J. and Amstutz, H.C., Results of the administration of diphosphonate for the prevention of heterotopic ossification after total hip arthroplasty. J. Bone Joint Surg. Am. 1985; 67: 400–403.

Abbreviations

1,25(OH)2D	1,25-dihydroxyvitamin D = calcitriol
99mTc	technetium-99-m-labelled
ADFR	activate-depress-free-repeat regimen
AHPrBP	APD
ALN	4-amino-1-hydroxybutylidene-1,1-bisphosphonic acid = alendronate
APD	ABDP = AHPrBP = 3-amino-1-hydroxypropylidene bisphosphonic acid = pamidronate
BGP	bone Gla protein = osteocalcin
BM 21.0955	methylpentylaminoprppylidene bisposphonci acid
BP	bisphosphonate
BPI	bisphosphinate
BSTFA	N,O-bis(trimethylsilyl)trifluoroacetamide
Cl2MBP	dichloromethylene bisphosphonic acid = Cl2MDP = clodronate
Cl2MDP	Cl2MBP
CT	calcitonin
DPMDP	methyleen bisphosphonate
DPyr	deoxypyrodinoline
EDTA	ethylenediaminetetracetic acid
EHDP	(1-hydroxyethylidene)-1,1-bisphosphonic acid = EHBP = HEBP = didronel = etidronate
HAP	hydroxyapatite
HEDP	= EHDP
HMDP	hydroxmethylene bisphosphonate
IL	interleukin
MIBG	meta-iodo-benzyl guanidine
NDA	naphtalene dicarboxyaldehyde
OCP	octacalcium phosphate
PAP	phosphonoalkylphosphinate
PPi	pyrophosphate acid
PTH	parathyroid hormone
PTHrP	parathyroid hormone related peptide
PTIC	phenylisothiocyanate
Pyr	pyridinoline
SPECT	single photon emission computed tomography
TGF	transforming growth factor
Th-DCTA	thorium-diaminocyclohexane tetracetate
tiludronate	chloro-4-phenylthiomethylidene-bisphosphonic acid
YM 175	cycloheptyl-aminomethylene-bisphosphonic acid

Subject Index